T0172899

Vascular Control of Hemostasis

Advances in Vascular Biology

A series of books bringing together important advances and reviewing all areas of vascular biology.

Edited by *Mathew A. Vadas, The Hanson Centre for Cancer Research, Adelaide, South Australia* and *John Harlan, Division of Hematology, University of Washington, Seattle, USA.*

Volume One

Vascular Control of Hemostasis
   edited by *V.W.M. van Hinsbergh*

Volumes in Preparation

Immune Functions of the Vessel Wall
   edited by *Göran K. Hansson* and *Peter Libby*

Platelets, Thrombosis and the Vessel Wall
   edited by *M.C. Berndt*

The Selectins: Initiators of Leukocyte-Endothelial Adhesion
   edited by *D. Vestweber*

Structure and Function of Endothelial Cell to Cell Junctions
   edited by *E. Dejana*

The Early Atherosclerotic Plaque: Viral, Mutagenic and Developmental Mechanisms

---

This book is part of a series. The publisher will accept continuation orders which may be cancelled at any time and which provide for automatic billing and shipping of each title in the series upon publication. Please write for details.

Vascular Control of Hemostasis

edited by

Victor W.M. van Hinsbergh

Gaubius Laboratory TNO-PG,
Leiden, The Netherlands

harwood academic publishers

Australia ● Canada ● China ● France ● Germany ● India ● Japan
Luxembourg ● Malaysia ● The Netherlands ● Russia ● Singapore
Switzerland ● Thailand ● United Kingdom

Emmaplein 5
1075 AW Amsterdam
The Netherlands

British Library Cataloguing in Publication Data

Vascular control of hemostasis. — (Advances in vascular
  biology; v. 1)
  1. Hemostasis 2. Blood-vessels 3. Cardiovascular system
  I. Series II. Hinsbergh, Victor van
  612. 1'34

  ISBN 3-7186-5796-1

CONTENTS

SERIES PREFACE

It is our privilege to live at a time when scientific discoveries are providing insights into human biology at an unprecendented rate. It is also a time when the sheer quantity of information tends to obscure underlying principles, and when hypotheses or insights that simplify and unify may be relegated to the shadow of hard data.

The driving force for editing a series of books on Vascular Biology was to partially redress this balance. In inviting editors of excellence and experience, it is our aim to draw together important facts, in particular areas of vascular biology, and to allow the generation of hypotheses and principles that unite an area and define newer horizons. We also anticipate that, as is often the case in biology, the formulation and application of these principles will interrelate with other disciplines.

Vascular biology is a frontier that has been recognised since at least the time of Cohnheim and Metchikoff, but has really come into prominence over the last 10–15 years, once the molecules that mediate the essential functions of the blood vessel started to be defined. The boundaries of this discipline are, however, not clear. There are intersections, for example, with hypertension and atherogenesis that bring in, respectively, neuroendocrine control of vessel tone and lipid biochemistry which exist as separate bodies of knowledge. Moreover, it would be surprising if some regional vascular biology (for example, pulmonary, renal, etc.) were not to emerge as subgroups in the future. Our aims for the moment, however, are to concentrate on areas of vascular biology that have wide impact.

It is our hope to publish two books each year for the next 3–4 years. Indeed the first five books have been commissioned and address areas primarily in endothelial biology (hemostasis and thrombosis), immunology, leukocyte adhesion molecules, platelet adhesion molecules, adhesion molecules that mediate cell–cell contact). Subsequent volumes will cover the physiology and pathology of other vascular cells as well as developmental vascular biology.

We thank the editors and contributors for their very hard work.

Mathew VADAS   John HARLAN

vii

LIST OF CONTRIBUTORS

Bauer, Kenneth A.
Molecular Medicine Unit
Beth Israel Hospital
330 Brookline Avenue
Boston MA 02215
USA

Brinkman, Herm-Jan M.
Department of Blood Coagulation,
Central Laboratory of the Netherlands Red
Cross Blood Transfusion Service
PO Box 9190
1006 AD Amsterdam
The Netherlands

Carmeliet, Peter
Center for Molecular and Vascular
Biology Campus Gasthuisberg,
Herestraat 49
University of Leuven
Leuven B-3000
Belgium

Collen, Désiré
Center for Molecular and Vascular
Biology Campus Gasthuisberg,
Herestraat 49
University of Leuven
Leuven B-3000
Belgium

de Groot, Philip G.
University Hospital Utrect
Department of Haematology
PO Box 85.500,
Utrect 3508 GA
The Netherlands

Emeis, Jef J.
Gaubius Laboratory TNO-PG
PO Box 430
Leiden 2300 AK
The Netherlands

Esmon, Charles T.
Oklahoma Medical Research
Foundation
Depts Pathology, Biochemistry and
Molecular Biology
University of Oklahoma Health Sciences
Center
Oklahoma OK 73104
USA

Fearns, Colleen
Department of Vascular Biology VB-3
The Scripps Research Institute
10666 North Torrey Pines Rd
La Jolla CA 92037
USA

Hajjar, David P.
Department of Pathology
Cornell University Medical College
1300 York Avenue
New York NY 10021
USA

Hop, Caroline
University of Amsterdam
Academic Medical Center,
Dept of Biochemistry
Meibergdreef 15
Amsterdam 1105 AZ
The Netherlands

Kao, Janet
Department of Physiology and Cellular
Biophysics
Columbia University
College of Physicians and Surgeons
630 West 168th Street
New York NY 10032
USA

Kooistra, Teake
Gaubius Laboratory TNO-PG
PO Box 430
Leiden 2300 AK
The Netherlands

Koolwijk, Pieter
Gaubius Laboratory TNO-PG
PO Box 430
Leiden 2300 AK
The Netherlands

Loskutoff, David J.
Department of Vascular Biology
VB-3
The Scripps Research Institute
10666 North Torrey Pines Rd
La Jolla CA 92037
USA

Nicholson, Andrew C.
Department of Biochemistry
Cornell University Medical College
1300 York Avenue
New York NY 10021
USA

Ogawa, Satoshi
Department of Physiology and Cellular
Biophysics
Columbia University
College of Physicians and Surgeons
630 West 168th Street
New York NY 10032
USA

Pannekoek, Hans
Academic Medical Center
Department of Biochemistry
Meibergdreef 15
Amsterdam 1105 AZ
The Netherlands

Pinsky, David
Department of Physiology and Cellular
Biophysics
Columbia University
College of Physicians and Surgeons
630 West 168th Street
New York NY 10032
USA

Preissner, Klaus T.
Haemostasis Research Unit,
Kerckhoff Klinik
Max-Plank-Institut
Sprudelhof 11
D-61231 Bad Nauheim
Germany

Quax, Paul H.A.
Gaubius Laboratory TNO-PG
PO Box 430
Leiden 2300 AK
The Netherlands

Reutelingsperger, Chris P.M.
Department of Biochemistry
Cardiovascular Research Institute
Maastrict (CARIM)
University of Limburg
PO Box 616
6200 MD Maastrict
The Netherlands

Rosenberg, Robert D.
Molecular Medicine Unit
Beth Israel Hospital
330 Brookline Avenue
Boston MA 02215
USA

Samad, Fahumiya
Department of Vascular Biology VB-3
The Scripps Research Institute
10666 North Torrey Pines Rd
La Jolla CA 92037
USA

Schmidt, Ann Marie
Department of Physiology and Cellular
Biophysics
Columbia University
College of Physicians and Surgeons
630 West 168th Street
New York NY 10032
USA

Sixma, Jan J.
University Hospital Utrect
Department of Haematology
PO Box 85.500
Utrect 3508 GA
The Netherlands

Stern, David
Department of Physiology and Cellular
Biophysics
Columbia University
College of Physicians and Surgeons
630 West 168th Street
New York NY 10032
USA

ten Cate, Hugo
Center of Hemostasis, Thrombosis,
Atherosclerosis and Inflammation
Research
Academic Medical Center, F4
Meibergdreef 9
Amsterdam 1105 AZ
The Netherlands

ten Cate, Jan W.
Center of Hemostasis, Thrombosis,
Atherosclerosis and Inflammation
Research
Academic Medical Center, F4
Meibergdreef 9
Amsterdam 1105 AZ
The Netherlands

van den Eijnden-Schrauwen, Yvonne
Gaubius Laboratory TNO-PG
PO Box 430
Leiden 2300 AK
The Netherlands

van der Poll, Tom
Center of Hemostasis, Thrombosis,
Atherosclerosis and Inflammation
Research
Academic Medical Center, F4
Meibergdreef 9
Amsterdam 1105 AZ
The Netherlands

van Deventer, Sander J.H.
Center of Hemostasis, Thrombosis,
Atherosclerosis and Inflammation
Research
Academic Medical Center, F4
Meibergdreef 9
Amsterdam 1105 AZ
The Netherlands

van Hinsbergh, Victor W.M.
Gaubius Laboratory TNO-PG
Zernikerdreef 9,
PO Box 2215
2301 CE Leiden
The Netherlands

van Mourik, Jan A.
Department of Blood Coagulation,
Central Laboratory of the Netherlands Red
Cross Blood Transfusion Service
PO Box 9190
1006 AD Amsterdam
The Netherlands

Verheijen, Jan H.
Gaubius Laboratory TNO-PG
PO Box 430
Leiden 2300 AK
The Netherlands

Wautier, Jean-Luc
Laboratoire de Recherche en Biologie
Vasculaire et Cellulaire
Unite d'Immunohematologie,
Hospital Lariboisière
Université Paris 7
Faculté de Medicine
Paris
France

Yan, Shi Du
Department of Physiology and Cellular
Biophysics
Columbia University
College of Physicians and Surgeons
630 West 168th Street
New York NY 10032
USA

1 Introduction: The Vessel Wall and Hemostasis

Victor W.M. van Hinsbergh

Gaubius Laboratory TNO-PG, Leiden, The Netherlands

INTRODUCTION

The circulatory system provides the tissues with oxygen, nutrients and hormones, and removes waste products and carbon dioxide therefrom. In mammalian species there is no alternative for the exchange of gasses, nutrients and metabolites. Therefore, a well functioning circulatory system, which can adapt regional blood flow according to the local needs, is essential. Disruption of the blood flow by wounding or by obstruction of the blood vessel causes ischemia and severe damage to the distal tissues and may cause death of the organism. During evolution a complex system has developed to guarantee blood fluidity, to limit blood loss after wounding, and to adapt this control system after exposure to infectious microorganisms. The functioning of this system represents hemostasis, a group of balanced activities that keeps the blood running.

THE VESSEL WALL AND HEMOSTASIS

The entire vascular system is lined by endothelial cells. Together these endothelial cells form a diffuse tissue of about 720 grams in an adult man (Wolinsky, 1980) covering a surface area which has been estimated to be up to 3500–6000 m^2. Most of these endothelial cells are in capillaries (>600 grams), which are highly exposed to the blood (up to 5000 cm^2/ml) (Busch and Owen, 1982). The exposure of large vessel endothelial cells to blood is much less (<10 cm^2/ml). Therefore, endothelial markers in the blood will preferentially reflect the products or actions of microvascular endothelial cells. Blood vessels also contain other cell types. Around the endothelial cells pericytes and, in larger vessels, multiple layers of smooth muscle cells are present. These cells mainly contribute to the vascular tone. Fibroblast are present in the adventitia of large vessels. Furthermore, nerve cell protrusions, mast cells and infiltrated leukocytes can be found in large vessels and may locally evoke responses of the vessel wall.

1

The fact that blood behaves as a fluid generates a certain risk. If the blood container, the circulatory system, is broken after wounding, blood is lost and tissues become devoid of nutrients. The body uses acute vasoconstriction, rapid formation of a hemostatic platelet plug and reinforcement of this plug by a fibrin meshwork, generated by the coagulation cascade, to prevent or reduce blood loss after wounding. Matrix proteins in the tissues as well as in the damaged vessel wall contribute to platelet adherence and activation. Activation of the coagulation cascade by tissue factor generates thrombin and causes fibrin polymerisation, by which the initial hemostatic plug is strengthened.

In the last two decades it has become increasingly clear that in particular the inner lining of the blood vessels, the endothelium, has profoundly characteristics that contribute to the maintenance of the fluidity of the blood. Living endothelium is necessary. After death, the blood will coagulate, albeit that the coagulated blood lyses again several hours later. If, in the living organism, the endothelium is damaged, platelets adhere to the damaged vessel wall or surrounding tissue, and coagulation is activated. These observations indicate that the continuous presence of living endothelium is crucial for the maintenance of blood fluidity.

ANTI-THROMBOTIC PROPERTIES OF THE ENDOTHELIUM

Closure of a wound must proceed rapidly and hence coagulation and platelet activation must be fast. The coagulation cascade and platelet activation are strongly catalyzed by proteins that become available after damage of a blood vessel. Such proteins include tissue factor, which triggers the extrinsic coagulation pathway, and collagen-bound von Willebrand factor, which plays an essential role in platelet activation. However, if such triggering molecules become available in intact vessels after injury of the endothelium at places distant from the wound or by activation of monocytes within the blood, intravascular coagulation or platelet aggregation can occur. Mural or obstructive thrombi may then impair the blood stream and cause ischemia and severe damage of the tissue distal to the occlusion. Therefore, a sofisticated machinery has been developed during evolution by which the intact vessel wall limits the extent of thrombus formation. This preventive action is realized by the endothelium by three types of anti-thrombotic mechanisms: interruption of the coagulation cascade, prevention of platelet activation and fibrinolysis (Table 1.1).

The coagulation pathway is a cascade of reactions which results in the formation of thrombin and subsequent fibrin formation. Activated components of the coagulation pathway activate new coagulation factors, by which a snowball-effect of activation occurs. Endothelial cells interrupt this snowball-effect by contributing to the inactivation of activated coagulation factors. They present heparan sulphates on their surface, which bind antithrombin III, the principal thrombin inhibitor at the luminal side of the vessel (Rosenberg and Bauer, chapter 3). Furthermore, endothelial cells express thrombomodulin, a surface protein, which catalyzes the activation of protein C by thrombin (Esmon, chapter 2). Protein C in its turn inactivates the coagulation factors Va and VIIIa. In addition, endothelial cells produce tissue factor pathway inhibitor (TFPI), an inhibitor that inhibits the start of the extrinsic coagulation pathway by forming a complex with tissue factor, factor VIIa and factor Xa. *In vitro*, endothelial cells also produce protein S, a co-factor for

Table 1.1 Hemostatic properties of endothelial cells

Antithrombotic Properties	*Thrombotic Properties*
Anticoagulant properties	*Procoagulant properties*
Surface heparan sulphates, which	Tissue factor synthesis
bind antithrombin III	Factor V synthesis
Expression thrombomodulin	Surface binding of clotting factors
Tissue Factor Pathway Inhibitor synthesis	
Synthesis and release of protein S	
Production of annexin V	
Prevention of platelet aggregation	*Platelet activating properties*
Proteoglycan surface (HS)	Synthesis von Willebrand factor
Prostacyclin and PGE_2 synthesis	Platelet Activating Factor synthesis
Nitric Oxide (NO) synthesis	Expression adhesive proteins
Ectonucleotidases (ADPase)	
Fibrinolysis	*Reduction fibrinolysis*
Synthesis and release of t-PA; u-PA synthesis	Synthesis PAI-1
Expression receptors for u-PA, t-PA and plasminogen	

Endothelial cells express a number of antithrombotic properties and synthesize and release von Willebrand factor. After activation by tumor necorsis factor-α, interleukin-1 or endotoxin, endothelial cells acquire several "prothrombotic" properties in addition, while the expression of thrombomodulin activity decreases.

activated protein C action, and vascular anticoagulant factor (annexin V), a protein that binds to negatively charged phospholipids (Reutelingsperger, chapter 4), but the function of which *in vivo* has still to be established.

Endothelial cells also prevent or limit thrombus formation by suppressing platelet activation (de Groot and Sixma, chapter 7). Platelet activation is counteracted by prostacyclin and prostaglandin E_2, which are liberated from the endothelial cells after stimulation by vasoactive substances, including thrombin. The effect of prostacyclin is enhanced by another endothelial release product nitric oxide (NO). In addition, endothelial cells contain large amounts of ectonucleotidases on their surface, which convert the platelet-stimulating agent ADP into adenosine. Finally, endothelial surface-bound proteoglycans, in particular the heparan-residues, prevent platelet adhesion to the endothelium. Endothelial cells also synthesize and store von Willebrand factor (Hop and Pannekoek, chapter 6). After its release from the endothelial cell, von Willebrand factor becomes incorporated in the subendothelial matrix. After damage of the endothelium, platelets adhere avidly to matrix-bound von Willebrand factor and become activated. Von Willebrand factor that — after stimulation of endothelial cells — is released from these cells will rapidly bind to the exposed collagen of a damaged vessel wall, and thus enhance platelet binding and activation and thus the formation of a platelet plug (Sixma and de Groot, chapter 8).

Endothelial cells express a third mechanism to maintain blood fluidity, if coagulation occurs despite all these anticoagulant mechanisms. They provide the regulatory components of fibrinolysis, in particular tissue-type plasminogen activator (t-PA). The fibrinolytic activity in blood is largely determined by the concentration of t-PA (Emeis *et al.*, chapter 10; Carmeliet and Collen, chapter 13), and is modulated by, amongst others, the plasminogen activator inhibitor PAI-1 (Fearns *et al.*, chapter 11). The concentration in blood is subject to changes in the synthesis and release of t-PA by the endothelium and to fluctuations in the liver blood flow, which influences the t-PA clearance by the liver. As the half-life of t-PA in plasma is very short, the t-PA concentration can vary rapidly. The production of t-PA comprises two mechanisms: a constitutive secretion of t-PA by the cells, and an immediate release of t-PA from a storage pool in endothelial cells, which is induced by vasoactive substances, such as platelet activating factor, bradykinin and thrombin (Emeis *et al.*, chapter 10). This acute release mechanism plays an important role in the effective protection of blood against a locally emerging thrombus, because t-PA present during thrombus generation and incorporated in the thrombus is much more effective than when added after thrombus formation.

ADAPTATION AND REGIONAL DIFFERENCES

The characteristics of the endothelial cells in various parts of the body can be markedly different. Liver, spleen and bone marrow contain sinusoids with fenestrated endothelial cells. Sinusoidal liver endothelial cells contribute together with Kupffer cells and hepatocytes, to selective clearance of plasma constituents in the liver. They bind large amounts of heparin on specific binding sites, contain receptors for modified proteins, such as oxidized low density lipoproteins, and are an important source of coagulation factor VIII. Endothelial cells of the microvessels in visceral beds often contain diaphragms, specialized structures at which the luminal and basolateral membrane contact each other. The endothelium of brain microvessels is much tighter than that in other parts of the body. Brain vessel endothelial cells contain relatively little thrombomodulin (Wong *et al.*, 1991) and may be protected by additional mechanisms against thrombosis. Local production of protease nexin 1 has been suggested to be important for inhibition of serine proteases in the brain. Relatively little is still known about how regional differences affect the hemostatic properties of the various vascular beds.

    One of the factors that contribute to the need of regional differences is the blood flow (Davies and Tripathi, 1993; Slack *et al.*, 1993). The shear forces generated by the flowing blood on the vessel wall depend on the shear rate and the viscosity of the blood. Shear rates vary as much as $270–2800$ sec^{-1} in capillaries, $1500–1900$ sec^{-1} in arterioles and small arteries, and $50–350$ sec^{-1} in large arteries. At an arterial stenosis the shear rate can be enhanced by 1 to 2 orders of magnitude (Slack *et al.*, 1993). The requirements for platelet adhesion and the kinetics of the activation of coagulation factors vary according to the shear forces generated by the flowing blood on the surface of blood cells and the vessel wall (Weiss *et al.*, 1986; Gemmell *et al.*, 1988; Ruggeri, 1993). Therefore, it is not surprising that quantitative differences exist in the production of anti-thrombotic factors by veins, arteries, postcapillary venules and capillaries. Such differences have been observed for example for the production of t-PA (Noordhoek Hegt, 1977; van Hinsbergh, 1988), nitric oxide (Vanhoutte and Miller, 1985), prostacyclin and prostaglandin E_2 (Gerritsen, 1987) by vein, artery and microvascular endothelial cells.

    In addition to these endogenous regional differences, the vessel wall, in particular the endothelium, may under challenging conditions, such as in inflammation or ischemia, rapidly change its contribution to the maintenance of hemostasis (Schmidt *et al.*, chapter 14; Nicholson and Hajjar, chapter 16). After inflammatory activation by endotoxin, IL-1 or TNFα, during hypoxia, and after exposure to the medium conditioned by certain tumors, endothelial cells *in vitro* start to express tissue factor, promote thrombin generation (Brinkman and van Mourik, chapter 5; Schmidt *et al.*, chapter 14), reduce their surface thrombomodulin activity and enhance their production of PAI-1 (Fearns *et al.*, chapter 11). In sepsis or after infusion of TNFα or endotoxin *in vivo*, increased thrombin generation, plasminogen consumption and increased circulating PAI-1 are observed (van der Poll *et al.*, chapter 15). This points to an activation of the coagulation pathway and modulation of the fibrinolytic system. Circulating thrombomodulin antigen has also been observed in certain inflammatory conditions *in vivo*, suggesting that part(s) of the thrombomodulin molecules are detached from the endothelial surface. Expression of tissue factor by endothelial cells *in vivo*, however, is still controversial. In intact vessels tissue factor has been demonstrated in the abluminal matrix of endothelial cells. As such it may play a role once the endothelial cell layer has become damaged. Although tissue factor has been reported to be present on endothelial cells *in vitro* after exposure to inflammatory mediators, no *in vivo* conformation has yet been obtained for a luminal expression of tissue factor on endothelial cells. However, if a low degree of controlled thrombin generation on the luminal surface of intact endothelium would occur, it might act more pronouncedly on the anti-thrombotic mechanisms than on the amplification of the coagulation pathway, because it would strongly contribute to the activation of protein C and stimulate the cells to release t-PA, NO and prostacyclin directly at the site where thrombin is present. Experiments by Hanson *et al.*, (1993), who found that preinfusion of an animal with low concentrations of thrombin reduced the formation of thrombi on arterial grafts via a protein C-dependent mechanism, provide evidence that small amounts of thrombin can indeed strongly stimulate the anti-thrombotic mechanisms provided by the endothelium.

Because chronic challenge of endothelial cells, eg. by hyperglycemia (Schmidt *et al.*, chapter 14) or homocysteinuria, can cause injury of endothelial cell functioning, such conditions may lead to a long lasting adaptation and impairment of the anti-thrombotic defence mechanisms of the vessel wall.

HEMOSTASIS AND TISSUE REPAIR

The hemostatic plug not only acts as an instant sealing after wounding, but also as a scaffold for invading cells during the subsequent repair process (Quax *et al.*, chapter 12; Carmeliet and Collen, chapter 13). The hemostatic plug not only consists of platelets and fibrin, but has also incorporated other adhesive proteins, such as fibronectin and vitronectin, which influence the behaviour of invading cells and, as has been nicely demonstrated for vitronectin, can directly or indirectly influence the action of several serine proteases (Preissner, chapter 9). Leukocytes, microvascular endothelial cells and tissue cells invade the fibrin matrix and convert it slowly into healthy tissue. Proteases of the coagulation system, in particular thrombin, as well as products released from activated platelets, such as platelet derived growth factor (PDGF), and the fibrin matrix itself, a scaffold for invading cells, all contribute to the subsequent healing process. Therefore, one may consider the stabilized hemostatic plug not only as a instant sealing reagent, but also as an important contributor to tissue repair (Colvin, 1986; van Hinsbergh, 1992). The contribution of the hemostatic system is not limited to the healing of open wounds, which causes contact of tissues with the outer world, but is also involved in healing the site of leakages within the body. Vascular leakage caused by inflammation is counteracted by coagulation via the extrinsic coagulation pathway. This causes a fibrinous exudate, which is subsequently invaded by inflammatory cells, capillaries and tissue cells (granulation tissue). Normally, the fibrinous material is degraded by fibrinolysis during healing of the injured area. Cell-associated fibrinolysis, which uses in particular urokinase-type plasminogen activator (u-PA) to generate plasmin (Quax *et al.*, chapter 12; Carmeliet and Collen, chapter 13) plays an important role in this process. Sometimes the fibrinous material is not degraded in a proper way and will provide a scaffold for scar tissue formation. The leaky vessels around many tumors will cause the formation of a stroma, a comparable fibrinous exudate area around the tumor. The tumor stroma provides a scaffold for the invasion of new blood vessels, which are necessary to nourish the growing tumor (Dvorak *et al.*, 1992). These examples indicate that the hemostatic plug is also an important contributor to tissue repair and tissue remodelling.

A similar contribution of products from the coagulation system and activated platelets is anticipated to contribute to the aggravation of atherosclerotic lesions, in addition to the well known contribution of lipoprotein-derived lipids. During atherosclerotic plaque formation, and during the formation of a stenosis after luminal angioplasty, migration and intimal accumulation of smooth muscle cells is induced by local factors, such as platelet-derived growth factor and fibrin accumulation (derived from incorporated mural thrombi and possibly from vascular leakage and macrophage-induced coagulation) in the intima. This enhances the risk for intra-intimal microvessel formation and hemorrhages within the vessel wall. In this case, apparently the repair mechanism overshoots and becomes a threat to the vessel itself.

SCOPE OF THE BOOK

This book deals with a number of aspects of the vascular control of hemostasis. It focuses on recent developments in this field, but does not intend to be or to replace a general handbook on hemostasis. The first chapters focus on the interaction of coagulation factors with the endothelium and their contribution to the anti-coagulant character of the endothelium. Subsequently, adherence of platelets to vascular matrix proteins and the contribution of the endothelium to prevent platelet activation are discussed. These chapters are followed by four chapters on the regulation and function of plasminogen activation, and the consequences of a genetically-induced defiency of plasminogen activators or their inhibitor PAI-1, in animals. The last three chapters deal with the effect of inflammation and other activating conditions on the hemostatic balance *in vitro* and *in vivo*.

References

Bush, P.C. and Owen, W.G. (1982). Interactions of thrombin with endothelium. In: *Pathobiology of the endothelial cell*, edited by H.L. Nossel and H.J. Vogel, pp. 97–101. New York: Academic Press.

Colvin, R.B. (1986). Wound healing processes in hemostasis and thrombosis. In: *Vascular endothelium in hemostasis and thrombosis*, edited by M.A. Gimbrone Jr, pp. 220–241. Edinburgh: Churchill Livingstone.

Davie, E.W., Fujikawa, K. and Kisiel, W. (1991). The coagulation cascade: initiation, maintenance, and regulation. *Biochemistry* **30**:10363–10370.

Davies, P.F. and Tripathi, S.C. (1993). Mechanical stress mechanisms and the cell. An endothelial paradigm. *Circulation Research* **72**:239–245.

Dvorak, H., Nagy, J.A., Berse, B., Brown, L.F., Yeo, K.-T., Yeo, T.-K., Dvorak, A.M., Van de Water, L., Sioussat, T.M. and Senger, D.R. (1982). Vascular permeability factor, fibrin, and the pathogenesis of tumor stroma formation. In: *Plasminogen activation in fibrinolysis, in tissue remodeling, and in development*, edited by P. Brakman and C. Kluft. Annals of the New York Academy of Sciences **667**:101–111.

Gemmell, C.H., Turitto, V.T. and Nemerson, Y. (1988). Flow as a regulator of the activation of factor X by tissue factor. *Blood* **72**:1404–1406.

Gerritsen, M.E. (1987). Functional heterogeneity of vascular endothelial cells. *Biochemical Pharmacology* **36**:2701–2711.

Hanson, S.R., Griffin, J.H., Harker, L.A., Kelly, A.B., Esmon, C.T. and Gruber, A. (1993). Antithrombotic effects of thrombin-induced activation of endogenous protein C in primates. *Journal of Clinical Investigation* **92**:2003–2012.

Rapaport, S.I. (1991). The extrinsic pathway inhibitor: a regulator of tissue factor-dependent blood coagulation. *Thrombosis and Hemostasis* **66**:6–15.

Ruggeri, Z.M. (1993) Mechanisms of shear-induced platelet adhesion and aggregation. *Thrombosis and Haemostasis* **70**: 119–123.

Slack, S.M., Cui, Y. and Turitto, V.T. (1993). The effect of flow on blood coagulation and thrombosis. *Thrombosis and Hemostasis* **70**:129–134.

Van Hinsbergh, V.W.M. (1988). Regulation of the synthesis and secretion of plasminogen activators by endothelial cells. *Hemostasis* **18**:307–327.

Van Hinsbergh, V.W.M. (1982). Impact of endothelial activation on fibrinolysis and local proteolysis in tissue repair. In: *Plasminogen activation in fibrinolysis, in tissue remodeling, and in development*, edited by P. Brakman and C. Kluft, Annals of the New York Academy of Sciences **667**:151–162.

Vanhoutte, P.M. and Miller, V.M. (1985). Heterogeneity of endothelium-dependent responses in mammalian blood vessels. *Journal of Cardiovascular Pharmacology* **7** (suppl. 3): S12–S23.

Weiss, H.J., Turitto, V.T. and Baumgartner, H.R. (1986). Role of shear rate and platelets in promoting fibrin formation on rabbit subendothelium. Studies utilizing patients with quantitative and qualitative platelet defects. *Journal of Clinical Investigation* **78**:1072–1082.

Wolinsky, H. (1980). A proposal linking clearance of circulating lipoproteins to tissue metabolic activity as a basis for understanding atherogenesis. *Circulation Research* **47**:301–311.

Wong, V.L.Y., Hofman, F.M., Ishii, H. and Fisher, M. (1991). Regional distribution of thrombomodulin in human brain. *Brain Research* **556**:1–5.

2 Anticoagulant Properties of Vascular Cells: Thrombomodulin and Protein C Activation Pathway

Charles T. Esmon

From the Oklahoma Medical Research Foundation, Departments of Pathology and Biochemistry and Molecular Biology, University of Oklahoma Health Sciences Center, and the Howard Hughes Medical Institute, Oklahoma City, OK 73104

Abbreviations — APC, activated protein C; EPCR, endothelial cell protein C receptor; TM, thrombomodulin, APA, antiphospholipid antibodies: LA, lupus anticoagulants; C4bBP, C4b binding protein; EGF, epidermal growth factor homology domain; DIC, disseminated intravascular coagulation; PE, phosphatidylethanolamine; TNF, tumor necrosis factor.

OVERVIEW

The protein C anticoagulant pathway provides a unique "on demand" anticoagulant, activated protein C (APC), in response to thrombin generation. The system has multiple components, many of which are modulated by inflammatory mediators or consumed during disseminated intravascular coagulation (DIC). Thus, acquired deficiencies can occur in selected clinical conditions that may contribute to thrombosis or DIC. Furthermore, abnormalities in the components or substrates of the protein C pathway appear to account for the majority of familial thrombophilia. To aid in understanding the basis for these observations, this chapter will focus on the currently understood mechanisms by which the pathway functions biochemically and physiologically. Several reviews covering the area in general or selected aspects of this complex pathway have been published (Comp, 1986; Esmon, 1989; Davie, Fujikawa, and Kisiel, 1991; Walker and Fay, 1992; Preissner, 1990; Rodgers and Chandler, 1992; Esmon, Taylor and Snow, 1991; Alving and Comp, 1992; Reitsma *et al.*, 1993; Esmon, 1993).

Known Interactions in the Protein C Pathway

A model of the known components of the protein C anticoagulant pathway is illustrated in Figure 2.1. The ability to deliver an on demand anticoagulant is due to the mechanism by which APC is generated. When thrombin, the terminal enzyme of the coagulation system, binds to the endothelial cell receptor thrombomodulin (TM), the formation of the anticoagulant enzyme, APC, is triggered. This interaction not only leads to APC formation, but

PROTEIN C PATHWAY-NORMAL FUNCTION

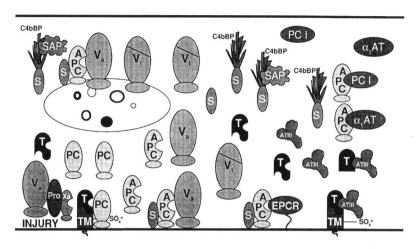

Figure 2.1   The protein C anticoagulant pathway under normal conditions. Vascular injury initiates prothrombin (Pro) activation that results in thrombin (T) formation. Prothrombin activation involves factor Va (Va) and factor Xa (Xa). Thrombin then binds to thrombomodulin (TM) on the lumen of the endothelium, illustrated by the heavy line, and the thrombin- TM complex converts protein C (PC) to activated protein C (APC). Thrombin bound to thrombomodulin can be inactivated very rapidly by antithrombin III (ATIII), at which time the thrombin-antithrombin III complex rapidly dissociates. Activated protein C then binds to protein S (S) on cellular surfaces. The activated protein C-protein S complex then converts factor Va to an inactive complex (Vi), illustrated by the slash through the larger part of the two-subunit factor Va molecule. Protein C and activated protein C (APC) interact with an endothelial cell protein C receptor (EPCR). This may concentrate the zymogen and enzyme near the cell surface and facilitate the function of the pathway, but this is yet to be shown directly. Protein S circulates in complex with C4bBP, which may in turn bind serum amyloid P (SAP). Activated protein C is inhibited by forming complexes with either the protein C inhibitor (PCI), α1-antitrypsin (α_1AT) or α_2-macroglobulin (not shown). See text for a more complete discussion. (Modified from Arterioscl. and Thromb. 12(2): 135–145, 1992, with permission of the American Heart Association.)

also reversibly blocks the ability of thrombin to carry out most of its procoagulant activities including fibrinogen clotting (Esmon, Esmon, and Harris, 1982) and platelet activation (Esmon, Carroll and Esmon, 1983). When thrombin is bound to TM, inhibition by antithrombin is enhanced due to the presence of a chondroitin sulfate moiety (Preissner, Delvos, and Muller-Berghaus, 1987; Parkinson *et al.,* 1992; Ye, Esmon, and Johnson, 1993; Bourin, Lundgren-Åkerlund, and Lindahl, 1990; Bourin and Lindahl, 1993; Lin *et al.,* 1994). This chondroitin sulfate moiety also increases the affinity of TM for thrombin (Parkinson *et al.,* 1992) by binding to a cluster of basic residues in anion binding exosite 2 of thrombin (Ye, Rezaie, and Esmon, 1994). Thrombin binding to TM also increases the rate of prourokinase inactivation by thrombin (de Munk, Groeneveld, and Rijken, 1991; Molinari *et al.,* 1992).

Formation of APC leads to the inactivation of two of the cofactors critical for thrombin formation, factors Va (Kalafatis and Mann, 1993) and VIIIa (Regan *et al.,* 1994) and may also enhance fibrinolysis either by interacting with plasminogen activator inhibitors (Heeb *et al.,* 1987) or by limiting prothrombin activation (Bajzar and Nesheim, 1993). Factor VIII is also a substrate for APC. With factor VIII, binding to von Willebrand factor protects the protein from inactivation (Fay, Coumans, and Walker, 1991; Koedam *et al.,*

1988). APC anticoagulant activity is facilitated by protein S (Walker, 1980). Very recent results suggest that factor V also facilitates APC dependent factor Va and VIIIa inactivation (Dahlbäck, Carlsson, and Svensson, 1993; Shen and Dahlbäck, 1994). Protein S and factor V appear to function synergistically in this process. Protein S serves as a cofactor for the inactivation of factors Va and VIIIa (Walker, 1980; Koedam *et al.,* 1988). Protein S also appears to have direct anticoagulant effects *in vitro* that are independent of APC, but protein S has very limited anticoagulant activity in plasma in the absence of APC (Hackeng *et al.,* 1993; Duchemin *et al.,* 1994). APC independent inhibition of prothrombin activation involves interaction with many of the proteins in the prothrombin activation complex (Heeb *et al.,* 1994; Hackeng *et al.,* 1993). Protein S circulates both free and in complex with C4bBP, a regulatory protein of the complement system (Dahlbäck, 1991). To function as a cofactor for APC, protein S must be in a free form (Dahlbäck, 1986; Comp *et al.,* 1984).

APC functions on several cellular surfaces, but the two that have been most analyzed are platelets (Tans *et al.,* 1991; Harris and Esmon, 1985; Dahlbäck, Wiedmer, and Sims, 1992; Mitchell and Salem, 1987) and endothelium (Hackeng *et al.,* 1993; Stern *et al.,* 1986). Protein C/APC binds specifically to the endothelium (Bangalore, Drohan, and Orthner, 1994; Fukudome and Esmon, 1994). This is mediated by a novel endothelial cell protein receptor, EPCR (Fukudome and Esmon, 1994). Protein C/APC can also interact with protein S (Dahlbäck, Wiedmer, and Sims, 1992) or TM (Hogg, Öhlin, and Stenflo, 1992; Olsen *et al.,* 1992). The role of EPCR in the protein C system remains unclear.

Once APC is formed, it is among the slowest of the proteases to be inhibited and cleared from the circulation. Inhibition of APC activity involves primarily the protein C inhibitor (Suzuki *et al.,* 1987), α_1-antitrypsin (Heeb and Griffin, 1988), or α_2-macroglobulin (Scully *et al.,* 1993; Heeb, Gruber, and Griffin, 1991). The half life for clearance from the circulation is approximately 10–20 min (España *et al.,* 1991; Comp and Esmon, 1981).

Unlike most clotting systems, the protein C pathway seems to be relatively species specific (Marciniak, 1972). For instance, compared to human APC, bovine APC is a poor anticoagulant of human plasma (Walker, 1981), but this problem can be corrected by addition of bovine protein S to the human plasma. Activation by the thrombin-TM complex does not show comparable species specificity.

Structural Organization of the Proteins of the Protein C Pathway

Considerable insight into the function of the protein C pathway can be gleaned from analysis of the key structural features of the proteins. A schematic of the structure of the proteins of the pathway is shown in Figure 2.2. Like most of the coagulation enzymes, protein C is a vitamin K dependent zymogen. The protease region of these proteins is located about 70 Å from the membrane surface (Husten, Esmon, and Johnson, 1987) as is thrombin when bound to TM (Lu *et al.,* 1989). The domain has homology to other serine proteases including trypsin and chymotrypsin. Molecular modelling of this domain has been done (Fisher, Greengard, and Griffin, 1994) and suggests that the active site of APC, like that of factor Xa (Padmanabhan *et al.,* 1993), is much more open to access of substrates than that of thrombin (Stubbs and Bode, 1993; Tulinsky and Qiu, 1993). For ease of comparison with mutations performed in other systems, amino acid substitutions will be referred to using the chymotrypsin numbering system described by Bode (Bode *et al.,*

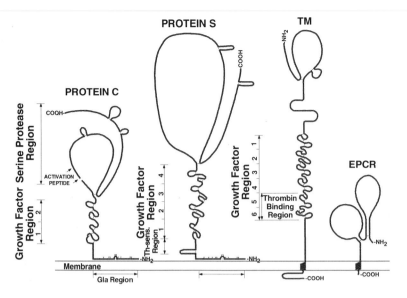

Figure 2.2   Schematic representation of protein C, protein S, the endothelial cell protein C receptor (EPCR) and thrombomodulin (TM). The vitamin K dependent Gla residues of protein C and protein S are indicated by small Y-shaped symbols. Formation of these vitamin K-dependent residues is essential to full activity of protein C and protein S. Gla, γ-carboxyglutamic acid; Th.-sens., thrombin sensitive. The EPCR domain structure is based on homology to the CD1 family and the disulfide pairing remains to be documented experimentally. (Modified and reprinted from J. Biol. Chem. 264: 4743–4746, 1989, with permission of the American Society for Biochemistry and Molecular Biology, Inc.)

1989). Between the protease domain and the membrane are two EGF like repeats. The one closest to the membrane surface in the diagram binds Ca^{2+} (Öhlin, Linse, and Stenflo, 1988; Stenflo, 1991) and contains a β hydroxy aspartic acid residue (Drakenberg *et al.*, 1983). The Gla domain, where the γ-carboxy glutamic acids are located, is responsible for membrane binding (Colpitts and Castellino, 1994; Jhingan *et al.*, 1994). Carboxylation is necessary for function (Jhingan *et al.*, 1994; D'Angelo *et al.*, 1986) and function is therefore blocked by oral anticoagulants like warfarin.

Protein S has a similar domain distribution, but unlike protein C, it is not a protease. Instead of a protease domain, the corresponding region in protein S has homology to the steroid binding proteins (Joseph and Baker, 1992; Gershagen, Fernlund, and Edenbrandt, 1991). This domain probably plays a role in C4bBP binding (Nelson and Long, 1992). Between this domain and the membrane are four EGF like domains and a thrombin sensitive loop. Ca^{2+} binding to protein S dramatically inhibits the ability of thrombin to cleave this region (Sugo *et al.*, 1986). The thrombin cleavage loop and the EGF domains may be involved in binding APC since antibodies to this region potently inhibit protein S function without preventing membrane binding. Protein S association with the membrane is mediated by the Gla domain since chemical modification of the Gla residues (Walker, 1986) blocks membrane binding and function, and the anticoagulant function of protein S is lost following oral anticoagulant treatment (D'Angelo *et al.*, 1988).

TM differs in its organization from protein C and protein S (Jackman *et al.*, 1987; Suzuki *et al.*, 1987; Wen *et al.*, 1987). The amino terminal domain is related distantly to lectin-like proteins including the asialoglycoprotein receptor (Petersen, 1988). The function of this domain is unknown. This region is followed by 6 EGF domains. The

EGF 4–6 domains play critical roles in protein C activation. EGF 5–6 contains the major-ity of the thrombin binding energy, can block fibrinogen clotting, but cannot accelerate activation of protein C (Kurosawa *et al.*, 1988). A synthetic peptide corresponding to the third loop of the 5th EGF domain can also bind to thrombin as can the regions of the 6th EGF 4 domain (Tsiang, Lentz, and Sadler, 1992).

When the EGF 4 domain is covalently associated with EGF 5–6, this small fragment accelerates protein C activation nearly as effectively as full length TM (Zushi *et al.*, 1989; Zushi *et al.*, 1991; Stearns, Kurosawa, and Esmon, 1989). Following the EGF domains is a region rich in O linked sugars. This site is also the location of a chondroitin sulfate attachment site (Bourin, Lundgren-Åkerlund, and Lindahl, 1990; Bourin and Lindahl, 1993; Bourin *et al.*, 1988; Parkinson *et al.*, 1990; Parkinson *et al.*, 1992; Ye, Rezaie, and Esmon, 1994; Lin *et al.*, 1994). The chondroitin sulfate moiety binds to thrombin at anion binding exosite 2 (the heparin binding site) (Ye, Rezaie, and Esmon, 1994), alters the Ca^{2+} dependence of protein C activation and enhances the affinity of thrombin for TM about 10–20 fold depending on the nature of the chondroitin and species of TM (Parkinson *et al.*, 1990). The O-linked sugar region, which apparently is a very extended structure rising rapidly from the membrane surface (Lu *et al.*, 1989), is fol-lowed by the transmembrane region of TM. The carboxy terminus of TM is located in the short cytosolic tail (36 residues).

EPCR is an integral membrane protein. It has structural homology to the MHC class 1/CD1 family of proteins. Based on this homology, the extra cellular domain has been tentatively drawn as a two domain structure with each domain having a single disulfide. Unlike TM, there is no extended O linked sugar region. The function of EPCR remains unknown except that it binds protein C and APC with equal affinity ($Kd \approx 30$ nM). To date, EPCR expression has only been detected at significant levels on endothelium, but cellular distribution studies remain incomplete. Since the molecule is structurally homol-ogous to the MHC/CD1 family of proteins, most of which have been shown to be associ-ated with inflammation, it is possible that EPCR constitutes the link between protein C and the anti-inflammatory activity associated with protein C/APC administration in septic shock (see section on **Acquired Deficiencies and Their Treatment with Protein C: Meningococcemia**).

Gene Structure

The gene structure of protein C (Foster, Yoshitake, and Davie, 1985), protein S (Schmidel *et al.*, 1990; Edenbrandt *et al.*, 1990; Ploos van Amstel *et al.*, 1990) and TM (Jackman *et al.*, 1987) have been determined. As might be expected from the domain structures, the different domains of protein C and protein S are in general separated by introns (14 in protein S and 7 in protein C). Protein S also has a pseudo gene (Schmidel *et al.*, 1990). Surprisingly, TM which also has many domains, lacks introns (Jackman *et al.*, 1987). The gene structure of EPCR is not yet known.

Regulation of the Protein C Pathway

Many lines of evidence suggest that abnormalities in the function of the pathway con-tribute to both hereditary and acquired thrombophilia. Furthermore, the pathway seems to be negatively regulated by a variety of inflammatory mediators.

Thrombomodulin is probably the best characterized of the components of the protein C pathway with respect to regulation. Down regulation can be accomplished by several mechanisms. In severe inflammatory conditions, soluble TM levels rise in the circulation due to proteolytic release, possibly by neutrophil elastase (Takano *et al.,* 1990). TM also has an exposed methionine that is sensitive to oxidative damage with a concomitant decrease in TM function (Glaser *et al.,* 1992). Oxidation could presumably occur when activated leukocytes adhere to endothelium releasing peroxides or superoxide. Finally, TM is down regulated by endotoxin (Moore *et al.,* 1987), tumor necrosis factor α (Nawroth and Stern, 1986), and interleukin 1 (Nawroth *et al.,* 1986), glycosylation (as might occur in diabetes) (Esposito *et al.,* 1989) or ischemia (Shreeniwas *et al.,* 1991). In cell culture, exposure of endothelium to TNF results in prolonged inhibition of transcription for more than 24 hr (Conway and Rosenberg, 1988) even if TNF is removed. TM antigen and activity then disappear from the cell surface due to internalization and degradation in lysosomes (Moore, Esmon, and Esmon, 1989; Lentz, Tsiang, and Sadler, 1991). Constitutive internalization of TM appears to involve both clathrin coated and uncoated pits (Conway *et al.,* 1987). TNF may not alter the turnover rate (Lentz, Tsiang, and Sadler, 1991).

Interestingly, while the transcriptional control, proteolytic sensitivity and oxidant sensitivity would suggest that TM would be readily down regulated in major inflammatory disease, the molecule seems to be more resistant *in vivo* than the *in vitro* data would predict. *In vivo,* endotoxin failed to down regulate TM in the rabbit aorta (Semeraro *et al.,* 1993) or in the rat kidney (Laszik *et al.,* 1994). In the rat model, the challenge was severe and thrombi were readily observed in the kidney. Thus, the thrombosis in the rat kidney could not be due to TM down regulation. A similar picture has emerged in the baboon. Baboon organs examined qualitatively by immunofluorescence failed to detect TM down regulation (Drake *et al.,* 1993). In contrast, organ rejection (Tsuchida *et al.,* 1992) and inflammatory disorders of the placenta (villitis) (Labarrere *et al.,* 1990) are associated with TM down regulation. Thus, some complex set of balancing reactions must exist *in vivo.*

Potential clues to the regulation come from factors that elevate TM expression or prevent TNF down regulation of TM. These include elevation of cyclic AMP (Tazawa *et al.,* 1994), interleukin 4 (Kapiotis *et al.,* 1991) and heat shock responses (Conway *et al.,* 1994). Perhaps a heat shock class response and/or the release of interleukin 4 may be responsible for the failure to observe TM down regulation *in vivo* when animals are challenged with endotoxin. Certainly, this is a clear example of the complex nature of regulatory events. It is interesting to speculate that inappropriate responses to the "balancing" factors could be responsible for certain forms of thrombotic disease.

TM also has an interesting developmental aspect. In the mouse, TM is expressed at very high concentrations in the neural crest early in development (Imada *et al.,* 1987). This is probably due to the presence of retinoic acid response elements in the TM promoter (Dittman *et al.,* 1994; Weiler-Guettler *et al.,* 1992) It is unclear what role TM plays in development.

Originally observed on endothelium, TM has now been identified on monocytes (McCachren *et al.,* 1991), smooth muscle cells in culture (Soff, Jackman, and Rosenberg, 1991), adherent synovial cells (Conway and Nowakowski, 1993), syncytiotrophoblasts of human placenta (Maruyama, Bell, and Majerus, 1985), neutrophils (Conway, Nowakowski, and Steiner-Mosonyi, 1992), mesothelial cells (Collins *et al.,* 1992), and platelets (Suzuki *et al.,* 1988). Based on immunofluorescence, however, the major site for

TM remains the endothelium. An early report suggested that human brain microvessels were devoid of TM (Ishii *et al.*, 1986), but recent reports have identified TM in these vessels (Wong *et al.*, 1991), but the levels seem to be relatively low. TM was earlier detected in rabbit brain microvessels (DeBault *et al.*, 1986; Boffa, Burke, and Haudenschild, 1987).

The other membrane associated protein in the pathway, EPCR, is like TM, down regulated by TNF α. The time course of down regulation of message and binding activity are somewhat faster than that of TM (Fukudome and Esmon, 1994). Like TM, EPCR synthesis remains depressed for 24 hr following exposure to TNF. Although the decrease in message is presumably due to inhibition of transcription, it is also possible that TNF alters message stability and that the decrease in EPCR function could be due to increased rates of EPCR internalization and degradation.

Protein S levels in vascular disease and thrombosis has been the subject of considerable clinical interest. Protein S cofactor activity is resident only in the free protein, i.e. not in the protein S-C4bBP complex (Dahlbäck, 1986; Comp *et al.*, 1984). Thus, free protein S levels are probably the clinically relevant values determining potential protein S contributions to a hypercoaguable state. Unfortunately, the affinity of free protein S for C4bBP is enhanced by physiological Ca^{2+} (Dahlbäck, Frohm, and Nelsestuen, 1990; Griffin, Gruber, and Fernandez, 1992), and this makes analysis of protein S distribution in patient plasma difficult. Free protein S and total protein S levels are often reported as low in patients with inflammatory diseases or following thrombotic complications (Comp *et al.*, 1986; Comp *et al.*, 1985; Sacco *et al.*, 1989; D'Angelo *et al.*, 1987; D'Angelo *et al.*, 1988; Heeb, Mosher, and Griffin, 1989; Girolami *et al.*, 1989; Sheth and Carvalho, 1991; Golub, Sibony, and Coller, 1990; Gouault-Heilmann *et al.*, 1988; Lauer *et al.*, 1990; Takahashi *et al.*, 1989; Engresser *et al.*, 1987; Fourrier *et al.*, 1992; Tsuchida *et al.*, 1992; Chafa *et al.*, 1992; Walker, 1992; Kemkes-Matthes, 1992; Alving and Comp, 1992; Alessi *et al.*, 1993; D'Angelo *et al.*, 1993; Anzola *et al.*, 1993; Carr and Zekert, 1993; Amster *et al.*, 1993). There are an extremely large number of papers published on this issue, with no obvious unifying consensus as to whether protein S is decreased in selected diseases or whether this is caused by decreased free or total protein S. In our experience in experimental animals, inflammatory stimuli increase C4bBP levels resulting in more protein S in complex and less free as assessed in citrated plasma. This would seem reasonable based on the fact that C4bBP is an acute phase reactant (Boerger *et al.*, 1987; Dahlbäck, 1991). This situation may be more complex, however (Garcia de Frutos *et al.*, 1994). C4bBP is composed of α and β chains. Some C4bBP is synthesized without β chains and β chains are required to bind protein S (Hillarp and Dahlbäck, 1988). In a recent study, Dahlback's group reported that inflammatory mediators enhance only α chain synthesis (Garcia de Frutos *et al.*, 1994). Thus, C4bBP may rise without increasing protein S binding capacity. It will be of future interest to confirm these studies and to examine whether some patients with thrombotic disease have an altered regulatory pathway that could allow enhanced β chain synthesis also. If this is the case, then it might explain some of the variability in the clinical results.

An alternative means of decreasing protein S function is through proteolytic cleavage (Sugo *et al.*, 1986; Dahlbäck, Lundwall, and Stenflo, 1986). Thrombin can cleave protein S in a protease sensitive loop, but this process is almost completely blocked by physiological Ca^{2+} (Sugo *et al.*, 1986), at least *in vitro*. The cleaved protein S has decreased cofactor activity, presumably due to decreased affinity for phospholipids at physiological

Ca^{2+} concentrations (Schwalbe *et al.,* 1990; Walker, 1984). Although Ca^{2+} blocks throm-bin inactivation of protein S, cleaved protein S has nevertheless been detected in the plasma from patients with disseminated intravascular coagulation (Heeb, Mosher, and Griffin, 1989). A possible means of rationalizing these apparently contradictory results is to invoke another protease in the inactivation of protein S. Indeed, neutrophil (Oates and Salem, 1991) and platelet membranes (Mitchell and Salem, 1987) have been shown by Salem's group to possess protease activity that cleaves protein S. It is quite possible that at regions of inflammation where neutrophils and platelets are recruited, protein S inacti-vation by these membrane proteases plays a significant role in allowing fibrin deposition to proceed.

Protein S is synthesized in the endothelium (Fair, Marlar, and Levin, 1986; Stern *et al.,* 1986), liver and several other organs (Maillard *et al.,* 1992) and is found in platelets (Schwarz *et al.,* 1985). Since severe liver disease depresses protein S levels much less than protein C levels (D'Angelo *et al.,* 1988), it is likely the extra-hepatic sources make significant contributions to the protein S pools. The endothelium is possibly the major other source of protein S based on rates of biosynthesis and the large amount of endothe-lium *in vivo.* Protein S biosynthesis, like TM and EPCR biosynthesis, is down regulated by TNF α (Hooper *et al.,* 1994).

Protein C levels can also decrease during intravascular coagulation (Griffin *et al.,* 1982), in response to vitamin K antagonists or due to liver disease (D'Angelo *et al.,* 1986). The relationship between protein C consumption and the clinical manifestations of septic shock will be discussed in greater detail later in the chapter.

Other Mechanisms for Down Regulating the Protein C Anticoagulant Pathway

Homocysteinurea is associated with vascular disease and thrombosis. Several studies have reported that homocysteine interferes with TM biosynthesis (Hayashi, Honda, and Suzuki, 1992; Lentz and Sadler, 1991). Another candidate is oxidized LDL. Like homo-cysteine, oxidized LDL has been shown to reduce TM activity (Weis *et al.,* 1991). I am unaware of any *in vivo* data related to whether TM is actually reduced in these clinical conditions. Given the multiplicity of regulatory events related to the control of TM biosynthesis, *in vivo* data to confirm these *in vitro* findings is especially relevant.

Viral infections can be associated with local thrombotic events (Key *et al.,* 1990; Visser *et al.,* 1988) and possibly with the onset of atherosclerosis (Benditt, Barrett, and McDougall, 1983). Herpes simplex virus 1 infection of endothelial cells *in vitro* leads to a procoagulant phenotype. Membrane surfaces become more available for assembly of pro-coagulant complexes (Visser *et al.,* 1988), tissue factor synthesis and expression is induced (Key *et al.,* 1990) and TM biosynthesis and expression is depressed (Key *et al.,* 1990). Again *in vivo* data is lacking. In one anecdotal and unpublished study, we did observe a young female athlete who began to develop superficial thrombosis that contin-ued to progress despite warfarin or heparin therapy. Vascular biopsy confirmed the pres-ence of herpes simplex 2 in or near the endothelium. Whether the virus was the cause of the unusual thrombotic response is unknown.

Promoting protein C activation, it has recently been observed that platelet factor 4 can stimulate protein C activation 4–25 fold (Slungaard and Key, 1994). This could enhance protein C activation and subsequent anticoagulant function in regions where significant platelet activation has occurred. In addition, factor Va has been shown to stimulate protein C activation on endothelium (Maruyama, Salem, and Majerus, 1984; Dittman and Majerus, 1990) suggesting that products of coagulation may enhance the anticoagulant pathway by multiple mechanisms.

Membrane Involvement in Protein C Pathway Functions

Like all vitamin K dependent proteins, the function of the protein C pathway is augmented by the presence of membrane surfaces composed of negatively charged phospholipids. In addition to stimulating the rate of factor Va inactivation (Kisiel *et al.,* 1977; Walker, Sexton, and Esmon, 1979), recent studies suggest that the membrane is required for complete inactivation of factor Va by APC (Kalafatis and Mann, 1993) (Figure 2.3). Another feature of membrane involvement is that phosphatidylethanolamine (PE), cardiolipin and phosphatidylinositol all facilitate APC dependent factor Va inactivation, with PE being the most effective (Smirnov and Esmon, 1994). As anticipated based on the literature, PE had little effect on the membrane dependent activation of prothrombin by the factor Xa-factor Va complex (Smirnov and Esmon, 1994). In plasma, the presence of PE in liposomes containing PS increased the anticoagulant activity of APC at least 10 fold. Thus, the assembly and function of the APC anticoagulant complex requires a phospholipid surface distinct from that of the prothrombinase complex. One obvious question is whether biologically relevant membranes that could be exposed to blood ever contain PE concentrations sufficient to accelerate APC dependent factor Va inactivation. Platelets are an obvious cellular source for this activity. Platelets and platelet microparticles (Harris and Esmon, 1985; Dahlbäck, Wiedmer, and Sims, 1992; Tans *et al.,* 1991) are known to support APC anticoagulant function. Once platelets are fully activated, the outer membrane leaflet contains approximately 38% PE (Bevers, Comfurius, and Zwaal, 1983), which approximates the amount needed for optimal APC anticoagulant function

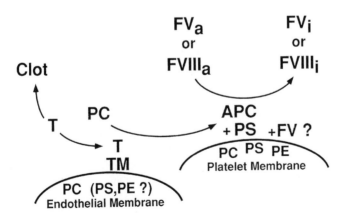

Figure 2.3   Membrane involvement in protein C activation and function. Optimal protein C activation and APC anticoagulant activity require PE in the membrane in addition to phosphatidylserine and phosphatidylcholine. Procoagulant reactions, at least prothrombinase, do not share a comparable requirement. In addition, membrane surfaces appear to be required for complete factor Va inactivation. FVi and FVIIIi are the APC inactivated forms of factor Va and VIIIa. See the text for a discussion.

(Smirnov and Esmon, 1994). Thus, PE appears to be both selective for APC function and available on biologically relevant membrane surfaces.

Endothelial cells appear to play an important role in both protein C activation and expression of APC anticoagulant activity. The role of the membrane phospholipids is of particular interest. *In vivo*, the endothelial membrane surface appears to be non-thrombogenic, although cultured cells do support prothrombin activation (Schoen, Reutelingsperger, and Lindhout, 1992; Hackeng *et al.*, 1994). Two classes of experiments support the contention that the surface is non thrombogenic *in vivo*. First, factor Xa infusion *in vivo* causes little fibrinogen consumption unless phospholipids were present (Taylor *et al.*, 1992, and references therein). Second, even when TNF is used to generate a hypercoaguable state, DIC was only detected when phospholipid vesicles were also infused (Taylor *et al.*, 1994). Thus, given the extraordinary amount of endothelial cell surface exposed to blood *in vivo* (Busch *et al.*, 1982), it is unlikely that these cells express significant procoagulant phospholipids.

Our current understanding of complex assembly suggests that negatively charged phospholipids are important and propagate both procoagulant and anticoagulant responses (Mann *et al.*, 1990). Since the endothelium is not thrombogenic *in vivo*, it must use other mechanisms to promote protein C activation and support APC anticoagulant activity. In solution, the Km for protein C activation by the thrombin-TM complex is very high (≈ 8 μM). Endothelial cell surface catalysis is characterized by a Km of ≈ 0.8 μM (Owen and Esmon, 1981). Incorporation of rabbit TM into neutral membranes composed of phosphatidylcholine decreased the Km to that observed on the endothelial cell surface (Galvin *et al.*, 1987). As one might expect, phosphatidylserine incorporation further decreases the Km.

With human TM incorporated into membranes by simple addition, an alternative set of observations have been made (Freyssinet, Gauchy, and Cazenave, 1986). In this study, phosphatidylserine appeared to be needed and it functioned by increasing Kcat. The basis for these differences is unknown, but it would seem that the rabbit data accounts for the experimental results with endothelium.

Interestingly, like APC dependent anticoagulant activity, recent studies have shown that activated endothelium expresses PE on the outer membrane leaflet and PE enhances protein C activation (Horie *et al.*, 1994). Thus, this phospholipid seems to play a role in both activation of protein C and the anticoagulant function of APC.

Endothelium can also support APC dependent factor Va inactivation *in vitro* (Stern *et al.*, 1986; Hackeng *et al.*, 1993). Whether this occurs *in vivo* is uncertain. If negatively charged phospholipids are not available on quiescent endothelium, then other mechanisms to promote assembly of functional complexes may be important. It is possible that EPCR plays a role in this process. If so, it would explain the observation that the capacity of endothelium to support APC dependent factor Va inactivation declined following exposure to certain cytokines (Nawroth *et al.*, 1986; Nawroth and Stern, 1986).

Possible Interaction of the Protein C System with Antiphospholipid Antibodies — A Potential Contribution to Thrombotic Risk

One of the curious aspects of *in vitro* coagulation results is that patients with lupus anticoagulants have increased clotting times *in vitro*, but seldom have bleeding complications.

Patients with lupus anticoagulants and antiphospholipid antibodies do have an increased risk of thrombosis (Triplett, 1993; Love and Santoro, 1990). It is possible that the antibodies are an epiphenomenon and not directly linked to thrombosis. Recent studies, however, suggest that they may actually promote a hypercoaguable state directly (Pierangeli *et al.,* 1994). These authors found that infusion of human IgG with antiphospholipid activity into mice promoted thrombus formation in a murine thrombosis model. Furthermore, markers of *in vivo* coagulation are elevated in patients with APAs (Ginsberg *et al.,* 1993).

APAs and LAs could inhibit coagulation and anticoagulation reactions at the level of blocking the membrane assembly of these complexes. Before discussing this possibility, it is necessary to consider the current information about the mechanisms of action of APAs and LAs. These antibodies have been reported to interact directly with phospholipids (see for instance Rauch *et al.,* 1986). Many of these antibodies react with PE and cardiolipin, both of which can adopt a hexagonal phase packing (Rauch *et al.,* 1986; Pryzdial and Mann, 1991). Other investigators have found that the antibodies bind only in the presence of β_2-glycoprotein 1 or prothrombin (Permpikul, Rao, and Rapaport, 1994; Bevers *et al.,* 1991; Keeling *et al.,* 1993), protein C (Keeling *et al.,* 1993) or protein S (Keeling *et al.,* 1993). Thus, it is not clear exactly what the target of these antibodies really is. In part, this probably reflects antibody heterogeneity. Alternatively, a unifying concept might be that all of these proteins insert into the membrane and/or reorient the membrane phospholipids in ways that allow recognition by these antibodies.

Several investigators, including ourselves, have suggested that the protein C pathway is a target for these antibodies and that they could elicit a thrombotic response either by inhibiting protein C activation or the anticoagulant activity of APC. Exactly how this might occur remains unknown. There is considerable disagreement in the literature as to whether LAs or APAs inhibit protein C activation and whether the inhibition involves binding to the membrane surface or to the protein. We described two patients with IgG antibodies that inhibited protein C activation by the thrombin-TM complex (Comp *et al.,* 1983). One of these has been further characterized, and found to bind heparin but not phospholipid membranes composed of PC:PS. The LA activity in one of these patients' plasmas was adsorbed onto this phospholipid without removing the inhibitory activity toward TM. We assume that the inhibitory activity in this patient is directed at the chondroitin sulfate moiety on TM. We (Carson *et al.,* 1994) and others (Oosting *et al.,* 1993) have identified a subset of patients with antibodies to TM that block protein C activation, while other investigators have failed to observe these antibodies (Nelson *et al.,* 1992). The role of auto-antibodies to TM in thrombosis is uncertain. It appears from initial studies that these antibodies are much more prevalent in patients with histories of thrombosis or lupus than in the general population, suggesting that they may contribute to the thrombotic tendency (Carson *et al.,* 1994).

Other investigators have observed that some LAs inhibit protein C activation by endothelial cell associated thrombin-TM complexes (Cariou *et al.,* 1986), or on negatively charged artificial membrane surfaces (Freyssinet *et al.,* 1986), while others have not observed this inhibition (Oosting *et al.,* 1991). Keeling *et al.,* (Keeling *et al.,* 1993) found that β_2-glycoprotein 1 could inhibit protein C activation, but LAs did not augment this activity.

APC anticoagulant activity has also been proposed to be blocked by LAs (Old, 1985; Borrell *et al.,* 1992; Oosting *et al.,* 1993; Marciniak and Romond, 1989; Bokarewa *et al.,*

1994), but no mechanism has been forwarded as to how to achieve a net hypercoaguable state merely by blocking the membrane surface with antibodies, a situation that would presumably mimic oral anticoagulant therapy in which all of the vitamin K dependent proteins lose affinity for membrane surfaces. This situation might be explained if the membrane requirements for the assembly of the anticoagulant complexes mimicked those of LA binding and were distinct from those of the procoagulant complexes. Since PE selectively augments APC anticoagulant activity and protein C activation, this is the role that we propose PE plays in linking the protein C pathway specifically to LAs and thrombosis. This raises the obvious question of whether anti-PE antibodies have ever been associated or identified in patients with thrombosis. In fact, several investigators have shown that these antibodies are present (Staub *et al.,* 1989; Falcon, Hoffer, and Carreras, 1990; Karmochkine *et al.,* 1992; Berrard *et al.,* 1993; Rauch *et al.,* 1986) and some have concluded that this specificity is associated with thrombosis (Karmochkine *et al.,* 1992). Given that PE augments protein C activation (Horie *et al.,* 1994) and APC anticoagulant activity selectively, PE may be a key to preferential inhibition of protein C activation by APAs on membranes.

We have recently completed an initial survey of patients with APAs to determine if these antibodies did inhibit APC anticoagulant activity and if so whether the inhibition was dependent on PE in the membrane (Smirnov *et al.,* 1995). In the group of patients we analyzed, lupus anticoagulant activity was enhanced by addition of PE to the membrane. The ability of the antibodies to inhibit APC anticoagulant activity was even more enhanced. As a result, in the presence of APC, some of the patients' plasmas with potent LAs actually clotted faster than the normal plasma. This only occurred with phospholipids containing PE. Perhaps more interestingly, another cohort of patients had APAs with little lupus anticoagulant activity, but still had potent inhibitory activity toward APC anticoagulant function. Many of these patients had histories of recurrent thrombosis, but it is not yet possible to determine whether this inhibition of APC function correlates with thrombotic risk in the general population. Illustrative examples of these two classes of patients responses are shown in Figure 2.4. In at least one of the patients, the inhibitory

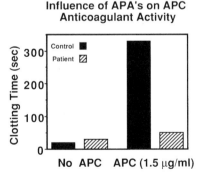

Figure 2.4 APAs can preferentially inhibit APC anticoagulant activity. Clotting of pooled plasma from normal donors (control) was compared to that of plasma from a patient with a history of thrombosis and APAs (patient). This particular patient did not have a potent LA. Clotting was initiated with the purified factor X activator from Russell's viper venom. Phospholipid liposomes (6 μg/ml containing 40% PE/ 20% phosphatidylcholine and 20% phosphatidyl serine) were present. Clotting was monitored in a V_{max} kinetic plate reader. Note that the clotting time was much faster in the patient plasma in the presence of APC than in the control plasma in the presence of APC.

activity toward APC function could be selectively adsorbed from the patient immunoglobulin on liposomes containing PE, but not on those devoid of the phospholipid.

The observation that PE enhances reactivity with APAs may be relevant to the discrepancies in the reports on the ability of LAs to inhibit protein C activation. Since PE is mobilized following endothelial cell activation, it is possible that under the conditions some investigators employed (higher thrombin, longer times for instance) that they mobilized PE and that the antibodies then reacted with that lipid. In addition, however, auto-antibodies directly to TM do exist and these are inhibitory (Carson *et al.*, 1994; Oosting *et al.*, 1993). Further studies will be required to clarify the role of phospholipid mobilization in the activation of protein C on the endothelium and its role in the inhibition of protein C activation by APAs.

APC Resistance Due to a Polymorphism in the Factor V Gene

Recently, a new phenomenon was observed in which patients were identified that responded poorly to APC and did not appear to have APAs (Dahlbäck, Carlsson, and Svensson, 1993) (see above). This situation was corrected by the addition of factor V (Dahlbäck and Hildebrand, 1994; Griffin *et al.*, 1993; Halbmayer *et al.*, 1994; Sun, Evatt, and Griffin, 1994; Zoller and Dahlbäck, 1994; Koeleman *et al.*, 1994). This defect has now been found to be due to a polymorphism that exists in about 3–8% of the general population. The polymorphism codes for a factor V molecule in which the Arg residue at 506 is replaced with a Gln (Bertina *et al.*, 1994; Greengard *et al.*, 1994; Zoller and Dahlbäck, 1994) (Figure 2.5). This Arg is the first bond cleaved during factor Va inactivation (Kalafatis and Mann, 1993). Initial clinical studies suggest that approximately 20% of patients with thrombosis may be APC resistant, thus making this a very significant risk factor (Halbmayer *et al.*, 1994; Lindblad, Svensson, and Dahlbäck, 1994; Koeleman *et al.*, 1994).

There are several unanswered questions with regard to APC resistance. Originally, factor V was shown to correct the resistance. How this occurs given that the cleavage site is altered is unclear. How factor Va carrying this mutation is actually inactivated is also unclear. Finally, the cofactor activity originally postulated to account for the deficiency

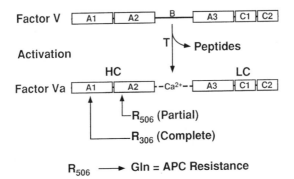

Figure 2.5   The current view of the molecular basis for APC resistance. Factor V is converted from a single chain molecule to a heterodimer held together by a Ca^{2+} ion. Several cleavage sites for APC are present in the molecule. In APC resistance, one of the Arg residues (506) is replaced with a Gln rendering this site inappropriate for cleavage by APC which is Arg specific for P1 residues. See the text for further discussion.

has not been fully explained. Toward the latter goal, it has, however, been found that factor V, but not factor Va, can enhance factor VIIIa inactivation by APC in the presence of protein S (Shen and Dahlbäck, 1994).

Clinical Ramifications of Deficiencies in the Protein C Pathway

Homozygous protein C deficiencies in which protein C levels are less than 5% of normal are associated with severe, life threatening thrombotic complications in infancy, often manifested by purpura fulminans, but patients with higher levels sometimes escape these problems until later life (Branson *et al.*, 1983; Sells *et al.*, 1984; Seligsohn *et al.*, 1984; Dreyfus *et al.*, 1991; Grundy *et al.*, 1991; Tuddenham *et al.*, 1989; Sharon *et al.*, 1986; Kakkar, Melissar, and Kakkar, 1987; Broekmans and Conard, 1988; Gladson, Groncy, and Griffin, 1987; Manco-Johnson *et al.*, 1991; Pabinger *et al.*, 1992; Marlar *et al.*, 1992). The skin lesions and thrombotic complications can be stopped by infusion of monoclonal antibody purified plasma protein C (Dreyfus *et al.*, 1991). Symptoms reappear when protein C levels drop. This clearly indicates that the thrombotic lesion is directly linked to protein C deficiency. Heterozygous individuals seem to have an increased risk of thrombosis (Allaart *et al.*, 1993; Bovill *et al.*, 1989).

Protein S deficiency is also associated with thrombotic disease. In general, the problems are similar to those of protein C deficiency and purpura fulminans has been observed in protein S deficient infants (Mahasandana *et al.*, 1990). A thrombotic risk is also observed in heterozygous individuals (Lauer *et al.*, 1990; Golub, Sibony, and Coller, 1990; Allaart *et al.*, 1990; Schwarz *et al.*, 1984; Kamiya *et al.*, 1986; Dolan, Ball, and Preston, 1989; Girolami *et al.*, 1989; Comp and Esmon, 1984; Comp *et al.*, 1986; Engresser *et al.*, 1987; Lefrancois *et al.*, 1991; Walker, 1992; Pabinger *et al.*, 1992; Melissari *et al.*, 1992; Alving and Comp, 1992; Pabinger *et al.*, 1994).

No deficiencies of TM nor EPCR have been reported. One would assume, at least in the homozygous state, that TM deficiency would be associated with severe thrombosis since blocking TM generates a hypercoaguable response (Kumada, Dittman, and Majerus, 1987).

Acquired Deficiencies and their Treatment with Protein C: Warfarin Induced Skin Necrosis

Protein C levels drop rapidly during oral anticoagulant therapy (D'Angelo *et al.*, 1986). Patients with heterozygous protein C deficiency are more commonly affected by this rare syndrome than normal individuals (Broekmans *et al.*, 1983). Recent studies suggest that the progress of the microvascular thrombosis associated with warfarin skin necrosis can be abruptly curtailed by administration of protein C concentrate (Muntean *et al.*, 1992; Schramm *et al.*, 1993).

Protein S deficiency has also been associated with warfarin induced skin necrosis (Goldberg *et al.*, 1991). Whether protein S, protein C or both could reverse this process in these patients is not known.

Acquired Deficiencies and their Treatment with Protein C: Meningococcemia

Severe acquired protein C deficiency is observed in some of the most severe cases of septic shock. In meningiococcemia, there is a good correlation between the more severity of the decrease in protein C levels, the severity of the appearance of skin lesions and a poor prognosis (Powars *et al.,* 1993). In addition, APC has been shown to block the lethal effects of E coli infusion in baboons (Taylor *et al.,* 1987) and inhibition of protein C (Taylor *et al.,* 1987) or protein S (Taylor *et al.,* 1991) exacerbate the response to E coli infusion. Blocking the protein C pathway *in vivo* increases TNF generation (Taylor *et al.,* 1991). Protein C/APC also has apparent anti-inflammatory activity *in vitro.* In addition to blocking experimental septic shock, protein C has been shown to inhibit neutrophil attachment to selectins (Grinnell, Hermann, and Yan, 1994) and to block cytokine (TNF) elaboration by mononuclear cells (Grey *et al.,* 1994). In our own experience, we have failed to obtain direct inhibition of TNF production (as assayed by direct ELISA methods) by mononuclear cells or in blood when we treat with APC despite multiple attempts. The molecular and cellular basis for the differences in results between two apparently similar experiments should prove interesting.

Given the anticoagulant and apparent anti-inflammatory activity of protein C, replacement therapy for acquired protein C deficiency in septic shock seems logical. To date, 8 patients with severe acquired protein C deficiency have been administered protein C concentrate (Rivard *et al.,* 1993). All patients were developing skin lesions at the time of administration. Skin lesion progression ceased following administration and patient vital signs improved. All patients survived. These results will need confirmation in a larger clinical trial.

Molecular Mechanisms of Protein C Activation

The intriguing property of TM is that it can accelerate the production of the anticoagulant APC, while at the same time inhibiting the procoagulant activity of thrombin. The ability of TM to block the procoagulant responses can be rationalized based on known interaction sites. Hirudin binds to thrombin and the carboxy terminal peptide, often referred to as hirugen, binds in anion binding exosite 1 (Rydel *et al.,* 1990; Stubbs *et al.,* 1992; Tulinsky and Qiu, 1993; Stubbs and Bode, 1993). Hirugen overlaps the fibrinogen binding site (on the P'side). The platelet has a similar site and peptides from the platelet receptor compete with hirugen for thrombin binding (Liu *et al.,* 1991). TM and TM fragments composed of EGF 5–6 also compete with hirugen. Hirugen and TM EGF 5–6 not only compete, but they elicit comparable changes in the conformation of the active center of thrombin (as assessed by active site fluorescent probes) and similar changes in synthetic substrate specificity. Mutations in anion binding exosite 1 have been shown to decrease TM interaction (Wu *et al.,* 1991). Finally, a peptide corresponding to a small region of EGF 5 has been shown to bind to thrombin anion binding exosite crystallographically (A. Tulinsky, personal communication). Based on mutation analysis, the major region involved in thrombin-TM interaction is probably EGF 5 (Tsiang *et al.,* 1990; Nagashima *et al.,* 1993; Wong *et al.,* 1991). Thus, TM, fibrinogen, the thrombin receptor and hirudin share common binding sites on thrombin. This not only identifies part of the TM binding domain, but adequately explains the fact that TM is a competitive inhibitor of fibrinogen clotting and hirudin interaction.

The question of how TM accelerates protein C activation is more complex. TM EGF 5–6 is insufficient to accelerate protein C activation, whereas TM fragments containing at least EGF 4–6 are sufficient (Zushi *et al.,* 1991; Zushi *et al.,* 1989; Stearns, Kurosawa, and Esmon, 1989). It has proven difficult to observe thrombin binding by fragments containing

EGF 4 (Stearns, Kurosawa, and Esmon, 1989), indicating that this EGF domain binds weakly if at all by itself. It is possible that the role of EGF 4 involves interaction with the substrate. TM binds weakly to protein C, but TM does not distinguish between protein C and APC (Olsen *et al.*, 1992; Hogg, Öhlin, and Stenflo, 1992). Asp 349 that is located in a connecting stretch between EGF 3 and 4 in TM is more important for protein C activation than for the activation of protein C derivatives lacking the first EGF domain. This would be consistent with TM interacting with the substrate. The EGF 4 domain probably contacts thrombin also, but at a site that is yet to be mapped. The basis for this conclusion stems from the fact that TM fragments containing EGF 4 elicit different effects on synthetic substrate specificities and the fluorescence properties of dyes attached to the catalytic center of TM (Ye *et al.*, 1991; Ye *et al.*, 1992). This suggests that EGF 4 does make direct contacts with thrombin and that these influence the conformation of the enzyme in ways that allow accommodation of protein C as a substrate.

Mutagenesis analysis has identified the P3 and P3′ Asp residues in the protein C molecule as being intimately involved in preventing rapid activation by thrombin. These inhibitory interactions involving these Asp residues are overcome by binding thrombin to TM. Conversion of Asp to Gly or other thrombin compatible residues enhances protein C activation by free thrombin at least 8 fold. Most of this difference is lost once thrombin is complexed with TM (Rezaie and Esmon, 1992; Ehrlich *et al.*, 1990; Richardson, Gerlitz, and Grinnell, 1992). These studies suggest that there should be key residues in thrombin that repel these acidic residues in protein C. Mutational analysis suggests that Glu[192] and Glu[39] are these two residues (Figure 2.6). Specifically, mutation of Glu[192] to Gln increases the rate of protein C activation by free thrombin approximately 20 fold, but is almost equivalent to wild type thrombin when in complex with TM. The influence of this mutation is relatively selective for protein C activation since it has little influence on fibrinogen clotting (Le Bonniec and Esmon, 1991). Analysis of cleavage of a peptide corresponding to the P7–P5′ residues of protein C reveals that this mutation overcomes the inhibitory influence of the P3 and P3′ Asp residues. Similar results were obtained by mutation of Glu[39] except that this residue was relatively specific for inhibiting cleavage

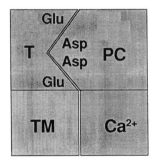 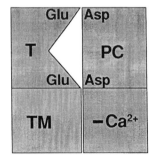

Figure 2.6   Schematic representation of a model for TM acceleration of protein C activation. The model accounts for the fact that the Asp residues in the P3 and P3′ sites potently inhibit protein C activation in the absence of TM, but not nearly as much in its presence. Likewise, the Glu residues at positions 192 and 39 have a selective inhibitory function on protein C activation in the absence but not the presence of TM. See the text for discussion. Reprinted from Arterioscl. and Thromb. 12(2): 135–145, 1992, with permission of the American Heart Association.

of peptides containing acidic residues in P3′ position. Again, when TM was present, the increased rate of protein C activation observed in the absence of TM was essentially eliminated (Le Bonniec, MacGillivray, and Esmon, 1991). It would appear that the conformational changes that occur in the extended binding pocket of thrombin upon complex formation with TM alleviate these inhibitory interactions. Interestingly, TM 4–6, but not TM 5–6, can elicit detectable conformational changes near the P3 binding site in thrombin (Ye *et al.*, 1991).

Ca^{2+} plays a critical role in protein C activation and function. As a vitamin K dependent factor, Ca^{2+} binding to Gla residues was assumed to play an important role. Deletion of the Gla domain proteolytically eliminated plasma anticoagulant activity, slowed the rate of protein C activation over endothelium, but was without significant effect on protein C activation by the soluble thrombin-TM complex (Esmon, DeBault, and Esmon, 1983). More recently the role of each of the Gla residues in protein C has been evaluated by mutational analysis (Jhingan *et al.*, 1994; Zhang and Castellino, 1993; Colpitts and Castellino, 1994). From these studies, it is clear that membrane binding and anticoagulant function are relatively well correlated and that some Gla residues are more important than others. Specifically, Gla 7, 16, 20, and 26 were essential, while Gla 6, 14, 19, 25 and 29 were not absolutely essential (Zhang, Jhingan, and Castellino, 1992). In addition, Leu at position 5 seems to play a significant role in membrane binding, possibly by making hydrophobic interactions with the membrane surface (Zhang and Castellino, 1994).

In solution, Ca^{2+} plays a different, but major role in protein C activation. Although relatively slow even in the absence of Ca^{2+}, free thrombin activation of protein C is decreased more than 10 fold further by the addition of physiological Ca^{2+} (Amphlett, Kisiel, and Castellino, 1981; Esmon, DeBault, and Esmon, 1983). The activation by the thrombin-TM complex, however, was almost entirely dependent on the presence of Ca^{2+}. The Ca^{2+} concentration dependence of both processes were virtually identical (Esmon, DeBault, and Esmon, 1983). Analysis of Ca^{2+} binding, protein C conformation and protein C activation rate with a protein C derivative lacking the Gla domain revealed that the three events were coincident and involved a single high affinity site (Kd ≈ 50 μM) (Johnson *et al.*, 1983). Binding of Ca^{2+} to this site also correlated with the binding of a Ca^{2+} dependent monoclonal antibody that bound to an epitope overlapping the cleavage site of protein C (Stearns *et al.*, 1988), indicating that Ca^{2+} binding to protein C caused a conformational change at or very near the scissile bond. The Ca^{2+} binding site was originally believed to be in the first EGF domain of protein C, but deletion mutagenesis eliminated this possibility (Rezaie, Esmon, and Esmon, 1992). An alternative site was identified by molecular modeling. Trypsin has a Ca^{2+} binding site (Bode and Schwager, 1975). In thrombin, which is not Ca^{2+} dependent, one of the acidic residues involved in Ca^{2+} chelation is replaced with Lys (residue 70). This forms an internal salt bridge that seems to stabilize this loop. Therefore, mutation of Glu → Lys at residues 70 or 80 was attempted in protein C to attempt to create a protein C molecule that no longer needed Ca^{2+} for activation by the thrombin-TM complex. Only the Glu80 to Lys mutation was successfully expressed, but this mutant activated rapidly with the thrombin-TM complex even in the absence of Ca^{2+}, Ca^{2+} no longer altered the rate of activation, and no Ca^{2+} binding to the mutant could be detected (Rezaie *et al.*, 1994). These results suggest that this site is entirely responsible for the Ca^{2+} dependence of protein C activation by the thrombin-TM complex in solution.

Regulation of APC Function

In plasma, protein S exerts a significant ($\approx$10 fold) enhancement of APC anticoagulant activity. In purified systems, most investigators observe about a two fold enhancement of factor Va inactivation. The ability to observe protein S stimulation is extremely dependent on the exact conditions employed (Walker and Fay, 1992). In our systems where APC and factor Va levels are extremely low, nearly a 10 fold stimulation can be observed with protein S. This variable and somewhat small dependence on protein S has slowed analysis of the mechanisms by which protein S functions.

One situation that is clear, however, is that APC inactivation of factor Va is inhibited by the presence of factor Xa (Walker, Sexton, and Esmon, 1979; Nesheim *et al.,* 1982; Solymoss, Tucker, and Tracy, 1988). Protein S serves to prevent the protection of factor Va by factor Xa (Solymoss, Tucker, and Tracy, 1988). A similar function for protein S in factor VIIIa inactivation has recently been described (Duchemin *et al.,* 1994). This function of protein S may be associated with the finding that it interacts directly with components of the prothrombin activation complex (Heeb *et al.,* 1993).

Another function for protein S is to facilitate APC binding to membrane surfaces (Walker, 1981). Interestingly, prothrombin which is much more abundant than APC binds to membranes with comparable affinity. This leads to very effective inhibition of APC function by prothrombin when analyzed on membranes lacking PE and in the absence of protein S. We recently observed that protein S and factor Va work together synergistically on PE containing membranes to provide a surface that is relatively insensitive to displacement of APC by prothrombin.

Taken together, these observations suggest that protein S differs from the other cofactors in that its primary role may be in allowing APC to function in conditions where either the substrate or the membrane surface might not be otherwise available.

Molecular basis for the slow inactivation of APC by plasma protease inhibitors

APC is slowly inactivated by several plasma protease inhibitors including protein C inhibitor, α_1-antitrypsin, and α_2-macroglobulin (Suzuki *et al.,* 1987; Heeb and Griffin, 1988; Scully *et al.,* 1993; Heeb, Gruber, and Griffin, 1991), but it does not react with antithrombin, tissue factor pathway inhibitors or pancreatic trypsin inhibitor. Based on the observations that protein C and thrombin both have Glu at position 192, that mutation of Glu $\rightarrow$ Gln in thrombin allows the enzyme to cleave substrates with acidic residues in the P3 and P3' sites more rapidly, and that factor Va has an acidic residue (Asp) in the P3 position (residue 504 i.e. near the APC resistance site), we mutated this Glu to Gln in APC (Rezaie and Esmon, 1993). As predicted, the enzyme inactivated factor Va approximately 3 fold better than wild type APC. Surprisingly, however, the mutant had less anticoagulant activity in plasma. This was due to the fact that the enzyme was now rapidly inhibited by α_1-antitrypsin, tissue factor pathway inhibitor and antithrombin. Thus, Glu at position 192 is a key to resistance of APC to inactivation by the proteinase inhibitors.

Interaction with inhibitors does not always involve residues near the active site. For instance, bovine APC, unlike its human counterpart, does not react with α_1-antitrypsin. This has been shown to be due to differences in the light chain of APC (Holly and Foster, 1994).

Summary

In the last 15 years, an appreciation of the complexity and clinical relevance of the protein C pathway has emerged. It is likely that additional protein components remain to be identified. Our appreciation of the roles of the pathway in controlling coagulation and inflammation in a variety of human disease states is still in its infancy. It is likely that the next 10 years will see even more rapid development of our understanding of the role of the protein C pathway in the pathophysiology of human disease.

Acknowledgements

The research which has been discussed in this chapter was funded in part by grants from the National Heart, Lung and Blood Institute of the National Institutes of Health (Nos. R01 HL 29807 and R37 HL30340). Dr. Esmon is an investigator of the Howard Hughes Medical Institute.

References

Öhlin, A-K., Linse, S. and Stenflo, J. (1988). Calcium binding to the epidermal growth factor homology region of bovine protein C. *J. Biol. Chem.*, **263**:7411–7417.

Alessi, M.C., Aillaud, M.F., Boyer-Neumann, C., Viard, L., Camboulives, J. and Juhan-Vague, I. (1993). Cutaneous necrosis associated with acquired severe protein S deficiency. *Thromb. Haemost.*, **69**:524–526.

Allaart, C.F., Aronson, D.C., Ruys, T. *et al.* (1990). Hereditary protein S deficiency in young adults with arterial occlusive disease. *Thromb. Haemost.*, **64**:206–210.

Allaart, C.F., Poort, S.R., Rosendaal, F.R., Reitsma, P.H., Bertina, R.M. and Briët, E. (1993). Increased risk of venous thrombosis in carriers of hereditary protein C deficiency defect. *Lancet*, **341**:134–138.

Alving, B.M. and Comp, P.C. (1992). Recent advances in understanding clotting and evaluating patients with recurrent thrombosis. *Am. J. Obstet. Gynecol.*, **167**:1184–1191.

Amphlett, G.W., Kisiel, W. and Castellino, F.J. (1981). Interaction of calcium with bovine plasma protein C. *Biochemistry*, **20**:2156–2161.

Amster, M.S., Conway, J., Zeid, M. and Pincus, S. (1993). Cutaneous necrosis resulting from protein S deficiency and increased antiphospholipid antibody in a patient with systemic lupus erythematosus. *J. Am. Acad. Dermatol.*, **29**:853–857.

Anzola, G.P., Magoni, M., Ascari, E. and Maffi, V. (1993). Early prognostic factors in ischemic stroke. The role of protein C and protein S. *Stroke*, **24**:1496–1500.

Bajzar, L. and Nesheim, M. (1993). The effect of activated protein C on fibrinolysis in cell-free plasma can be attributed specifically to attenuation of prothrombin activation. *J. Biol. Chem.*, **268**:8608–8616.

Bangalore, N., Drohan, W.N. and Orthner, C.L. (1994). High affinity binding sites for activated protein C and protein C on cultured human umbilical vein endothelial cells. Independent of protein S and distinct from known ligands. *Thromb. Haemost.*, **72**:465–474.

Benditt, E.P., Barrett, T. and McDougall, J.K. (1983). Viruses in the etiology of atherosclerosis. *Proc. Natl. Acad. Sci. (USA)*, **80**:6386–6389.

Berrard, M., Boffa, M.C., Karmochkine, M. *et al.* (1993). Plasma reactivity to hexagonal II phase phosphatidylethanolamine is more frequently associated with lupus anticoagulant than with antiphosphatidylethanolamine antibodies. *J. Lab. Clin. Med.*, **122**:601–605.

Bertina, R.M., Koeleman, B.P.C., Koster, T. *et al.* (1994). Mutation in blood coagulation factor V associated with resistance to activated protein C. *Nature*, **369**:64–67.

Bevers, E.M., Comfurius, P. and Zwaal, R.F.A. (1983). Changes in membrane phospholipid distribution during platelet activation. *Biochim. Biophys. Acta*, **736**:57–66.

Bevers, E.M., Galli, M., Barbui, T., Comfurius, P. and Zwaal, R.F.A. (1991). Lupus anticoagulant IgG's (LA) are not directed to phospholipids only, but to a complex of lipid-bound human prothrombin. *Thromb. Haemost.*, **66**:629–632.

Bode, W. and Schwager, P. (1975). The refined crystal structure of bovine beta-trypsin at 1•8 Å resolution. II. Crystallographic refinement, calcium binding site, benzamidine binding site and active site at pH 7•0. *J. Mol. Biol.*, **98** 693–717.

Bode, W., Mayr, I., Baumann, U., Huber, R., Stone, S.R. and Hofsteenge, J. (1989). The refined 1.9 Å crystal structure of human α-thrombin: interaction with D-Phe-Pro-Arg chloromeyhylketone and significance of the Tyr-Pro-Pro-Trp insertion segment. *EMBO J.*, **8**:3467–3475.

Boerger, L.M., Morris, P.C., Thurnau, G.R., Esmon, C.T. and Comp, P.C. (1987). Oral contraceptives and gender affect protein S status. *Blood*, **69**:692–694.

Boffa, M., Burke, B. and Haudenschild, C.C. (1987). Preservation of thrombomodulin antigen on vascular and extravascular surfaces. *J. Histochem. Cytochem.*, **35**:1267–1276.

Bokarewa, M.I., Blomback, M., Egberg, N. and Rosen, S. (1994). A new variant of interaction between phospholipid antibodies and the protein C system. *Blood Coagul. Fibrinol.*, **5**:37–41.

Borrell, M., Sala, N., de Castellarnau, C., Lopez, S., Gari, M. and Fontcuberta, J. (1992). Immunoglobulin fractions isolated from patients with antiphospholipid antibodies prevent the inactivation of factor Va by activated protein C on human endothelial cells. *Thromb Haemost*, **68**:268–272.

Bourin, M-C., Öhlin, A-K., Lane, D.A., Stenflo, J. and Lindahl, U. (1988). Relationship between anticoagulant activities and polyanionic properties of rabbit thrombomodulin. *J. Biol. Chem.*, **263**:8044–8052.

Bourin, M.C. and Lindahl, U. (1993). Glycosaminoglycans and the regulation of blood coagulation. *Biochem. J.*, **289**:313–330.

Bourin, M.C., Lundgren-Åkerlund, E. and Lindahl, U. (1990). Isolation and characterization of the glycosaminoglycan component of rabbit thrombomodulin proteoglycan. *J. Biol. Chem.*, **265**:15424–15431.

Bovill, E.G., Bauer, K.A., Dickerman, J.D., Callas, P. and West, B. (1989). The clinical spectrum of heterozygous protein C deficiency in a large New England kindred. *Blood*, **73**:712–717.

Branson, H., Katz, J., Marble, R. and Griffin, J.H. (1983). Inherited protein C deficiency and a coumarin-responsive chronic relapsing purpura fulminans syndrome in a neonate. *Lancet*, **2**:1165–1168.

Broekmans, A.W. and Conard, J.: Hereditary protein C deficiency; in Bertina RM (ed): Protein C and Related Proteins, p 160. New York, Churchill Livingstone, 1988.

Broekmans, A.W., Bertina, R.M., Loeliger, E.A., Hofman, V. and Klingeman, H.G. (1983). Protein C and the development of skin necrosis during anticoagulant therapy. *Thromb. Haemost.*, **49**, 251-Letter.

Busch, C., Cancilla, P., DeBault, L., Goldsmith, J. and Owen, W. (1982). Use of endothelium cultured on microcarriers as a model for the microcirculation. *Lab. Invest.*, **47**:498–504.

Cariou, R., Tobelem, G., Soria, C. and Caen, J. (1986). Inhibition of protein C activation by endothelial cells in the presence of lupus anticoagulant. *N. Engl. J. Med.*, **18**:1193–1194.

Carr, M.E., Jr. and Zekert, S.L. (1993). Protein S and C4b-binding protein levels in patients with stroke: Implications for protein S regulation. *Haemostasis*, **23**:159–167.

Carson, C.W., Comp, P.C., Esmon, N.L., Rezaie, A.R. and Esmon, C.T. (1994). Thrombomodulin antibodies are found in patients with lupus anticoagulant and unexplained thrombosis. *Circulation*, (October), (Abstract)

Chafa, O., Fischer, A.M. and Meriane, F. *et al.* (1992). Behçet syndrome associated with protein S deficiency. *Thromb. Haemost.*, **67**:1–3.

Collins, C.L., Fink, L.M., Hsu, S.-M., Schaefer, R. and Ordonez, N. (1992). Thrombomodulin staining of mesothelioma cells. *Hum. Pathol.*, **23**: 966.

Colpitts, T.L. and Castellino, F.J. (1994). Calcium and phospholipid binding properties of synthetic gamma-carboxyglutamic acid-containing peptides with sequence counterparts in human protein C. *Biochemistry*, **33**:3501–3508.

Comp, P.C. (1986). Hereditary disorders predisposing to thrombosis. *Prog. Haemost. Thromb.*, **8**:71–102.

Comp, P.C. and Esmon, C.T. (1981). Generation of fibrinolytic activity by infusion of activated protein C into dogs. *J. Clin. Invest.*, **68**:1221–1228.

Comp, P.C. and Esmon, C.T. (1984). Recurrent venous thromboembolism in patients with a partial deficiency of protein S. *N. Engl. J. Med.*, **311**:1525–1528.

Comp, P.C., DeBault, L.E., Esmon, N.L. and Esmon, C.T. (1983). Human thrombomodulin is inhibited by IgG from two patients with non-specific anticoagulants. *Blood*, **62**:309–1141. (Abstract)

Comp, P.C., Doray, D., Patton, D. and Esmon, C.T. (1986). An abnormal plasma distribution of protein S occurs in functional protein S deficiency. *Blood*, **67**:504–508.

Comp, P.C., Nixon, R.R., Cooper, M.R. and Esmon, C.T. (1984). Familial protein S deficiency is associated with recurrent thrombosis. *J. Clin. Invest.*, **74**:2082–2088.

Comp, P.C., Vigano, S., D'Angelo, A., Thurnau, G., Kaufman, C. and Esmon, C.T. (1985). Acquired protein S deficiency occurs in pregnancy, the nephrotic syndrome and acute systemic lupus erythematosus. *Blood*, **66**:348a–abstr. (Abstract)

Conway, E.M. and Nowakowski, B. (1993). Biologically active thrombomodulin is synthesized by adherent synovial fluid cells and is elevated in synovial fluid of patients with rheumatoid arthritis. *Blood*, **81**:726–733.

Conway, E.M. and Rosenberg, R.D. (1988). Tumor necrosis factor suppresses transcription of the thrombomodulin gene in endothelial cells. *Mol. Cell. Biol.*, **8**:5588–5592.

Conway, E.M., Bauer, K.A., Barzegar, S. and Rosenberg, R.D. (1987). Suppression of hemostatic system activation by oral anticoagulants in the blood of patients with thrombotic diatheses. *J. Clin. Invest.*, **80**:1535–1544.

Conway, E.M., Liu, L., Nowakowski, B., Steiner-Mosonyi, M. and Jackman, R.W. (1994). Heat shock of vascular endothelial cells induces an up-regulatory transcriptional response of the thrombomodulin gene that is delayed in onset and does not attenuate. *J. Biol. Chem.*, **269**:22804–22810.

Conway, E.M., Nowakowski, B. and Steiner-Mosonyi, M. (1992). Human neutrophils synthesize thrombomodulin that does not promote thrombin-dependent protein C activation. *Blood*, **80**:1254–1263.

D'Angelo, A., Valle, P.D., Crippa, L., Pattarini, E., Grimaldi, L.M.E. and D'Angelo, S.V. (1993). Brief report: Autoimmune protein S deficiency in a boy with severe thromboembolic disease. *N. Engl. J. Med.*, **328**:1753–1757.

D'Angelo, A., Vigano-D'Angelo, S., Esmon, C.T. and Comp, P.C. (1988). Acquired deficiencies of protein S: Protein S activity during oral anticoagulation, in liver disease and in disseminated intravascular coagulation. *J. Clin. Invest.*, **81**:1445–1454.

D'Angelo, S.V., Comp, P.C., Esmon, C.T. and D'Angelo, A. (1986). Relationship between protein C antigen and anticoagulant activity during oral anticoagulation and in selected disease states. *J. Clin. Invest.*, **77**:416–425.

D'Angelo, S.V., D'Angelo, A., Kaufman, C., Esmon, C.T. and Comp, P.C. (1987). Acquired functional protein S deficiency occurs in the nephrotic syndrome. *Ann. Intern. Med.*, **107**:42–47.

Dahlbäck, B. (1986). Inhibition of protein Ca cofactor function of human and bovine protein S by C4b-binding protein. *J. Biol. Chem.*, **261**:12022–12027.

Dahlbäck, B. (1991). Protein S and C4b-binding protein: Components involved in the regulation of the protein C anticoagulant system. *Thromb. Haemost.*, **66**:49–61.

Dahlbäck, B. and Hildebrand, B. (1994). Inherited resistance to activated protein C is corrected by anticoagulant cofactor activity found to be a property of factor V. *Proc. Natl. Acad. Sci. (USA)*, **91**:1396–1400.

Dahlbäck, B., Carlsson, M. and Svensson, P.J. (1993). Familial thrombophilia due to a previously unrecognized mechanism characterized by poor anticoagulant response to activated protein C: Prediction of a cofactor to activated protein C. *Proc. Natl. Acad. Sci. (USA)*, **90**:1004–1008.

Dahlbäck, B., Frohm, B. and Nelsestuen, G. (1990). High affinity interaction between C4b-binding protein and vitamin K-dependent protein S in the presence of calcium. *J. Biol. Chem.*, **265**:16082–16087.

Dahlbäck, B., Lundwall, A. and Stenflo, J. (1986). Localization of thrombin cleavage sites in the amino-terminal region of bovine protein S. *J. Biol. Chem.*, **261**:5111–5115.

Dahlbäck, B., Wiedmer, T. and Sims, P.J. (1992). Binding of anticoagulant vitamin K-dependent protein S to platelet-derived microparticles. *Biochemistry*, **31**:12769–12777.

Davie, E.W., Fujikawa, K. and Kisiel, W. (1991). The coagulation cascade: Initiation, maintenance and regulation. *Biochemistry*, **30**:10363–10370.

de Munk, G.A.W., Groeneveld, E. and Rijken, D.C. (1991). Acceleration of the thrombin inactivation of single chain urokinase-type plasminogen activator (pro-urokinase) by thrombomodulin. *J. Clin. Invest.*, **88**:1680–1684.

DeBault, L.E., Esmon, N.L., Smith, G.P. and Esmon, C.T. (1986). Localization of thrombomodulin antigen in rabbit endothelial cells in culture: An immunofluorescence and immunoelectron microscope study. *Lab. Invest.*, **54**:179–187.

Dittman, W.A. and Majerus, P.W. (1990). Structure and function of thrombomodulin: A natural anticoagulant. *Blood*, **75**:329–336.

Dittman, W.A., Nelson, S.C., Greer, P.K., Horton, E.T., Palomba, M.L. and McCachren, S.S. (1994). Characterization of thrombomodulin expression in response to retinoic acid and identification of a retinoic acid response element in the human thrombomodulin gene. *J. Biol. Chem.*, **269**:16925–16932.

Dolan, G., Ball, J. and Preston, F.E. (1989). Protein C and protein S., *Clin. Haematol.*, **2**:999–1042.

Drake, T.A., Cheng, J., Chang, A. and Taylor, F.B., Jr. (1993). Expression of tissue factor, thrombomodulin, and E-selectin in baboons with lethal E. coli sepsis. *Am. J. Pathol.*, **142**:1458–1470.

Drakenberg, T., Fernlund, P., Roepstorff, P. and Stenflo, J. (1983). β-Hydroxyaspartic acid in vitamin K-dependent protein C. *Proc. Natl. Acad .Sci. (USA)*, **80**:1802–1806.

Dreyfus, M., Magny, J.F., Bridey, F. *et al.* (1991). Treatment of homozygous protein C deficiency and neonatal purpura fulminans with a purified protein C concentrate. *N. Engl. J. Med.*, **325**:1565–1568.

Duchemin, J., Pittet, J.-L., Tartary, M. *et al.* (1994). A new assay based on thrombin generation inhibition to detect both protein C and protein S deficiencies in plasma. *Thromb. Haemost.*, **71**: 331–338.

Edenbrandt, C.-M., Lundwall, A., Wydro, R. and Stenflo, J. (1990). Molecular analysis of the gene for vitamin K-dependent protein S and its pseudogene. Cloning and partial gene organization. *Biochemistry*, **29**:7861–7868.

Ehrlich, H.J., Grinnell, B.W., Jaskunas, S.R., Esmon, C.T., Yan, S.B. and Bang, N.U. (1990). Recombinant human protein C derivatives: altered response to calcium resulting in enhanced activation by thrombin. *EMBO J.*, **9**:2367–2373.

Engresser, L., Broekmans, A.W., Briët, E., Brommer, E.J.P. and Bertina, R.M. (1987). Hereditary protein S deficiency: clinical manifestations. *Ann. Intern. Med.*, **106**:677–682.

Esmon, C.T. (1989). The roles of protein C and thrombomodulin in the regulation of blood coagulation. *J. Biol. Chem.*, **264**:4743–4746.

Esmon, C.T. (1993). Molecular events that control the protein C anticoagulant pathway. *Thromb. Haemost.*, **70**:1–5.

Esmon, C.T., Esmon, N.L. and Harris, K.W. (1982). Complex formation between thrombin and thrombomodulin inhibits both thrombin-catalyzed fibrin formation and factor V activation. *J. Biol. Chem.*, **257**:7944–7947.

Esmon, C.T., Taylor, F.B., Jr. and Snow, T.R. (1991). Inflammation and coagulation: Linked processes potentially regulated through a common pathway mediated by protein C. *Thromb. Haemost.*, **66**:160–165.

Esmon, N.L., Carroll, R.C. and Esmon, C.T. (1983). Thrombomodulin blocks the ability of thrombin to activate platelets. *J. Biol. Chem.*, **258**:12238–12242.

Esmon, N.L., DeBault, L.E. and Esmon, C.T. (1983). Proteolytic formation and properties of gamma-carboxyglutamic acid-domainless protein C. *J. Biol. Chem.*, **258**:5548–5553.

España, F., Gruber, A., Heeb, M.J., Hanson, S.R., Harker, L.A. and Griffin, J.H. (1991). *In vivo* and *in vitro* complexes of activated protein C with two inhibitors in baboons. *Blood*, **77**:1754–1760.

Esposito, C., Gerlach, H., Brett, J., Stern, D. and Vlassara, H. (1989). Endothelial receptor-mediated binding of glucose-modified albumin is associated with increased monolayer permeability and modulation of cell surface coagulant properties. *Journal of Experimental Medicine*, **170**:1387–1407.

Fair, D.S., Marlar, R.A. and Levin, E.G. (1986). Human endothelial cells synthesize protein S. *Blood*, **67**:68–71.

Falcon, C.R., Hoffer, A.M. and Carreras, L.O. (1990). Evaluation of the clinical and laboratory associations of antiphosphatidylethanolamine. *Thromb. Res.,* **59**:383–388.

Fay, P.J., Coumans, J.-V. and Walker, F.J. (1991). von Willebrand factor mediates protection of factor VIII from activated protein C-catalyzed inactivation. *J. Biol. Chem.*, **266**:2172–2177.

Fisher, C.L., Greengard, J.S. and Griffin, J.H. (1994). Models of the serine protease domain of the human antithrombotic plasma factor activated protein C and its zymogen. *Protein Sci.*, **3**:588–599.

Foster, D.C., Yoshitake, S. and Davie, E.W. (1985). The nucleotide sequence of the gene for human protein C. *Proc. Natl. Acad. Sci. (USA)*, **82**:4673–4677.

Fourrier, F., Chopin, C., Goudemand, J. *et al.* (1992). Septic shock, multiple organ failure, and disseminated intravascular coagulation. Compared patterns of antithrombin III, protein C, and protein S deficiencies. *Chest*, **101**:816–823.

Freyssinet, J., Gauchy, J. and Cazenave, J. (1986). The effect of phospholipids on the activation of protein C by the human thrombin-thrombomodulin complex. *Biochem. J.*, **238**:151–157.

Freyssinet, J., Wiesel, M.L., Gauchy, J., Boneu, B. and Cazenave, J.P. (1986). An IgM lupus anticoagulant that neutralizes the enhancing effect of phospholipid on purified endothelial thrombomodulin activity. A mechanism for thrombosis. *Thromb. Haemost.*, **55**:309–313.

Fukudome, K. and Esmon, C.T. (1994). Identification, cloning and regulation of a novel endothelial cell protein C/activated protein C receptor. *J. Biol. Chem.*, **269**:26486–26491.

Galvin, J.B., Kurosawa, S., Moore, K., Esmon, C.T. and Esmon, N.L. (1987). Reconstitution of rabbit thrombomodulin into phospholipid vesicles. *J. Biol. Chem.*, **262**:2199–2205.

Garcia de Frutos, P., Alim, R.I.M., Hardig, Y., Zoller, B. and Dahlbäck, B. (1994). Differential regulation of α and beta chains of C4b-binding protein during acute-phase response resulting in stable plasma levels of free anticoagulant protein S. *Blood*, **84**:815–822.

Gershagen, S., Fernlund, P. and Edenbrandt, C.-M. (1991). The genes for SHBG/ABP and the SHBG-like region of vitamin K-dependent protein S have evolved from a common ancestral gene. *J. Steroid Biochem. Molec. Biol.*, **40**:763–769.

Ginsberg, J.S., Demers, C., Brill-Edwards, P. *et al.* (1993). Increased thrombin generation and activity in patients with systemic lupus erythematosus and anticardiolipin antibodies: evidence for a prothrombotic state. *Blood*, **81**:2958–2963.

Girolami, A., Simioni, P., Lazzaro, A.R. and Cordiano, I. (1989). Severe arterial cerebral thrombosis in a patient with protein S deficiency (moderately reduced total and markedly reduced free protein S): A family study. *Thromb. Haemost.*, **61**:144–147.

Gladson, C.L., Groncy, P. and Griffin, J.H. (1987). Coumarin necrosis, neonatal purpura fulminans, and protein C deficiency. *Arch. Dermatol.*, **123**:1701a–1706a.

Glaser, C.B., Morser, J., Clarke, J.H. *et al.* (1992). Oxidation of a specific methionine in thrombomodulin by activated neutrophil products blocks cofactor activity. *J. Clin. Invest.*, **90**:2565–2573.

Goldberg, S.L., Orthner, C.L., Yalisove, B.L., Elgart, M.L. and Kessler, C.M. (1991). Skin necrosis following prolonged administration of coumarin in a patient with inherited protein S deficiency. *Am. J. Haematol.*, **38**:64–66.

Golub, B.M., Sibony, P.A. and Coller, B.S. (1990). Protein S deficiency associated with central retinal artery occlusion. *Arch. Ophthalmol.*, **108**:918.

Gouault-Heilmann, M., Gadelha-Parente, T., Levent, M., Intrator, L., Rostoker, G. and Lagrue, G. (1988). Total and free protein S in nephrotic syndrome. *Thromb. Res.*, **49**:37–42.

Greengard, J.S., Sun, X., Xu, X., Fernandez, J.A., Griffin, J.H. and Evatt, B. (1994). Activated protein C resistance caused by Arg506Gln mutation in factor Va. *Lancet*, **343**:1361–1362.

Grey, S.T., Tsuchida, A., Hau, H., Orthner, C.L., Salem, H.H. and Hancock, W.W. (1994). Selective inhibitory effects of the anticoagulant activated protein C on the responses of human mononuclear phagocytes to LPS, IFN-gamma, or phorbol ester. *J. Immunol.*, **153**:3664–3672.

Griffin, J.H., Evatt, B., Wideman, C. and Fernández, J.A. (1993). Anticoagulant protein C pathway defective in majority of thrombophilic patients. *Blood*, **82**:1989–1993.

Griffin, J.H., Gruber, A. and Fernandez, J.A. (1992). Reevaluation of total, free, and bound protein S and C4b-binding protein levels in plasma anticoagulated with citrate or hirudin. *Blood*, **79**:3203–3211.

Griffin, J.H., Mosher, D.F., Zimmerman, T.S. and Kleiss, A.J. (1982). Protein C, an antithrombotic protein, is reduced in hospitalized patients with intravascular coagulation. *Blood*, **60**:261–264.

Grinnell, B.W., Hermann, R.B. and Yan, S.B. (1994). Human protein C inhibits selectin-mediated cell adhesion: Role of unique fucosylated oligosaccharide. *Glycobiology*, **4**:221–226.

Grundy, C.B., Lindo, V., Kakkar, V.V., Melissari, E., Scully, M.F. and Cooper, D.N. (1991). Late-onset homozygous protein C deficiency. *Lancet*, **338**:575–576.

Hackeng, T.M., Hessing, M., van't Veer, C. *et al.* (1993). Protein S binding to human endothelial cells is required for expression of cofactor activity for activated protein C. *J. Biol. Chem.*, **268**:3993–4000.

Hackeng, T.M., van't Veer, C., Meijers, J.C.M. and Bouma, B.N. (1994). Human protein S inhibits prothrombinase complex activity on endothelial cells and platelets via direct interactions with factors Va and Xa. *J. Biol. Chem.*, **269**:21051–21058.

Halbmayer, W.-M., Haushofer, A., Schon, R. and Fischer, M. (1994). The prevalence of poor anticoagulant response to activated protein C (APC resistance) among patients suffering from stroke or venous thrombosis and among healthy subjects. *Blood Coagul. Fibrinol.*, **5**:51–57.

Harris, K.W. and Esmon, C.T. (1985). Protein S is required for bovine platelets to support activated protein C binding and activity. *J. Biol. Chem.*, **260**:2007–2010.

Hayashi, T., Honda, G. and Suzuki, K. (1992). An atherogenic stimulus homocysteine inhibits cofactor activity of thrombomodulin and enhances thrombomodulin expression in human umbilical vein endothelial cells. *Blood*, **79**:2930–2936.

Heeb, M.J. and Griffin, J.H. (1988). Physiologic inhibition of human activated protein C by α_1-antitrypsin. *J. Biol. Chem.*, **263**:11613–11616.

Heeb, M.J., España, F., Geiger, M., Collen, D., Stump, D.C. and Griffin, J.H. (1987). Immunological identity of heparin-dependent plasma and urinary protein C inhibitor and plasminogen activator inhibitor-3. *J. Biol. Chem.*, **262**:15813–15816.

Heeb, M.J., Gruber, A. and Griffin, J.H. (1991). Identification of divalent metal ion-dependent inhibition of activated protein C by alpha$_2$-macroglobulin and alpha$_2$-antiplasmin in blood and comparisons to inhibition of factor Xa, thrombin, and plasmin. *J. Biol. Chem.*, **266**:17606–17612.

Heeb, M.J., Mesters, R.M., Tans, G., Rosing, J. and Griffin, J.H. (1993). Binding of protein S to Factor Va associated with inhibition of prothrombinase that is independent of activated protein C. *J. Biol. Chem.*, **268**:2872–2877.

Heeb, M.J., Mosher, D. and Griffin, J.H. (1989). Activation and complexation of protein C and cleavage and decrease of protein S in plasma of patients with intravascular coagulation. *Blood*, **73**:455–461.

Heeb, M.J., Rosing, J., Bakker, H.M., Fernandez, J.A., Tans, G. and Griffin, J.H. (1994). Protein S binds to and inhibits factor Xa. *Proc. Natl. Acad. Sci. (USA)*, **91**:2728–2732.

Hillarp, A. and Dahlbäck, B. (1988). Novel subunit in C4b-binding protein required for protein S binding. *J. Biol. Chem.*, **263**:12759–12764.

Hogg, P.J., Öhlin, A.-K. and Stenflo, J. (1992). Identification of structural domains in protein C involved in its interaction with thrombin-thrombomodulin on the surface of endothelial cells. *J. Biol. Chem.*, **267**:703–706.

Holly, R.D. and Foster, D.C. (1994). Resistance to inhibition by alpha-1-anti-trypsin and species specificity of a chimeric human/bovine protein C. *Biochemistry*, **33**:1876–1880.

Hooper, W.C., Phillips, D.J., Ribeiro, M.J.A. *et al.* (1994). Tumor necrosis factor-α downregulates protein S secretion in human microvascular and umbilical vein endothelial cells but not in the HepG-2 hepatoma cell line. *Blood*, **84**:483–489.

Horie, S., Ishii, H., Hara, H. and Kazama, M. (1994). Enhancement of thrombin-thrombomodulin-catalysed protein C activation by phosphatidylethanolamine containing unsaturated fatty acids: Possible physiological significance of phosphatidylethanolamine in anticoagulant activity of thrombomodulin. *Biochem. J.*, **301**:683–691.

Husten, E.J., Esmon, C.T. and Johnson, A.E. (1987). The active site of blood coagulation factor Xa: its distance from the phospholipid surface and its conformational sensitivity to components of the prothrombinase complex. *J. Biol. Chem.*, **262**:12953–12962.

Imada, M., Imada, S., Iwasaki, H., Kume, A., Yamaguchi, H. and Moore, E.E. (1987). Fetomodulin: Marker surface protein of fetal development which is modulatable by cyclic AMP. *Dev. Biol.* **122**:483–491.

Ishii, H., Salem, H.H., Bell, C.E., Laposata, E.A. and Majerus, P.W. (1986). Thrombomodulin, an endothelial anticoagulant protein, is absent from the human brain. *Blood*, **67**:362–365.

Jackman, R.W., Beeler, D.L., Fritze, L., Soff, G. and Rosenberg, R.D. (1987). Human thrombomodulin gene is intron depleted: nucleic acid sequences of the cDNA and gene predict protein structure and suggest sites of regulatory control. *Proc. Natl. Acad. Sci. (USA)*, **84**:6425–6429.

Jhingan, A., Zhang, L., Christiansen, W.T. and Castellino, F.J. (1994). The activities of recombinant gamma-carboxyglutamic-acid-deficient mutants of activated human protein C toward human coagulation factor Va and Factor VIII in purified systems and in plasma. *Biochemistry*, **33**:1869–1875.

Johnson, A.E., Esmon, N.L., Laue, T.M. and Esmon, C.T. (1983). Structural changes required for activation of protein C are induced by Ca^{2+} binding to a high affinity site that does not contain gamma-carboxyglutamic acid. *J. Biol. Chem.*, **258**:5554–5560.

Joseph, D.R. and Baker, M.E. (1992). Sex hormone-binding globulin, androgen-binding protein, and vitamin K-dependent protein S are homologous to laminin A, merosin, and Drosophila crumbs protein. *FASEB J.*, **6**:2477–2481.

Kakkar, S., Melissar, E. and Kakkar, V.V. (1987). Congenital severe protein C deficiency in adults. *Thromb. Haemost.*, **58**:410. (Abstract)

Kalafatis, M. and Mann, K.G. (1993). Role of the membrane in the inactivation of factor Va by activated protein C. *J. Biol. Chem.*, **268**:27246–27257.

Kamiya, T., Sugihara, T., Ogata, K. *et al.* (1986). Inherited deficiency of protein S in a Japanese family with recurrent venous thrombosis: A study of three generations. *Blood*, **67**:406–410.

Kapiotis, S., Besemer, J., Bevec, D. *et al.* (1991). Interleukin-4 counteracts pyrogen-induced downregulation of thrombomodulin in cultured human vascular endothelial cells. *Blood*, **78**:410–415.

Karmochkine, M., Cacoub, P., Piette, J.C., Godeau, P. and Boffa, M.C. (1992). Antiphosphatidylethanolamine antibody as the sole antiphospholipid antibody in systemic lupus erythematosus with thrombosis. *Clin. Exp. Rheumatol.*, **10**:603–605.

Keeling, D.M., Wilson, A.J.G., Mackie, I.J., Isenberg, D.A. and Machin, S.J. (1993). Role of β_2-glycoprotein I and anti-phospholipid antibodies in activation of protein C *in vitro*. *J. Clin. Pathol.*, **46**:908–911.

Kemkes-Matthes, B. (1992). Acquired protein S deficiency. *Clin. Investig.*, **70**:529–534.

Key, N.S., Vercellotti, G.M., Winkelmann, J.C. *et al.* (1990). Infection of vascular endothelial cells with herpes simplex virus enhances tissue factor activity and reduces thrombomodulin expression. *Proc. Natl. Acad. Sci. (USA)*, **87**:7095–7099.

Kisiel, W., Canfield, W.M., Ericsson, L.H. and Davie, E.W. (1977). Anticoagulant properties of bovine plasma protein C following activation by thrombin. *Biochemistry*, **16**:5824–5831.

Koedam, J.A., Meijers, J.C.M., Sixma, J.J. and Bouma, B.N. (1988). Inactivation of human factor VIII by activated protein C. Cofactor activity of protein S and protective effect of von Willebrand factor. *J. Clin. Invest.*, **82**:1236–1243.

Koeleman, B.P.C., Reitsma, P.H., Allaart, C.F. and Bertina, R.M. (1994). Activated protein C resistance as an additional risk factor for thrombosis in protein C-deficient families. *Blood*, **84**:1031–1035.

Kumada, T., Dittman, W.A. and Majerus, P.W. (1987). A role for thrombomodulin in the pathogenesis of thrombin-induced thromboembolism in mice. *Blood*, **71**:728–733.

Kurosawa, S., Stearns, D.J., Jackson, K.W. and Esmon, C.T. (1988). A 10-kDa cyanogen bromide fragment from the epidermal growth factor homology domain of rabbit thrombomodulin contains the primary thrombin binding site. *J. Biol. Chem.*, **263**:5993–5996.

Labarrere, C.A., Esmon, C.T., Carson, S.D. and Faulk, W.P. (1990). Concordant expression of tissue factor and Class II MHC antigens in human placental endothelium. *Placenta*, **II**, 309–318.

Laszik, Z., Carson, C.W., Nadasdy, T. *et al.* (1994). Lack of suppressed renal thrombomodulin expression in a septic rat model with glomerular thrombotic microangiopathy. *Lab. Invest.*, **70**:862–867.

Lauer, C.G., Reid, T.J., III, Wideman, C.S., Evatt, B.L. and Alving, B.M. (1990). Free protein S deficiency in a family with venous thrombosis. *J. Vasc. Surg.*, **12**:541–544.

Le Bonniec, B.F. and Esmon, C.T. (1991). Glu-192 [to] Gln substitution in thrombin mimics the catalytic switch induced by thrombomodulin. *Proc. Natl. Acad. Sci. (USA)*, **88**:7371–7375.

Le Bonniec, B.F., MacGillivray, R.T.A. and Esmon, C.T. (1991). Thrombin Glu-39 restricts the P'3 specificity to nonacidic residues. *J. Biol. Chem.*, **266**:13796–13803.

Lefrancois, C., Derlon, A., Maurel, J., Le Querrec, A., Sillard, B. and Valla, A. (1991). Déficit constitutionnel en protéine S de type II. Rôle dans la survenue d'une thrombose artérioveineuse mésocolique. *Presse Méd.*, **20**:2106.

Lentz, S.R. and Sadler, J.E. (1991). Inhibition of thrombomodulin surface expression and protein C activation by the thrombogenic agent homocysteine. *J. Clin. Invest.*, **88**:1906–1914.

Lentz, S.R., Tsiang, M. and Sadler, J.E. (1991). Regulation of thrombomodulin by tumor necrosis factor-α: Comparison of transcriptional and posttranscriptional mechanisms. *Blood*, **77**:543–550.

Lin, J.-H., McLean, K., Morser, J. *et al.* (1994). Modulation of glycosaminoglycan addition in naturally expressed and recombinant human thrombomodulin. *J. Biol. Chem.*, **269**:25021–25030.

Lindblad, B., Svensson, P.J. and Dahlbäck, B. (1994). Arterial and venous thromboembolism with fatal outcome and resistance to activated protein C. *Lancet*, **343**:917.

Liu, L-W., Vu, T-K.H., Esmon, C.T. and Coughlin, S.R. (1991). The region of the thrombin receptor resembling hirudin binds to thrombin and alters enzyme specificity. *J. Biol. Chem.*, **266**:16977–16980.

Love, P.E. and Santoro, S.A. (1990). Antiphospholipid antibodies: Anticardiolipin, and the lupus anticoagulant in systemic lupus erythematosus (SLE) and in non-SLE disorders. Prevalence and clinical significance. *Ann. Intern. Med.*, **112**:682.

Lu, R., Esmon, N.L., Esmon, C.T. and Johnson, A.E. (1989). The active site of the thrombin-thrombomodulin complex: a fluorescence energy transfer measurement of its distance above the membrane surface. *J. Biol. Chem.*, **264**:12956–12962.

Mahasandana, C., Suvatte, V., Chuansumrit, A. *et al.* (1990). Homozygous protein S deficiency in an infant with purpura fulminans. *J. Pediatr.*, **117**:750–753.

Maillard, C., Berruyer, M., Serre, C.M., Dehavanne, M. and Delmas, P.D. (1992). Protein-S, a vitamin K-dependent protein, is a bone matrix component synthesized and secreted by osteoblasts. *Endocrinology*, **130**:1599–1604.

Manco-Johnson, M.J., Abshire, T.C., Jacobson, L.J. and Marlar, R.A. (1991). Severe neonatal protein C deficiency: Prevalence and thrombotic risk. *J. Pediatr.*, **119**:793–798.

Mann, K.G., Nesheim, M.E., Church, W.R., Haley, P. and Krishnaswamy, S. (1990). Surface-dependent reactions of the vitamin K-dependent enzyme complexes. *Blood*, **76**:1–16.

Marciniak, E. (1972). Inhibitor of human blood coagulation elicited by thrombin. *J. Lab. Clin. Med.*, **79**:924–934.

Marciniak, E. and Romond, E.H. (1989). Impaired catalytic function of activated protein C: A new *in vitro* manifestation of lupus anticoagulant. *Blood*, **74**:2426–2432.

Marlar, R.A., Sills, R.H., Groncy, P.K., Montgomery, R.R. and Madden, R.M. (1992). Protein C survival during replacement therapy in homozygous protein C deficiency. *Am. J. Haematol.*, **41**:24–31.

Maruyama, I., Bell, C.E. and Majerus, P.W. (1985). Thrombomodulin is found on endothelium of arteries, veins, capillaries, lymphatics, and on syncytiotrophoblast of human placenta. *J. Cel.l Biol.*, **101**:363–371.

Maruyama, I., Salem, H. and Majerus, P. (1984). Coagulation factor Va binds to human umbilical vein endothelial cells and accelerates protein C activation. *J. Clin. Invest.*, **74**:224–230.

McCachren, S.S., Diggs, J., Weinberg, J.B. and Dittman, W.A. (1991). Thrombomodulin expression by human blood monocytes and by human synovial tissue lining macrophages. *Blood*, **78**:3128–3132.

Melissari, E., Monte, G., Lindo, V.S. *et al.* (1992). Congenital thrombophilia among patients with venous thromboembolism. *Blood Coagul. Fibrinol.*, **3**:749–758.

Mitchell, C.A. and Salem, H.H. (1987). Cleavage of protein S by a platelet membrane protease. *J. Clin. Invest.*, **79**:374–379.

Molinari, A., Giogetti, C., Lansen, J. *et al.* (1992). Thrombomodulin is a cofactor for thrombin degradation of recombinant single-chain urokinase plasminogen activator *in vitro* and in a perfused rabbit heart model. *Thromb. Haemost.*, **67**:226–232.

Moore, K.L., Andreoli, S.P., Esmon, N.L., Esmon, C.T. and Bang, N.U. (1987). Endotoxin enhances tissue factor and suppresses thrombomodulin expression of human vascular endothelium *in vitro*. *J. Clin. Invest.*, **79**:124–130.

Moore, K.L., Esmon, C.T. and Esmon, N.L. (1989). Tumor necrosis factor leads to internalization and degradation of thrombomodulin from the surface of bovine aortic endothelial cells in culture. *Blood*, **73**:159–165.

Muntean, W., Finding, K., Gamillscheg, A. and Zenz, W. (1992). Multiple thromboses and coumarin-induced skin necrosis in a young child with antiphospholipid antibodies. *Thromb. Haemorrh. Disorders*, **5**:43–45.

Nagashima, M., Lundh, E., Leonard, J.C., Morser, J. and Parkinson, J.F. (1993). Alanine-scanning mutagenesis of the epidermal growth factor-like domains of human thrombomodulin identifies critical residues for its cofactor activity. *J. Biol. Chem.*, **268**:2888–2892.

Nawroth, P.P. and Stern, D.M. (1986). Modulation of endothelial cell hemostatic properties by tumor necrosis factor. *J. Exp. Med.*, **163**:740–745.

Nawroth, P.P., Handley, D.A., Esmon, C.T. and Stern, D.M. (1986). Interleukin-1 induces endothelial cell procoagulant while suppressing cell surface anticoagulant activity. *Proc. Natl. Acad. Sci. (USA)*, **83**:3460–3464.

Nelson, M., Gibson, J., Brown, R., Salem, H. and Kronenberg, H. (1992). A search for autoantibodies to thrombomodulin in patients with documented thrombosis. *Thromb. Haemost.*, **68**:477.

Nelson, R.M. and Long, G.L. (1992). Binding of protein S to C4b-binding protein. Mutagenesis of protein S. *J. Biol. Chem.*, **267**:8140–8145.

Nesheim, M.E., Canfield, W.M., Kisiel, W. and Mann, K.G. (1982). Studies on the capacity of factor Xa to protect factor Va from inactivation by activated protein C. *J. Biol. Chem.*, **257**:1443–1447.

Oates, A.M. and Salem, H.H. (1991). The binding and regulation of protein S by neutrophils. *Blood Coagul. Fibrinol.*, **2**:601–607.

Old, J.L. (1985). Tumor necrosis factor (TNF). *Science*, **230**:630–632.

Olsen, P.H., Esmon, N.L., Esmon, C.T. and Laue, T.M. (1992). The Ca^{2+}-dependence of the interactions between protein C, thrombin and the elastase fragment of thrombomodulin. Analysis by ultracentrifugation. *Biochemistry*, **31**:746–754.

Oosting, J.D., Derksen, R.H.W.M., Bobbink, I.W.G., Hackeng, T.M., Bouma, B.N. and de Groot, P.G. (1993). Antiphospholipid antibodies directed against a combination of phospholipids with prothrombin, protein C, or protein S: an explanation for their pathogenic mechanism? *Blood*, **81**:2618–2625.

Oosting, J.D., Derksen, R.H.W.M., Hackeng, T.M. *et al.* (1991). *In vitro* studies of antiphospholipid antibodies and its cofactor, β_2-glycoprotein I, show negligible effects on endothelial cell mediated protein C activation. *Thromb. Haemost.*, **66**:666–671.

Oosting, J.D., Preissner, K.T., Derksen, R.H.W.M. and de Groot, P.G. (1993). Autoantibodies directed against the epidermal growth factor-like domains of thrombomodulin inhibit protein C activation *in vitro*. *Br. J. Haematol.*, **85**:761–768.

Owen, W.G. and Esmon, C.T. (1981). Functional properties of an endothelial cell cofactor for thrombin-l catalyzed activation of protein C. *J. Biol. Chem.*, **256**:5532–5535.

Pabinger, I., Brucker, S., Kyrle, P.A. *et al.* (1992). Hereditary deficiency of antithrombin III, protein C and protein S: prevalence in patients with a history of venous thrombosis and criteria for rational patient screening. *Blood Coagul. Fibrinol.*, **3**:547–553.

Pabinger, I., Kyrle, P.A., Heistinger, M., Eichinger, S., Wittmann, E. and Lechner, K. (1994). The risk of thromboembolism in asymptomatic patients with protein C and protein S deficiency: a prospective cohort study. *Thromb. Haemost.*, **71**:441–445.

Padmanabhan, K., Padmanabhan, K.P., Tulinsky, A. *et al.* (1993). Structure of human des (1–45) factor Xa at 2.2 Å resolution. *J. Mol. Biol.*, **232**:947–966.

Parkinson, J.F., Grinnell, B.W., Moore, R.E., Hoskins, J., Vlahos, C.J. and Bang, N.U. (1990). Stable expression of a secretable deletion mutant of recombinant human thrombomodulin in mammalian cells. *J. Biol. Chem.*, **265**:12602–12610.

Parkinson, J.F., Koyama, T., Bang, N.U. and Preissner, K.T. (1992). Thrombomodulin: An anticoagulant cell surface proteoglycan with physiologically relevant glycosaminoglycan moiety. *Adv. Exp. Med. Biol.*, **313**:177–188.

Parkinson, J.F., Vlahos, C.J., Yan, S.C.B. and Bang, N.U. (1992). Recombinant human thrombomodulin: Regulation of cofactor activity and anticoagulant function by a glycosaminoglycan side chain. *Biochem. J.*, **283**:151–157.

Permpikul, P., Rao, L.V.M. and Rapaport, S.I. (1994). Functional and binding studies of the roles of prothrombin and β_2-glycoprotein I in the expression of lupus anticoagulant activity. *Blood*, **83**:2878–2892.

Petersen, T.E. (1988). The amino-terminal domain of thrombomodulin and pancreatic stone protein are homologous with lectins. *FEBS Letters*, **231**:51–53.

Pierangeli, S.S., Barker, J.H., Stikovac, D. *et al.* (1994). Effect of human IgG antiphospholipid antibodies on an *in vivo* thrombosis model in mice. *Thromb. Haemost.*, **71**:670–674.

Ploos van Amstel, H.K., Reitsma, P.H., van der Logt, C.P.E. and Bertina, R.M. (1990). Intron-exon organization of the active human protein S gene PS alpha and its pseudogene PSβ: Duplication and silencing during primate evolution. *Biochemistry*, **29**:7853–7861.

Powars, D., Larsen, R., Johnson, J. *et al.* (1993). Epidemic meningococcemia and purpura fulminans with induced protein C deficiency. *Clin. Infect. Dis.*, **17**:254–261.

Preissner, K.T. (1990). Biological relevance of the protein C system and laboratory diagnosis of protein C and protein S deficiencies. *Clin. Sci.*, **78**:351–364.

Preissner, K.T., Delvos, U. and Muller-Berghaus, G. (1987). Binding of thrombin to thrombomodulin accelerates inhibition of enzyme by antithrombin III. Evidence for a heparin-independent mechanism. *Biochemistry*, **26**:2521–2528.

Pryzdial, E.L.C. and Mann, K.G. (1991). The association of coagulation factor Xa and factor Va. *J. Biol. Chem.*, **266**:8969–8977.

Rauch, J., Tannenbaum, M., Tannenbaum, H. *et al.* (1986). Human hybridoma lupus anticoagulants distinguish between lamellar and hexagonal phase lipid systems. *J. Biol. Chem.*, **261**:9672–9677.

Regan, L.M., Lamphear, B.J., Huggins, C.F., Walker, F.J. and Fay, P.J. (1994). Factor IXa protects factor VIIIa from activated protein C. *J. Biol. Chem.*, **269**:9445–9452.

Reitsma, P.H., Poort, S.R., Bernardi, F. *et al.* (1993). Protein C deficiency: A database of mutations. For the Protein C & S Subcommittee of the Scientific and Standardization Committee of the International Society on Thrombosis and Haemostasis. *Thromb. Haemost.*, **69**:77–84.

Rezaie, A.R. and Esmon, C.T. (1992). The function of calcium in protein C activation by thrombin and the thrombin-thrombomodulin complex can be distinguished by mutational analysis of protein C derivatives. *J. Biol. Chem.*, **267**:26104–26109.

Rezaie, A.R. and Esmon, C.T. (1993). Conversion of Glu 192 to Gln in activated protein C changes the substrate specificity and increases reactivity toward macromolecular inhibitors. *J. Biol. Chem.*, **268**:19943–19948.

Rezaie, A.R., Esmon, N.L. and Esmon, C.T. (1992). The high affinity calcium-binding site involved in protein C activation is outside the first epidermal growth factor homology domain. *J. Biol. Chem.*, **267**:11701–11704.

Rezaie, A.R., Mather, T., Sussman, F. and Esmon, C.T. (1994). Mutation of Glu 80 [to] Lys results in a protein C mutant that no longer requires Ca^{2+} for rapid activation by the thrombin-thrombomodulin complex. *J. Biol. Chem.*, **269**:3151–3154.

Richardson, M.A., Gerlitz, B. and Grinnell, B.W. (1992). Enhancing protein C interaction with thrombin results in a clot-activated anticoagulant. *Nature*, **360**:261–264.

Rivard, G.E., David, M., Farrell, C. *et al.* (1993). Treatment of purpura fulminans in meningococcemia with protein C concentrate. *Thromb. Haemost.*, **69**:2338. (Abstract)

Rodgers, G.M. and Chandler, W.L. (1992). Laboratory and clinical aspects of inherited thrombotic disorders. *Am. J. Haematol.*, **41**:113–122.

Rydel, T.J., Ravichandran, K.G., Tulinsky, A. *et al.* (1990). The structure of a complex of recombinant hirudin and human α-thrombin. *Science*, **249**:277–280.

Sacco, R.L., Owen, J., Mohr, J.P., Tatemichi, T.K. and Grossman, B.A. (1989). Free protein S deficiency: A possible association with cerebrovascular occulsion. *Stroke*, **20**:1657–1661.

Schmidel, D.K., Tatro, A.V., Phelps, L.G., Tomczak, J.A. and Long, G.L. (1990). Organization of the human protein S genes. *Biochemistry*, **29**:7845–7852.

Schoen, P., Reutelingsperger, C. and Lindhout, T. (1992). Activation of prothrombin in the presence of human umbilical-vein endothelial cells. *Biochem. J.*, **281**:661–664.

Schramm, W., Spannagl, M., Bauer, K.A. *et al.* (1993). Treatment of coumarin-induced skin necrosis with a monoclonal antibody purified protein C concentrate. *Arch. Dermatol.*, **129**:753–756.

Schwalbe, R., Dahlbäck, B., Hillarp, A. and Nelsestuen, G. (1990). Assembly of protein S and C4b-binding protein on membranes. *J. Biol. Chem.*, **265**:16074–16081.

Schwarz, H.P., Fischer, M., Hopmeier, P., Batard, M.A. and Griffin, J.H. (1984). Plasma protein S deficiency in familial thrombotic disease. *Blood*, **64**:1297–1300.

Schwarz, H.P., Heeb, M.J., Wencel-Drake, J.D. and Griffin, J.H. (1985). Identification and quantitation of protein S in human platelets. *Blood*, **66**:1452–1455.

Scully, M.F., Toh, C.H., Hoogendoorn, H. *et al.* (1993). Activation of protein C and its distribution between its inhibitors, protein C inhibitor, β_1-antitrypsin and β_2-macroglobulin, in patients with disseminated intravascular coagulation. *Thromb. Haemost.*, **69**:448–453.

Seligsohn, U., Berger, A., Abend, M. *et al.* (1984). Homozygous protein C deficiency manifested by massive thrombosis in the newborn. *N. Engl. J. Med.*, **310**:559–562.

Sells, R.H., Marlar, R.A., Montgomery, R.R., Desphande, G.N. and Humbert, J.R. (1984). Severe homozygous protein C deficiency. *J. Pediatrics.*, **105**:409–413.

Semeraro, N., Triggiani, R., Montemurro, P., Cavallo, L.G. and Colucci, M. (1993). Enhanced endothelial tissue factor but normal thrombomodulin in endotoxin-treated rabbits. *Thromb. Res.*, **71**:479–486.

Sharon, C., Tirindelli, M., Mannucci, P.M., Tripodi, A. and Mariani, G. (1986). Homozygous protein C deficiency with moderately severe clinical symptoms. *Thromb. Res.*, **41**:483–488.

Shen, L. and Dahlbäck, B. (1994). Factor V and protein S as synergistic cofactors to activated protein C in degradation of factor VIIa. *J. Biol. Chem.*, **269**:18735–18738.

Sheth, S.B. and Carvalho, A.C. (1991). Protein S and C alterations in acutely ill patients. *Amer. J. Haematol.*, **36**:14–19.

Shreeniwas, R., Ogawa, S., Cozzolino, F. *et al.* (1991). Macrovascular and microvascular endothelium during long-term hypoxia: Alterations in cell growth, monolayer permeability, and cell surface coagulant properties. *Journal of Cellular Physiology*, **146**:8–17.

Slungaard, A. and Key, N.S. (1994). Platelet factor 4 stimulates thrombomodulin protein C-activating cofactor activity. A structure-function analysis. *J. Biol. Chem.*, **269**:25549–25556.

Smirnov, M.D. and Esmon, C.T. (1994). Phosphatidylethanolamine incorporation into vesicles selectively enhances factor Va inactivation by activated protein C. *J. Biol. Chem.*, **269**:816–819.

Smirnov, M.D., Triplett, D.T., Comp, P.C., Esmon, N.L. and Esmon, C.T. (1995). On the role of phosphatidylethanolamine in the inhibition of activated protein C activity by antiphospholipid antibodies. *J. Clin. Invest.*, **95**:309–316.

Soff, G.A., Jackman, R.W. and Rosenberg, R.D. (1991). Expression of thrombomodulin by smooth muscle cells in culture: Different effects of tumor necrosis factor and cyclic adenosine monophosphate on thrombomodulin expression by endothelial cells and smooth muscle cells in culture. *Blood*, **77**:515–518.

Solymoss, S., Tucker, M.M. and Tracy, P.B. (1988). Kinetics of inactivation of membrane-bound factor Va by activated protein C. *J. Biol. Chem.*, **263**:14884–14890.

Staub, H.L., Harris, E.N., Khamashata, M.H., Savidge, G. and Hughes, G.R.V. (1989). Antibody to phosphatidylethanolamine in a patient with lupus anticoagulant and thrombosis. *Ann. Rheum. Dis.*, **48**:166–169.

Stearns, D.J., Kurosawa, S. and Esmon, C.T. (1989). Micro-thrombomodulin: Residues 310–486 from the epidermal growth factor precursor homology domain of thrombomodulin will accelerate protein C activation. *J. Biol. Chem.*, **264**:3352–3356.

Stearns, D.J., Kurosawa, S., Sims, P.J., Esmon, N.L. and Esmon, C.T. (1988). The interaction of a Ca^{2+} dependent monoclonal antibody with the protein C activation peptide region: Evidence for obligatory Ca^{2+} binding to both antigen and antibody. *J. Biol. Chem.*, **263**:826–832.

Stenflo, J. (1991). Structure-function relationships of epidermal growth factor modules in vitamin K-dependent clotting factors. *Blood*, **78**:1637–1651.

Stern, D.M., Brett, J., Harris, K. and Nawroth, P. (1986). Participation of endothelial cells in the protein C-protein S anticoagulant pathway: The synthesis and release of protein S. *J. Cell. Biol.*, **102**:1971–1978.

Stern, D.M., Nawroth, P.P., Harris, K. and Esmon, C.T. (1986). Cultured bovine aortic endothelial cells promote activated protein C-protein S-mediated inactivation of Factor Va. *J. Biol. Chem.*, **261**:713–718.

Stubbs, M.T. and Bode, W. (1993). A player of many parts: The spotlight falls on thrombin's structure. *Thromb. Res.*, **69**:1–58.

Stubbs, M.T., Oschkinat, H., Mayr, I. *et al.* (1992). The interaction of thrombin with fibrinogen. A structural basis for its specificity. *Eur. J. Biochem.*, **206**:187–195.

Sugo, T., Dahlbäck, B., Holmgren, A. and Stenflo, J. (1986). Calcium binding of bovine protein S. Effect of thrombin cleavage and removal of the gamma-carboxyglutamic acid-containing region. *J. Biol. Chem.*, **261**:5116–5120.

Sun, X., Evatt, B. and Griffin, J.H. (1994). Blood coagulation factor Va abnormality associated with resistance to activated protein C in venous thrombophilia. *Blood*, **83**:3120–3125.

Suzuki, K., Deyashiki, Y., Nishioka, J. *et al.* (1987). Characterization of a cDNA for human protein C inhibitor. A new member of the plasma serine protease inhibitor superfamily. *J. Biol. Chem.*, **262**:611–616.

Suzuki, K., Kusumoto, H., Deyashiki, Y. *et al.* (1987). Structure and expression of human thrombomodulin, a thrombin receptor on endothelium acting as a cofactor for protein C activation. *EMBO J.*, **6**:1891–1897.

Suzuki, K., Nishioka, J., Hayashi, T. and Kosaka, Y. (1988). Functionally active thrombomodulin is present in human platelets. *J. Biochem. (Tokyo)*, **104**:628–632.

Takahashi, H., Tatewaki, W., Wada, K. and Shibata, A. (1989). Plasma protein S in disseminated intravascular coagulation, liver disease, collagen disease, diabetes mellitus, and under oral anticoagulant therapy. *Clinica Chimica Acta*, **182**:195–208.

Takano, S., Kimura, S., Ohdama, S. and Aoki, N. (1990). Plasma thrombomodulin in health and diseases. *Blood*, **76**:2024–2029.

Tans, G., Rosing, J., Thomassen, M.C.L.G.D., Heeb, M.J., Zwaal, R.F.A. and Griffin, J.H. (1991). Comparison of anticoagulant and procoagulant activities of stimulated platelets and platelet-derived microparticles. *Blood*, **77**:2641–2648.

Taylor, F., Chang, A., Ferrell, G. *et al.* (1991). C4b-binding protein exacerbates the host response to Escherichia coli. *Blood*, **78**:357–363.

Taylor, F.B. Jr., Chang, A., Esmon, C.T., D'Angelo, A., Vigano-D'Angelo, S. and Blick, K.E. (1987). Protein C prevents the coagulopathic and lethal effects of E coli infusion in the baboon. *J. Clin. Invest*, **79**:918–925.

Taylor, F.B. Jr., He, S.E., Chang, A.C.K. *et al.* (1994). Infusion of phospholipid vesicles amplifies the local thrombotic response to TNF and anti-protein C into a systemic consumptive response. *Blood*, (in press)

Taylor, F.B. Jr., Hoogendoorn, H., Chang, A.C.K. *et al.* (1992). Anticoagulant and fibrinolytic activities are promoted, not retarded, *in vivo* after thrombin generation in the presence of a monoclonal antibody that inhibits activation of protein C. *Blood*, **79**:1720–1728.

Tazawa, R., Yamamoto, K., Suzuki, K., Hirokawa, K., Hirosawa, S. and Aoki, N. (1994). Presence of functional cyclic AMP responsive element in the 3'-untranslated region of the human thrombomodulin gene. *Biochem. Biophys. Res. Commun.*, **200**:1391–1397.

Triplett, D.A. (1993). Antiphospholipid antibodies and thrombosis. A consequence, coincidence, or cause? *Arch. Pathol. Lab. Med.*, **117**:78–88.

Tsiang, M., Lentz, S. and Sadler, J.E. (1992). Functional domains of membrane-bound human thrombomodulin. EGF-like domains four to six and the serine/threonine-rich domain are required for cofactor activity. *J. Biol. Chem.*, **267**:6164–6170.

Tsiang, M., Lentz, S.R., Dittman, W.A., Wen, D., Scarpati, E.M. and Sadler, J.E. (1990). Equilibrium binding of thrombin to recombinant human thrombomodulin: Effect of hirudin, fibrinogen, factor Va, and peptide analogues. *Biochemistry*, **29**:10602–10612.

Tsuchida, A., Salem, H., Thomson, N. and Hancock, W.W. (1992). Tumor necrosis factor production during human renal allograft rejection is associated with depression of plasma protein C and free protein S levels and decreased intragraft thrombomodulin expression. *J. Exp. Med.*, **175**:81–90.

Tuddenham, E.G.D., Takase, T., Thomas, A.E. *et al.* (1989). Homozygous protein C deficiency with delayed onset of symptoms at 7 to 10 months. *Thromb. Res.*, **53**:475–484.

Tulinsky, A. and Qiu, X. (1993). Active site and exosite binding of alpha-thrombin. *Blood Coagul. Fibrinol.*, **4**:305–312.

Visser, M.R., Tracy, P.B., Vercellotti, G.M., Goodman, J.L., White, J.G. and Jacob, H.S. (1988). Enhanced thrombin generation and platelet binding on herpes simplex virus-infected endothelium. *Proc. Natl. Acad. Sci. (USA)*, **85**:8227–8230.

Walker, F.J. (1980). Regulation of activated protein C by a new protein: A role for bovine protein S. *J. Biol. Chem.*, **255**:5521–5524.

Walker, F.J. (1981). Regulation of activated protein C by protein S: The role of phospholipid in factor Va inactivation. *J. Biol. Chem.*, **256**:11128–11131.

Walker, F.J. (1981). Regulation of bovine activated protein C by protein S: the role of the cofactor protein in species specificity. *Thromb. Res.*, **22**:321–327.

Walker, F.J. (1984). Regulation of vitamin K-dependent protein S. Inactivation by thrombin. *J. Biol. Chem.*, **259**:10335–10339.

Walker, F.J. (1986). Properties of chemically modified protein S: effect of the conversion of gamma-carboxyglutamic acid to gamma-methyleneglutamic acid on functional properties. *Biochemistry*, **25**:6305–6311.

Walker, F.J. (1992). Protein S and thrombotic disease (43435). *Proc Soc Exp Biol Med*, **200**:285–295.

Walker, F.J. and Fay, P.J. (1992). Regulation of blood coagulation by the protein C system. *FASEB J*, **6**:2561–2567.

Walker, F.J., Sexton, P.W. and Esmon, C.T. (1979). Inhibition of blood coagulation by activated protein C through selective inactivation of activated factor V. *Biochem. Biophys. Acta.*, **571**:333–342.

Weiler-Guettler, H., Yu, K., Soff, G., Gudas, L.J. and Rosenberg, R.D. (1992). Thrombomodulin gene regulation by cAMP and retinoic acid in F9 embryonal carcinoma cells. *Proc. Natl. Acad. Sci. (USA)*, **89**:2155–2159.

Weis, J.R., Pitas, R.E., Wilson, B.D. and Rodgers, G.M. (1991). Oxidized low-density lipoprotein increases cultured human endothelial cell tissue factor activity and reduces protein C activation. *FASEB J.*, **5**:2459–2465.

Wen, D., Dittman, W.A., Ye, R.D., Deaven, L.L., Majerus, P.W. and Sadler, J.E. (1987). Human thrombomodulin: Complete cDNA sequence and chromosome localization of the gene. *Biochemistry*, **26**:4350–4357.

Wong, V.L.Y., Hofman, F.M., Ishii, H. and Fisher, M. (1991). Regional distribution of thrombomodulin in human brain. *Brain Res.*, **556**:1–5.

Wu, Q., Sheehan, J.P., Tsiang, M., Lentz, S.R., Birktoft, J.J. and Sadler, J.E. (1991). Single amino acid substitutions dissociate fibrinogen-clotting and thrombomodulin-binding activities of human thrombin. *Proc. Natl. Acad. Sci. (USA)*, **88**:6775–6779.

Ye, J., Esmon, C.T. and Johnson, A.E. (1993). The chondroitin sulfate moiety of thrombomodulin binds a second molecule of thrombin. *J. Biol. Chem.*, **268**:2373–2379.

Ye, J., Esmon, N.L., Esmon, C.T. and Johnson, A.E. (1991). The active site of thrombin is altered upon binding to thrombomodulin: Two distinct structural changes are detected by fluorescence, but only one correlates with protein C activation. *J. Biol. Chem.*, **266**:23016–23021.

Ye, J., Liu, L-W., Esmon, C.T. and Johnson, A.E. (1992). The fifth and sixth growth factor-like domains of thrombomodulin bind to the anion exosite of thrombin and alter its specificity. *J. Biol. Chem.*, **267**:11023–11028.

Ye, J., Rezaie, A.R. and Esmon, C.T. (1994). Glycosaminoglycan contributions to both protein C activation and thrombin inhibition involve a common arginine-rich site in thrombin that includes residues arginine 93, 97, and 101. *J. Biol. Chem.*, **269**:17965–17970.

Zhang, L. and Castellino, F.J. (1993). The contributions of individual gamma-carboxyglutamic acid residues in the calcium-dependent binding of recombinant human protein C to acidic phospholipid vesicles. *J. Biol. Chem*, **268**: 12040–12045.

Zhang, L. and Castellino, F.J. (1994). The binding energy of human coagulation protein C to acidic phospholipid vesicles contains a major contribution from leucine 5 in the gamma-carboxyglutamic acid domain. *J. Biol. Chem.*, **269**: 3590–3595.

Zhang, L., Jhingan, A. and Castellino, F.J. (1992). Role of individual Gamma-Carboxyglutamic acid residues of activated human protein C in defining its *in vitro* anticoagulant activity. *Blood*, **80**:942–952.

Zoller, B. and Dahlbäck, B. (1994). Linkage between inherited resistance to activated protein C and factor V gene mutation in venous thrombosis. *Lancet*, **343**:1536–1538.

Zushi, M., Gomi, K., Honda, G. *et al.* (1991). Aspartic acid 349 in the fourth epidermal growth factor-like structure of human thrombomodulin plays a role in its Ca^{2+}-mediated binding to protein C. *J Biol Chem*, **266**:19886–19889.

Zushi, M., Gomi, K., Yamamoto, S., Maruyama, I., Hayashi, T. and Suzuki, K. (1989). The last three consecutive epidermal growth factor-like structures of human thrombomodulin comprise the minimum functional domain for protein C-activating cofactor activity and anticoagulant activity. *J Biol. Chem.*, **264**:10351–10353.

3 The Heparan Sulfate-Antithrombin Pathway: A Natural Anticoagulant Mechanism of the Blood Vessel Wall

Robert D. Rosenberg and Kenneth A. Bauer

Department of Molecular Medicine, Beth Israel Hospital, Boston, USA, Department of Hematology/Oncology, Brockton-West Roxbury Department of Veterans Affairs Medical Center, USA

HISTORICAL INTRODUCTION

At the very end of the nineteenth century, thrombin was known to lose activity gradually when added to defibrinated plasma (Contejean, 1895; Morowitz, 1968). Based on this information, it was surmised that a specific inactivator of thrombin, antithrombin (AT), must be present in blood. In 1916, McLean purified heparin from the liver and discovered the anticoagulant properties of this polysaccharide (McLean, 1916). The mechanism of its inhibitory effect was clarified by Brinkhous and colleagues (1939), who showed that heparin was effective as an anticoagulant only in the presence of a plasma component termed *heparin cofactor* (HC). During the 1950's, kinetic studies conducted by several investigators indicated that plasma AT activity and plasma HC activity were intimately related (Waugh and Fitzgerald, 1956; Monkhouse *et al.*, 1955). In 1968, Abildgaard (1968) isolated small amounts of a human protein that functioned in both capacities. Subsequently, Rosenberg and Damus (1973) provided the first reproducible means of purifying large quantities of this human inhibitor and advanced convincing physiochemical evidence that plasma AT activity and plasma HC activity reside in the same molecule. In this chapter, we will discuss the structure of AT and its gene; the structure and biosynthesis of heparin and heparan sulfate; the molecular basis of the anticoagulant action of heparin and heparan sulfate; the synthesis of anticoagulantly active heparan sulfate proteoglycans (HSPG[act]) by endothelial cells; the physiologic role of the heparan sulfate-AT pathway; and functional defects in the heparan sulfate-AT pathway. Hence, we will provide a framework for evaluating the importance of the heparan sulfate-AT pathway as a natural anticoagulant mechanism of the blood vessel wall.

The Structure and Mechanism of Action of Antithrombin

Human antithrombin (AT) exhibits a molecular weight of 58,000 and an isoelectric point of 5.11 (Rosenberg and Damus, 1973). Its overall shape is best represented by a prolate

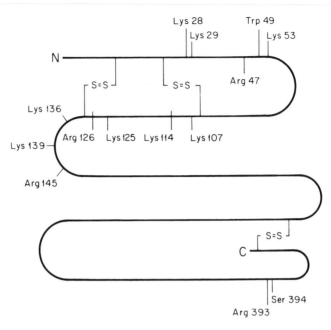

Figure 3.1 Critical sites within antithrombin. Arg-393-Ser-394 is the reactive site of antithrombin. Trp-49 is the conformation-sensitive aromatic residue. The various lysine and arginine residues are potential sites for the binding of the different domains of heparin to the protease inhibitor.

ellipsoid, with an axial ratio of 5 to 1 (Nordenman *et al.,* 1977). The concentration of the protease inhibitor in human plasma is about 140 μg/ml (Murano *et al.,* 1980). The complete amino acid sequence of AT has been reported by Petersen and co-workers (1979). The location of functionally important domains such as the enzyme binding region (reactive site), the heparin binding sites, the conformation-sensitive tryptophan residue, and the S-S crosslinks are depicted in Figure 3.1.

The human gene that codes for AT is 16 kb in size and contains x exons and x introns (Prochownik *et al.,* 1983b; Prochownik and Orkin, 1984). We note that the promoter region does not exhibit a TATA box at –25 to –30. However, the 5′ flanking region possesses an 8 base pair segment that is homologous to the $J_K – C_K$ enhancer of murine and human IgC_K genes. This control element is critical for the efficient synthesis of protease inhibitor and IgC_K light chains within tissue-specific environments. The transcription of the AT gene is initiated at a unique site 72 base pairs upstream from the ATG translation initiation codon, and the resultant mRNA contains 96 bases that code for the signal peptide, 1296 bases that code for the amino acid sequence of AT, and about 175 base pairs of 3′ untranslated region including a polyadenylation segment. It is worth pointing out that alternate splicing of the primary transcripts take place at two sites within the first intron. This process generates either a native AT with its signal peptide or a drastically truncated product consisting of the N-terminal 14 amino acids of the signal peptide as well as the five C-terminal amino acids encoded by a segment of the first intron. This small polypeptide appears to remain within the cell, but its function is known (Prochownik *et al.,* 1983b; Prochownik and Orkin, 1984).

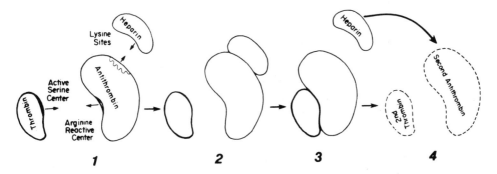

Figure 3.2   The overall mechanism of action of heparin and antithrombin.

The overall mechanism by which thrombin is inhibited by AT was initially elucidated by Rosenberg and Damus (1973). These investigators demonstrated that AT neutralizes thrombin by forming a 1:1 stoichiometric complex between the two components via a reactive site (arginine)-active center (serine) interaction. It was surmised that the above process involves generation of a stable tetrahedral intermediate between enzyme and inhibitor which resists bond cleavage as would normally occur with substrate. Complex formation occurs at a relatively slow rate in the absence of heparin. However, when the polysaccharide is present, it binds to lysyl residues on AT and dramatically accelerates the rate of generation of interaction product (Rosenberg and Damus, 1973). These studies suggest that the heparin-induced acceleratory phenomenon is due to an allosteric alteration in the protease inhibitor which renders it more readily available for interaction with thrombin or other coagulation enzymes (Figure 3.2) (Jordan *et al.*, 1979). Over the past two decades, the above model has been refined with regard to the position and nature of the reactive site, and the regions which bind heparin.

The structure-function relationships of the reactive site have been investigated in considerable detail. Bjork and collaborators (1982) have demonstrated that the AT reactive site is positioned near the carboxy terminal end of the protein at Arg-393 (P1 site)-Ser-394 (P1′ site). This conclusion has been confirmed by isolating natural mutants of AT and generating recombinant forms of the protease inhibitor which possess alterations of this region (Stephens *et al.*, 1987; Stephens *et al.*, 1988; Erdjument *et al.*, 1988a; Owen *et al.*, 1988; Erdjument *et al.*, 1989; Lane *et al.*, 1989a; Lane *et al.*, 1989b; Austin *et al.*, 1990). The characterization of these mutant protease inhibitors demonstrates that alterations of the P1 site have a profound suppressive effect on activity, whereas modifications of the P1′ site reduce potency in a variable manner depending upon the size and hydrophobicity of the substitution. These results are expected based upon bond specificity of coagulation enzymes. However, until recently, it remained unclear why the reactive site of AT traps hemostatic proteases rather than merely functioning as a substrate for these enzymes. The resolution of this conundrum was provided by X-ray crystallography of alpha 1 antitrypsin and AT in which the reactive bond had been cleaved (Huber and Carrell, 1989; Engh *et al.*, 1990; Mourey *et al.*, 1990; Schulze *et al.*, 1990; Bjork *et al.*, 1992). The three dimensional structures revealed that both P1–P16 regions (N-terminal to the cleaved reactive site) represent central beta strands of six-membered beta sheets within the central core of both proteins. Based upon modeling studies, it appears that the native structure of the two protease inhibitors could be reconstructed by extracting the P1–P16 region from the beta strand complex and reattaching it to the P1′ residue. This surprising result suggested that partial insertion of the same region into the central core of both proteins might be involved in stabilizing a reactive bond conformation which traps proteases in a tetrahedral intermediate rather than permitting bond cleavage as occurs with substrates. This hypothesis was confirmed by adding P1–P14 peptides to several plasma protease inhibitors which block insertion of the different reactive site loops, allow the reactive site bonds to be cleaved by added proteases, and prevent these proteins from functioning as inhibitors. Thus, the available evidence indicates that the serine active center of thrombin binds to the reactive site residues of AT. The interaction induces an insertion of a portion of the amino terminal region of the reactive site into the core of the inhibitor which arrests cleavage of the reactive site bond and thereby traps the hemostatic enzyme in a stable complex with protease inhibitor.

The two major heparin binding domains of AT have been defined by several techniques. The first region (residues 28–53) was pinpointed by investigating naturally occurring variants of AT, as well as variously chemically modified protease inhibitors with regard to heparin interaction, and examining proteolytic cleavage patterns of AT in the presence and absence of polysaccharide. The initial data obtained from natural variants reveal that mutations at Pro-41 and Arg-47 significantly decrease interaction of AT with heparin (Bjork *et al.*, 1989; Olson and Bjork, 1991). Blackburn and Sibley (1980), as well as other investigators, (Bjork and Nordling, 1979; Villanueva *et al.*, 1980) also claim that Trp-49 lies within the polysaccharide binding site of the protease inhibitor. Their conclusion is based on the fact that chemical modification of Trp-49 prevents AT from binding to heparin-Sepharose and produces a dramatic reduction in the polysaccharide induced acceleration of thrombin-protease inhibitor interactions. Karp and co-workers (1984) have shown that this chemical alteration causes only a modest reduction (~tenfold) in the avidity of heparin for AT but a much larger decrease (~500 fold) in the heparin-dependent acceleration of coagulation enzyme-protease inhibitor interactions. These data suggest that Trp-49 lies close to, but not within, a major binding region of AT and may be involved in a conformational transition required for polysaccharide-dependent acceleration of hemostatic enzyme-antithrombin interactions. Chang and coworkers have also shown that protease V8 preferentially attacks Glu 34-Gly 35, Glu 42-Ala 43, and Glu 50-Leu 51 of AT and that heparin protects against cleavage of these bonds (Liu and Chang, 1987a; Liu and Chang, 1987b). We note that Lys-28, Lys-29, and Lys-53 lie within this region and could serve as positive binding sites for heparin. In general, NMR studies support the importance of the above region with regard to interaction of protease inhibitor with polysaccharide (Horne and Gettins, 1992).

The second region (residues 107–156) was identified by studying selectively reduced or chemically modified AT as well as examining the biologic effects of antibodies directed against specific regions of the protease inhibitor. Chang and coworkers demonstrated that selective reduction of the Cys-8-Cys-128 bridge causes a dramatic decrease in the binding of AT to heparin, suppresses the polysaccharide dependent conformational change of the protease inhibitor, and prevents rapid inhibition of factor X_a or thrombin by AT and heparin (Sun and Chang, 1989; Chang, 1989). The positively charged residues involved in heparin interaction, Lys 107, Lys 114, Lys 125, Lys 136, and possibly

Arg 129 or Arg 145, were identified by chemical modification of AT in the presence and absence of polysaccharide. Knauer and coworkers reached a similar conclusion by proteolytically cleaving AT and then isolating a peptide (residues 107–156) which binds tightly to heparin (Smith *et al.*, 1990). These investigators prepared antibodies against the above region and then showed that a heterologous antibody directed against residues 138–145 inhibited heparin binding as well as served as a mimic for polysaccharide with regard to accelerating thrombin inhibition by AT. It is of interest to emphasize that the above domain contains Lys 139 as well as Arg 145. Using a computer generated model of antithrombin based upon the known structure of alpha 1-antitrypsin, Huber and Carrell (1989) have suggested that a subset of the positively charged resides of region I and region II are aligned to form a stretch of positive residues which could bind sulfate groups of heparin.

The coagulation cascade is composed of a series of linked proteolytic reactions (Mcfarlane, 1964; Davie and Ratnoff, 1964). At each step, a zymogen is converted to its corresponding serine protease, which is responsible for a subsequent zymogen-protease transition. Rosenberg and co-workers (Rosenberg *et al.*, 1975; Stead *et al.*, 1976), as well as other investigators (Kurachi *et al.*, 1976; Summana *et al.*, 1977), have shown that hemostatic enzymes of the intrinsic coagulation cascade — factors IX_a, X_a, XI_a, and XII_a — are inactivated by AT in a manner similar to that outlined for thrombin. Heparin is able to dramatically accelerate each of these protease-protease inhibitor interactions. It is of interest to note that the magnitude of the polysaccharide dependent acceleration of factor XI_a-AT interactions has been the subject of considerable debate (Beeler *et al.*, 1976). The available information suggests that saturation of AT with heparin accelerates the above interaction to a very considerable extent. The addition of high molecular weight kininogen allows this cofactor to bind to factor XI_a which further augments the rate of enzyme neutralization by the heparin AT complex via interactions of bound cofactor with bound polysaccharide (Scott *et al.*, 1982). Indeed, under these conditions, the extent of acceleration of factor XI_a inhibition by AT and heparin approaches that of thrombin (Olson and Shore, 1989). Thus, the current data indicate that upon addition of heparin the AT system described above is the major pathway of neutralization for most of the activated factors of the intrinsic coagulation cascade except possibly for Factor XII_a where C_l inhibitor may play an important role, even in the presence of polysaccharide and protease inhibitor. Careful studies of the interaction between purified Factor VII_a or activated protein C and AT upon addition of heparin reveal that these enzymes are only slowly inactivated (Godal *et al.*, 1974; Broze and Majerus, 1980). Other steps of the coagulation cascade that do not involve serine proteases are only minimally affected by heparin. These include the binding of activated cofactors such as Factor V_a to platelets and the polymerization or crosslinking of fibrin.

The Structure and Biosynthesis of Heparin and Heparan Sulfate

Heparin is a sulfated glycosaminoglycan which is found in all animals above horseshoe crabs. Within mammalian species, it is present in mast cells and therefore widely distributed throughout a variety of organs (Engelberg, 1963). The biosynthesis of the polysaccharide has been extensively studied over the past three decades employing a mast cell tumor system. It has been observed that synthesis of the heparin is initiated by attachment of a carbohydrate-protein linkage region to the serine residues of a specific polypeptide chain. This core protein, termed serglycin, contains extended sequences of alternating residues of serine and glycine, with virtually all of the former moieties bearing carbohydrate-protein connecting segments (Ruoslahti, 1988). The synthesis of this linkage region is dependent on the sequential action of four specific glycosyltransferases that utilize UDP sugars as their substrates. The structures of the core protein and its linkage region are depicted in Figure 3.3 (Engelberg, 1963; Silbert, 1967; Lindahl *et al.,* 1977; Roden and Horowitz, 1977; Robinson *et al.,* 1978; Yurt *et al.,* 1978; Jacobson *et al.,* 1979).

After formation of the carbohydrate-protein connecting sequence, the polymer chain of the polysaccharide is assembled by the alternate attachment of *N*-acetylglucosamine and glucuronic acid. This is accomplished through the action of a single specific glycosyltransferase that utilizes UDP-*N*-acetylglucosamine and UDP-glucuronic acid (Lind *et al.,* 1993). Thereafter, this simple copolymer is modified by a concerted process which leads

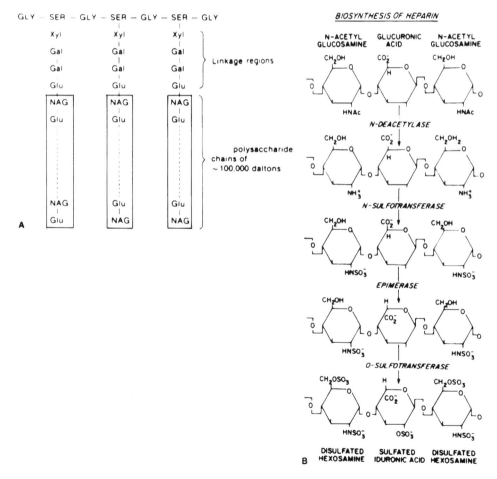

Figure 3.3   (A) Structure of the heparin proteoglycan. (B) Biosynthesis of the mucopolysaccharide chains.

to different modifications in various segments of the polysaccharide chain, as shown in Figure 3.3. For the purposes of discussion, these modifications can be divided into four major categories which are under the control of specific enzymes. First, glucosamine residues are partially *N*-deacetylated, and the exposed amino groups serve as acceptors of sulfate ions in a transfer reaction with PAPS. Second, glucuronic acid residues are variably epimerized to iduronic acid moieties. Third, the iduronic acid residues and, to a lesser extent, glucuronic acid residues are partially ester-sulfated at the C-2 position. Fourth, the glucosamine moieties are ester-sulfated to a variable extent at the C-3 and the C-6 positions (Silbert, 1967; Lindahl *et al.*, 1977; Roden and Horowitz, 1977; Jacobson *et al.*, 1979). The final product of the above pathway, the heparin proteoglycan, contains variable numbers of polysaccharide chains of molecular weight 30,000 to 100,000 (Robinson *et al.*, 1978; Yurt *et al.*, 1978).

The complex series of modification events appear to be regulated in at least two major ways. On the one hand, the *N*-deacetylase and *N*-sulfotransferase are physically linked as two activities on the same enzyme (Pettersson *et al.*, 1991; Wei *et al.*, 1993; Eriksson *et al.*, 1994; Mandon *et al.*, 1994). This situation allows tight coupling between *N*-deactylation and *N*-sulfation reactions. The placement of a *N*-sulfate moiety on the reducing end of the uronic acid permits epimerization of that residue as well as *O*-sulfation of neighboring glucosamine and uronic acid residues. On the other hand, a precise sequence of sulfated and nonsulfated uronic acid and glucosamine residues is apparently essential for 3-*O*-sulfation of glucosamine residues which is required for anticoagulant properties. This region occurs relatively infrequently in the heparin chain and is thought to include a glucuronic acid residue on the reducing end of the glucosamine to be 3-*O*-sulfated and a sulfated iduronic acid residue on the nonreducing end of the same residue (Kusche *et al.*, 1988). The availability of this precursor for 3-*O*-sulfation may in part regulate the abundance of the AT binding sequence within heparin (Kusche *et al.*, 1990; Linhardt *et al.*, 1992).

Physical methods have been used to study the three-dimensional conformation of porcine and bovine heparin. The techniques employed include viscometry, low-angle x-ray scattering, optical rotary dispersion of dye complexes, ^{13}C nuclear magnetic resonance, and X-ray diffraction of oriented films (Stone, 1964; Stivala *et al.*, 1968; Yuan and Stivala, 1972; Nieduszynski and Atkins, 1973; Atkins *et al.*, 1974; Fransson *et al.*, 1978). The experimental data are most consistent with the view that the polysaccharide is present within aqueous solutions as a loose helical coil. The sulfate and carboxyl groups are placed peripherally and are directed outward. Of course, the precise molecular structure of a given segment of the helical coil depends critically on the monosaccharide sequence present within that region.

Mammalian cells other than mast cells synthesize a second type of heparinlike proteoglycan — a heparan sulfate proteoglycan — which consists of a core protein of specific structure with covalently attached glycosaminoglycans of 50-150 disaccharide units. The glycosaminoglycan sidechains exhibit a structural diversity similar to heparin which arises from differing arrangements of disaccharide units composed of alternating *N*-sulfate or *N*-acetylglucosamine residues with or without 6-*O* and/or 3-*O* ester groups and glucuronic acid or iduronic acid residues with or without 2-*O*-ester sulfate groups. The distinction between heparin and heparan sulfate proteoglycans is based upon the structure of the core protein, the location of the glycoconjugate within the cell, and the relative amounts of *N*-sulfated and *O*-sulfated glucosamine and glucuronic acid present in the carbohydrate chains. Firstly, the heparin core protein is small and relatively simple in structure with extended runs of ser-gly attachments sites, whereas heparan sulfate core proteins are large and more diverse in structure with isolated ser-gly attachments sites and membrane spanning regions or glycolipid anchors. Secondly, the heparin proteoglycan is found within mast cell granules, whereas heparan sulfate proteoglycans are located on cell surfaces or in the surrounding matrix. Thirdly, heparin is more extensively modified with larger amounts of *N*-sulfate glucosamine residues with and without 3-*O*- and 6-*O*-ester sulfate groups and iduronic acid residues with and without 2-*O*-ester sulfate groups, whereas heparan sulfate is less extensively modified with more *N*-acetylglucosamine residues and glucuronic acid residues. As outlined in subsequent sections, endothelial cell heparan sulfate proteoglycans with regions of defined monosaccharide structure regulate coagulation system function via interaction with AT.

The biosynthesis of heparan sulfate proteoglycans is conducted in a similar overall manner to heparin except that the pathway is more complex and the final products more structurally diverse. These events have been examined in great detail by somatic cell genetic techniques which utilize cloned animal cells. This approach involves isolation of cell mutants with specific defects in the pathway which are then investigated to learn more about the regulation of these events. To this end, the animal cells are mutagenized, screened for reduced glycosaminoglycan content or decreased capacity to bind antithrombin or fibroblast growth factor, isolated at clonal purity and characterized biochemically as well as functionally (Esko *et al.*, 1985). The above approach has identified critical genetic loci involved in sulfate transport (Esko *et al.*, 1986), carbohydrate linkage region attachment (Esko *et al.*, 1987), linkage of *N*-acetylglucosamine and glucuronic acid (Lidholt *et al.*, 1992), co-ordination of *N*-deacetylation and *N*-sulfation (Bame and Esko, 1989), and production of the antithrombin binding region (de Agostini *et al.*, 1990).

The above analyses of cell mutants in conjunction with the isolation and expression of cDNAs has revealed that the characteristic reduced modification of heparan sulfate, compared to heparin, in part results from two different forms of the enzyme *N*-deacetylase/ *N*-sulfotransferase. Heparan sulfate producing liver cells express a form which is distinct from the enzyme found in heparin producing mast cells (Hashimoto *et al.*, 1992; Eriksson *et al.*, 1994). Over-expression studies indicate that the liver enzyme can only generate the relatively lower level of *N*-sulfates found in heparan sulfate (Ishihara *et al.*, 1993). The decreased availability of *N*-sulfates limits the placement of additional modifications on the heparan chain since the presence of this moiety is a prerequisite for the subsequent epimerization and ester sulfation steps (Bame *et al.*, 1991). The eventual identification of additional genes will reveal whether regulation of heparan sulfate biosynthesis employs further pathway specific isoforms.

It is obvious from the above information that substantial progress has been made in defining the biosynthesis and linear sequence of heparin and heparan sulfate. However, the precise relationship between the structure of glycosaminoglycans and their anticoagulant properties remained elusive until the past decade. Indeed, it had been tacitly assumed that the polysaccharide might exhibit numerous alternative structures equally capable of activating antithrombin and accelerating hemostatic enzyme-protease inhibitor interactions. The following section summarizes investigations on the kinetics of hemostatic enzyme-antithrombin-heparin interaction and the structure-function relationships of heparin that have served as an essential foundation for elucidating the physiologic role of heparan sulfate proteoglycans as a natural anticoagulant mechanism of the blood vessel wall.

The Molecular Basis of the Anticoagulant Action of Heparin

The overall mechanism by which heparin accelerates hemostatic enzyme-AT complex formation was initially investigated by determining the binding parameters and steady state kinetic constants of the various heparin-AT-hemostatic enzyme interactions (Jordan *et al.*, 1980a; Jordan *et al.*, 1980b). Based on these data, Rosenberg and coworkers assessed the relative importance of the binding of heparin to either protease inhibitor or enzyme or both (Broze and Majerus, 1980; Jordan *et al.*, 1980a; Jordan *et al.*, 1980b). The results suggest that heparin-dependent enhancement in the rates of neutralization of thrombin, factor IX_a, or factor X_a by AT requires binding of the polysaccharide to the protease inhibitor but not necessarily to the enzyme. Comparisons of the various kinetic constants indicate that direct binding of heparin to AT is responsible for an approximate 1000-fold acceleration of enzyme-inhibitor complex formation. The approximation interaction between free thrombin or free factor IX_a and polysaccharide bound to AT appears to provide only an additional approximate 10-fold enhancement in the rate of enzyme neutralization. The complexing of free factor X_a by polysaccharide bound to AT leads to essentially no augmentation in the velocity of enzyme inactivation. Therefore, the acceleration of AT action appears to be mainly due to the direct binding of heparin to the protease inhibitor, whereas the approximation phenomenon between heparin and hemostatic enzymes is of lesser importance (Jordan *et al.*, 1980a; Jordan *et al.*, 1980b). The above model of heparin action has been confirmed and extended by the work of Evans *et al.*, (1992) who investigated the effects of different sizes and types of heparin on the rates of neutralization of hemostatic enzymes by AT as well as polysaccharide dependent changes in other physical/biochemical parameters. These studies indicate that the binding of heparin to AT is responsible for a major portion of the polysaccharide dependent enhancement in the rate of thrombin neutralization and virtually all of the polysaccharide dependent enhancement in the rate of factor X_a inhibition (Bjork *et al.*, 1989).

The above view of the relative importance of the direct binding of heparin to AT versus the approximation of enzyme to protease inhibitor is not completely shared by all investigators in the field. Shore and coworkers have conducted fast reaction kinetic analysis of the heparin dependent neutralization of thrombin or factor X_a by AT (Olson and Shore, 1982; Shore *et al.*, 1989; Craig *et al.*, 1989; Bjork *et al.*, 1989). They conclude that heparin induces a 1000-fold enhancement in the affinity of thrombin for AT in the intermediate encounter complex, but possesses no accelerating effect on the limiting rate of conversion to the stable thrombin-AT complex. These investigators state that the above results could be due either to a pure approximation mechanism or a direct effect of heparin on AT or to a mixed mechanism as outlined above. The above investigators then attempted to discriminate between these potential mechanisms by carrying out kinetic studies at varying ionic strengths (Bjork *et al.*, 1989). The reaction rates under these conditions could be accounted for by changes in the ionic strength dependent interaction of thrombin with heparin bound to AT. However, it is quite clear that ionic strength changes may also exert effects on the type of direct binding of heparin to AT. Shore and coworkers have also carried similar studies on the heparin dependent acceleration of factor X_a inhibition by AT. The data show that polysaccharide enhances both the rate of formation of the intermediate encounter complex and the limiting rate of conversion to the stable thrombin-AT complex. No effect of heparin with regard to approximation of enzyme could be documented. Therefore, the relative importance of the direct binding of heparin to AT or thrombin in the acceleration of the protease-protease inhibitor interaction is disputed. However, the effect of heparin on the acceleration of the factor X_a-AT interaction is clearly due to the direct effect of the polysaccharide on the protease inhibitor.

It should be noted that investigations of Rosenberg and coworkers were carried out with heparin molecules of molecular weight ~6500, whereas other investigators studied the kinetic effects of polysaccharides of greater sizes (Jordan *et al.,* 1982; Nesheim, 1983; Hoylaerts *et al.,* 1984). The larger complex carbohydrates are able to accelerate certain of the hemostatic enzyme-protease inhibitor interactions to a greater degree than that outlined above, which appears to be due to multiple binding sites for antithrombin as well as more potent approximation phenomena. Thus, the somewhat different conclusions about reaction mechanism outlined above may also reflect the use of different heparin preparations. It should also be pointed out that in the case of factor XI_a, high molecular weight kininogen appears to function as an adapter molecule to augment approximation phenomena (see above). These approximation events with regard to thrombin and factor IX_a may be of great significance with respect to anticoagulantly active heparan sulfates of the endothelium of blood vessels.

Throughout the studies cited above, Jordan and co-workers (1980b) noted that trace amounts of heparin catalyze the interaction of large quantities of hemostatic enzyme and AT. In addition, these investigators observed that neutralization of hemostatic enzyme by the heparin-AT complex results in the release of the polysaccharide from the protease inhibitor on a one-to-one molar basis (Jordan *et al.,* 1980b). Furthermore, it was also evident that the binding of heparin to the hemostatic enzyme-AT complex is 100- to 1000-fold weaker than the interaction of polysaccharide with free protease inhibitor (Jordan *et al.,* 1980b). These data indicate that heparin is able to function as a catalyst in the above interactions and to initiate multiple rounds of protease-protease inhibitor complex formation (see Figure 3.2).

Heparin is the only complex carbohydrate that is capable of binding to AT, activating the protease inhibitor, and accelerating the neutralization of hemostatic enzymes. However, the nature of the critical groups on the polysaccharide that are responsible for this unique property was completely enigmatic until recently. During the past decade, biochemical studies of the detailed structure-function relationships of heparin have resolved much of this mystery. Lam and co-workers (1976) showed that only a small fraction of commercial polysaccharide is able to bind to AT but is responsible for virtually all of the anticoagulant activity of the complex carbohydrate. Thus, it appeared likely that the failure of previous studies to uncover any relationship between heparin structure and anticoagulant activity was due to the employment of polysaccharide preparations that contain large amounts of complex carbohydrates with monosaccharide sequences that are inappropriate for interacting with AT. These findings were rapidly confirmed by Hook and associates (1976), as well as Andersson and colleagues (1976), and kindled intense interest in defining the critical regions on heparin that are involved in its unique anticoagulant function. To accomplish this goal, Oosta and co-workers (1981) randomly cleaved anticoagulantly active heparin with chemical techniques and isolated polysaccharide fragments of varying size that bind tightly to the protease inhibitor. These data revealed that oligosaccharides of eight or more monosaccharide units accelerate factor X_a-AT interactions but do not catalyze the rates of neutralization of other hemostatic enzymes by the protease inhibitor. This region of the polysaccharide, which is required for enhancing the interactions of factor X_a with AT, will be termed Domain 1 (see below). However, larger oligosaccharides of approximately 16 or more residues accelerate thrombin-AT as well as factor X_a-AT interactions. Kinetic examination of these species (Oosta *et al.*, 1981) suggests that oligosaccharides of approximately 16 residues display the capacity to neutralize thrombin rapidly by directly activating AT, whereas larger oligosaccharides contain an additional structural element(s) required for approximating free enzyme with protease inhibitor. These two regions of the heparin molecule that are required for enhancing the interactions of thrombin with AT have been termed Domains 2 and 3 (see below). These latter segments of the polysaccharide are also needed to accelerate factor IX_a-AT as well as factor XI_a-AT (Oosta *et al.*, 1981). The above results strongly suggest that heparin contains several discrete structural domains that are responsible for its ability to complex with AT and modulate the biologic activities of the protease inhibitor.

Rosenberg and colleagues (Rosenberg *et al.*, 1978; Rosenberg and Lam, 1979) utilized highly active heparin as well as fragments of the polysaccharide to conduct structural studies of Domain 1. These investigators revealed that this region contains a critical tetrasaccharide sequence composed of a nonsulfated iduronic acid residue on the nonreducing end, followed by an *N*-acetylglucosamine 6-*O*-sulfate group, a glucuronic acid moiety, and an *N*-sulfated/*O*-sulfated glucosamine residue on the reducing end of the oligosaccharide. Anticoagulantly inactive heparin does not contain this unique structure and consequently does not bind the protease inhibitor (Rosenberg *et al.*, 1978; Rosenberg and Lam, 1979). Leder (1980) isolated a sulfatase that removes this moiety from the 3-*O* position of glucosamine and postulated that this substituent could be a critical functional group within the heparin molecule. Lindahl and co-workers (1979) confirmed this supposition by showing with the above enzyme that a 3-*O*-sulfate substituent exists on the reducing-end glucosamine residue of the above tetrasaccharide. These observations were substantiated by Choay and colleagues who synthesized a pentasaccharide with anticoagulant activity (Choay *et al.*, 1980). The various investigations outlined above have also demonstrated that an octasaccharide that contains the unique tetrasaccharide region constitutes Domain 1 of the heparin molecule (Figure 3.4) (Choay *et al.*, 1983; Atha *et al.*, 1984a).

Direct studies of the interaction of the above octasaccharide with the protease inhibitor reveal that it is responsible for about 8.7 kcal/mol to 10.2 kcal/mol of binding energy (Atha *et al.*, 1984a; Atha *et al.*, 1985). The contributions of individual residues of Domain 1 have been evaluated by comparing the avidity of synthetic oligosaccharides as well as deaminative and enzyme cleavage fragments of the natural octasaccharide for AT. Based on these data, the relative importance of individual residues has been estimated and is provided at the bottom of Figure 4 (Lindahl *et al.*, 1983; Atha *et al.*, 1984a; Atha *et al.*, 1984b; Atha *et al.*, 1985).

The contributions of the nonreducing-end iduronic acid, residue 1, and the glucuronic acid, residue 3, to the binding energy of the octasaccharide are minimal. However, it should be noted that sulfation of the glucuronic acid residue never occurs within the natural oligosaccharide although it has been claimed that sulfated iduronic acid may occasionally be found at the nonreducing-end position (Loganathan *et al.,* 1990). The contributions of the 6-*O*-sulfate group of *N*-acetylglucosamine (residue 2) and the 3-*O*-sulfate group of the *N*-sulfated, 6-*O*-sulfated glucosamine (residue 4) to the binding energy of the octasaccharide are each about 4 kcal/mol to 5 kcal/mol. However, the 3-*O*-sulfate group of residue 4 is functionally linked to the 6-*O*-sulfate group of residue 2, such that both of these moieties appear to be required for the binding of octasaccharide to the protease inhibitor. This hypothesis is suggested by noting that the loss of either the 6-*O*-sulfate group of residue 2 or the 3-*O*-sulfate group of residue 4 leads to the same 4-kcal/mol to 5-kcal/mol loss in binding energy. It should be emphasized that the lack of an apparent contribution by residues 1 and 3 to the interaction of the octasaccharide with antithrombin does not indicate that these moieties are without importance. It is likely that these two uronic acid units function as critical spacers in orientating the 6-*O* sulfate group of residue 2 and the 3-*O*-sulfate group of residue 4 and that sulfation of, at least, the glucuronic acid residue would interfere with the binding of this region of the oligosaccharide to antithrombin. The contributions of the 2-*O*-sulfated iduronic acid (residue 5) and the *N*-sulfate group of the glucosamine 6-*O*-sulfate (residue 6) to the binding of octasaccharide to antithrombin is approximately 1.7 kcal/mol and 2.8 kcal/mol, respectively, whereas that of residues 7 and 8 is only about 0.6 kcal/mol.

The data presented above clearly indicate that the structure of Domain 1 of the heparin molecule has been almost completely defined. Unfortunately, the state of our knowledge about the structure of Domains 2 and 3 is quite primitive. Indeed, little is currently known about the presence of critical groups within these regions except that they may also contain minimally sulfated uronic acid moieties (Stone, 1985).

Growing knowledge of the structure of the various domains of anticoagulantly active heparin prompted investigators to attempt to define how these regions of the polysaccharide accelerate the function of AT. The initial studies of Einarsson and Andersson (1977), Nordenman and Bjork (1978), Olson and co-workers (1981) and Villanueva and Danishefsky (1977) revealed that the binding of heparin to AT induced a conformational transition within the protease inhibitor. There is a rapid alteration in the positioning of the exposed tryptophan and tyrosine groups, (Einarsson and Andersson, 1977; Villanueva and Danishefsky, 1977; Nordenman and Bjork, 1978; Olson *et al.,* 1981) whereas buried tryptophan residues undergo a subsequent slow change in location (Olson *et al.,* 1981). Stone and colleagues (1982) subsequently showed that most of the conformational alterations described above are induced by the interactions of Domain 1 with the protease inhibitor.

How can the binding of Domain 1 to AT lead to conformational changes within AT, as well as acceleration of factor X_a-protease inhibitor interactions? Rosenberg and Damus (1973) initially demonstrated that heparin binds to AT via a limited number of lysyl residues. Subsequent experimental data revealed that positively charged lysine and arginine residues present within residues 28-53 as well as residues 107–156 of AT may serve as binding sites for heparin (see previous discussion). Using a computer generated model of AT based upon the crystal structure of reactive site cleaved alpha 1-antitrypsin, Huber and Carrell (1989) suggest that certain critical positively charged sites in residues 28–53 align with other positively charged sites in residues 114–156 to form a long stretch of positive moieties which could bind sulfate groups of heparin. It appears that lysine and arginine residues within the helical region from 107–150 might interact with the 6-O-sulfate of residue 2, the N-sulfate of residue 4, the O-sulfate of residue 5 and the N-sulfate of residue 6 of the octasaccharide. Atha and co-workers (1987) provide evidence that the first and third of these sulfate groups are important for binding Domain 1 to AT but also reveal that the 3-O-sulfate group of residue 4 is critical for complex formation. It is possible that the 3-O-sulfate group of residue 4 interacts with residues 28–53 and thereby induces a conformational transition of the protease inhibitor, as evidenced by the spectral alteration in the protease inhibitor. This hypothesis is suggested by the lack of a fluorescence enhancement when Domain 1 does not contain a 3-O-sulfate group (Atha *et al.*, 1987). It is also consistent with the investigations of Blackburn and Sibley (1980) and Karp and associates (1984) in which modification of Trp-49 near the N-terminal end of AT blocks the heparin-enhanced inhibition of factor X_a, and would also explain the fluorescence transfer studies of Pecon and Blackburn (Pecon and Blackburn, 1984), which indicate that 1–2 lysines such as Lys-28, Lys-29, and/or Lys-53 located near Trp-49, are essential for polysaccharide binding. If such is the case, the interactions of the 6-O-sulfate group of residue 2 and 3-O-sulfate group of residue 4 with separate domains on AT could induce a conformational change in the protease inhibitor involving the region about Trp-49 that would functionally link the binding of these two residues. This transition could also lead to the repositioning of the Arg-393-Ser-394 locale or the formation of a secondary enzyme complexing site that is ultimately responsible for the acceleration of factor X_a neutralization.

Domain 2 of the heparin molecule appears to interact with a separate area of AT and triggers a conformational transition of the protease inhibitor distinct from that induced by Domain 1 of the polysaccharide. Stone and associates (1982) employed ultraviolet circular dichroism spectroscopy to examine the interaction of AT with oligosaccharides that ranged from approximately 8 to 18 monosaccharide. The first type of heparin induced conformation was apparent when oligosaccharides of 8 to 14 residues interact with AT and was identical to Domain 1-AT interactions outlined above. The second type of heparin-induced conformation was apparent when oligosaccharides of approximately 18 or more monosaccharide units bound to the protease inhibitor. The circular dichroism spectra of these interaction products, when compared to those of Domain 1-protease inhibitor complexes, are similar except for distinct chiral alterations that may be due to conformational changes about a disulfide bridge(s). It should be noted that these additional transitions are strongly correlated with the binding of Domain 2 of the polysaccharide to AT. Indeed, the extension of the approximately 14-monomer oligosaccharide by 4 monosaccharide units permits this species to accelerate thrombin-AT interactions as well as to induce the second type of spectral transition. These observations provide direct experimental evidence that Domain 2 of the heparin molecule may exert its effect by binding to an area of AT somewhat distinct from that of Domain 1 and by inducing an additional set of conformational changes within the protease inhibitor that are critical for the acceleration of thrombin-AT interactions. It is possible that Domain 2 of the heparin molecule binds to positively charged residues such as Lys 139 and/or Arg 145 which might induce the additional conformation transition monitored above. In this regard, we note that antibody directed against residues 138–145 is able to bind to AT and mimic the action of heparin in accelerating inhibition of thrombin (Smith *et al.*, 1990). This result

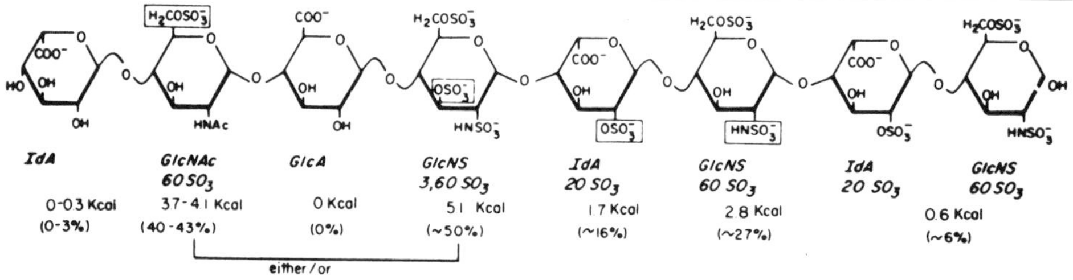

Figure 3.4 Structure of domain 1 of anticoagulantly active heparin. The relative importance of the various residues is provided with regard to binding to antithrombin.

suggests that the above antibody may be triggering the second conformational transition required for rapid neutralization of thrombin. Alternately, Domain 2 of heparin might interact with other positively charged residues within the reactive site loop (Cys 239-Cys 422) and play a similar role. These interactions could either reposition the Arg 393-Ser 394 locale or trigger the formation of a secondary binding site such that thrombin, factor IX_a, and factor XI_a can complex more quickly with the protease inhibitor. The investigations of Evans *et al.,* (1992) have confirmed the importance of Domain 2, but suggest that the function of this region of heparin molecule could be to neutralize positive charges on AT which suppress the rate of interaction with thrombin.

In summary, Domain 1 of the heparin molecule appears to bind to a discrete region of AT that induces a conformational transition of the protease inhibitor required for accelerating factor X_a-AT interactions. Furthermore, Domains 1 and 2 of the heparin molecule interact with separate areas of AT that trigger a second conformational alteration/charge neutralization of the protease inhibitor needed for enhancing the rate of neutralization of factor IX_a, factor XI_a, and thrombin by AT. As outlined above, this latter conclusion is disputed by some investigators. It is also certain that Domain 3 of the heparin molecule aids in the approximation of certain of the hemostatic enzymes during interactions with the protease inhibitor (see above; Figure 3.4). Recent data would suggest that Lys 174 and Lys 252 of the B chain of thrombin may serve as important sites for interaction of enzyme with heparin bound to protease inhibitor (Church *et al.,* 1989).

Heparin and heparan sulfate are also able to express their anticoagulant action via a second plasma protease inhibitor termed heparin co-factor II. This protein was first identified by Briginshaw and Shanberge (1974) and was subsequently isolated in homogeneous form by Tollefsen and co-workers (1981). The primary amino acid structure of heparin cofactor II is quite distinct from that of AT, including a reactive site with a leucine-x bond (Church *et al.,* 1985). The protease inhibitor also possesses an affinity for heparin/heparan sulfate that is significantly less than that of AT (Tollefsen and Blank, 1981). However, the rate of thrombin neutralization by heparin cofactor II approaches that of AT at saturating levels of polysaccharide (Tollefsen and Blank, 1981). It is of interest that the specificity of heparin cofactor II is narrowly restricted to thrombin and that other polysaccharides, especially dermatan sulfate, are able to accelerate dramatically the action of this protease inhibitor. Indeed, it appears likely that the observed anticoagulant effects of polysaccharides other than heparin/heparan sulfate are primarily due to interactions with heparin cofactor II (Ofosu *et al.,* 1984). This protease inhibitor probably plays a minimal role when heparin is utilized clinically as an anticoagulant. Tollefsen and co-workers (1981) have suggested that heparin cofactor II functions as an inhibitor of thrombin after its activation by dermatan sulfate present within the vessel wall.

Dermatan sulfate binds to heparin cofactor II via a unique hexasaccharide sequence composed of three disulfated disaccharides with iduronic acid 2-*O*-sulfate alternating with *N*-acetyl galactosamine 4-*O*-sulfate (Maimone and Tollefsen, 1990). Heparin/heparan sulfate and dermatan sulfate interact with two overlapping, but distinct sets, of positively charged residues on the protease inhibitor (Blinder *et al.*, 1989; Blinder and Tollefsen, 1990; Whinna *et al.*, 1991). Heparin cofactor II contains an N-terminal acidic domain which is homologous to a region on hirudin involved in ionic and hydrophobic interactions with thrombin (Hortin *et al.*, 1989; Van Deerlin and Tollefsen, 1991). Current data suggest that binding of polysaccharide to heparin cofactor II accelerates neutralization of thrombin by inducing the acidic domain of the protease inhibitor to complex with enzyme as well as functioning in approximating heparin cofactor II to thrombin. Indeed, dermatan sulfate dependent liberation of the acidic domain is responsible for a 50- to 100-fold acceleration of thrombin neutralization, whereas the approximation of enzyme to protease inhibitor by polysaccharide augments the above reaction rate by an additional 50- to 100-fold. Thus, polysaccharide dependent acceleration of thrombin-heparin cofactor II interactions exhibit both conformational as well as approximation effects similar to that observed with heparin/heparan sulfate and AT.

The Synthesis of Anticoagulantly Active Heparan Sulfate Proteoglycans by Endothelial Cells

The preceding sections outline the detailed structure-function relationships of anticoagulantly active heparin and directed attention to whether this polysaccharide could serve as a physiologic regulator of the hemostatic mechanism. Until recently, mast cells were thought to be the sole site of synthesis of anticoagulantly active polysaccharide (Galli *et al.*, 1984). These specialized cells are located beneath the endothelium, possess intracellular granules which contain heparin, and do not continuously discharge polysaccharide under *in vivo* conditions. Therefore, one must postulate a complex set of events in which mast cell release of heparin would be linked to the activity of the hemostatic mechanism and the released polysaccharide would eventually come in contact with blood. This unlikely scenario led Damus and co-workers (Damus *et al.*, 1973) to suggest that endothelial cells might synthesize heparan sulfate proteoglycans (HSPG) which are endowed with the critical structures required to bind AT and activate protease inhibitor.

The early investigations of Thein and associates (1977) and Thomas and colleagues (1979) showed that heparan sulfate present in the aorta possesses trace amounts of anticoagulant activity. However, it was possible that the anticoagulant activity might be due either to contamination with mast cell heparin or the nonspecific inhibitory effects of a highly charged polysaccharide. Subsequently, Marcum and Rosenberg (1984) purified heparan sulfate from aortae and calf cerebral microvessels by standard chromatographic techniques. These polysaccharides were then affinity fractionated by employing AT bound to a matrix which revealed the presence of two distinct subpopulations of components. The aortic heparan sulfate species that complexed with AT exhibited an enhancement in the specific thrombin inhibitory and factor X_a inhibitory activities of 80-fold and

120-fold, respectively. This subpopulation constitutes approximately 0.3% of the mass of the complex carbohydrate and accounts for approximately 60% of the anticoagulant activity of the starting material. The cerebral microvascular heparan sulfate species that interact avidly with protease inhibitor exhibited an augmentation in the specific thrombin inhibitory and factor X_a inhibitory activities of 13-fold and 15-fold, respectively. This subpopulation constitutes approximately 4.2% of the chemical mass of the complex carbohydrate and is responsible for approximately 75% of the anticoagulant activity of the starting material. These data indicate that anticoagulantly active heparan sulfate molecules exist within the vasculature and express their biologic activities by means of interactions with AT.

The presence of endothelial cells within the above aortic and cerebral microvascular preparations was confirmed by visualization of surface-bound von Willebrand factor protein. However, additional examination of these products revealed the existence of a small population of metachromically staining granulated cells (<1% of the total nucleated cells) that resembled mast cells. Further study of these tissue samples by histamine radioisotopic assay confirmed the presence of these cells. Therefore, it was possible that some of the anticoagulantly active polysaccharide found within blood vessel wall preparations is synthesized by mast cells (Marcum and Rosenberg, 1984). In an attempt to define the cellular source of anticoagulantly active heparan sulfate molecules, Marcum and co-workers (1983) isolated retinal microvessels, which are believed to be free of mast cells by previously reported techniques (Meezan *et al.,* 1974). These preparations consisted of fragments of small blood vessels, capillaries, and single endothelial cells with little nonvascular contamination. The presence of endothelial cells was established with antisera directed against von Willebrand factor protein. The absence of mast cells was confirmed by light microscopic examination (Ellison *et al.,* 1978) as well as by the lack of histamine. The heparan sulfate components were then isolated from the above preparations, and significant levels of AT accelerating activity were detected (Marcum *et al.,* 1983). The above observations suggest that endothelial cells synthesize heparan sulfate proteoglycans with anticoagulant activity (HSPG^{act}).

To prove unequivocally that endothelial cells are able to produce HSPG^{act}, Marcum and associates (Marcum and Rosenberg, 1985) isolated cloned microvascular endothelial cells from the rat epididymal fat pad. The polysaccharides were extracted from the above cells and assayed for AT accelerating activity. The data showed that these cells produced about 4×10^{-4} USP units of heparinlike activity per 10^6 cells, which could be completely eliminated with purified *Flavobacterium* heparinase. This estimate of heparan sulfate components would correspond to about 500,000 AT binding sites per endothelial cell. In addition, virtually all of these macromolecules could be harvested by a brief exposure to dilute trypsin, which suggests that these components are located on the surface of these endothelial cells. Furthermore, these complex carbohydrates were metabolically radiolabeled with ^{35}S, harvested by a brief trypsinization, affinity fractionated with AT, and then examined with respect to oligosaccharide structure. The biochemical data indicate that the critical tetrasaccharide present in the anticoagulantly active commercial heparin (see above) is also found within these polysaccharides of endothelial cell origin (Marcum and Rosenberg, 1985). Studies of this type have also been conducted with cloned bovine aortic endothelial cells with virtually identical results except that the level of anticoagulantly active heparan sulfate species present would correspond to about 50,000 AT binding sites per endothelial cell. This latter estimate of surface-bound anticoagulantly active polysaccharide is in excellent agreement with data generated by characterizing the interactions of AT with bovine aortic tissue sections (Stern *et al.,* 1985).

The endothelial cell core proteins that are endowed with anticoagulantly active heparan sulfate chains have only recently been characterized. Kojima and associates isolated intact HSPG from rat microvascular endothelial cells using a combination of ion exchange chromatography, affinity fractionation with AT, and gel filtration in denaturating solvents (Kojima *et al.,* 1992a). The HSPG^{act} which binds to AT constitute approximately 5% of total HSPG and are endowed almost entirely with anticoagulantly active heparan sulfate chains. The anticoagulantly inactive heparan sulfate proteoglycans (HSPG^{inact}) which do not interact with protease inhibitor represent about 95% of total HSPG and bear anticoagulantly inactive heparan sulfate chains. The two types of carbohydrate chains exhibit the same molecular size of about 25–30 Kd with the anticoagulantly active carbohydrate chains possessing multiple AT binding sites. The core proteins of HSPG^{act} and HSPG^{inact} were isolated after treatment with *Flavobacterium* heparitinase and purification by ion exchange chromatography. The molecular sizes of the core proteins were established by SDS gel electrophoresis, and their primary structures were examined by cleavage with proteolytic enzymes as well as separation by reverse phase HPLC. The results show that HSPG^{act} and HSPG^{inact} core proteins contain the same two major components with molecular sizes of 50 Kd and 30 Kd, respectively, and possess virtually identical primary structures as judged by the peptide mapping procedures.

The primary sequences of internal peptides derived from HSPG^{inact} core proteins were utilized to molecularly clone two cDNAs from a microvascular endothelial cell library. The first cDNA constitutes a previously unidentified species, termed ryudocan, whereas the second cDNA represents the rat homolog of syndecan. The latter species is a known HSPG which was originally thought to be limited in its distribution to epithelial cells (Kojima *et al.,* 1992b). The two cDNAs encode integral membrane proteins of 202 amino acids (ryudocan) and 313 amino acids (syndecan), respectively, which have extraordinarily homologous transmembrane and intracellular domains but very distinct extracellular regions. Ryudocan exhibits three potential glycosaminoglycan attachment sites within the extracellular domain, whereas syndecan has five potential glycosaminoglycan attachment sites within the same region. Both species are expressed at high levels (0.1% to 0.5% of total mRNA) in primary endothelial cells and primary smooth muscle cells as well as primary fibroblasts. The possibility that slightly different core proteins direct the synthesis of HSPG^{act} and HSPG^{inact} was excluded by stably expressing epitope tagged ryudocan in cells which synthesize anticoagulantly active and anticoagulantly inactive heparan sulfate chains, recovering the proteoglycan with specific antibody against the epitope, and demonstrating that both types of chains are present (Shworak *et al.,* 1994). These two core proteins constitute major integral membrane components which bear anticoagulatively active heparan sulfate chains synthesized by endothelial cells. Latter studies revealed that fibroglycan, glypican, and perlican can also bear HSPG^{act} and HSPG^{inact} (Mertens *et al.,* 1992).

The availability of expression vectors coupled to epitope tagged core protein cDNAs allowed a more detailed exploration of the intracellular biosynthetic pathway by which HSPG^{act} is synthesized (Shworak *et al.,* 1994). To this end, ryudocan was stably expressed at varying levels in L cells and human endothelial cells which are able to generate both HSPG[act] and HSPG[inact]. It was noted in both cell types that production of HSPG[inact] increased linearly as a function of expression of epitope tagged ryudocan which indicates that the overall synthesis of glycosaminoglycan is limited by the availability of core protein and not biosynthetic enzymes. Indeed, the detailed examination of the structure of HS[inact] at high levels of core protein expression failed to reveal any changes in chain size or type of sulfation or epimerization. It was also observed in both cell types that generation of HSPG[act] decreased as a function of expression of ryudocan which suggests that the production of this particular glycosaminoglycan is limited by factors other than core protein. Indeed, the detailed study of the structure of HS[act] at high levels of core protein expression failed to show any alterations in chain size or type of sulfation or epimerization. This discordant relationship is a general property of the biosynthetic machinery since in both cell types HS[act] production was reduced to an equal extent on protein cores of either exogenous (epitope tagged ryudocan) or endogenous origins. The suppression of HS[act] was also observed with a secreted form of the core protein lacking transmembrane and cytoplasmic domains or by a glycosaminoglycan acceptor site mutated form of the core protein which cannot be glycanated.

These above results strongly suggest that elevated intracellular levels of core protein saturate the capacity of critical components of the HS[act] biosynthetic machinery. The critical components are not members of the common set of biosynthetic enzymes involved in the production of HS[act] and HS[inact] since no compositional changes were observed in either glycosaminoglycan during overexpression of core protein. Based upon the above data, it appears likely that increased intracellular levels of ryudocan probably act by saturating the capacity of regulatory components which coordinate the action of the common set of biosynthetic enzymes that carry out the appropriate sequence of epimerization/sulfation reactions required to generate HS[act]. For example, these regulatory components might position the 6-*O*-sulfotransferase and the 3-*O*-sulfotransferase so that neighboring glucosamine residues are modified and thereby favor production of HS[act]. Of course, no change would be expected in the overall numbers of 6-*O*- or 3-*O*-sulfated disaccharides. These regulatory components might constitute separate proteins or specific modifications of biosynthetic enzymes or post-translational alterations of core proteins which facilitate interactions between a specific subset of biosynthetic enzymes. The potential complexity of the coordination mechanism is suggested by the absolute decrease in the generation of HS[act] as a function of core protein expression. The kinetics of this response suggests that the coordination mechanism is not characterized by a single limiting component, but requires the action of multiple regulatory components and/or the production of glycosaminoglycan sequences that inhibit synthesis of the AT binding domain. The presence of these regulatory components has also been demonstrated by the isolation of mutant L cell clones which generate greatly decreased amounts of HSPG[act], but normal levels of HSPG[inact], without any change in the biochemical structure of the glycosaminoglycans (Colliec-Jouault *et al.*, 1994).

We should emphasize the potential importance of the above observations with regard to the overall regulation of the heparan sulfate-AT pathway. The cultured endothelial cells appear to be generating maximum amounts of HSPG[act] which are limited by the existing levels of specific regulatory factors. If a similar situation exists under *in vivo* conditions, then the regulatory factors are likely to ultimately determine the relative importance of the heparan sulfate-AT pathway to the overall natural anticoagulant mechanisms of the

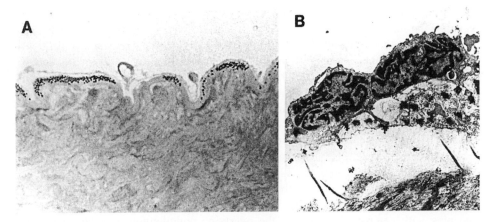

Figure 3.5 Light and electron micrographs as well as light and EM level autoradiographs of perfused normal and damaged rat aorta. (A) Light microscopic autoradiograph of rat aorta after perfusion with ^{125}I-AT. The intense labeling is noted in the basement membrane beneath the endothelial cells (arrows). Bar, μm. (B) EM level autoradiograph of rat aorta after perfusion with ^{125}I-AT. The labeling is clearly evident beneath the endothelial cells. Bar, 1.0 μm

blood vessel wall. Furthermore, the up or down regulation of the heparan sulfate-AT pathway by biologic mediators is likely to function by altering the properties of these regulatory components.

The Physiologic Role of Anticoagulantly Active Heparan Sulfate Proteoglycans of the Blood Vessel Wall

Given the above results, it was important to pinpoint the actual location of HSPG^{act}. These investigations were carried out by de Agostini and coworkers who perfused normal rat aorta for short periods of time with ^{125}I-AT and then determined the location of labelled protease inhibitor (de Agostini *et al.*, 1990). It is readily apparent that ^{125}I-AT is bound to the aortic subendothelium (Figure 3.5A). This finding is particularly evident with light microscopy which shows that only small quantities of protease inhibitor interact with the luminal side of the endothelium or are found within smooth muscle cells or connective tissue. This localization of AT binding is more clearly defined at the electron microscopic level which demonstrates that labelled protease inhibitor is present beneath the endothelial cells (Figure 3.5B). Quantitation of the above data reveal that about 1% of the bound ^{125}I-AT is associated with the luminal surface of the endothelium. The labelled protease inhibitor is also noted to bind to regions around capillaries especially in the subendothelium associated with the basal lamina/basement membrane. The above experiments were repeated by perfusing the aorta with ^{125}I-bovine serum albumin which produced no detectable labelling in any locale. This latter observation demonstrates that binding of ^{125}I-AT within the aorta is not due to non-specific interactions or trapping of labelled protease inhibitor. To ensure that ^{125}I-AT specifically interacts with anticoagulantly active heparan sulfate chains, the vasculature was infused with *Flavobacterium* heparinase before perfusion with labelled protease inhibitor. This treatment leaves the endothelial cell layer intact but effectively eliminates any binding of ^{125}I-AT to all regions including the subendothelium.

These data suggest that endothelial cells produce HSPG^{act} which are initially positioned within cell membranes, proteoglycans are liberated intact or cleaved by plasmalemmal proteases, and free HSPG^{act} then accumulate predominantly in basement membranes. This conclusion is consistent with the known synthesis of HSPG^{act} by cultured endothelial cells and HSPG^{inact} by cultured smooth muscle cells as well as the previous isolation of HSPG^{act} from the aortic intima and HSPG^{inact} from aortic media (Marcum and Rosenberg, 1984). It is likely that coagulation system activity could be regulated in two separate ways by blood vessel wall HSPG^{act}. On the one hand, the small amounts of luminal HSPG^{act} could be critically placed to bind AT, accelerate the action of the protease inhibitor, and regulate hemostatic mechanism activity at the blood-vessel wall interface. The much larger quantities of abluminal HSPG^{act} could serve as a reservoir which could be brought into play with extensive damage to the overlying endothelium. On the other hand, HSPG^{act} which accumulates on the abluminal surface of the endothelial cells could also act to modulate the function of the coagulation cascade. Plasma AT should have relatively free access to this region as suggested by numerous studies which document the extraordinary permeability of the endothelial cell layer (Simionescu, 1983). Indeed, the presence of ^{125}I-AT bound to subendothelium after *ex vivo* perfusion indicates the ready accessibility of this area to protease inhibitor. This subendothelial concentration of HSPG^{act} would also explain kinetic tracer data which suggests that a significant amount of labelled protease inhibitor is located in a unique extravascular compartment (Carlson *et al.,* 1985). This interaction of coagulation enzymes with AT bound to subendothelium might constitute the heparan sulfate dependent acceleration of protease inhibitor action observed in animal models described below. This postulated interaction would imply that inhibition of coagulation enzymes is quite active within the subendothelial region and would expand our present notions of the critical biologic surfaces in contact with blood.

Marcum and associates confirmed the physiologic relevance of the above model by showing that intact blood vessels possess HSPG^{act} which accelerate blood AT function (Marcum *et al.,* 1984). To accomplish this goal, rat hindlimb preparations were perfused with purified thrombin at a constant level, and purified AT was infused at several different concentrations. The amount of thrombin-AT complex produced within the vasculature was determined by a specific radioimmunoassay for the interaction product. The rate of enzyme-inhibitor complex formation was enhanced as much as 19-fold in the animal with respect to the uncatalyzed amount of interaction product that might be expected to be generated without polysaccharide (Table 3.1). The AT accelerating activity detected in the hindlimb vasculature is due to HSPG^{act}. A physically homogeneous preparation of *Flavobacterium* heparinase that did not exhibit proteolytic or chondroitinase activities was recirculated through the hindlimb vasculature prior to perfusion of the hemostatic components. The amount of enzyme-inhibitor complex generated within the animal was reduced to uncatalyzed levels (Table 3.2). The location of HSPG^{act} within the hemicorpus preparation has also been investigated. Buffer was recirculated through the hindlimb preparation for extended periods, and the presence of HSPG^{act} was ascertained by quantitating the acceleration of thrombin-AT complex formation. Heparan sulfate components were not detected within the buffer, which indicates that HSPG^{act} are tightly associated with the endothelium (Marcum *et al.,* 1984).

Table 3.1 Generation of thrombin-antithrombin complex during constant infusion of native or modified antithrombin through the rat hindlimb preparation

Antithrombin Infused (μM)	Thrombin-antithrombin complex (pmol/20 sec)*			Acceleration of Antithrombin action	
	Antithrombin			*Native*	*Modified*
	Native	*Modified*	*Uncatalyzed*		
0.03	0.26 ± 0.1 (n = 3)	ND† (n = 2)	0.014	18.6	
0.09	0.48 ± 0.12 (n = 6)	ND† (n= 5)	0.043	11.2	
0.18	0.94± 0.17 (n = 13)	0.22 ± 0.04 (n = 4)	0.086	10.9	2.6

* Mean ± SE, enzyme-inhibitor complex formation within the cannuli at antithrombin concentrations of 0.03 μM, 0.09 μM, and 0.18 μM were 0.154 ± 0.46 (n = 2), 0.26 ± 0.18 (n = 6), and 0.283 ± 0.59 (n = 5) pmol/20 sec, respectively. These values were subtracted from the original data to obtain the amount of complex generated within 20 seconds in the vasculature of the animal.
† ND, not detected.

Table 3.2 Generation of thrombin-antithrombin complex during constant infusion of antithrombin through the rat hindlimb preparation

Proteins perfused through hindlimb preparation	Thrombin-antithrombin complex* (pmol/20 sec)
Thrombin (5.4 nM) followed by native antithrombin (0.18 μM)	0.94 ± 0.17 (n = 13)
Thrombin (5.4 nM) + PF$_4$ (3 nM) followed by native antithrombin (0.18 μM)	0.080 ± 0.02 (n = 4)
Thrombin (5.4 nM) after treatment with purified heparinase followed by native antithrombin (0.18 μM)	0.074 ± 0.013 (n = 4)
Uncatalyzed amount	0.086

* Mean ± SE. See footnote to Table 41–2 for details.
PF$_4$, platelet factor 4.

To show that endothelial cell HSPG[act] function as expected, AT modified at Trp 49 was substituted for native protease inhibitor during studies employing the hindlimb perfusion. This change in components resulted in a reduction of thrombin-AT complex formation to uncatalyzed levels (see Table 3.2). These observations indicate that HSPG[act] potentiates thrombin-AT complex formation via a mechanism dependent on the same critical tryptophan residue that is required for heparin-dependent acceleration of the protease inhibitor (Marcum *et al.*, 1984). This conclusion is strengthened by the finding that native and modified AT are able to interact with thrombin at a virtually identical rate under conditions in which commercial heparin is absent. Furthermore, an enhancement of enzyme-inhibitor interactions due solely to binding of thrombin to endothelial sites was not observed, as suggested by Lollar and Owen (1980).

We wondered whether platelet factor 4 (PF$_4$) released from the alpha-granules of platelets could modulate the above acceleratory phenomena. Therefore, purified human PF$_4$ was added to an AT bolus prior to injection into the enzyme perfusion stream. The addition of PF$_4$ to AT was responsible for a decrease in enzyme-inhibitor complex formation to the uncatalyzed rate (see Table 3.2). This platelet peptide has been shown to interfere with binding of heparin molecules to AT, thereby inhibiting the acceleration of enzyme-inhibitor complex formation. These data suggest that PF$_4$, after expulsion from activated platelets, may play a role in thrombogenesis by neutralizing blood vessel wall HSPG[act] (Marcum *et al.,* 1984).

Marcum and associates (1985) have also conducted perfusion experiments similar to those outlined above with normal mice and litter mates who are genetically deficient in mast cells. These data show that both strains of mice exhibit an identical 20-fold acceleration of thrombin-AT interactions, which can be eliminated by the prior infusion of *Flavobacterium* heparinase or the use of AT modified at Trp 49. These latter findings strongly suggest that endothelial cell HSPG[act] are wholly responsible for the acceleration of AT action and that mast cell heparin plays little, if any, role in this phenomenon.

In summary, it appears probable that a small fraction of plasma AT is normally bound to HSPG[act] associated with endothelial cells of the blood vessel wall. As discussed above, it is unclear whether the functionally critical HSPG[act] is mainly present on the luminal surface of the blood vessel wall and/or within the subendothelial region. The above components, independent of location, would permit the protease inhibitor to be selectively activated at blood-surface interfaces, where enzymes of the intrinsic coagulation cascade are commonly generated. Thus, AT would be critically placed to neutralize these hemostatic enzymes and thereby protect natural surfaces against thrombus formation. Furthermore, the catalytic nature of anticoagulantly active heparan sulfate species would ensure the continual regeneration of the nonthrombogenic properties of the endothelial cell layer. Potential defects in the above mechanism in humans that might lead to arterial or venous thrombosis are considered in the last section of this chapter.

Functional Defects in Heparan Sulfate-AT Pathway

The experimental data outlined in previous sections suggest that the heparan sulfate-AT pathway serves as a major natural anticoagulant mechanism in humans and that inherited defects in this inhibitory process could lead to thrombotic complications. In 1965, Egeberg reported a Norwegian family whose members exhibited plasma AT concentrations that were 40–50% of normal values with an associated history of repeated thrombotic events. Additional kindreds were then described with similar clinical and laboratory abnormalities (Egeberg, 1965; Van der Meer *et al.,* 1973; Shapiro *et al.,* 1973; Marciniak *et al.,* 1974; Filip *et al.,* 1975; Gruenberg *et al.,* 1975; Carvalho and Ellman, 1976; Stathakis *et al.,* 1977; Gyde *et al.,* 1978; Johansson *et al.,* 1978; Mackie *et al.,* 1978; Matsuo *et al.,* 1979; Ambruso *et al.,* 1980; Beukes and Heyns, 1980; Boyer *et al.,* 1980; Pitney *et al.,* 1980; Scully *et al.,* 1981; Winter *et al.,* 1982). The above reports demonstrated that AT deficiency is inherited as an autosomal dominant trait with a frequency of about one in 2000 to 5000 (Rosenberg, 1975; Odegard and Abildgaard, 1978). Based on studies in the United Kingdom, the prevalence of AT deficiency in the general population is 0.2–0.4 percent (Meade *et al.,* 1990; Tait *et al.,* 1990). The majority of AT-deficient patients identified in these investigations did not report a personal or familial history of thrombosis and were noted to have a functional deficiency of the inhibitor (type II with a mutation at the heparin-binding site) (Tait *et al.,* 1992).

The published case histories of individuals with familial AT deficiency reveal that approximately 65 percent experience at least one thrombotic event during their lifetime (Thaler and Lechner, 1981). However, patients rarely report thrombotic episodes before the age of 10 years, and increasing numbers experience these phenomena as they reach the age of 50. The initial clinical manifestations occur spontaneously in about 42 percent of patients, but are related to pregnancy, delivery, oral contraceptive ingestion, surgery, or trauma in 58 percent of patients. The most common sites of disease are the deep veins of the leg and the mesenteric veins. Approximately 60 percent of individuals develop recurrent thrombotic episodes, and clinical signs of pulmonary embolism are evident in 40 percent.

Two major types of inherited AT deficiency have been delineated. The type I deficiency state is caused by decreased production of biologically normal protease inhibitor molecules (Scully *et al.*, 1981; Ambruso *et al.*, 1982). Therefore, the immunological and biological activity of plasma AT is reduced to the same extent. The molecular basis of this disorder is either a deletion of a large segment of the gene, or more commonly the occurrence of small deletions, insertions, or single base substitutions often generating a premature stop codon (Winter *et al.*, 1982; Prochownik *et al.*, 1983; Bock and Prochownik, 1987; Olds *et al.*, 1990b; Gandrille *et al.*, 1991; Grundy *et al.*, 1991; Olds *et al.*, 1991; Vidaud *et al.*, 1991). The type II AT deficiency state is caused by a specific molecular defect. Under these circumstances, the plasma levels of AT are greatly reduced as judged by biologic activity measurements but are normal as measured by immunologic determinations. Data obtained from small numbers of AT deficient cohorts that exhibit venous thromboembolism prior to the age of 40 years or recurrent venous thrombosis suggest that approximately equal numbers of patients have type I and types II defects (Harper *et al.*, 1991).

Sas reported the first family with a functional deficiency of AT (Sas *et al.*, 1974). Subsequently, other investigators have described additional affected cohorts which have been categorized on the basis of two different types of biologic assays (Bauer *et al.*, 1983). The first test employed is the heparin cofactor assay which measures the ability of heparin to bind to the inhibitor and catalyze neutralization of coagulation enzymes such as thrombin and factor X_a. The second test utilized is the progressive AT activity assay which measures the capacity of the inhibitor to neutralize the enzymatic activity of thrombin in the absence of heparin. The two functional assays have identified AT-deficient patients with reductions in heparin cofactor activity with or without a proportional decrease in progressive AT activity. The patients with reductions in heparin cofactor activity, but not progressive AT activity, have abnormalities at the heparin-binding site or in a region essential for the polysaccharide dependent conformational alteration. These individuals usually exhibit mutations at the amino terminal end of the molecule (Table 3.3). In one variant, the substitution of asparagine for isoleucine at residue 7 generates a new glycosylation site and the resultant protease inhibitor has reduced avidity for heparin (Brennan *et al.*, 1988). The patients with proportional reductions in heparin cofactor activity and progressive AT activity generally have mutations near the thrombin binding site at the carboxy terminal end of the molecule (Table 3.3). However, certain AT variants cannot be characterized by this approach since single amino acid substitutions can affect both functional domains of the molecule. This is illustrated by a mutation in which arginine is replaced by histidine at residue 393 (Table 3.3). The reactive site mutation markedly decreases the ability of the protein to inhibit thrombin but also leads to a conformational alteration such that the abnormal molecule has increased heparin affinity. In a similar manner, the replacement of a proline by leucine at residue 429 leads to a molecular defect that affects both the heparin and thrombin binding sites (Table 3.3).

Table 3.3 Point Mutations in Antithrombin III

City or Region of Propositus	Substitution	Effect of Mutation
Rouen 3[1]	Ile 7 — Asn	Defective heparin binding, new carbohydrate attachment site
Rouen 4[2]	Arg 24 — Cys	Defective heparin binding
Basel[3], Clichy[4], Dublin II[5], Franconville[6]	Pro — 41 Leu	Defective heparin binding
Toyama[7], Tours[8], Alger[9], Paris 1[10], Paris 2[10], Barcelona 2[11], Kumamoto[12], Padua 2[13], Amiens[14]	Arg 47 — Cys	Defective heparin binding
Rouen 1[5], Padua 1[15], Bligny[16]	Arg 47 — His	Defective heparin binding
Rouen 2[17]	Arg 47 — Ser	Defective heparin binding
Budapest 3[18]	Leu 99 — Phe	Defective heparin binding
Geneva[19]	Arg 129 — Gin	Defective heparin binding
Hamilton[20], Glasgow-II[21]	Ala 382 — Thr	Defective serine protease inhibition
Charleville[10], Cambridge 1[22], Vicenza[23], Sudbury[24]	Ala 384 — Pro	Defective serine protease inhibition
Cambridge 2[25]	Ala 384 — Ser	Defective serine protease inhibition
Stockholm[26]	Gly 392 — Asp	Defective serine protease inhibition
Glasgow[27,28], Sheffield[29], Chicago[30], Avranches[10]	Arg 393 — His	Defective serine protease inhibition
Northwick Park[27], Milano 1[36], Frankfurt 1[33]	Arg 393 — Cys	Defective serine protease inhibition
Pescara[33]	Arg 393 — Pro	Defective serine protease inhibition
Denver[34], Milano 2[35]	Arg 394 — Ser	Defective serine protease inhibition
Oslo[36]	Ala 404 — Thr	These mutations result in the
Kyoto[37]	Arg 406 — Met	presence of trace amounts of the
Utah[25]	Pro 407 — Leu	abnormal antithrombin III in patient's plasma
Budapest[38]	Pro 429 — Leu	Mutation produces altered conformation of antithrombin III resulting in abnormal heparin binding and reduced thrombin inhibitory activity

References: [1] Brennan *et al.*, 1988; [2] Borg *et al.*, 1990; [3] Chang and Tran, 1986; [4] Molho-Sabatier *et al.*, 1989; [5] Daly *et al.*, 1989; [6] de Roux *et al.*, 1990; [7] Koide *et al.*, 1984; [8] Duchange *et al.*, 1987; [9] Brunel *et al.*, 1987; [10] Mohlo-Sabatier *et al.*, 1989; [11] Owen *et al.*, 1989; [12] Ueyama *et al.*, 1990; [13] Aiach *et al.*, 1987; [14] Roussel *et al.*, 1991; [15] Caso *et al.*, 1990; [16] Wolf *et al.*, 1990; [17] Borg *et al.*, 1988; [18] Sambrano *et al.*, 1986; [19] Stephens *et al.*, 1987; [20] Devraj-Klzuk *et al.*, 1988; [21] Ireland *et al.*, 1991; [22] Perry *et al.*, 1989; [23] Caso *et al.*, 1991; [24] Cosgriff *et al.*, 1983; [25] Bock *et al.*, 1988; [26] Blajchman *et al.*, 1992; [27] Erdjument *et al.*, 1988b; [28] Owen *et al.*, 1988; [29] Lane *et al.*, 1989a; [30] Erdjument *et al.*, 1989; [31] Erdjument *et al.*, 1988a; [32] Bock *et al.*, 1985; [33] Lane *et al.*, 1989b; [34] Stephens *et al.*, 1987; [35] Olds *et al.*, 1989; [36] Bock *et al.*, 1989; [37] McDonald *et al.*, 1982; [38] Olds *et al.*, 1992.

The clinical history of thrombosis in type II patients with defects in heparin cofactor activity, but not progressive AT function, is particularly interesting with regard to the physiology of protease inhibitor action (Finazzi *et al.*, 1987). It has been noted that heterozygous individuals with a 50% reduction in plasma heparin cofactor activity, but normal progressive AT activity, have infrequent thrombotic episodes (Sakuragawa *et al.*, 1983; Chasse *et al.*, 1984; Fischer *et al.*, 1986; Finazzi *et al.*, 1987; Borg *et al.*, 1988; Daly *et al.*, 1989; Okajima *et al.*, 1989). These individuals are brought to clinical attention when they enter consanguinious unions and produce homozygous children who develop severe venous and/or arterial thrombosis (Sakuragawa *et al.*, 1983; Boyer *et al.*, 1986; Fischer *et al.*, 1986; Okajima *et al.*, 1989). Thus, individuals with a plasma heparin cofactor level of less than 10 percent and a virtually normal plasma progressive AT activity exhibit profound arterial and venous thrombotic episodes early in life. These clinical observations emphasize the importance of the interaction of AT with blood vessel wall heparan sulfate proteoglycans.

It is interesting that congenital reductions in AT lead to the development of profound venous thromboembolic disease in humans. However, only occasional families with this malady experience multiple episodes of arterial thrombosis. It is not surprising that the initial manifestations of this diffuse systemic hypercoagulable state occur within the deep veins of the lower extremity since blood flow is relatively slow in this segment of the circulation. The reasons for the apparent absence of a dramatic increase in arterial thrombosis are less clear. The traditional view of this matter is that the development of thrombi in the systemic circulation requires excessive activation of coagulation proteins in conjunction with gross defects in platelet or endothelial cell function. A more speculative possibility is that inherited or acquired local abnormalities in the heparan sulfate proteoglycans of the vessel wall might result in the emergence of arterial thrombotic disorders. This situation should be expected since the appearance of such alterations would constitute a more profound localized defect than would be experienced with a 50% reduction in the systemic levels of antithrombin. Detailed studies are needed to resolve this critical issue.

It should be apparent that investigations of the heparan sulfate-AT pathway have entered a new and exciting stage. Great progress has been made over the past two decades. The primary structures of AT and heparin/heparan sulfate have been defined in large measure, and the molecular mechanism of their action has been partially unraveled. The structure of the gene that encodes AT has been elucidated, and the tissue-specific processes that regulate the synthesis of the protease inhibitor are under active investigation. The importance of the heparan sulfate-AT pathway as a natural anticoagulant mechanism has been revealed, and molecular defects in its function have been shown to lead to a hypercoagulable state in humans. We can look forward to the continuing application of biochemical, molecular, biological, and clinical investigative approaches to this area of research. These efforts should result in a more precise understanding of how the synthesis of blood vessel wall HSPG[act] is regulated, a more profound knowledge of the interrelationships between the heparan sulfate-AT pathway and other biologic macromolecules that alter its function, and a greater appreciation of the molecular defects in the above natural anticoagulant mechanism that lead to venous and arterial vascular disorders in humans.

References

Abildgaard, U. (1968). Highly purified antithrombin III with heparin cofactor activity prepared by disc gel electrophoresis. *Scand. J. Clin. Lab. Invest.,* **21**:89–91.

Aiach, M., Francois, D., Priollet, P., Capron, L., Roncato, M, Alhenc-Gelas, M. and Fiessinger, J. (1987). An abnormal antithrombin III (AT III) with low heparin affinity. *Br. J. Haematol.,* **66**:515–522.

Ambruso, D., Jacobson, L. and Hathaway, W. (1980). Inherited antithrombin III deficiency and cerebral thrombosis in a child. *Pediatrics,* **65**:125–131.

Ambruso, D., Leonard, B., Bies, R., Jacobson, L., Hathaway, W. and Reeve, E. (1982). Antithrombin III deficiency: decreased synthesis of a biochemically normal molecule. *Blood,* **60**:78–83.

Andersson, L.O., Barrowcliffe, T.W., Holmer, E. *et al.* (1976). Anticoagulant properties of heparin fractionated by affinity chromatography on matrix-bound antithrombin III and by gel filtration. *Thromb. Res.,* **9**:575–583.

Atha, D.H., Stephens, A.W., Rimon, A. and Rosenberg, R.D. (1984a). Sequence variation in heparin octasaccharides with high affinity for antithrombin III. *Biochemistry,* **23**:5801–5812.

Atha, D.H., Stephens, A.W. and Rosenberg, R.D. (1984b). Evaluation of critical groups required for binding of heparin to antithrombin. *Proc. Natl. Acad. Sci. USA,* **81**:1030–1034.

Atha, D.H., Lormeau, J.C., Petitou, M. *et al.* (1985). Contribution of monosaccharide residues in heparin binding to antithrombin III. *Biochemistry,* **24**:6723–6729.

Atha, D.H., Lormeau, J-C., Petitou, M., Rosenberg, R.D. and Choay, J. (1987). Contribution of 3-0- and 6-0-sulfated glucosamine residues in the heparin-induced conformational change in antithrombin III. *Biochemistry,* **26**:6454–6461.

Atkins, E.D.T., Nieduszynski, I.A. and Horner, A.A. (1974). Crystallizahon of macromolecular heparin. *Biochem. J.,* **143**:251–252.

Austin, R.C., Rachubinski, R.A., Fernandez-Rachubinski, F. and Blajchman, M.A. (1990). Expression in a cell-free system of normal and variant forms of human antithrombin III. Ability to bind heparin and react with a-thrombin. *Blood,* **76**:1521–1529.

Bame, K.J. and Esko, J.D. (1989). Undersulfated heparan sulfate in a Chinese hamster ovary cell mutant defective in heparan sulfate *N*-sulfotransferase. *J. Biol. Chem.,* **264**:8059–8065.

Bame, K.J., Lidholt, K., Lindahl, U. and Esko, J.D. (1991). Biosynthesis of heparan sulfate: Coordination of polymer-modification reactions in a chinese hamster ovary cell mutant defective in *N*-sulfotransferase. *J. Biol. Chem.,* **266**:10287–10293.

Bauer, K., Teitel, J. and Rosenberg, R.D. (1983). Assays for the quantitation of antithrombin III thrombin-antithrombin complex and prothrombin activation fragments. In *Disorders of thrombin formation.* edited by Colman, pp. 142–155 New York: Churchill Livingstone.

Bauer, K., Ashenhurst, J., Chediak, J. and Rosenberg, R.D. (1983). Antithrombin "Chicago" a functionally abnormal molecule with increased heparin affinity causing familial thrombophilia. *Blood,* **62**:1242–1250.

Beeler, D.L., Marcum, J.A., Schiffman, S. and Rosenberg, R.D. (1986). Interaction of factor XIa and antithrombin the presence and absence of heparin. *Blood,* **67**:1488–1492.

Bertina, R., van der Linden, I., Engesser, L., Muller, H. and Brommer, E. (1987). Hereditary heparin cofactor II deficiency and the risk of development of thrombosis. *Thromb. Haemostas.,* **57**:196–200.

Beukes, C. and Heyns, A. (1980). A South African family with antithrombin III deficiency. *S. Afr. Med. J.,* **58**:528–530.

Bjork, I. and Nordling, K. (1979). Evidence of a chemical modification for the involvement of one or more tryptophanyl residues of bovine antithrombin in the binding of high affinity heparin. *Eur. J. Biochem.,* **102**:497.

Bjork, I., Jackson, C.M., Jornvall, H. *et al.* (1982). The active site of antithrombin. *J. Biol. Chem.,* **257**:2406–2411.

Bjork, I., Olson, S.T. and Shore, J.D. (1989). Molecular Mechanisms of the accelerating effect of heparin on the reactions between antithrombin and clotting proteinases In *Heparin. Chemical and Biological Properties. Clinical Applications,* edited by D.A. Lane and U. Lindahl, pp. 229–255 London: Edward Arnold.

Bjork, I., Ylinenjarvi, K., Olson, S.T. and Bock, P.E. (1992). Conversion of antithrombin from an inhibitor of thrombin to a substrate with reduced heparin affinity and enhanced conformational stability by binding of a tetradecapeptide corresponding to the P_1 to P_{14} region of the putative reactive-bond loop of the inhibitor. *J. Biol. Chem.,* **267**:1976–1982.

Blackburn, M.N. and Sibley, C.C. (1980). The heparin binding site of antithrombin III. *J. Biol. Chem.,* **255**:824–826.

Blinder, M.A., Andersson, T.R., Abildgaard, U. and Tollefsen, D.M. (1989). Heparin cofactor II Oslo. Mutation of Arg-189 to His decreases the affinity for dermatan sulfate. *J. Biol. Chem.,* **264**:5128–5133.

Blinder, M.A. and Tollefsen, D.M. (1990). Site directed mutagenesis of arginine 103 and lysine 185 in the proposed glycosaminoglycan-binding site of heparin cofactor II. *J. Biol. Chem.,* **265**:286–291.

Bock, S., Harris, J., Schwartz, C., Ward, J., Hershgold, E. and Skoinick, M. (1985). Hereditary thrombosis in a Utah kindred is caused by a dysfunctional antithrombin III gene. *Am. J. Hum. Genet.,* **37**:32–41.

Bock, S. and Prochownik, E. (1987). Molecular genetic survey of 16 kindreds with hereditary antithrombin III deficiency. *Blood,* **70**:1273–1278.

Bock, S., Marrinan, J. and Radziejewska, E. (1988). Antithrombin III Utah: proline-407 to leucine mutation in a highly conserved region near the inhibitor reactive site. *Biochemistry,* **27**:6171–6178.

Bock, S., Silbermann, J., Wikoff, W., Abildgaard, U. and Hultin, M. (1989). Identification of a threonine for alanine substitution at residue 404 of antithrombin III Oslo suggests integrity of the 404–407 region is important for maintaining normal plasma inhibitor levels. *Thromb. Haemostas.,* **62**:494.

Borg, J., Owen, M., Soria, C., Soria, J., Caen, J. and Carrell, R. (1988). Proposed heparin binding site in antithrombin based on arginine 47. A new variant Rouen-II, 47 arg to ser. *J. Clin. Invest.,* **81**:1292–1296.

Borg, J., Brennan, S., Carrell, R., Perry, D. and Shaw, J. (1990). Antithrombin Rouen-IV 24Arg Cys. The amino terminal contribution to heparin binding. *FEBS Lett.,* **266**:163–166.

Boyer, C., Wolf, M., Lavergne, J. and Larrieu, M. (1980). Thrombin generation and formation of thrombin-antithrombin III complexes in congenital antithrombin deficiency. *Thromb. Res.,* **20**:207–218.

Boyer, C., Wolf, M., Vedrenne, J., Meyer, D. and Larrieu, M. (1986). Homozygous variant of antithrombin III: AT III Fountainebleau. *Thromb. Haemostas.,* **56**:18–22.

Brennan, S., Borg, J., George, P., Soria, C., Soria, J., Caen ,J. and Carrell, R. (1988). New carbohydrate site in mutant antithrombin (7 Ile — Asn) with decreased heparin affinity. *FEBS Lett.,* **237**:118–122.

Briginshaw, G.F. and Shanberge, J.N. (1974). Identification of two distinct heparin cofactors in human plasma: Separation and partial purification. *Arch. biochem. Biophys.,* **161**:683–690.

Brinkhous, K.M., Smith, H.P., Warner, E.D. and Seegers, W.H. (1939). The inhibition of blood clotting: An unidentified substance which acts in conjunction with heparin to prevent the conversion of prothrombin to thrombin. *Am. J. Physiol.,* **125**:683–687.

Broze, G.J. Jr. and Majerus, P.W. (1980). Purification and properties of human coagulation factor VII. *J. Biol. Chem.,* **225**:1242–1242.

Brunel, F., Duchange, N., Fischer, A., Cohen, G. and Zakin, M. (1987). Antithrombin III Alger: a new case of Arg47-Cys mutation. *Am. J. Haematol.,* **25**:223–224.

Carlson, T.H., Simon, T.L. and Atencio, A.C. (1985). *In vivo* behavior of human radioiodinated antithrombin III: distribution between three physiologic pools. *Blood,* **66**:13–19.

Carvalho, A. and Ellman, L. (1976). Hereditary antithrombin III deficiency: effect of antithrombin III deficiency on platelet function. *Am. J. Med.,* **61**:179–183.

Caso, R., Lane, D., Thompson, E., Zangouras, D., Panico, M., Morris, H., Olds, R., Thein, S. and Girolami, A. (1990). Antithrombin Padua I: Impaired heparin binding caused by an Arg47 to His (CGT to CAT) substitution. *Thromb. Res.,* **58**:185–190.

Chang, J-Y. (1989). Binding of heparin to human antithrombin III activates selective chemical modification at Lysine 236. *J. Biol. Chem.,* **264**:3111–3115.

Chang, J. and Tran, T. (1986). Antithrombin III Bassel. Identification of a Pro-Leu substitution in a hereditary abnormal antithrombin with impaired heparin cofactor activity. *J. Biol. Chem.,* **261**:1174–1176.

Chasse, J., Esnard, F., Guitton, J., Mouray, H., Perigois, F., Fauconneau, G. and Gaullthier, F. (1984). An abnormal plasma antithrombin with no apparent affinity for heparin. *Thromb. Res.,* **34**:297–302.

Choay, I., Petitou, M., Lormeau, I.C. *et al.* (1983). Structure-activity relationship in heparin: A synthetic pentasacchande with high affinity for antithrombin III and factor Xa activity. *Biochem. Biophys. Res. Commun.,* **116**:492–499.

Choay, J., Lormeau, I.C., Petitou, M. *et al.* (1980). Anb-Xa active heparin oligosacchandes. *Thromb. Res.,* **18**:573–578.

Church, F.C., Pratt, C.W., Noyes, C.M., Kalayanamit, T., Sherrill, G.B., Tobin, R.B. and Meade, J.B. (1989). Structural and functional properties of human alpha-thrombin, phosphopyridoxylated alpha-thrombin, and alpha$_T$-thrombin. *J. Biol. Chem.,* **264**:18419–18422.

Church, F.C., Noyes, C.M. and Griffith, M.J. (1985). Inhibition of chymotrypsin by heparin, cofactor II. *Proc. Natl.. Acad.. Sci.. USA,* **82(19)**:6431–6434.

Colliec-Jouault, S., Shworak, N.W., Liu, J. and Rosenberg, R.D. (1994). Characterization of a cell mutant specifically defective in the synthesis of anticoagulantly active heparan sulfate. *J. Biol. Chem.,* **269**:24953–24958.

Contejean, C. (1895). Recherches sur les injections intraveineuses de peptone et leur influence sur la coagulabilite du sang chez le chien. *Archives de Physiologie Normale et Pathologique,* **7**:45.

Cosgriff, T., Bishop, D., Hershgold, E., SKoinick, M., Martin, B., Baty, B. and Carlson, K. (1983). Familial antithrombin III deficiency: its natural history, genetics, diagnosis and treatment. *Medicine,* **62**:209–220.

Craig, P.A., Olson, S.T. and Shore, J.D. (1989). Characterization of assembly, product formation, and heparin dissociation steps in the FActor Xa reaction *J. Biol. Chem.,* **264**:5452–5461.

Daly, M., Ball, R., O'Meara, A. and Hallinan, F.: Identification and characterization of an antithrombin III mutant (AT Dublin 2) with marginally decreased heparin activity. *Thromb. Res.,* **56**:503–513, 1989.

Damus, P.S., Hicks, M. and Rosenberg, R.D. (1973). A generalized view of heparin's anticoagulant action. *Nature* **246**:355–357

Davie, E.W. and Ratnoff, O.D. (1964). Waterfall sequence for intrinsic blood clotting. *Science,* **145**:1310–1312.

de Agostini, A.L., Lau, H.K., Leone, C., Youssoufian, H. and Rosenberg, R.D. (1990). Cell mutants defective in synthesizing a heparan sulfate protoglycan with regions of defined monosaccharide sequence. *Proc. Natl. Acad. Sci. USA,* **87**:9784–9788.

de Agostini, A.I., Watkins, S.C., Slayter, H.S., Youssoufian, H. and Rosenberg, R.D. (1990). Localization of anticoagulantly active heparan sulfate proteoglycans in vascular endothelium: Antithrombin binding on cultured endothelial cells and perfused rat aorta. *J. Cell. Biol.,* **111**:1293–1304.

de Moerloose, P., Reber, G., Vernet, P., Minazio, P. and Bouvier, C. (1987). Antithrombin III Geneva: a hereditary abnormal antithrombin III with defective heparin cofactor activity. *Thromb. Haemostas.,* **57**:154–157.

de Roux, N., Chadeuf, G., Molho-Sabatier, P., Plouin, F. and Alach, M. (1990). Clinical and biochemical characterization of antithrombin III Franconville, a variant with Pro 41 Leu mutation. *Br. J. Haematol.,* **75**:222–227.

Devraj-Klzuk, R., Chu, I.D., Prochownik, E., Carter, C., Ofosu, F. and Blajchman, M. (1988). Antithrombin-III-Hamilton: a gene with a point mutation (guanine to adeninine) in codon 382 causing impaired serine protease reactivity. *Blood,* **72**:1518–1523.

Duchange, N., Chasse, J., Cohen, G. and Zakin, M. (1987). Molecular characterization of the antithrombin III Tours deficiency. *Thromb. Res.,* **45**:115–121.

Egeberg, O. (1965). Inherited antithrombin deficiency causing thrombophilia. *Thromb. Diath. Haemorrh.,* **13**:516–530.

Einarsson, R. and Andersson, L.O. (1977). 8incling of heparin to human antithrombin III as studied by measurements of tryptophan fluorescence. *Biochim. Biophys. Acta,* **490**:104–111.

Ellison, N., Edmunds, L.H. Jr. and Colman, R.W. (1978). Platelet aggregation following heparin and protamine administration. *Anesthesiology,* **48**:65–68.

Engelberg, H. (1963). *Heparin: Metabolism, Physiology and Clinical Application.* Springfield, I.L., Charles C. Thomas.

Engh, R.A., Wright, H.T. and Huber, R. (1990). Modeling of the intact form of the a_1-proteinase inhibitor. *Protein Engng.,* **3**:469–477.

Erdjument, H., Lane, D., Ireland, H., Di Marzo, V., Panico, M., Morris, H., Tripodi, A. and Mannucci, P. (1988a). Antithrombin Milano, single amino acid substitution at the reactive site, Arg 393 to Cys. *Thromb. Haemostas.,* **60**:471–475.

Erdjument, H., Lane, D., Di Marzo, V. and Morris, H. (1988b). Single amino acid substitutions in the reactive site of antithrombin leading to thrombosis. Congenital substitution of arginine 393 to cysteine in antithrombin Northwick Park and to histidine in antithrombin Glasgow. *J. Biol. Chem.,* **263**:5589–5593.

Erdjument, H., Lane, D.A., Panico, M., Di Marzo, V., Morris, H.R., Bauer, K. and Rosenberg, R.D. (1989). Antithrombin Chicago, amino acid substitution of arginine 393 to histidine. *Thromb. Res.,* **54**:613–619.

Eriksson, I., Sandback, D., Ek, B., Lindahl, U. and Kjellen, L. (1994). cDNA cloning and sequencing of mouse mastocytoma glucosaminyl *N*-deacetylase/*N*-sulfotransferase, an enzyme invovled in the biosynthesis of heparin. *J. Biol. Chem.,* **269**:10438–10443.

Esko, J.D., Stewart, T.E. and Taylor, W.H. (1985). Animal cell mutants defective in glycosaminoglycan biosynthesis. *Proc. Natl. Acad. Sci. USA,* **82**:3197–3201.

Esko, J.D., Elgavish, A., Prasthofer, T., Taylor, W.H. and Weinke, J.L. (1986). Sulfate transport-deficient mutants of Chinese hamster ovary cells. *J. Biol. Chem.,* **261**:15725–15733.

Esko, J.D., Weinke, J.L., Taylor, W.H., Ekborg, G., Roden, L., Anantharamaiah, G. and Gawish, A. (1987). Inhibition of chondroitin and heparan sulfate biosynthesis in chinese hamster ovary cell mutants defective in galactosyltransferase I. *J. Biol. Chem.,* **262**:12189–12195.

Evans, D.L., Marshall, C.J., Christey, P.B. and Carrell, R.W. (1992). Heparin binding site, conformational change, and activation of antithrombin. *Biochemistry,* **31**:12629–12642.

Filip, D., Eckstein, J. and Veltkamp, J. (1976). Hereditary antithrombin III deficiency and thromboembolic disease. *Am. J. Haematol.,* **2**:343–349.

Finazzi, G., Caccia, R. and Barbui, T. (1987). Different prevalence of thromboembolism in the subtypes of congenital antithrombin deficiency: review of 404 cases (letter). *Thromb. Haemostas.,* **58**:1094.

Fischer, A., Beguin, S., Sternberg, C. and Dautzenberg, M. (1987). Comparative effect of heparin and heparan sulphate on two abnormal antithrombin III type 3 variants. *Br. J. Haemotol.,* **66**:213–217.

Fischer, A., Cornu, P., Sternberg, C., Meriane, F., Dautzenberg, M., Chafa, O., Beguin, S. and Desnos, M. (1986). Antithrombin III Alger: a new homozygous AT III variant. *Thromb. Haemostas.,* **55**:218–221.

Fransson, L-A, Huckerby, T.N. and Nieduszynski, I.A. (1978). a-L-iduronate ring conformations in heparin and heparin derivatives. *Biochem. J.,* **175**:299–309.

Galli, S.J., Orenstein, N.S., Gill, P.J. *et al.* (1984). In *The Mast Cell: Its Role in Health and Disease,* editor J. Pepys and A.M. Edwards A.M., pp. 842–852, Kent, England, Pitman Medical Publishers.

Gandrille, S., Vidaud, D., Emmerich, J., Clauser, E., Sie, P., Flessinger, J., Alhenc-Gelas, M., Priollet, P., and Alach, M. (1991). Molecular basis for hereditary antithrombin III quantitative deficiencies: a stop codon in exon IIIa and a frameshift in exon VI. *Br. J. Haematol.,* **78**:414–420.

Girolami, A., Fabris, F., Cappellato, G., Sainati, L. and Boeri, G. (1983a). Antithrombin III Padua 2: a new congenital abnormality with defective heparin co-factor activities but no thrombotic disease. *Blut,* **47**:93–103.

Girolami, A., Pengo, V., Patrassi, G., Cappelatto, G., Vianello, C. and Cartei, L. (1983b). Antithrombin III Padua: a "new" congenital antithrombin III abnormality with normal or near normal activity, normal antigen, abnormal migration and no thrombotic disease. *Folia Haematol., (Leipz)* **110**:98–111.

Godal, H.C., Rygh, M. and Laake, K. (1974). Progressive inactivation of purified factor VII by heparin and anhthrombin III. *Thromb. Res.,* **5**:773–775.

Gruenberg, J., Smallridge, R. and Rosenberg, R.D. (1975). Inherited antithrombin-III dificiency causing mesenteric venous infarction: a new clinical entity. *Ann. Surg.,* **181**:791–794.

Grundy, C., Thomas, F., Millar, D., Krawczak, M., Melissari, E., Lindo, V., Moffat, E., Kakkar, V. and Cooper, D. (1991). Recurrent deletion in the human antithrombin III gene. *Blood,* **78**:1027–1032.

Gyde, O., Middleton, M., Vaughan, G. and Fletcher, D. (1978). Antithrombin III deficiency, hypertriglyceridaemia and venous thrombosis. *Br. Med. J.,* **1**:621–622.

Harper, P., Luddington, R., Daly, M., Bruce, D., Williamson, D., Edgar, P., Perry, D. and Carrell, R. (1991). The incidence of dysfunctional antithrombin variants: four cases in 210 patients with thromboembolic disease. *Br. J. Haematol.*, **77**:360–364.

Hashimoto, Y., Orellana, A., Gil, G. and Hirschberg, C.B. (1992). Molecular cloning and expression of rat liver *N*-heparan sulfate sulfotransferase. *J. Biol. Chem.*, **267**:15744–15750.

Hook, M., Bjork, I., Hopwood, J. and Lindahl, U. (1976). Anticoagulant activity of heparin: Separation of high-activity and low-activity heparin species by affinity chromatography on immobilized antithrombin. *Fed. Eur. Biochem. Soc. Letters*, **66**:90–93.

Horne, A. and Gettins, P.H. (1992). NMR spectroscopic studies on the interactions between human plasma antithrombin III and defined low molecular weight heparin fragments. *Biochemistry* **31**:2286–2294

Hortin, G.L., Tollefsen, D.M. and Benutto, B.M. (1989). Antithrombin activity of a peptide corresponding to residues 54–75 of heparin cofactor II. *J. Biol. Chem.*, **264**:13979–13982.

Hoylaerts, M., Owen, W.G. and Collen, D. (1984). Involvement of heparin chain length in the heparin-catalyzed inhibition of thrombin by antithrombin III. *J. Biol. Chem.*, **259**:5670–5677.

Huber, R. and Carrell, R.W. (1989). Implications of the three-dimensional structure of a_1-antitrypsin for structure and function of serpins. *Biochemistry*, **28**:8951–8965.

Ishihara, M., Guo, Y., Wei, Z., Yang, Z., Swiedler, S.J., Orellana, A. and Hirschberg, C.B. (1993). Regulation of biosynthesis of the basic fibroblast growth factor binding domains of heparin sulfate by heparan sulfate-*N*-deacetylase/*N*-sulfotransferase expression. *J. Biol. Chem.*, **268**:20091–20095.

Jacobson, I., Backstrom, E., Hook, M. *et al.* (1979). Biosynthesis of heparin: Assay and properties of the microsomal uronosyl C5 epimerase. *J. Biol. Chem.*, **254**:2975–2982.

Johansson, L., Hedner, U. and Nilsson, I. (1978). Familial antithrombin III deficiency as pathogenesis of deep venous thrombosis. *Acta Med. Scand.*, **204**:491–495.

Jordan, R.E., Beeler, D. and Rosenberg, R.D. (1979). Fractionation of low molecular weight heparin species and their interaction with antithrombin. *J. Biol. Chem.*, **254**:2902–2913.

Jordan, R.E., Oosta, G.M., Gardner, W.T. and Rosenberg, R.D. (1980a). The binding of low-molecular-weight heparin to hemostatic enzymes. *J. Biol. Chem.*, **255**:10073–10080.

Jordan, R.E., Oosta, G.M., Gardner, W.T. and Rosenberg, R.D. (1980b). The kinetics of hemostatic enzyme-antithrombin interactions in the presence of low-molecular-weight heparin. *J. Biol. Chem.*, **255**:10081–10090.

Jordan, R.E., Favreau, L.V., Braswell, E.H. and Rosenberg, R.D. (1982). Heparin with two binding sites for antithrombin or platelet factor 4. *J. Biol. Chem.*, **277**:400–406.

Karp, G.I., Marcum, J.A. and Rosenberg, R.D. (1984). The role of tryptophan residues in heparin-antithrombin interactions. *Arch. Biochem. Biophys.*, **233**:712–720.

Koide, T., Takahashi, K., Ono, T. and Sakuragawa, N. (1983). Isolation and characterization of a hereditary abnormal antithrombin III: "antithrombin III Toyama". *Thromb. Res.*, **31**:319–328.

Koide, T., Odani, S., Takahashi, K., Ono, T. and Sakuragawa, N. (1984). Antithrombin III Toyama: replacement of arginine-47 by cysteine in hereditary abnormal antithrombin III that lacks heparin-binding ability. *Proc. Natl. Acad. Sci. USA*, **81**:289–293.

Kojima, T., Leone, C.W., Marchildon, G.A., Marcum, J.A. and Rosenberg, R.D. (1992a). Isolation and characterization of heparan sulfate proteoglycans produced by cloned rat microvascular endothelial cells. *J. Biol. Chem.*, **267**:4859–4869.

Kojima, T., Shworak, N.W. and Rosenberg, R.D. (1992b). Molecular cloning and expressions of two distinct cDNA-encoding heparan sulfate proteoglycan core proteins from a rat endothelial cell line. *J. Biol. Chem.*, **267**:4870–4877.

Kurachi, F., Fujikawa, K., Schmier, G. and Davie, E.W. (1976). Inhibihon of bovine factor IX_a and factor X_a by antithrombin III. *Biochemistry*, **15**:373–377.

Kusche, M., Backstrom, G., Riesenfeld, J., Petitou, M., Choay, J. and Lindahl, U. (1988). Biosynthesis of heparin: *O*-sulfation of the antithrombin-binding region. *J. Biol. Chem.*, **263**:15474–15484.

Kusche, M., Torri, G., Casu, B. and Lindahl, U. (1990). Biosynthesis of heparin: Availability of glucosaminyl 3-*O*-sulfation sites. *J. Biol. Chem.*, **265**:7292–7300.

Lam, L.H., Silbert, J.E. and Rosenberg, R.D. (1976). The separation of active and inactive forms of heparin. *Biochem. Biophys. Res. Commun.*, **69**:570–577.

Lane, D.A., Erdjument, H., Flynn, A., DeMarzo, V., Panico, M., Morris, H.R., Greaves, M., Dolan, G. and Preston, F.E. (1989a). Antithrombin Sheffield: amino acid substitution at the reactive site (Arg 393 to His) causing thrombosis. *Brit. J. Haematol.*, **71**:91–96.

Lane, D., Erdjument, H., Thompson, E., Panico, M., Di Marzo, V., Morris, H., Leone, G., De Stefano, V. and Thein, S. (1989b). A novel amino acid substitution in the reactive site of a congenital antithrombin. Antithrombin Pescara Arg393 to Pro, caused by a CGT to CCT mutation. *J. Biol. Chem.*, **264**:10200–102004.

Leder, I.G. (1980). A novel 3-*0* sulfatase from human urine acting on methyl-2-deoxy-2-sulfamino- alpha- D-glucopyranoside-3-sulfate. *Biochem. Biophys. Res. Commun.*, **94**:1183–1189.

Lidholt, K., Weinke, J.L., Kiser, C.S., Lugemwa, F.N., Bame, K.J., Cheifetz, S., Massague, J., Lindahl, U. and Esko, J.D. (1992). A single mutation affects both *N*-acetylglucosaminyltransferase and glucuronosyltransferase activities in a Chinese hamster ovary cell mutant defective in heparan sulfate biosynthesis. *Proc. Natl. Acad. Sci. USA,* **89**:2267–2271.

Lind, T., Lindahl, U. and Lidholt, K. (1993). Biosynthesis of heparin/heparan sulfate. Identification of a 70kDa protein catalyzing both the D-glucuronosyl- and the *N*-acetyl-D-glucosaminyltransferase reactions. *J. Biol. Chem.,* **268**:20705–20708, 1993.

Lindahl, U., Hook, M., Backstrom, G. *et al.* (1977). Structure and biosynthesis of heparin-like polysaccharides. *Fed. Proc.,* **36**:19–24.

Lindahl, U., Backstrom, G., Hook, M. *et al.* (1979). Structure of the antithrombin-binding site of heparin. *Proc. Natl. Acad. Sci. USA,* **76**:3198–3202.

Lindahl, U., Backstrom, G. and Thunberg, L. (1983). The antithrombin-binding sequence in heparin: Identification of an essential 6-0 sulfate group. *J. Biol. Chem.,* **258**:9826–9830.

Linhardt, R.J., Wang, H., Loganathan, D. and Bae, J. (1992). Search for the heparin antihthrombin III-binding site precursor. *J. Biol. Chem.,* **267**:2380–2387.

Liu, C-S. and Chang J-Y. (1987a). The heparin binding site of human antithrombin III. Selective chemical modification at Lys114, Lys125, and Lys287 impairs its heparin cofactor activity. *J. Biol. Chem.,* **262**:17356–17361.

Liu, C-S. and Chang, J-Y. (1987b). Probing the heparin-binding domain of human antithrombin III with V8 protease. *Eur. J. Biochem.,* **167**:247–252.

Loganathan, D., Wang, H.M., Mallis, L.M. and Linhardt, R.J. (1990). *Biochemistry,* **29**:2611–2617.

Lollar, P. and Owen, W.G. (1980). Clearance of thrombin from the circulation in rabbits by high-affinity binding sites on the endothelium: Possible role in the inactivation of thrombin by antithrombin III. *J. Clin. Invest.,* **66**:1222–1230.

Mackie, M., Bennett, B., Ogston, D. and Douglas, A. (1978). Familial thrombosis: inherited deficiency of antithrombin III. *Br. Med. J.,* **1**:136–138.

Maimone, M.M. and Tollefsen, D.M. (1990). Structure of a dermatan sulfate hexasaccharide that binds to heparin cofactor II with high affinity. *J. Biol. Chem.,* **265**:18263–18271.

Mandon, E., Kempner, E.S., Ishihara, M. and Hirschberg, C.B. (1994). A monomeric protein in the golgi membrane catalyzes both *N*-deacetylation and *N*-sulfation of heparan sulfate. *J. Biol. Chem.,* **269**:11729–11733.

Marciniak, E., Farley, C. and DeSimone, P. (1974). Familial thrombosis due to antithrombin III deficiency. *Blood,* **43**:219–231.

Marcum, J.A., Fritze, L., Galli, S.J. *et al.* (1983). Microvascular heparinlike species with anticoagulant activity. *Am. J. Physiol.,* **245**:H725–733.

Marcum, J.A. and Rosenberg, R.D. (1984). Anticoagulantly active heparin-like molecules from vascular tissue. *Biochemistry,* **23**:1730–1737.

Marcum, J.A., McKenney, J.B. and Rosenberg, R.D. (1984). The acceleration of thrombin-antithrombin complex formation in rat hindquarters via naturally occurring heparin-like molecules bound to the endothelium. *J. Clin. Invest.,* **74**:341–350.

Marcum, J.A. and Rosenberg, R.D. (1985). Heparinlike molecules with anticoagulant activity are synthesized by cultured endothelial cell. *Biochem. Biophys. Res. Commun.,* **126**:365–372, 1985.

Marcum, J.A., McKenney, J.B., Galli, S.J., Jackman, R.W. and Rosenberg, R.D. (1986). Anticoagulantly active heparin-like molecules from mast cell deficient mice. *Am. J. Physiol.,* **250**:H879–H888.

Matsuo, T., Ohki, Y., Kondo, S. and Matsuo, O. (1979). Familial antithrombin III deficiency in a Japanese family. *Thromb. Res.,* **16**:815–823.

McDonald, M., Hathaway, W., Reeve, E. and Leonard, B. (1982). Biochemical and functional study of antithrombin III in newborn infants. *Thromb. Haemostas.,* **47**:56–58.

Mcfarlane, R.G. (1984). An enzyme cascade in blood clotting mechanism, and its function as a biochemical amplifier. *Nature,* **202**:498–499.

McLean, J. (1916). The thromboplastic action of cephalin. *Am. J. Physiol.,* **41**:250–257.

Meezan, E., Brendel, K. and Carlson, E.C. (1974). Isolation of a purified preparation of metabolically active retinal blood vessels. *Nature,* **251**:65–67.

Mertens, G., Cassiman, J-J., Van den Berghe, H., Vermylen, J. and David, G. (1992). Cell surface heparan sulfate proteoglycan from human vascular endothelial cells. Core protein characterization and antithrombin III binding properties. *J. Biol. Chem.,* **267**:20435–20443.

Molho-Sabatier, P., Aiach, M., Gaillard, I., Fiessinger, J., Fischer, A., Chadeuf, G. and Clauser, E. (1989). Molecular characterization of antithrombin III (ATIII) variants using polymerase chain reaction. Identification of the ATIII Charleville as an Ala 384 Pro mutation. *J. Clin. Invest.,* **84**:1236–1242.

Monkhouse, F.C., France, E.S. and Seegers, W.H. (1955). Studies on the antithrombin and heparin cofactor activities of a fraction absorbed from plasma by aluminum hydroxide. *Circ. Res.,* **3**:397–402.

Morowitz, P. (1968). The Chemistry of Blood Coagulation. Springfield, IL, Charles C Thomas.

Mourey, L., Samama, J.P., Delarue, M., Choay, J., Lormeau, J.C., Petitou, M. and Moras, D. (1990). Antithrombin III: structural and functional aspects. *Biochimie, 72*:599–608.

Murano, G., Williams, L., Miller-Andersson, M. *et al.* (1980). Some properties of antithrombin III and its concentration in human plasma. *Thromb. Res., 18*:259–262.

Nesheim, M.E. (1983). A simple rate law that describes the kinetics of heparin catalyzed reaction between antithrombin III and thrombin. *J. Biol. Chem., 258*:14708–14717.

Nieduszynski, I.A. and Atkins, E.D.T. (1973). Conformation of the mucopolysaccharides — x-ray fibre diffraction of heparin. *Biochem. J., 135*:729–733.

Nordenman, B., Nystrom, C. and Bjork, I. (1977). The size and shape of human bovine antithrombin III. *Eur. J. Biochem., 78:195–203.*

Nordenman, B. and Bjork, I. (1978). Binding of low-affinity and high-affinity heparin to antithrombin: Ultraviolet difference spectroscopy and circular dichroism studies. *Biochemistry, 17*:3339–3344.

Odegard, O. and Abildgaard, U. (1978). Antithrombin III: critical review of assay methods. Significance of variations in health and disease. *Haemostasis, 7*:127–134.

Meade, T., Dyer, S., Howarth, D., Imeson, J. and Stirling, Y. (1990). Antithrombin III and procoagulant activity: sex differences and effects of the menopause. *Br. J. Haematol., 74*:77–81.

Ofosu, F.A., Modi, G.J., Smith, L.M. *et al.* (1984). Heparin sulfate and dermatan sulfate inhibit the generation of thrombin activity in plasma by complementary pathways. *Blood, 64*:742–747.

Okajima, K., Ueyama, H., Hashimoto, Y., Sasaki, Y., Matsumoto, K., Okabe, H., Inoue, M., Araki, S. and Takatsuki, K. (1989). Homozygous variant of antithrombin III that lacks affinity for heparin, AT III Kumamato. *Thromb. Haemostas., 61*:20–24.

Olds, R., Lane, D., Caso, R., Girolami, A. and Thein, S. (1990a). Antithrombin III Padua 2: a single base substitution in exon 2 detected with PCR and direct genomic sequencing. *Nucl. Acids Res., 18*:1926.

Olds, R., Lane, D., Finazzi, G., Barbui, T. and Thein, S. (1990b). A frameshift mutation leading to type I antithrombin deficiency and thrombosis. *Blood, 76*:2182–2186.

Olds, R., Lane, D., Ireland, H., Leone, G., De Stefano, V., Wiesel, M., Cazenave, J. and Thein, S. (1991). Novel point mutations leading to type 1 antithrombin deficiency and thrombosis. *Br. J. Haematol., 78* 408–413.

Olson, S.T., Srinivasant, K.R., Bjork, I. and Shore, J.D. (1981). Binding of high affinity heparin to antithrombin III: Stopped flow kinetic studies of the binding interaction. *J. Biol. Chem., 256*:11073–11079.

Olson, S.T. and Shore, J.D. (1982). Demonstration of a two step reaction mechanism for inhibition of alpha thrombin by antithrombin III and identification of the step affected by heparin. *J. Biol. Chem., 257*:14891–14895.

Olson, S.T. and Shore, J.D. (1989). High molecular weight-kininogen and heparin acceleration of factor XIa inactivation by plasma proteinase inhibitors. *Thromb. Haemostas., 62*:381.

Olson, S.T. and Bjork, I. (1991). Regulation of thrombin by antithrombin and heparin cofactor II, In *Thrombin: Structure and Function*, edited by L.J. Berliner LJ, New York City: Plenum.

Oosta, G.M., Gardner, W.T., Beeler, D.L. and Rosenberg, R.D. (1981). Multiple functional domains of the heparin molecule. *Proc. Natl. Acad. Sci. USA, 78*:829–833.

Owen, M., Borg, J., Soria, J., Caen, J. and Carrell, R. (1987). Heparin binding defect in a new antithrombin III variant: rouen, 47Arg to His. *Blood, 69*:1275–1279, 1987.

Owen, M., Beresford, C. and Carrell, R. (1988). Antithrombin Glasgow, 393 Arg to His: a P1 reactive site variant with increased heparin affinity but no thrombin inhibitory activity. *FEBS Lett., 231*:317–320.

Owen, M., Shaw, G., Grau, E., Foncuberta, J., Carrell, R. and Boswell, D. (1989). Molecular characterization of antithrombin Barcelona-2: 47 arginine to cysteine. *Thromb. Res., 55*:451–457.

Pecon, I.M. and Blackburn, M.N. (1984). Pyndoxylation of essential lysines in the heparin-binding site of antithrombin III. *J. Biol. Chem., 259*:935–938.

Petersen, E.E., Dudek-Wojciechowska, G., Sottrup-Jensen, L. and Magnusson, S. (1979). The primary structure of antithrombin 111 (heparin-cofactor): Partial homology between alpha$_1$, -antitrypsin and antithrombin III. In *The Physiological Inhibitors of Coagulation and Fibrinolysis*, edited by D. Collen, B. Wiman, M. Verstraete, p. 43–56, Amsterdam: Elsevier/North-Holland Biomedical Press.

Pettersson, I., Kusche, M., Unger, E., Wlad, H., Nylund, L., Lindahl, U. and Kjellen, L. (1991). Biosynthesis of heparin: Purification of a 110-kDa mouse mastocytoma protein required for both glucosaminyl N-deacetylation and N-sulfation. *J. Biol. Chem., 266*:8044–8049.

Pitney, W., Manoharan, A. and Dean, S. (1980). Antithrombin III deficiency in an Australian family. *Br. J. Haematol., 46*:147–149.

Prowchownik, E., Antonarkis, S., Bauer, K., Rosenberg, R.D., Fearon, E. and Orkin, S. (1983). Molecular heterogeneity of inherited antithrombin III deficiency. *New Engl. J. Med., 308*:1549–1552, 1983.

Prochownik, E.V. and Orkin, S.H. (1984). *In vivo* transcription of a human antithrombin III "minigene". *J. Biol. Chem., 259*:15386–15392.

Robinson, H.C., Horner, A.A., Hook, M. *et al.* (1978). A proteoglycan form of heparin and its degradation to single chain molecules. *J. Biol. Chem., 253*:6687–6693.

Roden, L. and Horowitz, M.I. (1977). Structure and biosynthesis of connective tissue proteoglycans. In The Glycoconjugates, Vol 11, p. 3, edited by M.I. Horowitz, W. Pigman, New York: Academic Press

Rosenberg, R.D. and Damus, P.S. (1973). The purification and mechanism of action of human antithrombin-heparin cofactor. *J. Biol. Chem.,* **248**:6490–6505.

Rosenberg, R.D. (1975). Actions and interaction of antithrombin and heparin. *N. Eng. J. Med.,* **292**:146–151.

Rosenberg, J.S., McKenna, P. and Rosenberg, R.D. (1975). Inhibition of human factor IX$_a$ by human antithrombin-heparin cofactor. *J. Biol. Chem.,* **250**:8883–8888.

Rosenberg, R.D., Armand, G. and Lam, L. (1978). Structure-function relationship of heparin species. *Proc. Natl. Acad. Sci. USA,* **75**:3065–3069.

Rosenberg, R.D. and Lam, L.H. (1979). Correlation between structure and function of heparin. *Proc. Natl. Acad. Sci. USA,* **76**:1218–1222.

Roussel, B., Dieval, J., Delobel, J., Fernandez-Rachubinski, F., Eng, B., Rachubinski, R. and Blajchman, M. (1991). Antithrombin III-Amiens: a new family with an Arg47-Cys inherited variant of antithrombin III with impaired heparin cofactor activity. *Am. J. Haematol.,* **36**:25–29.

Ruoslahti, E. (1988). Structure and biology of proteoglycans. *Annu. Rev. Cell. Biol.,* **4**:229–255.

Sakuragawa, N., Takahashi, K., Kondo, S. and Koide, T. (1983). Antithrombin III Toyama: a hereditary abnormal antithrombin III of a patient with recurrent thrombophlebitis. *Thromb. Res.,* **31**:305–317.

Sas, G., Blasko, G., Banhegyi, D., Jako, J. and Palos, L. (1974). Abnormal antithrombin II (antithrombin III "Budapest II") as a cause of familial thrombophilia. *Thromb. Diathes. Haemorrh.,* **32**:105–115.

Schulze, A.J., Baumann, U., Knof, S., Jaeger, E., Huber, R. and Laurell, C-B. (1990). Structural transition of α_1-antitrypsin by a peptide sequentially similar to β-strand s4A. *Eur. J. Biochem.,* **194**:51–56.

Scott, C.F., Schapira, M. and Colman, R.W. (1982). Effect of heparin on the inactivation rate of human factor XI$_a$ by antithrombin III. *Blood,* **60** 940–947.

Scully, M., De Haas, H., Chan, P. and Kakkar, V. (1981). Hereditary antithrombin III deficiency in an English family. *Br. J. Haematol.,* **47**:235–240.

Shapiro, S., Prager, D. and Martinez, J. (1973). Inherited antithrombin III deficiency associated with multiple thromboembolic phenomena. *Blood,* **42** 1001 (abstract).

Shore, J.D., Olson, S.T., Craig, P.A., Choay, J. and Bjork, I. (1989). Kinetics of heparin action. *Ann. NY. Acad. Sci.,* **556**:75–80.

Shworak, N.W., Colliec-Jouault, S., Liu, J., Shirakawa, M., Mulligan, R.C., Birinyi, L.K. and Rosenberg, R.D. (1994). Pathway-specific regulation of the synthesis of anticoagulantly active heparan sulfate. *J. Biol. Chem.,* **269**:24941–24952.

Silbert, J.E. (1967). Biosynthesis of heparin. Formation of a sulfated glycosaminoglycan with a microsomal preparation from mast cell tumors. *J. Biol. Chem.,* **242**:5146–5152.

Simionescu, N. (1983). Cellular aspects of transcapillary exchange. *Physiol. Rev.,* **63**:1536–1579.

Smith, J.W., Dey, N. and Knauer, D.J. Heparin binding domain of antithrombin III (1990). Characterization using a synthetic peptide directed polyclonal antibody. *Biochemistry,* **29**:8950–8957.

Stathakis, N., AG, P., Antonopoulos, M. and Gardikas, C. (1977). Familial thrombosis due to antithrombin III deficiency in a Greek family. *Acta Haemat.,* **57**:47–54.

Stead, N., Kaplan, A.P. and Rosenberg, R.D. (1976). Inhibition of activated factor XII by antithrombin-heparin cofactor. *J. Biol. Chem.,* **251**:6481–6488.

Stephens, A.W., Thalley, B.S. and Hirs, C.H.W. (1987). Antithrombin III Denver, a reactive site variant. *J. Biol. Chem.,* **262**:1044–1048.

Stephens, A.W. Siddiqui, A. and Hirs, C.H.W. (1988). Site-directed mutagenesis of the reactive center (serine 394) of antithrombin III. *J. Biol. Chem.,* **263**:15849–15852.

Stern, D., Nawroth, P., Marcum, J.A. et al. (1985). Interaction of antithrombin III with bovine aortic segments: Role of heparin in binding and enhanced anticoagulant activity. *J. Clin. Invest.,* **75**:272–279.

Stivala, S.S., Herbst, N., Kratky, O. and Pilz, I. (1968). Physico-chemical studies of fractionated bovine heparin. *Arch. Biochem. Biophys.,* **127**:795–802.

Stone, A.L. (1964). Anomalous rotary dispersion of melachromatic mucopolysaccharide-dye complexes. 1. Heparin. *Biopolymers,* **2**:315.

Stone, A.L. (1985). Far-ultra violet circular dichroism and uronic acid components of anticoagulant deca-, dodeca-, tetradeca-, and octadecasaccharide heparin fractions. *Biochem. Biophys. Res. Commun.,* **236**:342–353.

Stone, A.L., Beeler, D., Oosta, G. and Rosenberg, R.D. (1982). Circular dichroism spectroscopy of heparin-antithrombin interactions. *Proc. Natl. Acad. Sci. USA,* **79**:7190–7194.

Summaria, L., Boreisha, I.G., Arzadon, L. and Robbins, K. (1977). Activation of human glu-plasminogen to glu-plasmin by urokinase in presence of plasmin inhibitors: Streptomyces leuteptin and human plasma alpha-l-anhtrypsin and antithrombin III. *J. Biol. Chem.,* **252**:3945–3951.

Sun, X-J. and Chang, J-Y. (1989). Heparin binding domain of human antithrombin III inferred from the sequential reduction of its three disulfide linkages. *J. Biol. Chem.,* **264**:11288–11293.

Tait, R., Walker, I., Davidson, J., Islam, S. and Mitchell, R. (1990). Antithrombin III activity in healthy blood donors: age and sex related changes and the prevalence of asymptomatic deficiency (letter). *Br. J. Haematol.,* **75**:141–142.

Tait, R., Walker, I., Perry, D., Carrell, R., Islam, S., McCall, F., Mitchell, R. and Davidson, J. (1992). Prevalence of antithrombin III deficiency subtypes in 4000 healthy blood donors. *Thromb. Haemostas.,* **65**:839 (abstract).

Thaler, E. and Lechner, K. (1981). Antithrombin III deficiency and thromboembolism. In *Clinics in Hematology,* edited by. Prentice, pp. 369–390, London: Saunders.

Thein, A.N., Abildgaard, U., Hook, M. and Lindahl, U. (1977). The anticoagulant effect of heparan sulfate and dermatan sulfate. *Thromb. Res.,* **11**:107–117.

Thomas, D.P., Merton, R.E., Barrowcliffe, T.W. *et al.* (1979). Anti-factor X_a activity of heparan sulfate. *Thromb. Res.,* **14**:501–506.

Tollefsen, D.M. and Blank, M.K. (1981). Detection.of a new heparin-dependent inhibitor of thrombin in human plasma. *J. Clin. Invest.,* **68**:589–596.

Tollefsen, D.M., Majerus, D.W. and Blank, M.K. (1981). Heparin cofactor II. *J. Biol. Chem.,* **257** 2162–2169.

Tran, T., Bondell, C., Marbet, G. and Duckert, F. (1980a). Reactivity of a hereditary abnormal antithrombin III fraction in the inhibition of thrombin and factor X_a. *Thromb. Haemostas.,* **44**:92–95.

Tran, T., Bounameaux, H., Bondeli, C., Honkanen, H., Marbet, G. and Duckert, F. (1980b). Purification and partial characterization of a hereditary abnormal antithrombin III fraction of a patient with recurrent thrombophlebitis. *Thromb. Haemostas.,* **44**:87–91.

Ueyama, H., Murakami, T., Nishiguchi, S., Maeda, S., Hashimoto, Y., Okajima, K., Shimada, K. and Araki, S. (1990). Antithrombin III Kumamoto: identification of a point mutation and genotype analysis of the family. *Thromb. Haemostas.,* **63**:231–234.

Van der Meer, J., Stoepman-van, Dalen, E. and Jansen, J. (1973). Antithrombin-III deficiency in a Dutch family. *J. Clin. Path.,* **26**:532–538.

Van Deerlin, V.M. and Tollefsen, D.M. (1991). The N-terminal acidic domain of heparin cofactor II mediates the inhibition of a-thrombin in the presence of glycosaminoglycans. *J. Biol. Chem.,* **266**:20223–20231.

Vidaud, D., Emmerich, J., Sirieix, M., Sie, P., Alhenc-Gelas, M. and Aiach, M. (1991). Molecular basis for antithrombin III type I deficiency: three novel mutations located in exon IV. *Blood,* **78**:2305–2309.

Villaneuva, G.B. and Danishefsky, I. (1977). Evidence for a heparin-induced conformational change in antithrombin lll. *Biochem. Biophys. Res. Commun.,* **74**:803–809.

Villaneuva, G.B., Perret, V. and Danishefsky, I. (1980). Tryptophan residue at the heparin binding site in antithrombin III. *Arch. Biochem. Biophys.,* **203**:453–457.

Waugh, D.F. and Fitzgerald, M.A. (1956). Quantitative aspects of antithrombin and heparin in plasma. *Am. J. Physiol.,* **184**:627–639.

Wei, Z., Swiedler, S.J., Ishihara, M., Orellana, A. and Hirschberg, C.B. (1993). A single protein catalyzes both N-deacetylation and N-sulfation during the biosynthesis of heparan sulfate. *Proc. Natl. Acad. Sci. USA,* **90**:3885–3888.

Whinna, H.C., Blinder, M.A., Szewczyk, M., Tollefsen, D.M. and Church, F.C. (1991). Role of lysine 173 in heparin binding to heparin cofactor II. *J. Biol. Chem.,* **266**:8129–8135.

Winter, J., Bennet, B., Watt, J., Brown, T., San Roman, C., Schinzel, A., King, J. and Cook, P. (1982a). Confirmation of linkage between antithrombin III and duffy blood group and assignment of AT3 to 1q22–q25. *Ann. Hum. Genet,* **46**:29–34.

Winter, J., Fenech, A., Ridley, W., Bennett, B., Cumming, A.M., Mackie, M. and Douglas, A. (1982b). Familial antithrombin III deficiency. *Quart. J. Med.,* **204**:373–395.

Wolf, M., Boyer, C., Lavergne, J. and Larrieu, M. (1982). A new familial variant of antithrombin III: "Antithrombin III Paris". *Br. J. Haemat.,* **51**:285–295.

Wolf, M., Boyer-Neumann, C., Molho-Sabatier, P., Neumann, C., Meyer, D. and Larrieu, M. (1990). Familial varient of antithrombin III (AT III Bligny, 47Arg to His) associated with protein C deficiency. *Thromb. Haemostas.,* **63**:215–219.

Yuan, L. and Stivala, S.S. (1972). Viscosity of heparin as a function of dielectric constant of desulfation. *Biopolymers,* **11**:2079–2089.

Yurt, R.W., Leid, R.W., Austen, K.F. and Silbert, J.E. (1978). Native heparin from rat peritoneal mast cell. *J. Biol. Chem.,* **252**:518–521.

4 Role of Annexins in Vascular Hemostasis

Chris P.M. Reutelingsperger

Department of Biochemistry, Cardiovascular Research Institute Maastricht (CARIM), University of Limburg, The Netherlands. P.O. Box 616, 6200 MD Maastricht, Tel: (31) 43 88 15 33, Fax: (31) 43 67 09 88

Since our understanding of the existence of the Annexin family a vast amount of data dealing with structural and functional aspects of Annexins has appeared in the literature. This chapter describes beside a limited introduction only those data that concern the interaction of Annexins with the hemostatic system in the extracellular space. It is not within the scope of this chapter to deal with the hypotheses concerning the intracellular physiological functions of Annexins. The chapter neither describes the intracellular actions of Annexins on signal transduction and synthesis of biological compounds, that may influence cellular behaviour in the hemostatic system. For more comprehensive treatises of these subjects, the reader is referred to other reviews (Crompton, 1988; Klee, 1988; Creutz, 1992; Raynal and Pollard, 1994; Swairjo and Seaton, 1994).

The Annexin Family

Annexins constitute a multigene family of proteins that share structural and functional features. They contain a conserved amino acid sequence, initially termed the endonexin loop (Geisow, 1986), which is four or eight fold repeated in the polypeptide chain. This chain can be organized in an N-terminal tail, that precedes a core of four or eight homologous domains each of which contains the endonexin loop motif. This structural motif forms the basis for their shared biological property to bind to phospholipids in a Ca^{2+}-dependent manner (Huber, 1990).

Annexins have been discovered in the kingdoms of plants and animals. Within the latter they occur in widely separated phyla such as Poriphera (Robitzki, 1990), Cnidaria (Schlaepfer, 1992), Arthropoda (Johnston, 1990) and Chordata (Huang, 1986; Wallner, 1986; Pepinsky, 1988; Funakoshi, 1987; Crompton, 1988; Burns, 1989; Hauptmann, 1989; Towle, 1992; Wice, 1992). In mammals almost all cell types express at least two different Annexin proteins, which make up more then 1% of total cellular protein. To date 13 different Annexins have been found in animals and their primary sequences have been fully elucidated. These sequences show that the different Annexins share 40–60% structural homology. Within the phylum of vertebrates the individual Annexins are highly conserved between the different species. This has led to the hypothesis that the family has evolved from gene duplications of an ancestral gene encompassing the endonexin loop motif (Crompton, 1988). Diversification of the family may then have occurred under the selection pressure to diverse on the theme of Ca^{2+}-dependent phospholipid binding.

Meanwhile the organisations of the genes of human Annexin I, II, III, V, and VI (Kovacic, 1991; Spano, 1990; Tait, 1993; Cookson, 1994; Smith, 1994) have been eluci-dated. They show an almost exact conservation of the exonic organisation. There are almost no variations in the positions of the introns-exons boundaries. Interestingly, the exon organisation does not reflect the repeat structure of the polypeptide chain. Moreover, the endonexin loop at the amino acid level is encoded by two exons. This renders the hypothesis of gene duplication somewhat difficult to reconcile.

In spite of the large amount of structural and functional information, the physiological significance of the family as a whole and the individual members in particular remains puzzling. This is not caused by a lack of hypotheses. At date the number of proposed physiological functions exceeds the number of observed *in vitro* biological activities. Amongst them is the ability of Annexins to inhibit the phospholipid dependent reactions of the coagulation cascade. This biological property and the interaction with the hemosta-tic system is described in more detail in the next sections.

Annexins in Blood Cells, Endothelial cells and the Extracellular Space

Annexin proteins are found in all human tissues and every cell type expresses at least two different members of the family. Which Annexin genes are activated and the level of the Annexin proteins depend on the genotype and environmental factors, such as the pres-ence of growth factors and hormones (Raynal and Pollard, 1994).

The cells that are circulating in the human blood also contain Annexin proteins as has been determined mostly by immunological techniques (Hirata and Iwata, 1983; Creutz, 1987; Meers, 1987; Comera, 1989; Rothhut, 1989; Flaherty, 1990; Fujimagari, 1990; Goulding, 1990; Murphy, 1992; Eldering, 1993; Ferrieres, 1994; Sjolin, 1994). Römisch and co-workers have measured the levels of Annexin I thru VI in blood cells by ELISA and Annexin specific antibodies (Römisch, 1992). The anucleated platelets and erythrocytes contain very low levels of Annexin proteins (<0.1% of total cellular protein). These low levels were also found by other groups (Flaherty, 1990; Trotter, 1994; Ferrieres, 1994). It is not yet clear whether the Annexins in platelets and erythrocytes originate from synthesis by the megakaryocyte and the erythroblast or from uptake during circulation of the anucleated cells in the blood. The nucleated blood cells contain much higher levels of Annexin proteins. Neutrophils, lymphocytes and monocytes express Annexins respectively at levels around 0.3%, 0.7% and 3.4% of their total cellular protein. The levels of the indi-vidual Annexins vary with the cell type (Table 4.1). These data suggest that the cells employ the various Annexins at different sites of the cellular machinery to accomodate dif-ferent (patho)physiological functions, which remain to be elucidated.

The endothelial cells, which interface between the blood and vascular structures, express Annexin proteins at a high level (approximately 4% of total cellular protein).

Table 4.1 Annexin Repertoire of Circulating Blood Cells and Endothelial Cells.

Cell	*Annexins (% of total amount of Annexins per cell)*					*Total Amount of Annexins (ng/10^{7}cells)*
	I+II	*III*	*IV*	*V*	*VI*	
platelet	11	16	9	64	n.d.[1]	11.4
erythrocyte	58	n.d.	12	30	n.d.	9.1
lymphocyte/monocyte	74	n.d.	1	8	16	13148
lymphocyte	81	1	1	9	8	4573
PMN[2]	36	61	2	n.d.	1	1211
HUVEC	85	1	1	12	2	115357

[1] Not Detectable.
[2] Polymorphonuclear Cells.
The data are extracted from (Römisch, 1992).

Data on Annexin expression in these cells mainly stem from studies with cultured human umbilical vein endothelial cells. These cells contain Annexin I thru VI (Raynal, 1993; Flaherty, 1990; Römisch, 1992; Table 4.1). Immunohistochemical studies have shown that *in vivo* endothelial cells from various arterial as well as venous blood vessels contain Annexin proteins also (Giambanco, 1991; Doubell, 1993; Rambotti, 1993). Interestingly, endothelial cells *in vivo* appear to have a tissue specific expression of Annexin. This has been shown for Annexin VIII, which is tissue-specifically expressed by lung endothelium (Reutelingsperger, 1994). The physiological significance of such tissue specific Annexin expression by a cell type *in vivo* remains obscure.

Annexins are found in the intracellular compartment as well as in the extracellular space. Extracellularly they have been detected in blood plasma (Flaherty, 1990; Nakao, 1990; Römisch, 1992; Uemura, 1992; van Heerde, 1994a), seminal plasma (Christmas, 1991) in peritoneal exudates (Pepinsky, 1986), in amniotic fluid (Flaherty, 1990; Nakao, 1990), in cell conditioned medium (Jacquot, 1990; Violette, 1990; Solito, 1991; Ma, 1994; Serres, 1994), and associated with the external site of the plasma membrane (Hertogs, 1993; Tressler, 1993; Yeatman, 1993; Chung, 1994; Hajjar, 1994; Kojima, 1994; Wright, 1994; Figure 4.1). The discovery of extracellular localisation created another Annexin enigma since Annexins bear none of the classic biochemical features of extracellular proteins (Raynal and Pollard, 1994): i) They are synthesized without a hydrophobic signal sequence; and ii) they have no or very low grades of glycosylation. Explanations for externalisation range from unselective events during cell injury to selective secretion by as yet unknown pathways, which may be responsible for the secretion of proteins like fibroblast growth factor and blood coagulation factor XIII. Christmas and co-workers published data indicative for selective externalisation of Annexin I (Christmas, 1991). Moreover, recent publications show that endothelial cell surface associated Annexin II fulfils a specific receptor function for proteins of the fibrinolytic pathway, indicating a physiological purpose of externalising Annexins (Hajjar, 1994). A proposed pathway for selective externalisation is the extrusion of Annexin containing microvesicles from the plasma membrane (Genge, 1989; Wu, 1991; Lee, 1993). The existence of such a route has been demonstrated for chondrocytes and fibroblasts. Endothelial cells may utilize a similar pathway to secrete Annexins, since these cells have been shown to generate microvesicles in cell culture (Ryan, 1992; Hamilton, 1990). It has also been proposed that

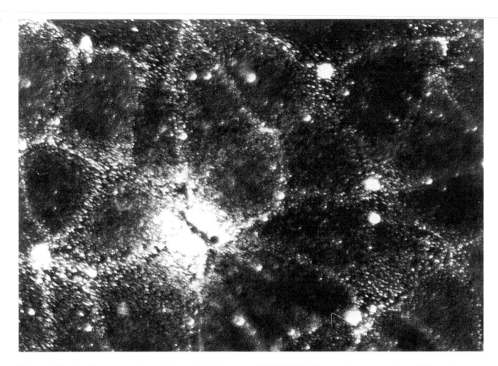

Figure 4.1 Surface expression of Annexins by cultured HUVEC. The surface expression of Annexins was assessed with confluent viable and non-fixed HUVEC by indirect immunofluorescence using the monoclonal antibody RUU-WAC11, that recognizes a common epitope of Annexins.

in vivo endothelial plasma membranes may become transiently permeable to high molecular weight constituents of the cytoplasm (Yu and McNeil, 1992). This mechanism could be responsible for the basal and elevated levels of Annexins in blood plasma of healthy people and patients, respectively. Basal levels in healthy people as measured by ELISA are in most cases less then 20 ng/ml for Annexins I thru VI (Flaherty, 1990; Nakao, 1990; Römisch, 1992; Van Heerde 1994a). Levels of Annexins III, IV and V around 100 ng/ml have been detected in plasmas of myocardial patients (Römisch, 1992). The sustained Annexin levels in these patients after infarction argue against an acute phase phenomenon and suggest active secretion of the Annexins into the blood. Elevated Annexin V has been detected in the plasmas of patients with a variety of clinical diagnoses (Flaherty, 1990; Nakao, 1990). This is not in favour of the straight forward explanation of tissue injury as the cause of externalisation. Systemic lupus erythematosus patients have elevated Annexin V levels, which in some cases go above 200 ng/ml, as measured by ELISA (Van Heerde, 1994a). Interestingly, this circulating Annexin V possesses full phospholipid binding capacity as measured by a functional assay (Van Heerde, 1994a). And hence, this circulating Annexin V has the potency to inhibit the phospholipid dependent reactions of the hemostatic system (see the next section). The circulating Annexin does not possess in all cases full phospholipid binding capacity as has been shown for Annexin I, the antigen levels of which are similar in serum and EDTA plasma (Uemura, 1992).

Circulating Annexins, which have lost their phospholipid binding property, may be considered as irrelevant to the phospholipid dependent part of the hemostatic system.

The Interaction of Annexins with the Hemostatic System

Annexin V was first described as a protein of the human umbilical arterial wall, that inhibits strongly the phospholipid dependent activation of prothrombin by factors Xa and Va (Reutelingsperger, 1985). The mechanism of its anticoagulant action is based on the high affinity binding to the procoagulant phosphatidylserine (Tait, 1989; Andree, 1990). This binding results in a shielding of the phospholipid surface such that the phospholipid dependent procoagulant complexes fail to assemble functionally on it (Reutelingsperger, 1988; Tait, 1988; Andree, 1992). Considering the role of phospholipids in hemostasis (Mann, 1990; Esmon, 1993) it is without surprise that this mechanism of action makes Annexin V not only an inhibitor of the phospholipid dependent enzyme complexes factors IXa/VIIIa and Xa/Va (Funakoshi, 1987; Maurer-Fogy, 1988; Tait, 1989; Römisch, 1990a; Rao, 1992; Van Heerde, 1994b) but also an inhibitor of the phospholipid dependent part of the protein C anticoagulant pathway (Freyssinet, 1991; Sun, 1993a).

The initial data on its phospholipid binding properties and its anticoagulant action were obtained by *in vitro* studies employing synthetic phospholipids. It is believed that *in vivo* endothelial cells and activated platelets form the principle source for supplying a phospholipid surface, that catalyzes the propagation and amplification of the biochemical signal, that results in thrombin formation (Esmon, 1993; Zwaal, 1992; Walsh, 1994; Kirchhofer, 1994; Chapter 9 of this book). Other blood cells like monocytes (Robinson, 1992) and neutrophils (Fadok, 1992) may under certain conditions generate procoagulant surfaces as well.

Binding studies have shown that Annexin V not only binds to synthetic phospholipids but also to biological surfaces. Binding is observed to activated platelets (Thiagarajan and Tait, 1990; Dachary, 1993; Sun, 1993b), stimulated monocytes (Römisch, 1990a), ageing erythrocytes (Tait and Gibson, 1994a), apoptotic lymphocytes and neutrophils (Koopman, 1994; Homburg), endothelial cells in culture (Van Heerde, 1994b) and extracellular matrix of cultured endothelial cells (Van Heerde, 1994c). Binding to these cells resembles binding to synthetic phospholipid surfaces in that it requires Ca^{2+}-ions and is fully reversible. However, the observed dissociation constants for binding to cells (k_d is in the nM range) is at least one order of magnitude higher compared to the dissociation constants for binding to synthetic phospholipid surfaces (Tait, 1989; Andree, 1990). This discrepancy in binding behaviour is not explained as yet. Interestingly, the binding of Annexin V to the circulating blood cells is not a constitutively expressed property of these cells but is an acquired one. Endothelial cells in culture on the other hand bind significant amounts of Annexin V under quiescent and unperturbed conditions. Activation and perturbation do not result in a measurable increase of the number of binding sites (Van Heerde, 1994b). Whether this property of endothelial cells to bind Annexin V in a quiescent state reflects the *in vivo* situation or results from the culture conditions needs to be further investigated.

The circulating blood cells neither bind significant amounts of Annexin V nor catalyze procoagulant reactions under quiescent and unperturbed conditions. Activation and/or perturbation of the cells are required to expose Annexin V binding sites and to generate procoagulant catalytic activity (Thiagarajan, 1991; Dachary, 1993; Sun, 1993b; Koopman, 1994; Homburg; Reutelingsperger unpublished results).

In addition to the close correlation between Annexin V binding and the catalytic capacity of the cell, Annexin V inhibits the tenase and prothrombinase complexes, that are assembled on these cells (Römisch, 1990; Thiagarajan 1991; Rao, 1992; Ravanat, 1992; Schoen, 1992; Almus, 1993; Van Heerde 1994b). Moreover, the IC_{50} values of Annexin V for the various reactions correlate nicely with the k_d of binding to the cell (Andree, 1992; Van Heerde 1994b). All these data strongly suggest that Annexin V binds to sites at the cellular surface, that exhibit catalytic activity for the phospholipid dependent procoagulant reactions, and that the mechanism of Annexin V mediated anticoagulation in a cellular system is identical to its anticoagulant mechanism as elucidated for the synthetic phospholipid system (see above). In addition to its action on tenase and prothrombinase, Annexin V can also inhibit the Tissue Factor/VIIa complex (Kondo, 1987; Gramziski, 1989; Andree, 1994; Van Heerde 1994b). This complex involves membrane structures somewhat differently. This probably causes the observed differential effects of Annexin V on Tissue Factor/VIIa activity in various systems (Kondo, 1987; Rao, 1992; Ravanat, 1992; Almus, 1993; Van Heerde 1994b). These differences can be explained by differences in the ratio of Tissue Factor and negatively charged phospholipids (Andree, 1994).

The studies mentioned sofar in this section show that Annexin V is an inhibitor of procoagulant and anticoagulant reactions in *in vitro* systems involving model membranes as well as cells. *In vivo* exogenously added Annexin V appears to be a potent antithrombotic compound in various animal thrombosis models (Römisch 1991; Chollet, 1992; Van Ryn-McKenna, 1993). Annexin V, that enters the blood stream, likely binds to cells, that have the potency to catalyze procoagulant reactions. These cells are present in an intravascular thrombus (Tait, 1994b). Bound Annexin V prevents the assembly of functional procoagulant processes on these surfaces and inhibits thereby the localised generation of thrombin. The results of the *in vivo* studies suggest that in a situation of ongoing thrombus formation, the action of Annexin V on the procoagulant arm dominates its action on the anticoagulant arm of the hemostatic system.

Whether the other Annexins exhibit similar antithrombotic properties *in vivo* is not known as yet. The anticoagulant and antithrombotic action of Annexin V is based on its phospholipid binding property, which is common to all Annexins. Accordingly, all Annexins exhibit anticoagulant activities *in vitro* (Chap, 1988; Tait, 1988; Hauptmann, 1989; Römisch, 1990b; Römisch and Heimburger, 1990; Yoshizaki, 1992; Cirino and Cicala, 1993). But Annexin V appears to be the most potent anticoagulant within the Annexin family. Differential behaviour of the various Annexins in the extracellular blood compartment *in vivo* has to be expected and is indicated by the findings that Annexin I binds specifically to quiescent monocytes and neutrophils and that this binding is lost during a perturbing state of disease, which contrasts Annexin V binding to these cells (Goulding, 1992; Perretti, 1993; Reutelingsperger unpublished results).

The (patho)physiological significance of Annexins to the hemostatic system

To date the number of postulated physiological functions of Annexins equals or exceeds the number of discovered *in vitro* biological activities. The individual Annexin can exhibit various biological activities (Raynal and Pollard, 1994). The search for the true physiological role tends to centre around one specific biological activity per Annexin. This may be too restricting and perhaps one should consider its true physiological significance as a function of its spatiotemporal coördinates in the organism.

Annexins, that are present in the extracellular compartment of the blood and still posses phospholipid binding capacity, inhibit coagulation and consequently thrombus formation. There are two compelling aspects of Annexin interaction with the hemostatic system: i) The anticoagulant action is localised to the sites of injury; And ii) the efficacy of the anticogulant action is determined by the balance between Annexin concentration and amounts of exposed procoagulant phospholipid. Studies with Annexin V indicate that these aspects translate *in vivo* in inhibition of intravascular thrombus formation without a concomitant risk of bleeding.

From this point of view extracellular Annexins with phospholipid binding properties have (patho)physiological significance to the hemostatic system. The major question now concentrates on how and when do Annexins enter functionally the extracellular space. Elevated levels of Annexins have been observed in the plasmas of patients with various clinical diagnoses. These Annexins can be functional or not in respect to phospholipid binding. No data exist as yet that allow correlation between disease and the level of functional Annexins. The circulating nucleated blood cells and the endothelial cells are the most likely sources for these extracellular Annexins. But it is still unclear via which routes these cells externalise Annexins and how the process of externalisation is influenced, if at all, by an activated hemostatic system.

A recent study unravels Annexin II as a constitutively expressed protein on the surface of endothelial cells in culture. It appears to be a cryptic receptor for tPA and plasminogen. It is hypothesized that limited proteolytic action, by e.g. plasmin, activates Annexin II to function as a catalyst for the cleavage of plasminogen by tPA (Cesarman, 1994; Hajjar, 1994). This opens new and stimulating avenues for the interaction of extracellular Annexins with vascular hemostasis.

References

Almus, F.E., Rao, L.V. and Rapaport, S.I. (1993). Regulation of factor VIIa/tissue factor functional activity in an umbilical vein model. *Arteriosclerosis and Thrombosis*, **13**:105–111.

Andree, H.A., Reutelingsperger, C.P.M., Hauptmann, R., Hemker, H.C., Hermens, W.T. and Willems, G.M. (1990). Binding of vascular anticoagulant alpha (VAC alpha) to planar phospholipid bilayers. *Journal of Biological Chemistry*, **265**:4923–4928.

Andree, H.A., Stuart, M.C., Hermens, W.T., Reutelingsperger, C.P.M., Hemker, H.C., Frederik, P.M. and Willems, G.M. (1992). Clustering of lipid-bound annexin V may explain its anticoagulant effect. *Journal of Biological Chemistry*, **267**:17907–17912.

Andree, H.A.M., Contino, P.B., Repke, D., Gentry, R. and Nemerson, Y. (1994). Transport Rate Limited Catalysis on Macroscopic Surfaces — The Activation of Factor-X in a Continuous Flow Enzyme Reactor. *Biochemistry*, **33**:4368–4374.

Cesarman, G.M., Guevara, C.A. and Hajjar, K.A. (1994). An endothelial cell receptor for plasminogen/tissue plasminogen activator (t-PA). 2. Annexin II-mediated enhancement of t-PA-dependent plasminogen activation. *Journal of Biological Chemistry*, **269**: 21198–21203.

Chap, H., Comfurius, P., Bevers, E.M., Fauvel, J., Vicendo, P., Douste, B.L. and Zwaal, R.F. (1988). Potential anticoagulant activity of lipocortins and other calcium/phospholipid binding proteins. *Biochemical Biophysical Research Communication*, **150**:972–978.

Chollet, P., Malecaze, F., Hullin, F., Raynal, P., Arne, J.L., Pagot, V., Ragab, T.J. and Chap, H. (1992). Inhibition of intraocular fibrin formation with annexin V. *British Journal of Ophthalmology*, **76**:450–452.

Christmas, P., Callaway, J., Fallon, J., Jones, J. and Haigler, H.T. (1991). Selective secretion of annexin 1, a protein without a signal sequence, by the human prostate gland. *Journal of Biological Chemistry*, **266**:2499–2507.

Chung, C.Y. and Erickson, H.P. (1994). Cell surface annexin II is a high affinity receptor for the alternatively spliced segment of tenascin-C. *Journal of Cell Biology*, **126**:539–548.

Cirino, G. and Cicala, C. (1993). Human recombinant lipocortin 1 (annexin 1) has anticoagulant activity on human plasma in vitro. *Journal of Lipid Mediators*, **8**:81–86.

Comera, C., Rothhut, B., Cavadore, J.C., Vilgrain, I., Cochet, C., Chambaz, E. and Russo, M.F. (1989). Further characterization of four lipocortins from human peripheral blood mononuclear cells. *Journal of Cellular Biochemistry*, **40**:361–370.

Cookson, B.T., Engelhardt, S., Smith, C., Bamford, H.A., Prochazka, M. and Tait, J.F. (1994). Organization of the Human Annexin V (Anx5) Gene. *Genomics*, **20**:463–467.

Creutz, C.E., Zaks, W.J., Hamman, H.C., Crane, S., Martin, W.H., Gould, K.L., Oddie, K.M. and Parsons, S.J. (1987). Identification of chromaffin granule-binding proteins. Relationship of the chromobindins to calelectrin, synhibin, and the tyrosine kinase substrates p35 and p36. *Journal of Biological Chemistry*, **262**:1860–1868.

Creutz, C.E. (1992). The annexins and exocytosis. *Science*, **258**:924–931.

Crompton, M.R., Moss, S.E. and Crumpton, M.J. (1988). Diversity in the lipocortin/calpactin family. *Cell*, **55**:1–3.

Dachary, P.J., Freyssinet, J.M., Pasquet, J.M., Carron, J.C. and Nurden, A.T. (1993). Annexin V as a probe of aminophospholipid exposure and platelet membrane vesiculation: a flow cytometry study showing a role for free sulfhydryl groups. *Blood*, **81**:2554–2565.

Doubell, A.F., Lazure, C., Charbonneau, C. and Thibault, G. (1993). Identification and immunolocalisation of annexins V and VI, the major cardiac annexins, in rat heart. *Cardiovascular Research*, **27**:1359–1367.

Eldering, J.A., Kocher, M., Clemetson, J.M., Clemetson, K.J., Frey, F.J. and Frey, B.M. (1993). Presence of lipocortins I and IV, but not II and VI, in human platelets. *Febs Letters*, **318**:231–234.

Esmon, C.T. (1993). Cell mediated events that control blood coagulation and vascular injury. *Annual Review of Cell Biology*, **9**:1–26.

Fadok, V.A., Savill, J.S., Haslett, C., Bratton, D.L., Doherty, D.E., Campbell, P.A. and Henson, P.M. (1992). Different populations of macrophages use either the vitronectin receptor or the phosphatidylserine receptor to recognize and remove apoptotic cells. *Journal of Immunology*, I **149**, 4029–4035.

Ferrieres, J., Simon, M.F., Fauvel, J. and Chap, H. (1994). Virtual lack of annexins in human platelets argues against a role in phospholipase A(2), regulation and platelet secretion. *Journal of Lipid Mediators and Cell Signalling*, **9**:155–165.

Flaherty, M.J., West, S., Heimark, R.L., Fujikawa, K. and Tait, J.F. (1990). Placental anticoagulant protein-I: measurement in extracellular fluids and cells of the hemostatic system. *Journal of Laboratory and Clinical Medicine*, **115**:174–181.

Freyssinet, J.M., Toti, O.F., Ravanat, C., Grunebaum, L., Gauchy, J., Cazenave, J.P. and Wiesel, M.L. (1991). The catalytic role of anionic phospholipids in the activation of protein C by factor X_a and expression of its anticoagulant function in human plasma. *Blood Coagulation and Fibrinolysis*, **2**:691–698.

Fujimagari, M., Williamson, P.L. and Schlegel, R.A. (1990) Ca2(+)-dependent membrane-binding proteins in normal erythrocytes and erythrocytes from patients with chronic myelogenous leukemia. *Blood*, **75**:1337–1345.

Funakoshi, T., Heimark, R.L., Hendrickson, L.E., McMullen, B.A. and Fujikawa, K. (1987). Human placental anticoagulant protein: isolation and characterization. *Biochemistry*, **26**:5572–5578.

Geisow, M.J., Fritsche, U., Hexham, J.M., Dash, B. and Johnson, T. (1986). A consensus amino-acid sequence repeat in Torpedo and mammalian Ca^{2+}-dependent membrane-binding proteins. *Nature*, **320**:636–638.

Genge, B.R., Wu, L.N. and Wuthier, R.E. (1989). Identification of phospholipid-dependent calcium-binding proteins as constituents of matrix vesicles. *Journal of Biological Chemistry*, **264**:10917–10921.

Giambanco, I., Pula, G., Ceccarelli, P., Bianchi, R. and Donato, R. (1991). Immunohistochemical localization of annexin V (CaBP33) in rat organs. *Journal of Histochemistry and Cytochemistry*, **39**:1189–1198.

Goulding, N.J., Godolphin, J.L., Sharland, P.R., Peers, S.H., Sampson, M., Maddison, P.J. and Flower, R.J. (1990). Anti-inflammatory lipocortin 1 production by peripheral blood leucocytes in response to hydrocortisone. *Lancet*, **335**:1416–1418.

Goulding, N.J., Jefferiss, C.M., Pan, L., Rigby, W.F. and Guyre, P.M. (1992). Specific binding of lipocortin-1 (annexin I) to monocytes and neutrophils is decreased in rheumatoid arthritis. *Arthritis and Rheumatology*, **35**:1395–1397.

Gramzinski, R.A., Broze, G.J. and Carson, S.D. (1989). Human fibroblast tissue factor is inhibited by lipoprotein-associated coagulation inhibitor and placental anticoagulant protein but not by apolipoprotein A-II. *Blood*, **73**:983–9.

Hajjar, K.A., Jacovina, A.T. and Chacko, J. (1994). An endothelial cell receptor for plasminogen tissue plasminogen activator. 1. Identity with annexin II. *Journal of Biological Chemistry*, **269**:21191–21197.

Hamilton, K.K., Hattori, R., Esmon, C.T. and Sims, P.J. (1990). Complement proteins C5b-9 induce vesiculation of the endothelial plasma membrane and expose catalytic surface for assembly of the prothrombinase enzyme complex. *Journal of Biological Chemistry*, **265**:3809–3814.

Hauptmann, R., Maurer, F.I., Krystek, E., Bodo, G., Andree, H. and Reutelingsperger, C.P. (1989). Vascular anticoagulant beta: a novel human Ca^{2+}/phospholipid binding protein that inhibits coagulation and phospholipase A2 activity. Its molecular cloning, expression and comparison with VAC-alpha. *European Journal of Biochemistry*, **185**:63–71.

Hertogs, K., Leenders, W.P., Depla, E., De, B.W., Meheus, L., Raymackers, J., Moshage, H. and Yap, S.H. (1993). Endonexin II, present on human liver plasma membranes, is a specific binding protein of small hepatitis B virus (HBV) envelope protein. *Virology*, **197**:549–557.

Hirata, F. and Iwata, M. (1983). Role of lipomodulin, a phospholipase inhibitory protein, in immunoregulation by thymocytes. *Journal of Immunology*, **130**:1930–1936.

Homburg, H.E., de Haas, M., von dem Borne, A.E.G.Kr., Verhoeven, A.J., Reutelingsperger, C.P.M. and Roos, D. (1995). Human neutrophils lose their surface FcγRIII and acquire Annexin V binding sites during apoptosis *in vitro*. *Blood*, **85**:532–540.

Huber, R., Schneider, M., Mayr, I., Römisch, J. and Paques, E.P. (1990). The calcium binding sites in human annexin V by crystal structure analysis at 2.0 A resolution. Implications for membrane binding and calcium channel activity. *Febs Letters*, **275**:15–21.

Jacquot, J., Dupuit, F., Elbtaouri, H., Hinnrasky, J., Antonicelli, F., Haye, B. and Puchelle, E. (1990). Production of lipocortin-like proteins by cultured human tracheal submucosal gland cells. *Febs Letters*, **274**:131–135.

Johnston, P.A., Perin, M.S., Reynolds, G.A., Wasserman, S.A. and Sudhof, T.C. (1990). Two novel annexins from Drosophila melanogaster. Cloning, characterization, and differential expression in development. *Journal of Biological Chemistry*, **265**:11382–11388.

Kirchhofer, D., Tschopp, T.B., Hadvary, P. and Baumgartner, H. (1994). Endothelial cells stimulated with tumor necrosis factor-a express varying amounts of tissue factor resulting in inhomogenous fibrin deposition in a native blood flow system. *Journal of Clinical Investigations*, **93**:2073–2083.

Klee, C.B. (1988). Ca^{2+}-dependent phospholipid- (and membrane-) binding proteins. *Biochemistry*, **27**:6645–6653.

Kojima, K., Utsumi, H., Ogawa, H. and Matsumoto, I. (1994). Highly Polarized Expression of Carbohydrate-Binding Protein P33/41 (Annexin IV) on the Apical Plasma Membrane of Epithelial Cells in Renal Proximal Tubules. *Febs Letters*, **342**:313–318.

Kondo, S., Noguchi, M., Funakoshi, T., Fujikawa, K. and Kisiel, W. (1987). Inhibition of human factor VIIa-tissue factor activity by placental anticoagulant protein. *Thrombosis Research*, **48**:449–459.

Koopman, G., Reutelingsperger, C.P.M., Kuijten, G.A.M., Keehnen, R.M.J., Pals, S.T. and Vanoers, M.H.J. (1994). Annexin V for flow cytometric detection of phosphatidylserine expression on B cells undergoing apoptosis. *Blood*, **84**:1415–1420.

Kovacic, R.T., Tizard, R., Cate, R.L., Frey, A.Z. and Wallner, B.P. (1991). Correlation of gene and protein structure of rat and human lipocortin I. *Biochemistry*, **30**:9015–9021.

Lee, T.L., Lin, Y.C., Mochitate, K. and Grinnell, F. (1993). Stress-relaxation of fibroblasts in collagen matrices triggers ectocytosis of plasma membrane vesicles containing actin, annexins II and VI, and beta 1 integrin receptors. *Journal of Cell Science*, **105**:167–177.

Ma, A.S.P., Bell, D.J., Mittal, A.A. and Harrison, H.H. (1994). Immunocytochemical detection of extracellular annexin II in cultured human skin keratinocytes and isolation of annexin II isoforms enriched in the extracellular pool. *Journal of Cell Science*, **107**:1973–1984.

Mann, K.G., Nesheim, M.E., Church, W.R., Haley, P. and Krishnaswamy, S. (1990). Surface-dependent reactions of the vitamin K-dependent enzyme complexes. *Blood*, **76**:1–16.

Maurer-Fogy, I., Reutelingsperger, C.P.M., Pieters, J., Bodo, G., Stratowa, C. and Hauptmann, R. (1988). Cloning and expression of cDNA for human vascular anticoagulant, a Ca^{2+}-dependent phospholipid-binding protein. *European Journal of Biochemistry*, **174**:585–592.

Meers, P., Ernst, J.D., Duzgunes, N., Hong, K.L., Fedor, J., Goldstein, I.M. and Papahadjopoulos, D. (1987). Synexin-like proteins from human polymorphonuclear leukocytes. Identification and characterization of granule-aggregating and membrane-fusing activities. *Journal of Biological Chemistry*, **262**:7850–7858.

Murphy, C.T., Peers, S.H., Forder, R.A., Flower, R.J., Carey, F. and Westwick, J. (1992). Evidence for the presence and location of annexins in human platelets. *Biochemical Biophysical Research Communication*, **189**:1739–1746.

Nakao, H., Nagoya, T., Iwasaki, A., Suda, M., Hattori, Y., Saino, Y., Shidara, Y. and Maki, M. (1990). An enzyme-linked immunosorbent assay system for quantitative determination of calphobindin I, a new placental anticoagulant protein, and its application to various specimens. *Chemical and Pharmaceutical Bulletin Tokyo*, **38**:1957–1960.

Perretti, M., Flower, R.J. and Goulding, N.J. (1993). The ability of murine leukocytes to bind lipocortin 1 is lost during acute inflammation. *Biochemical Biophysical Research Communication*, **192**:345–350.

Pepinsky, R.B., Sinclair, L.K., Browning, J.L., Mattaliano, R.J., Smart, J.E., Chow, E.P., Falbel, T., Ribolini, A., Garwin, J.L. and Wallner, B.P. (1986). Purification and partial sequence analysis of a 37-kDa protein that inhibits phospholipase A2 activity from rat peritoneal exudates. *Journal of Biological Chemistry*, **261**:4239–4246.

Rambotti, M.G., Spreca, A. and Donato, R. (1993). Immunocytochemical Localization of Annexins-V and Annexins-VI in Human Placentae of Different Gestational Ages. *Cellular and Molecular Biology Research*, **39**:579–588.

Rao, L.V., Tait, J.F. and Hoang, A.D. (1992). Binding of annexin V to a human ovarian carcinoma cell line (OC–2008). Contrasting effects on cell surface factor VIIa/tissue factor activity and prothrombinase activity. *Thrombosis Research*, **67**:517–531.

Ravanat, C., Archipoff, G., Beretz, A., Freund, G., Cazenave, J.P. and Freyssinet, J.M. (1992). Use of annexin-V to demonstrate the role of phosphatidylserine exposure in the maintenance of haemostatic balance by endothelial cells. *Biochemical Journal*, **282**:7–13.

Raynal, P., Hullin, F., Ragab, T.J., Fauvel, J. and Chap, H. (1993). Annexin 5 as a potential regulator of annexin 1 phosphorylation by protein kinase C. In vitro inhibition compared with quantitative data on annexin distribution in human endothelial cells. *Biochemical Journal*, **292**:759–765.

Raynal, P. and Pollard, H.B. (1994). Annexins: the problem of assessing the biological role for a gene family of multifunctional calcium- and phospholipid-binding proteins. *Biochimica et Biophysica Acta*, **1197**:63–93.

Reutelingsperger, C.P.M., Hornstra, G. and Hemker, H.C. (1985). Isolation and partial purification of a novel anticoagulant from arteries of human umbilical cord. *European Journal of Biochemistry*, **151**:625–629.

Reutelingsperger, C.P.M., Kop, J.M., Hornstra, G. and Hemker, H.C. (1988). Purification and characterization of a novel protein from bovine aorta that inhibits coagulation. Inhibition of the phospholipid-dependent factor-Xa-catalyzed prothrombin activation, through a high-affinity binding of the anticoagulant to the phospholipids. *European Journal of Biochemistry*, **173**:171–178.

Reutelingsperger, C.P.M., Vanheerde, W., Hauptmann, R., Maassen, C., Vangool, R.G.J., Deleeuw, P. and Tiebosch, A. (1994). Differential tissue expression of Annexin VIII in human. *Febs Letters*, **349**:120–124.

Robitzki, A., Schroder, H.C., Ugarkovic, D., Gramzow, M., Fritsche, U., Batel, R. and Muller, W.E. (1990). cDNA structure and expression of calpactin, a peptide involved in Ca2(+)-dependent cell aggregation in sponges. *Biochemical Journal*, **271**:415–420.

Robinson, R.A., Worfolk, L. and Tracy, P.B. (1992). Endotoxin enhances the expression of monocyte prothrombinase activity. *Blood* , **79**:406–416.

Römisch, J., Schorlemmer, U., Fickenscher, K., Paques, E.P. and Heimburger, N. (1990a). Anticoagulant properties of placenta protein 4 (annexin V). *Thrombosis Research*, **60**:355–366.

Römisch, J., Grote, M., Weithmann, K.U., Heimburger, N. and Amann, E. (1990b). Annexin proteins PP4 and PP4-X. Comparative characterization of biological activities of placental and recombinant proteins. *Biochemical Journal*, **272**:223–229.

Römisch, J. and Heimburger, N. (1990). Purification and characterization of six annexins from human placenta. *Biological and Chemical Hoppe Seyler*, **371**:383–388.

Römisch, J., Seiffge, D., Reiner, G., Paques, E.P. and Heimburger, N. (1991). *In-vivo* antithrombotic potency of placenta protein 4 (annexin V). *Thrombosis Research*, **61**:93–104.

Römisch, J., Schuler, E., Bastian, B., Burger, T., Dunkel, F.G., Schwinn, A., Hartmann, A.A. and Paques, E.P. (1992). Annexins I to VI: quantitative determination in different human cell types and in plasma after myocardial infarction. *Blood Coagulation and Fibrinolysis*, **3**:11–17.

Rothhut, B., Comera, C., Cortial, S., Haumont, P.Y., Diep, L.K., Cavadore, J.C., Conard, J., Russo, M.F. and Lederer, F. (1989). A 32 kDa lipocortin from human mononuclear cells appears to be identical with the placental inhibitor of blood coagulation. *Biochemical Journal*, **263**:929–935.

Ryan, J., Brett, J., Tijburg, P., Bach, R.R., Kisiel, W. and Stern, D. (1992). Tumor necrosis factor-induced endothelial tissue factor is associated with subendothelial matrix vesicles but is not expressed on the apical surface. *Blood*, **80**:966–974.

Schlaepfer, D.D., Fisher, D.A., Brandt, M.E., Bode, H.R., Jones, J.M. and Haigler, H.T. (1992). Identification of a novel annexin in Hydra vulgaris. Characterization, cDNA cloning, and protein kinase C phosphorylation of annexin XII. *Journal of Biological Chemistry*, **267**:9529–9539.

Schoen, P., Reutelingsperger, C.P.M. and Lindhout, T. (1992). Activation of prothrombin in the presence of human umbilical-vein endothelial cells. *Biochemical Journal*, **3**:661–664.

Serres, M., Comera, C. and Schmitt, D. (1994). Annexin I regulation in human epidermal cells. *Cellular and Molecular Biology*, **40**:701–706.

Sjolin, C., Stendahl, O. and Dahlgren, C. (1994). Calcium-induced translocation of annexins to subcellular organelles of human neutrophils. *Biochemical Journal*, **300**:325–330.

Smith, P.D., Davies, A., Crumpton, M.J. and Moss, S.E. (1994). Structure of the Human Annexin-VI Gene. *Proceedings of the National Academy of Sciences of the United States of America*, **91**:2713–2717.

Solito, E., Raugei, G., Melli, M. and Parente, L. (1991). Dexamethasone induces the expression of the mRNA of lipocortin 1 and 2 and the release of lipocortin 1 and 5 in differentiated, but not undifferentiated U-937 cells. *Febs Letters*, **291**:238–244.

Spano, F., Raugei, G., Palla, E., Colella, C. and Melli, M. (1990). Characterization of the human lipocortin-2-encoding multigene family: its structure suggests the existence of a short amino acid unit undergoing duplication. *Gene*, **95**:243–251.

Sun, J., Bird, P. and Salem, H.H. (1993a). Effects of annexin V on the activity of the anticoagulant proteins C and S. *Thrombosis Research*, **69**:279–287.

Sun, J., Bird, P. and Salem, H.H. (1993b). Interaction of annexin V and platelets: effects on platelet function and protein S binding. *Thrombosis Research*, **69**:289–296.

Swairjo, M.A. and Seaton, B.A. (1994). Annexin structure and membrane interactions: A molecular perspective. *Annual Review of Biophysics and Biomolecular Structure*, **23**:193–213.

Tait, J.F., Sakata, M., McMullen, B.A., Miao, C.H., Funakoshi, T., Hendrickson, L.E. and Fujikawa, K. (1988). Placental anticoagulant proteins: isolation and comparative characterization four members of the lipocortin family. *Biochemistry*, **27**:6268–6276.

Tait, J.F., Gibson, D. and Fujikawa, K. (1989). Phospholipid binding properties of human placental anticoagulant protein-I, a member of the lipocortin family. *Journal of Biological Chemistry*, **264**:7944–7949.

Tait, J.F., Smith, C., Xu, L. and Cookson, B.T. (1993). Structure and polymorphisms of the human annexin III (ANX3) gene. *Genomics*,**18**: 79–86.

Tait, J.F. and Gibson, D. (1994a). Measurement of membrane phospholipid asymmetry in normal and sickle-cell erythrocytes by means of annexin V binding. *Journal of Laboratory and Clinical Medicine*, **123**:741–748.

Tait, J.F., Cerqueira, M.D., Dewhurst, T.A., Fujikawa, K., Ritchie, J.L. and Stratton, J.R. (1994b). Evaluation on annexin V as a platelet-directed thrombus targeting agent. *Thrombosis Research*, **75**:491–501.

Thiagarajan, P. and Tait, J.F. (1990). Binding of annexin V/placental anticoagulant protein I to platelets. Evidence for phosphatidylserine exposure in the procoagulant response of activated platelets. *Journal of Biological Chemistry*, **265**:17420–17423.

Thiagarajan, P. and Tait, J.F. (1991). Collagen-induced exposure of anionic phospholipid in platelets and platelet-derived microparticles. *Journal of Biological Chemistry*, **266**:24302–24307.

Tressler, R.J., Updyke, T.V., Yeatman, T. and Nicolson, G.L. (1993). Extracellular annexin II is associated with divalent cation-dependent tumor cell-endothelial cell adhesion of metastatic RAW117 large-cell lymphoma cells. *Journal of Cellular Biochemistry*, **53**:265–276.

Trotter, P.J., Orchard, M.A. and Walker, J.H. (1994). Thrombin stimulates the intracellular relocation of annexin V in human platelets. *Biochimica et Biophysica Acta — Molecular Cell Research*, **1222**:135–140.

Uemura, K., Inagaki, H., Wada, Y., Nakanishi, K., Asai, K., Kato, T., Ando, Y. and Kannagi, R. (1992). Identification of immuno-reactive lipocortin 1-like molecules in serum and plasma by an enzyme immunoassay for lipocortin 1. *Biochimica et Biophysica Acta*, **1119**:250–255.

Van Ryn-McKenna, J., Merk, H., Muller, T.H., Buchanan, M.R. and Eisert, W.G. (1993). The effects of heparin and annexin V on fibrin accretion after injury in the jugular veins of rabbits. *Thrombosis and Haemostasis*, **69**:227–230.

Van Heerde. (1994a). Annexin V. Localization, plasma levels and anticoagulant properties. Thesis, University of Utrecht.

Van Heerde, W.L., Poort, S., Vantveer, C., Reutelingsperger, C.P.M. and Degroot, P.G. (1994b). Binding of recombinant annexin V to endothelial cells: Effect of annexin V binding on endothelial-cell-mediated thrombin formation. *Biochemical Journal*, **302**:305–312.

Van Heerde, W.L., Sakariassen, K.S., Hemker, H.C., Sixma, J.J., Reutelingsperger, C.P.M. and Degroot, P.G. (1994c). Annexin V inhibits the procoagulant activity of matrices of TNF-stimulated endothelium under blood flow conditions. *Arteriosclerosis and Thrombosis*, **14**:824–830.

Violette, S.M., King, I., Browning, J.L., Pepinsky, R.B., Wallner, B.P. and Sartorelli, A.C. (1990). Role of lipocortin I in the glucocorticoid induction of the terminal differentiation of a human squamous carcinoma. *Journal of Cellular Physiology*, **142**:70–77.

Walsh, P.N. (1994). Platelet-Coagulant protein interactions. In *Haemostasis and Thrombosis*, 3rd edn, R.W. Colman, J. Hirsch, V.J. Marder and E.W. Salzman (eds.), pp. 629-651. Philadelphia: J.B. Lippincot Company.

Wright, J.F., Kurosky, A. and Wasi, S. (1994). An Endothelial Cell-Surface Form of Annexin II Binds Human Cytomegalovirus. *Biochemical and Biophysical Research Communications*, **198**:983–989.

Wu, L.N., Genge, B.R., Lloyd, G.C. and Wuthier, R.E. (1991). Collagen-binding proteins in collagenase-released matrix vesicles from cartilage. Interaction between matrix vesicle proteins and different types of collagen. *Journal of Biological Chemistry*, **266**:1195–1203.

Yeatman, T.J., Updyke, T.V., Kaetzel, M.A., Dedman, J.R. and Nicolson, G.L. (1993). Expression of annexins on the surfaces of non-metastatic and metastatic human and rodent tumor cells. *Clinical and Experimental Metastasis*, **11**:37–44.

Yoshizaki, H., Tanabe, S., Arai, K., Murakami, A., Wada, Y., Ohkuchi, M., Hashimoto, Y. and Maki, M. (1992). Effects of calphobindin II (annexin VI) on procoagulant and anticoagulant activities of cultured endothelial cells. *Chemical and Pharmaceutical Bull Tokyo*, **40**:1860–1863.

Yu, Q.C. and McNeil, P.L. (1992). Transient disruptions of aortic endothelial cell plasma membranes. *American Journal of Pathology*, **141**:1349–1360.

Zwaal, R.F.A., Comfurius, P. and Bevers, E. (1992). Platelet procoagulant activity and microvesicle formation. Its putative role in hemostasis and thrombosis. *Biochimica et Biophysica Acta*, **1180**:1–8.

5 Vessel Wall Mediated Activation of the Blood Coagulation System

Herm-Jan M. Brinkman and Jan A. van Mourik

Department of Blood Coagulation, Central Laboratory of the Netherlands Red Cross Blood Transfusion Service, The Netherlands

1. INTRODUCTION

Hemostasis is classically described as a delicate and co-ordinate interaction between platelets, the humoral coagulation system, and procoagulant constituents of the vessel wall. Upon vessel wall damage the coagulation system is triggered by tissue factor, expressed by perivascular cells such as smooth muscle cells and fibroblasts. Simultaneously platelets adhere and aggregate at sites of injury and, by translocation of negatively charged phospholipids from the inner leaflet to the outer leaflet of the plasma membrane, expose a procoagulant surface. This procoagulant surface participates in a number of activation steps within the coagulation cascade (Figure 5.1), ultimately leading to the formation of thrombin, the enzyme which converts soluble fibrinogen into an insoluble fibrin network. There is little doubt that these events serve an essential role in preventing excessive extravasation of blood after vascular injury. Experiments of nature, including observations from studies on the pathophysiology and molecular basis of both inherited or acquired platelet abnormalities and coagulation factor deficiencies, provide ample evidence that this view is correct.

Although less well understood, accumulated data indicate that also the endothelium, the anticoagulant lining of the vasculature (for a review, see elsewhere in this book), could participate in the regulation and amplification of the primary hemostatic response. At the plasma membrane of the endothelial cell coagulation factors may assemble, a process which could provide a mechanism for localization of the coagulation reaction at sites requiring a hemostatic response. In this review we will focus on two questions: 1, are endothelial cells unique in this respect or are the coagulant properties of these cells common features for perivascular cells as well, and 2, what is the mechanism underlying the procoagulant properties of the endothelium. Finally, we will speculate about the physiological role of the endothelial cell-mediated coagulation response, one of the major questions that remains to be answered.

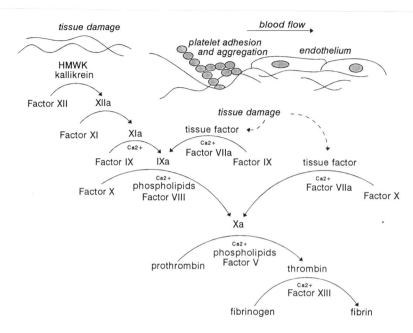

Figure 5.1 Simplified scheme of the blood coagulation system. Damage of the vascular wall leads to the exposure of tissue factor and other, as yet unidentified procoagulant molecules, which trigger the coagulation cascade. This process eventually leads to the formation of thrombin, which subsequently catalyses the conversion of fibrinogen into fibrin.

2. THE ENDOTHELIUM, A PROCOAGULANT BLOOD-TISSUE INTERFACE

Hemostasis requires a rapid and localized generation of thrombin. Conversion of coagulation factor X into its enzymatically active form, factor Xa, is a key event in this process. It is well established that biological membranes essentially participate in factor X activation in a factor VII-dependent (extrinsic) and a factor VIII/IXa-dependent (intrinsic) pathway (Mann *et al.*, 1992). However, the membrane requirements for these two pathways are notably different. Factor VII-mediated factor X activation requires the presence of tissue factor, a transmembrane glycoprotein that is constitutively expressed by perivascular cells. Tissue factor specifically bind factor VII and its activated form factor VIIa, thereby localizing factor VIIa-mediated factor X activation to the cell membrane (Nemerson, 1988; Edgington *et al.*, 1991). On the other hand, factor VIII/IXa-dependent factor X activation requires complex formation between the cofactor factor VIII and the serine protease factor IXa (activated factor IX) on a procoagulant surface (van Dieijen *et al.*, 1981a; Mertens *et al.*, 1985). Also prothrombin activation requires the assembly of a functional complex, consisting of the cofactor factor V and the enzyme factor Xa on a procoagulant membrane (Rosing *et al.*, 1980). *In vitro* the procoagulant surface for factor VIII/IXa-dependent factor X activation, as well as for factor V/Xa-dependent prothrombin activation can be supplied by negatively charged phospholipid vesicles, whereas the activated platelet is considered as the physiological procoagulant counterpart (Rosing

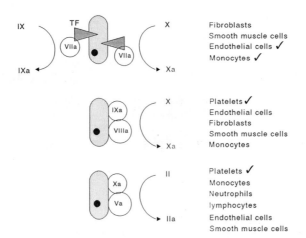

Figure 5.2 Factor X and prothrombin (factor II) activating properties of hematopoietic cells and cells of the vasculature. Cells are schematically depicted as oval structures. The receptor for factor VIIa, tissue factor (TF) is represented by the triangle. As the membrane constituents involved in functional factor VIIIa/IXa- and factor Va/Xa complex assembly have not been clearly identified, these structures are not depicted. Some cells exhibit their procoagulant property only after perturbation (✓).

et al., 1985a and 1985b; Rawala-Sheikh *et al.*, 1990). In addition, leucocytes and cells constituting the vessel wall, especially endothelial cells, may provide appropriate binding sites for both enzymes and cofactors involved in the activation of factor X and prothrombin. Figure 5.2 summarises our current knowledge of cell types likely to be involved in factor X and/or prothrombin activation. It should be noted that certain cell types do not support the indicated events of the coagulation cascade, unless these cells are exposed to stimuli which induce upregulation of synthesis or translocation of procoagulant molecules (e.g. tissue factor, negatively charged phospholipids).

2.1 Cellular specificity of tissue factor expression

Both *in vivo* (Wilcox *et al.*, 1989; Drake *et al.*, 1989; Fleck *et al.*, 1990) and *in vitro* (Maynard *et al.*, 1977; Bach and Rifkin, 1990) experiments revealed that tissue factor is constitutively expressed on perivascular cells, such as fibroblasts and smooth muscle cells. On the other hand, cells that are in direct contact with the blood stream, including endothelial cells and leucocytes, do normally not express tissue factor. However, tissue factor expression can be induced on endothelial cells and monocytes by inflammatory mediators such as lipopolysacharides and cytokines as well as by phorbolesters and thrombin (Carlsen *et al.*, 1988; Archipoff *et al.*, 1991; Bom *et al.*, 1991; Schwager and Jungi, 1994).

2.2 Cellular specificity of factor VIII/IXa-mediated activation of factor X

It is generally accepted that, *in vivo*, the membrane of the activated platelet serves a major role in controlling VIII/IXa-dependent activation of factor X. It has been reported that monocytes also provide a catalytic surface for factor VIII/IXa-dependent activation

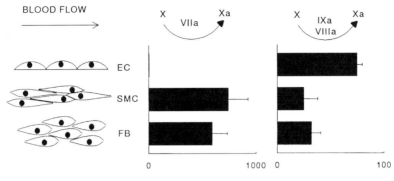

FACTOR X ACTIVATION (FMOL/CM².MIN)

Figure 5.3   Intrinsic and extrinsic factor X activation by human endothelial and perivascular cells. Factor X activation by the factor VIIa/tissue factor-dependent (extrinsic) and factor VIIIa/IXa-dependent (intrinsic) pathway was examined on unperturbed human umbilical vein endothelial cells (EC), human vascular smooth muscle cells (SMC) and human fibroblasts (FB). Data given are mean values (± s.e.m.) of 3–9 observations done on different cell isolations (data taken from Brinkman *et al.*, 1994). These data suggests that the first step in blood coagulation (activation of factor X and IX by tissue factor/factor VIIa complexes) occurs on perivascular cells, while the second step (activation of factor X by factor VIIIa/IXa complexes) predominantly occurs on the vascular lining.

of factor X (McGee and Li, 1991), with kinetic constants similar to that of blood platelets (McGee *et al.*, 1992). However, the purified monocyte preparations used in our laboratory were consistently much less potent in promoting factor VIII/IXa-dependent factor X activation than platelets (Brinkman *et al.*, 1994). These discrepant observations might be due to differences in the procedures used to purify the monocytes. Pertinent to this view is the observation that purification of monocytes may affect the expression of membrane antigens and consequently may alter the functional properties of these cells (Kuijpers *et al.*, 1993).

Evidence is accumulating that, in addition to the activated platelet, the vascular endothelium also may actively participate in the factor VIII/IXa-dependent pathway of coagulation. It has been shown that segments of bovine aortas support the activation of factor X (Stern *et al.*, 1984b). Furthermore, on cultured endothelial cells isolated from bovine aortas (Stern *et al.*, 1985), human umbilical veins (Varadi and Elodi, 1987; Brinkman *et al.*, 1994; Koppelman *et al.*, 1994), human aortas and microvessels (Brinkman *et al.*, 1994) functional factor VIII/IXa complexes can be assembled. Endothelial cells, in contrast to platelets, do not require perturbation to expose a procoagulant surface (see Figure 5.4B). In addition, the endothelial cells distinguish themselves from perivascular cells, including fibroblasts and smooth muscle cells, in that they are more effective in supporting factor VIII/IXa-dependent factor X activation (Figure 5.3).

2.3 Cellular specificity of factor V/Xa-mediated activation of prothrombin

Prothrombin activation, like intrinsic factor X activation, requires complex formation between the cofactor, factor V, and the enzyme, factor Xa on negatively charged membranes, *in vivo* provided by activated platelets. Evidence is accumulating that also endothelial cells (Rodgers and Kane, 1986; Visser *et al.*, 1988; Hamilton *et al.*, 1990; Tijburg *et al.*, 1991; Schoen *et al.*, 1992), smooth muscle cells (Rodgers, 1988a) and leucocytes (Tracy *et al.*, 1985; McGee and Rothberger, 1986; Altieri and Edgington, 1989; Robinson *et al.*, 1992) are able to support factor V/Xa-dependent prothrombin activation. As for the factor VIII/IXa-dependent activation of factor X, also prothrombin activation can be observed on unperturbed endothelial cells (see Figure 5.4C). Fibroblasts do not provide appropriate membrane constituents for functional factor V/Xa complex assembly (Maruyama *et al.*, 1984; Rodgers and Shuman, 1983).

3. MECHANISM OF ENDOTHELIAL CELL MEDIATED ACTIVATION OF FACTOR X AND PROTHROMBIN

Both the factor VIII/IXa-dependent and the tissue factor/factor VIIa-dependent activation of factor X as well as the factor V/Xa-dependent activation of prothrombin can be readily observed on cultured endothelial cells (Figure 5.4). We will now discuss the mechanisms underlying these coagulation reactions on the endothelial cell membrane.

3.1 Assembly of the tissue factor/factor VII(a) complex on endothelial cells

3.1.1 Interaction of factor VII(a) with the endothelial cell

Factor VII is a zymogen and has to be converted into its active form, factor VIIa, by limited proteolysis (Williams *et al.*, 1989; Wildgoose *et al.*, 1990), for instance by endothelial cell bound factor Xa (Rao *et al.*, 1988). Binding of factor VII as well as its activated form, factor VIIa, to endothelial cells has been observed (Reuning *et al.*, 1993). This binding was inhibited by other vitamin K-dependent coagulation factors, suggesting

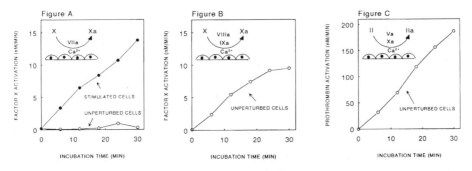

Figure 5.4 Time-dependent activation of factor X and prothrombin on endothelial cells. Monolayers of human umbilical vein endothelial cells were incubated with purified human coagulation factors in the presence of 5 mM Ca^{++}. A: 1 nM activated factor VII (VIIa) and 200 nM of the substrate factor X. B: 0.3 nM activated factor IX (IXa), 0.3 nM activated factor VIII (VIIIa) and 200 nM of the substrate factor X. C: 0.01 nM activated factor X (Xa), 0.1 nM activated factor V (Va) and 1 μM of the substrate prothrombin (II). Factor X and prothrombin activation is expressed as the amount of factor Xa or thrombin (IIa) detectable in the supernatant. Only after perturbation (in this experiment with the phorbolester myristate acetate during 4 hours) tissue factor-dependent activation of factor X was observed. In contrast, the second (factor VIIIa/IXa-dependent) pathway of factor X activation as well as prothrombin activation can be observed on unperturbed endothelial cells. (Brinkman *et al.*, unpublished observations).

that negatively charged lipids are involved in the association of factor VII(a) with the endothelial cell membrane.

Activated factor VII displays virtually no proteolytic activity unless the protein is bound to tissue factor (Ruf *et al.*, 1991; Wildgoose *et al.*, 1992; Krishnaswamy, 1992; Lawson *et al.*, 1992). Integrated into biological membranes, tissue factor/factor VIIa complexes effectively catalyse the activation of the coagulation factors IX and X (Nemerson and Gentry, 1986; Komiyama *et al.*, 1990; Bom and Bertina, 1990). Both factor VII and factor VIIa bind to tissue factor expressed on activated endothelial cells (Reuning *et al.*, 1993). Thus, a dual interaction of both factor VII and its activated form with the endothelial cell surface can be observed: a tissue factor-dependent interaction and an interaction in which negatively charged lipids are involved. The tissue factor-dependent interaction is essential for the activation of factor X (and factor IX) by activated factor VII.

3.1.2 Synthesis and expression of tissue factor

No or little factor X activation by activated factor VII can be observed on monolayers of cultured endothelial cells, unless these cells are stimulated and the synthesis of tissue factor is upregulated (see Figure 5.4A). The stimulus induced tissue factor expression on endothelial cells is transient, with a maximum after 4–8 hours, returning to basal levels within 24–48 hours. Induced tissue factor expression on endothelial cells is preceded by an increase in tissue factor-mRNA levels, and can be blocked by protein synthesis inhibitors (Galdal *et al.*, 1985; Conway *et al.*, 1989; Scarpati and Sadler, 1989; Busso *et al.*, 1991). This indicates that the induced tissue factor expression on the endothelial cell membrane is a result of de novo synthesis rather than a release of tissue factor from intracellular storage pools. The transient nature of tissue factor expression in endothelial cells indicates efficient inhibition of tissue factor gene transcription and decay of both tissue factor mRNA and protein. The precise nature of these control mechanisms remains to be determined.

After stimulation, endothelial cells express tissue factor both on the luminal and abluminal site of the cell. It is not clear if abluminal expressed tissue factor is deposited into the extracellular matrix (Ryan *et al.*, 1992) or remains cell associated (Mulder *et al.*, 1994). Irrespective of the exact location of tissue factor, it appears that most of the tissue factor, synthesized by endothelial cells upon stimulation, is associated with the abluminal side of the cell, and is not directly accessible to blood proteins.

3.1.3 Role of lipids

From studies with purified human brain- or recombinant tissue factor relipidated into lipid vesicles (Wildgoose *et al.*, 1992; Krishnaswamy, 1992; Lawson *et al.*, 1992) as well as from studies employing a recombinant tissue factor mutant deleted of the membrane spanning and intracellular domain (Ruf *et al.*, 1991), it appears that negatively charged phospholipids are involved in factor X binding to the factor VIIa/tissue factor complex rather than in the interaction of factor VIIa with tissue factor. Data have been provided suggesting the exposure of negatively charged lipids on the endothelial cell membrane (Ravanat *et al.*, 1992; Reuning *et al.*, 1993; Brinkman *et al.*, 1994; van Heerde *et al.*, 1994). Therefore, a similar phospholipid-dependent interaction of factor X with the tissue factor/factor VIIa complex might occur on the endothelial cell membrane. Negatively charged phospholipids, however, are known to be localised primarily at the inner leaflet of membranes of eukaryotic cells (Op den Kamp, 1979). As negatively charged phospholipids are of importance in binding the substrate to the tissue factor/factor VIIa complex, these lipids might have an important regulatory role in tissue factor mediated activation of factor IX and factor X upon cell damage (Rao *et al.*, 1992).

3.2 Assembly of factor VIII(a)/IXa complexes on endothelial cells

3.2.1 Role of lipids

It is well established that exposure of negatively charged phospholipids on the outer leaflet of the plasma membrane of activated platelets is essential for functional factor VIII/IXa complex formation (Rosing *et al.*, 1985a and 1985b). As also endothelial cells may expose negatively charged phospholipids on the outside of the plasma membrane (see 3.1.3), these anionic phospholipids could play a role in endothelium-mediated factor VIII/IXa-dependent factor X activation as well. The observation that annexin V, an anticoagulant protein by virtue of its high affinity binding properties to procoagulant phospholipids, inhibits the factor VIII/IXa-dependent activation of factor X on endothelial

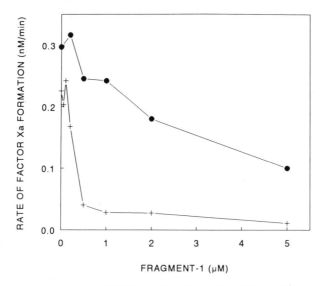

FRAGMENT-1 (μM)

Figure 5.5 Dependence of factor VIII/IXa-mediated activation of factor X on vascular endothelial cells by endogenous anionic phospholipids. Factor VIII/IXa-dependent activation of factor X on cultured human umbilical vein endothelial cells (●) was compared with that on 5 μM phospholipid vesicles (+) composed of phosphatidylserine/phosphatidylcholine 1/1. Factor X activation was examined in the presence of increasing concentrations of prothrombin fragment 1, the phospholipid binding fragment of prothrombin, in order to discriminate between negatively charged lipids and other cellular compounds involved in factor X activation on the endothelial surface. In the absence of prothrombin fragment 1, the rate of factor X activation on the lipid vesicles was similar to that on endothelial cells. Upon addition of prothrombin fragment 1, the factor VIII/IXa-dependent activation was inhibited on phospholipid vesicles but also on endothelial cells, although to a lesser extent. Therefore, anionic phospholipids as well as other cell membrane constituents are involved in the factor VIII/IXa-dependent activation of factor X on endothelial cells. Reprinted with permission from Brinkman *et al.*, 1994.

cells, suggests that negatively charged lipids indeed are involved (van Heerde *et al.*, 1994). Similarly, prothrombin fragment 1, the phospholipid binding polypeptide region of prothrombin (Jackson, 1987), inhibits factor VIII/IXa-dependent activation of factor X on endothelial cells in a dose-dependent manner (Brinkman *et al.*, 1994). However, at least a ten-fold higher concentration of this fragment is required to obtain the same degree of inhibition as found on lipid vesicles (Figure 5.5). This observation suggests that on endothelial cells also membrane constituents other than negatively charged phospholipids serve a role in controlling factor VIII/IXa-dependent activation of factor X.

3.2.2 Binding of factor IX and IXa to endothelial cells.

It has been shown that the zymogen factor IX can be activated on the surface of unperturbed endothelial cells by factor XIa (Stern *et al.*, 1984a; Berrettini *et al.*, 1992). In turn, this activated, cell associated factor IX is able to activate factor X in the presence of factor VIII (Stern *et al.*, 1984a). Studies have demonstrated specific Ca^{2+}-dependent binding of factor IX and its activated form, factor IXa, to the endothelial cell surface. Both zymogen and enzyme share the same binding site on endothelial cells (Stern *et al.*, 1983; Heimark and Schwartz, 1983). Efforts were made to elucidate the polypeptide region of factor IX defining the specific interaction of this coagulation factor with the endothelial cell membrane. It is generally accepted that the Ca^{2+}-dependent interaction of factor IX and factor IXa with negatively charged lipids, like that of other vitamin K-dependent coagulation factors, is mediated by γ-carboxyglutamic acid (Gla) residues (Jones *et al.*, 1985). These Ca^{2+}-binding Gla residues are located in the amino-terminal region of the protein, the Gla domain (for a review see: Furie and Furie, 1988 and Ichinose and Davie, 1994). As the various vitamin K-dependent coagulation factors share the same mechanism of interaction with negatively charged phospholipids, they are able to displace each other from the lipid surface (Van Dieijen *et al.*, 1981b; Mertens *et al.*, 1984). In contrast, the binding of both factor IX and factor IXa to the endothelial surface

Table 5.1 Inhibition of binding of ^{125}I-labelled factor IX to monolayers of cultured bovine endothelial cells by native factor IX and isolated domains of factor IX, X and prothrombin.

	Inhibition of ^{125}I-factor IX binding to endothelial cells		
unlabelled competitor	*IC$_{50}$ (nM)*	*Ki (nM)*	*reference*
factor IX	8–25		1,2
factor IXa	3–8		1,2
Gla-domainless factor IX	400–10000		1,2
EGF domain of factor IX	10000	.	2
EGF+Gla domain of factor IX	30		2
Gla domain of factor IX	30–100	60	1,3
Gla domain of factor X		50000	3
Gla domain of prothrombin		15000	3

Data taken from:1: Derian *et al.*, 1989; 2: Astermark and Stenflo, 1991; 3: Ryan *et al.*, 1989. IC$_{50}$, concentration of competitor required to obtain half maximal binding of 4–5 nM radiolabeled factor IX to endothelial cells. K$_i$, inhibition constant.

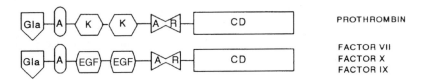

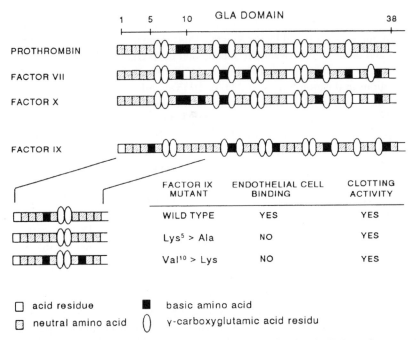

| acid residue | ■ basic amino acid |
| neutral amino acid | ( ) γ-carboxyglutamic acid residu |

Figure 5.6 Primary structure of the amino-terminal Gla-region of vitamin K-dependent coagulation factors; their role in endothelial cell interaction. Domain structure of the vitamin K-dependent coagulation factors and the amino acid composition of the γ-carboxyglutamic acid rich n-terminal part of the protein (Gla domain), are according to Furie and Furie (1988) and Ichinose and Davie (1994). Data about endothelial cell-binding properties and negatively charged phospholipid-dependent clotting activities of native factor IX and recombinant variants are taken from Cheung *et al.*, (1992). Abbreviations used: Gla, Gla domain; A, aromatic amino acid stack domain; K, kringle domain; EGF, epidermal growth factor domain; AR, zymogen activation region; CD, catalytic domain.

has been defined as specific, as no competition by other vitamin K-dependent coagulation factors was observed (Stern *et al.*, 1983; Heimark and Schwartz, 1983). Attempts were therefore made to discriminate between specific and aspecific, Gla-mediated interactions of factor IX with the endothelial cell. It was observed that Gla-domainless factor IX did not inhibit the interaction of natural factor IX with endothelial cells, while this interaction was markedly inhibited by peptides comprising the Gla domain of factor IX (Table 5.1).

These data suggests that the Gla domain of factor IX is not only important for the interaction between factor IX and negatively charged lipids, but is also essential for the interaction of factor IX with the endothelial cell membrane. Interestingly, the Gla domain of factor X or prothrombin was much less effective in inhibiting factor IX binding to endothelial cells (see Table 5.1). Thus, it appears that the Gla domain of factor IX both mediates the (aspecific) interaction of factor IX with negatively charged phospholipids as well as the specific interaction with the endothelial cell membrane. In addition, a chimeric protein of factor IX in which the Gla domain was substituted for that of factor VII, did not compete for binding of wild type factor IX to endothelial cells (Toomey *et al.*, 1992). This observation underscored the importance of the Gla domain of factor IX in defining the specific interaction of factor IX with the endothelial cell membrane. As shown in Figure 5.6, major differences between the Gla domain of factor IX and that of prothrombin, factor VII and factor X can be found in the region heading the first Gla residu (neutral in prothrombin, factor VII and factor X, while this region contains charged amino acids in factor IX) and the region between the second and third Gla residue (neutral in factor IX, while this region contains charged amino acids in prothrombin, factor VII and factor X). Point mutations at position 5 (Lys → Ala) or 10 (Val → Lys) in human factor IX resulted in loss of the endothelial binding property while the phospholipid-dependent clotting activity was not affected (Cheung *et al.*, 1992). Thus, as suggested previously (Stern *et al.*, 1983; Heimark and Schwartz, 1983), it seems that the binding of factor IX to endothelial cells is independent of negatively charged membrane phospholipids.

Carboxylate oxygen atoms of Gla residues are able to bind Ca^{2+} ions. Crystallographic studies (Soriano-Garcia *et al.*, 1992) have revealed that Ca^{2+} ions are involved in intermolecular interactions between Gla residues within the Gla domain. Therefore, Ca^{2+} ions are essential for proper folding of the Gla domain. It has been shown that noncarboxylated factor IX is not able to compete for binding of native factor IX to endothelial cells (Derian *et al.*, 1989). It appears therefore that the Ca^{2+}-dependency of the interaction between factor IX with the endothelial cell membrane resides, at least in part, in a Ca^{2+}-dependent native conformation of the Gla peptide.

Both factor IX and factor IXa bind to the same site on the endothelial cell membrane with a K_d of 2–5 nM (Heimark and Schwartz, 1983; Stern *et al.*, 1985). As the plasma concentration of the zymogen, factor IX, is about 100 nM, it might be expected that the zymogen will effectively compete for the binding of factor IXa to the endothelial cell membrane under physiological conditions. However, in competition studies (see Table 5.1), factor IXa was about 3 times more effective in inhibiting binding of factor IX to endothelial cells than the zymogen itself. This observation suggests that activated factor IX has a somewhat higher affinity for the receptor than the zymogen factor IX. In addition, factor X enhances the binding of factor IXa (K_d 0.1 nM), while the affinity of factor IX for the endothelium remains unaltered (Stern *et al.*, 1985). Apparently, the integration of factor IXa in the enzyme/cofactor/substrate complex on the endothelial cell surface originates both from the interaction of factor IXa with its putative 140 kDa binding protein on the endothelial cell membrane (Rimon *et al.*, 1987) and from the interaction of factor IXa with its substrate.

3.2.3 Interaction of factor VIII(a) with endothelial cells

The catalytic efficiency of the activation of factor X by factor IXa is dramatically increased when factor IXa is assembled with factor VIII on negatively charged phospholipid surface (van Dieijen *et al.*, 1981a). The observation that the endothelial cell-mediated activation of factor X by factor IXa depends on factor VIII (Stern *et al.*, 1985; Brinkman *et al.*, 1994) suggests that also factor VIII interacts with factor IXa on the endothelial cell membrane. Activation of factor VIII, achieved by limited proteolysis by thrombin or factor Xa (Eaton *et al.*, 1986; see also Figure 5.8A), is required for appropriate cofactor function in the factor X activating complex. Activation of factor VIII by factor Xa requires the presence of an appropriate procoagulant surface like negatively charged phospholipid vesicles or activated platelets (Neuenschwander and Jesty, 1988). The endothelial cell membrane also mediates the activation of factor VIII by factor Xa (Brinkman *et al.*, unpublished observation) Activation of factor VIII by thrombin is independent of a procoagulant membrane (Neuenschwander and Jesty, 1988). The dual mechanism of factor VIII activation is shown in Figure 5.7.

Within the factor X activating complex on endothelial cells, factor VIII is saturable with a $K_{1/2}$ (i.e. the concentration of factor VIII at which the rate of factor X activation is half of maximal) of 0.1 nM for factor VIIIa (Stern *et al.*, 1985) and 0.1–0.2 nM for factor VIII in its non-activated state (Brinkman *et al.*, 1994). These parameters are below the plasma concentration of factor VIII (0.3 nM) and suggest that, together with the high affinity binding site for factor IXa on endothelial cells (Stern *et al.*, 1985), the formation of the enzyme-cofactor complex that catalyses factor X activation can occur at physiological conditions on the endothelium.

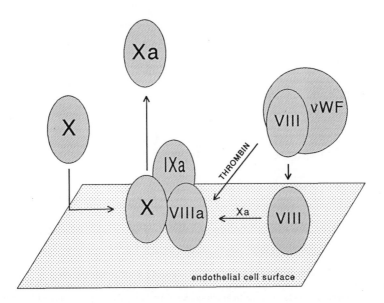

Figure 5.7   Assembly of functional factor VIII(a)/IXa complexes on the endothelial cell membrane. Model of functional complex assembly between factor VIII and factor IXa in which enzyme (factor IXa), substrate (factor X) and cofactor (factor VIIIa) all bind to specific sites on the endothelial cell membrane in proximity of each other. Alternative models can be proposed in which only specific sites on the endothelial cell membrane for factor IXa or factor VIIIa or both are required for functional complex assembly. The cofactor in its not activated form, factor VIII, is activated by thrombin or factor Xa. The activation of factor VIII by factor Xa requires a procoagulant surface, for instance the endothelial cell membrane. Von Willebrand factor may affect the interaction of factor VIII with the endothelial surface.

The mechanism of the factor VIII-endothelial cell interaction, however, is much less understood than the factor IXa-endothelial cell interaction. One can only speculate about the constituents of the endothelial cell membrane involved in factor VIII binding (Figure 5.8). As endothelial cells may expose negatively charged lipids on their cell membrane (see 3.1.3) and factor VIII can bind to negatively charged phospholipids (Arai et al., 1989; Foster et al., 1990), the interaction of factor VIII with the endothelial surface may be mediated by these phospholipids. Furthermore, factor IXa both bind to endothelial cells (Cheung et al., 1992) and factor VIII (Fay et al., 1994; Lenting et al., 1994). Therefore, endothelial cell-bound factor IXa might mediate the binding of factor VIII to the endothelial cell membrane. In addition, similar to blood platelets (Nesheim et al., 1988), endothelial cells might expose a specific factor VIII binding constituent. As endothelial cells synthesize and secrete von Willebrand factor (Jaffe et al., 1974; Verweij, 1988), and factor VIII can bind to von Willebrand factor (see Figure 5.8A), the interaction of factor VIII with the endothelial cell might also be mediated by cell membrane-associated von Willebrand factor. It is unlikely, however, that endothelial cell-bound von Willebrand factor is the recognition site for factor VIII involved in functional complex assembly between factor IXa and factor VIII on the surface of the endothelial cell, since

fig A   FACTOR VIII STRUCTURE

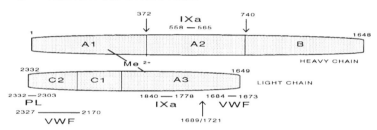

fig B   POSSIBLE FACTOR VIII BINDING SITES ON
        THE ENDOTHELIAL CELL MEMBRANE

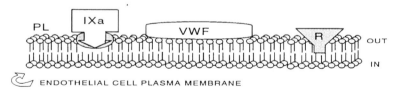

ENDOTHELIAL CELL PLASMA MEMBRANE

Figure 5.8   Binding of factor VIII to endothelial cells; role of putative binding sites. A: A schematic representation of the polypeptide structure of factor VIII heterodimer. The heavy chain (A1–A2–B domains) is linked by divalent metal ions (Me^{2+}) to the light chain (A3–C1–C2 domains). Upon proteolytic activation by factor Xa or thrombin, factor VIII is cleaved at the positions indicated by the arrows (Eaton et al., 1986). On the light chain of factor VIII binding sites for negatively charged phospholipids (Foster et al., 1990), factor IXa (Lenting et al., 1994) and von Willebrand factor (Foster et al., 1988; Leyte et al., 1989 and 1991; Shima et al., 1993) has been identified. In addition, a binding site for factor IXa on the heavy chain of factor VIII has been identified (Fay et al., 1994). Some of these binding sites might be of importance in defining the interaction of factor VIII with the endothelial cell membrane. B: Potential binding sites for factor VIII on the endothelial cell membrane. PL, phospholipid bilayer. IXa, factor IXa. VWF, von Willebrand Factor. R, hypothetical receptor for factor VIII.

the activated cofactor lacks the for von Willebrand factor binding essential sulphated tyrosine at position 1680 (Leyte *et al.*, 1991).

3.2.4 Role of von Willebrand factor

In plasma, factor VIII circulates as an inactive precursor, bound to von Willebrand factor. Von Willebrand factor inhibits processes required for proper factor VIII cofactor function such as binding of factor VIII to procoagulant surfaces (Andersson and Brown, 1981; Nesheim *et al.*, 1991) and the association of factor VIII with factor IXa (Lenting *et al.*, 1994). Furthermore, von Willebrand factor inhibits the factor VIII dependent activation of factor X by factor IXa on phospholipid vesicles (Koedam *et al.*, 1990; Koppelman *et al.*, 1994) as well as on endothelial cells (Koppelman *et al.*, 1994; Brinkman *et al.*, 1994). It is noteworthy that von Willebrand factor exerts its inhibitory properties only on factor VIII and not on its activated form. The latter lacks the for von Willebrand factor binding essential sulphated tyrosine at position 1680 (Leyte *et al.*, 1991).

In Figure 5.7, the complex assembly between factor VIIIa, factor IXa and factor X on the endothelial cell membrane is depicted. The activation of factor VIII by factor Xa requires a procoagulant surface (see 3.2.3). As von Wilebrand factor inhibits the interaction of factor VIII with procoagulant surfaces (see above), the activation of factor VIII by factor Xa is also inhibited by von Willebrand factor. As a consequence, also the factor VIIIa/IXa-dependent activation of factor X on the endothelial cell membrane is inhibited by von Willebrand factor (Brinkman *et al.*, 1994; Koppelman *et al.*, 1994). Activation of factor VIII by thrombin is independent of a procoagulant surface (see 3.2.3). Therefore, as for negatively charged lipid vesicles (Koedam *et al.*, 1990), von Willebrand factor will be without effect on the endothelial cell-mediated activation of factor X by the factor VIIIa/IXa complex, if thrombin is the activator of factor VIII.

3.2.5 Influence of endothelial cell perturbation

As factor VIII/IXa-mediated factor X activation takes place on the endothelial cell surface, changes in the composition of the outside of the endothelial cell membrane might affect endothelial cell-mediated activation of factor X. It seems likely that upon perturbation the composition of the endothelial cell membrane is altered. For instance, a characteristic feature of endothelial cell perturbation is the secretion of von Willebrand factor (Figure 5.9), stored in endothelial cell specific secretory vesicles, the Weibel Palade bodies (reviewed by Wagner, 1993). As a consequence of exocytosis of the Weibel Palade bodies, a process which is accompanied with fusion of the plasma membrane with the membrane of these secretory vesicles (Burgoyne and Morgan, 1993), it is expected that the plasma membrane composition is altered. Upon perturbation, also the synthesis and expression of a number of cellular adhesion molecules on the endothelial surface is modulated (McEver, 1991). In addition, data has been reported suggesting the exposure of procoagulant phospholipids on the surface of unperturbed endothelial cells (Reuning *et al.*, 1993; Brinkman *et al.*, 1994; Van Heerde *et al.*, 1994) which might be enhanced upon perturbation (Ravanat *et al.*, 1992). Furthermore, in addition to tissue factor, other hemostatic properties of the endothelium, including factor V/Xa-dependent prothrombin activation, thrombomodulin expression and fibrinolytic activities, are modulated upon

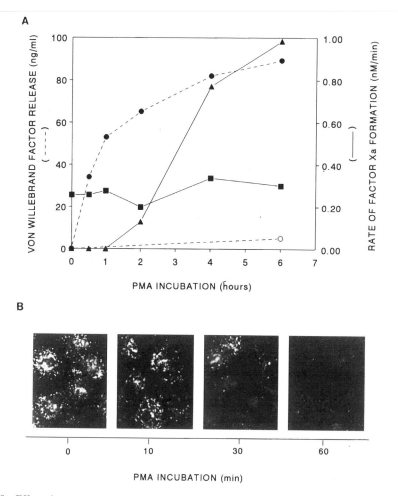

Figure 5.9   Effect of perturbation on the procoagulant activity of endothelial cells. Cultures of endothelial cells were incubated with the perturbing agent PMA (phorbol myristate acetate) for the time periods indicated. A characteristic feature of stimulated endothelial cells is the induced rapid secretion of von Willebrand factor, stored in specific secretory vesicles, the Weibel Palade bodies. This feature can be demonstrated by the accumulation of von Willebrand factor in the culture medium (Figure A, preincubation with ● and without ○ PMA) and by the disappearance of immunofluorescent staining of von Willebrand factor in the cell (Figure B). An other characteristic feature of endothelial cell perturbation is the induction of tissue factor synthesis and expression. This is demonstrated by the tissue factor/factor VIIa-dependent activation of factor X, which became perceptible only after 2 hours exposure to PMA (Figure A, ▲). The factor VIII/IXa-dependent activation of factor X, however, is not affected upon perturbation (Figure A, ■). Apparently, the membrane constituents involved in functional factor VIII/IXa-complex assembly are constitutively expressed on the endothelial cell membrane. Reprinted with permission from Brinkman *et al.*, 1994.

perturbation as well (Rodgers, 1988b; Scarpati and Sadler, 1989; Archipoff *et al.*, 1991). Interestingly, we observed no changes in intrinsic factor X activation after perturbation of endothelial cells with the phorbolester myristate acetate, lipopolysacharide (Brinkman *et al.*, 1994), or thrombin (Brinkman *et al.*, unpublished observation). Thus, the membrane constituents of endothelial cells involved in factor VIII/IXa-dependent activation of factor X are apparently constitutively expressed. Table 5.2 summarises the effect of perturbing agents on the procoagulant properties of endothelial cells.

Table 5.2   Effect of perturbing agents on endothelial cell-mediated factor X and Prothrombin activation

| | *factor X activation* | | *prothrombin activation* | |
| | | | *factor Xa dependent* | |
perturbing compound	*tissue factor/factor VIIa-dependent*	*factor VIII/IXa dependent*	*exogenous factor Va*	*endogenous factor V(a)*
Phorbolesters	↑(2,6,11,13,15)	— (17)		
Thrombin	↑ (4,5,13)	— (18)	↑ (12)	↑ (3)
Interleukin-1	↑ (7,9,13,15)			— (8)
Lipopolysacharide	↑ (1,2,4,6,14,15)	— (17)	— (10)	↑ (8)
Homocysteine				↑ (8,16)
Complement C5b-9			↑ (12)	

A summary of the effects of various perturbing agents on endothelium-mediated factor X and prothrombin activation. The list of perturbing agents enhancing tissue factor/factor VIIa-dependent factor X activation is far from complete; only agents also examined in factor VIII/IXa-dependent factor X activation and prothrombin activation are listed. ↑, enhanced or induced factor X or prothrombin activation; —, no influence of perturbation. Numbers between parentheses correspond with the following references: (1) Colucci *et al.*, 1983; (2) Lyberg *et al.*, 1983; (3) Rodgers and Shuman, 1983; (4) Brox *et al.*, 1984; (5) Galdal *et al.*, 1985; (6) Nawroth *et al.*, 1985b; (7) Bevilacqua *et al.*, 1986; (8) Rodgers and Kane, 1986; (9) Carlsen *et al.*, 1988; (10) Visser *et al.*, 1988; (11) Scarpati and Sadler, 1989; (12) Hamilton *et al.*, 1990; (13) Archipoff *et al.*, 1991; (14) Bom *et al.*, 1991; (15) Busso *et al.*, 1991; (16) Tijburg *et al.*, 1991; (17) Brinkman *et al.*, 1994; (18) Brinkman *et al.*, unpublished observation.

3.3 Assembly of the factor V(a)/Xa complex on endothelial cells

3.3.1 Binding of factor Xa to endothelial cells

Both factor X (Heimark and Schwartz, 1983; Nawroth *et al.*, 1985a; Persson *et al.*, 1991) and its activated form, factor Xa (Nawroth *et al.*, 1985a; Rodgers and Shuman, 1985; Dryjski *et al.*, 1988; Friedberg *et al.*, 1988; Rao *et al.*, 1988), bind to endothelial cells. There are no biochemical data available about factor Xa binding sites on the endothelial cell membrane participating in factor V/Xa complex assembly. Evidence to date implies that the binding of factor Xa to the platelet surface is promoted by factor Va, such that factor Va provides the equivalent for a receptor of the proteolytic enzyme (Kane *et al.*, 1980; Tracy *et al.*, 1981). In contrast, it has been shown that an anti-factor V antibody, known to inhibit to the same extent the rate of thrombin generation and the binding of factor Va and factor Xa to the platelet surface (Tracy *et al.*, 1981), was ineffective in the inhibition of endothelial cell-factor Xa interaction while endothelial cell-mediated prothrombin activation was markedly inhibited (Stern *et al.*, 1984b; Rodgers and Shuman, 1985). In addition, evidence was obtained that the vascular endothelial cell-mediated activation of factor VII by factor Xa is independent of factor Va (Rao *et al.*, 1988). These data indicate that the interaction of factor Xa with the endothelial cell membrane is, at least partially, factor Va-independent. The biochemical nature of this binding site as well as the involvement of this site in prothrombin activation on the endothelial cell membrane remains to be established.

3.3.2 Factor V and the endothelial cell

Like factor VIII, factor V also circulates in blood as an inactive cofactor. In order to exert its cofactor activity, factor V must be activated. Factor V can be activated both by factor Xa and thrombin (Kane and Davie, 1988). Bovine aortic endothelial cells are able to bind factor V (Rodgers and Kane, 1986), while human umbilical vein endothelial cells apparently do not possess this property. These cells bind only factor Va (k_d 3.7 nM), but not factor V in its inactive form (Maruyama *et al.*, 1984; Annamalai *et al.*, 1986).

Factor Va-dependent activation of prothrombin has been observed to occur on human umbilical vein endothelial cells (Visser *et al.*, 1988; Hamilton *et al.*, 1990; Schoen *et al.*, 1992). On the other hand, it has been reported that the activation of prothrombin can be supported by human umbilical vein endothelial cells as well as bovine aortic endothelial cells, only in the presence of Ca^{2+} ions. Endogenous factor V(a) seems to be involved, as this process was inhibited by antibodies directed against factor V (Rodgers and Shuman, 1983; Tijburg *et al.*, 1991). Apparently, factor V is produced by endothelial cells. Indeed, synthesis of factor V in bovine endothelial cells have been demonstrated by immune pre-cipitation of metabolically labelled factor V (Cerveny *et al.*, 1984). In human umbilical vein endothelial cells however, no factor V mRNA could be detected (Jenny *et al.*, 1987). Although it is clear that prothrombin can be activated on the endothelial surface, the contribution of (endogenous) factor V from endothelial origin, thus remains controversial. Data have been reported, suggesting that only injured cells express factor V on their surface (Annamalai *et al.*, 1986). Although this observation might, in part, explain the discrepant results concerning the factor Va requirement in endothelial cell mediated prothrombin activation, the synthesis of factor V by endothelial cells remains to be established.

3.3.3 Influence of endothelial cell perturbation

Table 5.2 summarises the effect of perturbing agents on the procoagulant properties of endothelial cells. Both endogenous- and exogenous factor V-dependent activation of pro-thrombin by factor Xa on the endothelial cell membrane is slightly increased (up to 30%) upon preincubation of endothelial cells with thrombin (Rodgers and Shuman, 1983; Hamilton *et al.*, 1990). Upon treatment of endothelial cells with complement proteins C5b–9, the exogenous factor Va-dependent prothrombin activation is enhanced more than 2 fold (Hamilton *et al.*, 1990). It has been shown that C5b–9 induces vesiculation of the plasma membrane of platelets. On these shedded membrane particles functional factor V/Xa complexes may assembly (Sims *et al.*, 1989). A similar process have been reported for endothelial cells (Hamilton *et al.*, 1990). In addition to the complement-induced vesiculation, it has been reported that perturbation of human umbilical vein endothelial cells with thrombin, either formed *in situ* or added, induce shedding of a procoagulant phospholipid surface, which supports the assembly of a functional factor V/Xa complex in the fluid phase (Schoen *et al.*, 1992). At this moment it is not clear to which extent this thrombin-induced vesiculation is of physiological relevance, as from other studies (Stern *et al.*, 1984b; Visser *et al.*, 1988) it appears that prothrombin activation is associated with the endothelial cell layer rather than with released cellular compounds.

Lipopolysacharides do not affect the prothrombin activation dependent on factor Va in the proximity of the vascular endothelial cells (Visser *et al.*, 1988). In contrast, endogenous factor V-dependent activation of prothrombin is enhanced 3–5 times upon exposure of endothelial cells with lipopolysacharides (Rodgers and Kane, 1986) or homocysteine (Rodgers and Kane, 1986; Tijburg *et al.*, 1991). Data have been provided suggesting that treatment of vascular endothelial cells with homocysteine induces activation of endogenous factor V (Rodgers and Kane, 1986). As no consensus exists concerning the synthesis of factor V by endothelial cells, the physiological significance of lipopolysacharide and homocysteine enhanced prothrombin activation remains to be established.

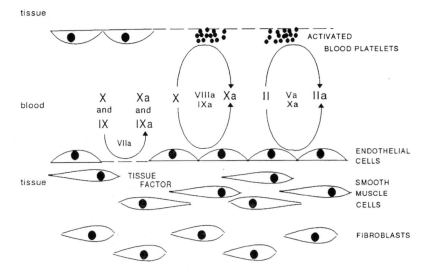

Figure 5.10 Hemostasis and the procoagulant properties of the endothelium. Under normal physiological conditions, tissue factor is sequestered from the blood stream. Upon vessel wall injury, blood coagulation is initiated by complex assembly between tissue factor and activated factor VII (VIIa). This tissue factor/factor VIIa complex readily activates the factors X and IX. Activated factor X (Xa) than activates factor VIII and V. Complex assembly between activated factor IX (IXa) and activated factor VIII (VIIIa) on the endothelial cell membrane results in the activation of additional amounts of factor X. Meanwhile, upon complex assembly between activated factor V (Va) and factor IXa on the endothelial cell membrane, prothrombin (II) is activated. In turn, the thrombin (IIa) generated will activate additional amounts of the factors VIII and V, resulting in enhanced prothrombin activation. Simultaneously, platelets adhere and aggregate at sites of vascular injury and, by translocation of negatively charged phospholipids, expose a procoagulant surface on which functional factor VIIIa/IXa- and Va/Xa complex assembly occurs. The procoagulant activity of the platelet membrane is further increased upon exposure to thrombin. This, self-amplifying cascade of activation of coagulation factors ultimately leads to the formation of an insoluble fibrin network, essential in the formation of a blood clot.

4. PHYSIOLOGICAL SIGNIFICANCE OF ENDOTHELIAL CELL MEDIATED COAGULATION

As summerized in Figure 5.10, endothelial cells may effectively participate in the regulation and amplification of the coagulation system at sites of vascular injury. The endothelial cell seems unique, in that it is the only cell type in direct contact with blood, able to support factor VIII/IXa-dependent activation of factor X, without cell perturbation. Furthermore, unperturbed vascular endothelial cells are also able to support prothrombin activation. In addition, endothelial *in vitro* cells can be stimulated to produce tissue factor, a process which requires *de novo* protein synthesis and, therefore, is probably not involved in the rapid primary hemostatic response. Endothelial tissue factor could rather be involved in pathological conditions associated with disordered coagulation and thrombosis.

It is evident that on the surface of cultured endothelial cells both functional factor VIII/IXa- and factor V/Xa complexes can be assembled. The question arises whether indeed these endothelium-mediated reactions are of physiological significance. Only indirect and limited evidence is available suggesting that these endothelial cell-mediated coagulation reactions observed *in vitro* could also play a role *in vivo*. For instance, evidence for intravascular binding sites for factor IX has been gained in baboons, as infusion of excess of bovine factor IX, but not prothrombin, resulted in a dose-dependent rise in the plasma level of endogenous, baboon factor IX. These observations suggest that baboon factor IX was displaced from binding sites on the vasculature by bovine factor IX. Evidence that indeed infused factor IX was bound to the vessel wall was obtained by the observation that after infusion, ^{125}I-factor IX could be detected on the luminal surface of baboon artery and aortic segments (Stern *et al.*, 1987). Furthermore, it has been suggested that a correlation exists between high risk factors for thrombosis and the expression of a prothrombotic phenotype of endothelial cells. For instance, endothelial cells isolated from areas of human aortas at high risk for atherosclerosis demonstrated a slight but significant enhanced prothrombin activation as compared to cells isolated from areas of human aortas at low risk of atherosclerosis (Antonov *et al.*, 1992). In addition, on aortic segments obtained from fat-fed rabbits an increased factor X and prothrombin activation has been observed (Lupu *et al.*, 1993). Thus, although ample evidence exists that endothelial cells are able to support activation of the coagulation system *in vitro*, it remains to be established whether also *in vivo* these cells significantly contribute to the primary hemostatic response upon vascular injury. These data, than, could facilitate our understanding of the role of the endothelium in maintaining the hemostatic balance under physiological and pathophysiological conditions.

Acknowledgments

We thank Dr. K. Mertens for the inspiring discussions and for reviewing this manuscript. We also thank Dr. C. Reutelingsperger (Department of Biochemistry, University of Limburg, The Netherlands) for providing factor Va. This work was financially supported by the Netherlands Organization for Scientific Research (NWO) (grand no. 900-526-191)

References

Altieri, D.C. and Edgington, T.S. (1989). Sequential receptor cascade for coagulation proteins on monocytes. *J. Biol. Chem.*, **264**:2969–2972.

Annamalai, A.E., Stewart, G.J., Hansel, B., Memoli, M., Chiu, H.C., Manuel, D.W., Doshi, K. and Colman, R.W. (1986). Expression of factor V on human umbilical vein endothelial cells is modulated by cell injury. *Arteriosclerosis*, **6**:196–202.

Andersson, L.O. and Brown, J.E. (1981). Interaction of factor VIII-von Willebrand factor with phospholipid vesicles. *Biochem. J.*, **200**:161–167.

Antonov, A.S., Key, N.S., Smirnov, M.D., Jacob, H.S., Vercellotti, G.M. and Smirnov, V.N. (1992). Prothrombotic phenotype diversity of human aortic endothelial cells in culture. *Thromb. Res.*, **67**:135–145.

Arai, M., Scandella, D. and Hoyer, L.W. (1989). Molecular basis of factor VIII inhibition by human antibodies. *J. Clin. Invest.*, **83**:1978–1984.

Archipoff, G., Beretz, A., Freyssinet, J.M., Klein-Soyer, C., Brisson, C. and Cazenave, J.P. (1991). Heterogeneous regulation of constitutive thrombomodulin or inducible tissue-factor activities on the surface of human saphenous-vein endothelial cells in culture following stimulation by interleukin-1, tumor necrosis factor, thrombin or phorbol ester. *Biochem. J.*, **273**:679–684.

Astermark, J. and Stenflo, J. (1991). The epidermal growth factor-like domains of factor IX. *J. Biol. Chem.*, **266**:2438–2443.

Bach, R. and Rifkin, D.B. (1990). Expression of tissue factor procoagulant activity: Regulation by cytosolic calcium. *Proc. Natl. Acad. Sci. USA*, **87**:6995–6999.

Berrettini, M., Schleef, R.R., Heeb, M.J., Hopmeier, P. and Griffin, J.H. (1992). Assembly and expression of an intrinsic factor IX activator complex on the surface of cultured human endothelial cells. *J. Biol. Chem.*, **267**:19833–19839.

Bevilacqua, M.P., Pober, J.S., Majeau, G.R., Fiers, W., Cotran, R.S. and Gimbrone Jr, M.A. (1986). Recombinant tumor necrosis factor induces procoagulant activity in cultured human vascular endothelium; Characterization and comparison with the actions of interleukin 1. *Proc. Natl. Acad. Sci. USA*, **83**:4533–4537.

Bom, V.J.J. and Bertina, R.M. (1990). The contributions of Ca²⁺, phospholipids and tissue-factor apoprotein to the activation of human blood-coagulation Factor X by activated Factor VII. *Biochem. J.*, **265**:327–336.

Bom, V.J.J., Van Hinsbergh, V.W.M., Reinalda-Poot, H.H., Mohanlal, R.W. and Bertina, R.M. (1991). Extrinsic activation of human blood coagulation factors IX and X on the endothelial surface. *Thromb. Haemost.*, **66**:283–291.

Brinkman, H.J.M., Mertens, K., Holthuis, J., Zwart-Huinink, L.A., Grijm, K. and Van Mourik, J.A. (1994). The activation of blood coagulation factor X on the surface of endothelial cells: a comparison with various vascular cells, platelets and monocytes. *Br. J. Hematol.*, **87**:332–342.

Brox, J.H., Osterud, B., Bjorklid, E. and Fenton, J.W. (1984). Production and availability of thromboplastin in endothelial cells: the effects of thrombin, endotoxin and platelets. *Br. J. Hematol.*, **57**:239–246.

Burgoyne, R.D. and Morgan, A. (1993). Regulated exocytosis. *Biochem. J.*, **293**:305–316.

Busso, N., Huet, S., Nicodeme, E., Hiernaux, J. and Hyafil, F. (1991). Refractory perion phenomenon in the induction of tissue factor expression on endothelial cells. *Blood*, **78**:2027–2035.

Carlsen, E., Flatmark, A. and Prydz, H. (1988). Cytokine-induced procoagulant activity in monocytes and endothelial cells. *Transplantation*, **46**:575–580.

Cerveny, T.J., Fass, D.N. and Mann, K.G. (1984). Synthesis of coagulation factor V by cultured aortic endothelium. *Blood*, **63**:1467–1474.

Cheung, W.-F., Hamaguchi, N., Smith, K.J. and Stafford, D.W. (1992). The binding of human factor IX to endothelial cells is mediated by residues 3–11. *J. Biol. Chem.*, **267**:20529–20531.

Colucci, M., Balconi, G., Lorenzet, R., Pietra, A. and Locati, D. (1983). Cultured human endothelial cells generate tissue factor in response to endotoxin. *J. Clin. Invest.*, **71**:1893–1896.

Conway, E.M., Bach, R., Rosenberg, R.D. and Koningsberg, W.H. (1989). Tumor necrosis factor enhances expression of tissue factor mRNA in endothelial cells. *Thromb. Res.*, **53**:231–241.

Derian, C.K., van Dusen, W., Przysiecki, C.T., Walsh, P.N., Berkner, K.L., Kaufman, R.J. and Friedman, P.A. (1989). Inhibitors of 2-ketoglutarate-dependent dioxygenases block aspartyl β-hydroxylation of recombinant human factor IX in several mammalian expression systems. *J. Biol. Chem.*, **264**:6615–6618.

Drake, T.A., Morrissey, J.H. and Edgington, T.S. (1989). Selective cellular expression of tissue factor in human tissues. *Am. J. Pathol.*, **134**:1087–1097.

Dryjski, M., Kuo, B-S. and Bjornsson, T.D. (1988). Interaction of thrombin and factor Xa with bovine vascular endothelial cells, smooth muscle cells and rat hepatoma cells. *Thromb. Haemostas.*, **60**:148–152.

Eaton, D., Rodriguez, H. and Vehar, G.A. (1986). Proteolytic processing of human factor VIII. Correlation of specific cleavages by thrombin, factor Xa and activated protein C with activation and inactivation of factor VIII coagulant activity. *Biochemistry*, **25**:505–512.

Edgington, T.S., Mackman, N., Brand, K. and Ruf, W. (1991). The structural biology of expression and function of tissue factor. *Thromb. Haemostas.*, **66**:67–79.

Fay, P.J., Beattie, T., Huggins, C.F. and Regan, L.M. (1994). Factor VIIIa A2 subunit residues 558–565 represent a factor IXa interactive site. *J. Biol. Chem.*, **269**:20522–20527.

Fleck, R.A., Rao, L.V.M., Rapaport, S.I. and Varki, N. (1990). Localization of human tissue factor antigen by immunostaining with monospecific, polyclonal anti-human tissue factor antibody. *Thromb. Res.*, **57**:765–781.

Foster, P.A., Fulcher, C.A., Houghten, R.A. and Zimmerman, T.S. (1988). An immunogenic region within residues val [1670]-glu**1684** of the factor VIII light chain induces antibodies which inhibit binding of factor VIII to von Willebrand factor. *J. Biol. Chem.*, **263**:5230–5234

Foster, P.A., Fulcher, C.A., Houghten, R.A. and Zimmerman, T.S. (1990). Synthetic factor VIII peptides with amino acid sequences contained within the C2 domain of factor VIII inhibit factor VIII binding to phosphatidylserine. *Blood*, **75**:1999–2004.

Friedberg, R.C., Hagen, P-O. and Pizzo, S.V. (1988). The role of endothelium in factor Xa regulation: The effect of plasma proteinase inhibitors and hirudin. *Blood*, **71**:1321–1328.

Furie, B. and Furie, B.C. (1988). The molecular basis of blood coagulation. *Cell*, **53**:505–518.

Galdal, K.S., Lyberg, T., Evensen, S.A., Nilsen, E. and Prydz, H. (1985). Thrombin induces thromboplastin synthesis in cultured vascular endothelial cells. *Thromb. Haemost.*, **54**:373–376.

Hamilton, K.K., Hattori, R., Esmon, C.T. and Sims, P.J. (1990). Complement proteins C5b–9 induce vesiculation of the endothelial plasma membrane and expose catalytic surface for assembly of the prothrombinase enzyme complex. *J. Biol. Chem.*, **265**:3809–3814.

Heimark, R.L. and Schwartz, S.M. (1983). Binding of coagulation factors IX and X to the endothelial cell surface. *Biochem. Biophys. Res. Commun.*, **111**:723–731.

Ichinose, A. and Davie, E.W. (1994). The blood coagulation factors: Their cDNAs, genes and expression. In: Hemostasis and Thrombosis: Basic principles and clinical practice. R.W. Colman, J. Hirsh, V.J. Marder, and E.W. Salzman (eds.), 3th edn, chapter 2, pp. 19–54. Philadelphia: J.B. Lippincott Company.

Jackson, C.M. (1987) Mechanisms of prothrombin activation. In: Hemostasis and thrombosis; Basic principles and clinical practice. R.W. Colman, J. Hirsh, V.J. Marder, and E.W. Salzman (eds.), 2nd edn, chapter 9, pp. 135–146. Philadelphia: J.B. Lippincott Company.

Jaffe, E.A., Hoyer, L.W., Nachman, R.L. (1974). Synthesis of von Willebrand factor by cultured human endothelial cells. *Proc. Natl. Acad. Sci. USA*. **71**:1906–1909

Jenny, R.J., Pittman, D.D., Toole, J.J., Kriz, R.W., Aldape, R.A., Hewick, R.M., Kaufman, R.J. and Mann, K.G. (1987). Complete cDNA and derived amino acid sequence of human factor V. *Proc. Natl. Acad. Sci. USA*, **84**:4846–4850.

Jones, M.E., Griffith, M.J., Monroe, D.M., Roberts, H.R. and Lentz, B.R. (1985). Comparison of lipid binding and kinetic properties of normal, variant and γ-carboxyglutamic acid modified human factor IX and Factor IXa. *Biochemistry*, **24**:8064–8069.

Kane, W.H. and Davie, E.W. (1988). Blood coagulation factors V and VIII: Structural and functional similarities and their relationship to hemorrhagic and thrombotic disorders. *Blood*,**71**: 539–555.

Kane, W.H., Lindhout, M.J., Jackson, C.M. and Majerus, P.W. (1980). Factor Va-dependent binding of factor Xa to human platelets. *J. Biol. Chem.*, **255**:1170–1174.

Koedam, J.A., Hamer, R.J., Beeser-Visser, N.H., Bouma, B.N. and Sixma, J.J. (1990). The effect of von Willebrand factor on activation of factor VIII by factor Xa. *Eur. J. Biochem.*, **189**:229–234.

Komiyama, Y., Pedersen, A.H. and Kisiel, W. (1990). Proteolytic activation of human factors IX and X by recombinant human factor VIIa: effects of calcium, phospholipids and tissue factor. *Biochemistry*, **29**:9418–9425.

Koppelman, S.J., Koedam, J.A., van Wijnen, M., Stern, D.M., Nawroth, P.P., Sixma, J.J. and Bouma, B.N. (1994). Von Willebrand factor as a regulator of intrinsic factor X activation. *J. Lab. Clin. Med.*, **123**:585–593.

Krishnaswamy, S. (1992). The interaction of human factor VIIa with tissue factor. *J. Biol. Chem.*, **267**:23696–23706.

Kuijpers, T.W., Hakkert, B.C., Knol, E.F. and Roos, D. (1993). Membrane surface antigen expression on human monocytes: changes during purification, *in vitro* activation and transmigration across monolayers of endothelial cells. In: Mononuclear Phagocytes. R. van Furth (ed), pp. 188–192. The Netherlands: Kluwer Academic Publishers.

Lawson, J.H., Butenas, S. and Mann, K.G. (1992). The evaluation of complex-dependent alterations in human factor VIIa. *J. Biol. Chem.*, **267**:4834–4843.

Lenting, P.J., Donath, M.J.S.H., Van Mourik, J.A. and Mertens, K. (1994). Identification of a binding site for blood coagulation factor IXa on the light chain of human factor VIII. *J. Biol. Chem.*, **269**:7150–7155.

Leyte, A., Verbeet, M.P., Brodniewicz-Proba, T., Van Mourik, J.A. and Mertens, K. (1989). The interaction between human blood-coagulation factor VIII and von Willebrand factor. Characterization of a high-affinity binding site on factor VIII. *Biochem. J.*, **257**:679–683

Leyte, A., Van Schijndel, H.B., Niehrs, C., Huttner, W.B., Verbeet, M.P., Mertens, K. and Van Mourik, J.A. Sulfation of Tyr[1680] of human blood coagulation factor VIII is essential for the interaction of factor VIII with von Willebrand factor (1991). *J. Biol. Chem.*, **266**:740–746

Lupu, F., Moldovan, N., Ryan, J., Stern, D. and Simionescu, N. (1993). Intrinsic procoagulant surface induced by hypercholesterolaemia on rabbit aortic endothelium. *Blood Coagul Fibrinolysis*, **4**:743–752.

Lyberg, T., Galdal, K.S., Evensen, S.A. and Prydz, H. (1983). Cellular cooperation in endothelial cell thromboplastin synthesis. *Br. J. Hematol.*, **53**:85–95.

Mann, K.G., Krishnaswamy, S. and Lawson, J.H. (1992). Surface-dependent hemostasis. Seminars in *Hematology*, **29**:213–226.

Maruyama, I., Salem, H.H. and Majerus, P.W. (1984). Coagulation factor Va binds to human umbilical vein endothelial cells and accelerates protein C activation. *J. Clin. Invest.*, **74**:224–230.

Maynard, J.R., Dreyer, B.E., Stemerman, M.B. and Pitlick, F.A. (1977). Tissue factor coagulant activity of cultured human endothelial and smooth muscle cells and fibroblasts. *Blood*, **50**:387–396.

McEver, R.P. (1991). Leukocyte interactions mediated by selectins. *Thromb. Haemostas.*, **66**:80–87.

McGee, M.P. and Li, L.C. (1991). Functional difference between intrinsic and extrinsic coagulation pathways. Kinetics of factor X activation on human monocytes and alveolar macrophages. *J. Biol. Chem.*, **266**:8079–8085.

McGee, M.P., Li, L.C. and Hensler, M. (1992). Functional assembly of intrinsic coagulation proteases on monocytes and platelets. Comparison between cofactor activities induced by thrombin and factor Xa. *J. Exp. Med.*, **176**:27–35.

McGee, M.P. and Rothberger, H. (1986). Assembly of the prothrombin activator complex on rabbit alveolar macrophage high-affinity factor Xa receptors. *J. Exp. Med.*, **164**:1902–1914.

Mertens, K., Cuperus, R., Van Wijngaarden, A. and Bertina, R.M. (1984). Binding of human blood-coagulation factors IXa and X to phospholipid membranes. *Biochem. J.*, **223**:599–605.

Mertens, K., Van Wijngaarden, A. and Bertina, R.M. (1985). The role of factor VIII in the activation of human blood coagulation factor X by activated factor IX. *Thromb. Haemostas.*, **54** 654–660.

Mulder, A.B., Hegge-Paping, K.S.M., Magielse, C.P.E., Blom, N.R., Smit, J.W., van der Meer, J., Halie, M.R. and Bom, V.J.J. (1994). Tumor necrosis factor a-induced endothelial tissue factor is located on the cell surface rather than in the subendothelial matrix. *Blood*, **84**:1559–1566.

Nawroth, P.P., McCarthy, D., Kisiel, W., Handley, D. and Stern, D.M. (1985a). Cellular processing of bovine factors X and Xa by cultured bovine aortic endothelial cells. *J. Exp. Med.*, **162**:559–572.

Nawroth, P.P., Stern, D.M., Kisiel, W. and Bach, R. (1985b). Cellular requirements for tissue factor generation by bovine aortic endothelial cells in culture. *Thromb. Res.*, **40**:677–691.

Nemerson, Y. (1988). Tissue factor and hemostasis. *Blood*, **71**:1–8.

Nemerson, Y. and Gentry, R. (1986). An ordered addition, essential activation model of the tissue factor pathway of coagulation: evidence for a conformational Cage. *Biochemistry*, **25**:4020–4033.

Nesheim, M., Pittman, D.D., Giles, A.R., Fass, D.N., Wang, J.H., Slonosky, D. and Kaufman, R.J. (1991). The effect of plasma von Willebrand factor on the binding of human Factor VIII to thrombin-activated human platelets. *J. Biol. Chem.*, **266**:17815–17820.

Nesheim, M.E., Pittman, D.D., Wang, J.H., Slonosky, D., Giles, A.R. and Kaufman, R.J. (1988). The binding of ^{35}S-labeled recombinant factor VIII to activated and unactivated human platelets. *J. Biol. Chem.*, **263**:16467–16470.

Neuenschwander, P. and Jesty, J. (1988). A comparison of phospholipid and platelets in the activation of human factor VIII by thrombin and factor Xa, and in the activation of factor X. *Blood*, **72**:1761–1770.

Op den Kamp, J.A.F. (1979). Lipid asymmetry in membranes. *Ann. Rev. Biochem*, **48**:47–71

Persson, E., Valcarce, C. and Stenflo, J. (1991). The y-carboxyglutamic acid and epidermal growth factor-like domains of factor X. Effect of isolated domains on prothrombin activation and endothelial cell binding of Factor X. *J. Biol. Chem.*, **266**:2453–2458.

Rao, L.V.M., Rapaport, S.I. and Lorenzi, M. (1988). Enhancement by human umbilical vein endothelial cells of factor Xa-catalysed activation of factor VII. *Blood*, **71**:791–796.

Rao, L.V.M., Robinson, T. and Hoang, A.D. (1992). Factor VIIa/tissue factor-catalysed activation of factors IX and X on a cell surface and in suspension: a kinetic study. *Thromb. Haemost.*, **67**:654–659.

Ravanat, C., Archipoff, G., Beretz, A., Freund, G., Cazenave, J.P. and Freyssinet, J.M. (1992). Use of annexin-V to demonstrate the role of phosphatidylserine exposure in the maintenance of hemostatic balance by endothelial cells. *Biochem. J.*, **282**:7–13.

Rawala-Sheikh, R., Ahmad, S.S., Ashby, B. and Walsh, P.N. (1990). Kinetics of coagulation factor X activation by platelet-bound factor IXa. *Biochemistry*, **29**:2606–2611.

Reuning, U., Preissner, K.T. and Muller-Berghaus, G. (1993). Two independent binding sites on monolayers of human endothelial cells are responsible for interaction with coagulation factor VII and Factor VIIa. *Thromb. Haemost.*, **69**:197–204.

Rimon, S., Melamed, R., Savion, N., Scott, T., Nawroth, P.P. and Stern, D.M. (1987). Identification of a factor IX/IXa binding protein on the endothelial cell surface. *J. Biol. Chem.*, **262**:6023–6031.

Robinson, R.A., Worfolk, L. and Tracy, P.B. (1992). Endotoxin enhances the expression of monocyte prothrombinase activity. *Blood*, **79**:406–416.

Rodgers, G.M. (1988a). Vascular smooth muscle cells synthesize, secrete and express coagulation factor V. *Biochim. Biophys. Acta*, **968**:17–23.

Rodgers, G.M. (1988b). Hemostatic properties of normal and perturbed vascular cells. *FASEB J.*, **2**:116–123.

Rodgers, G.M. and Kane, W.H. (1986). Activation of endogenous factor V by a homocysteine-induced vascular endothelial cell activator. *J. Clin. Invest.*, **77**:1909–1916.

Rodgers, G.M. and Shuman, M.A. (1983). Prothrombin is activated on vascular endothelial cells by factor Xa and calcium. *Proc. Natl. Acad. Sci. USA*, **80**:7001–7005.

Rodgers, G.M. and Shuman, M.A. (1985). Characterization of the interaction between Factor Xa and bovine aortic endothelial cells. *Biochim. Biophys. Acta*, **844**:320–329.

Rosing, J., Bevers, E.M., Comfurius, P., Hemker, H.C., van Dieijen, G., Weiss, H.J. and Zwaal, R.F.A. (1985a). Impaired factor X and prothrombin activation associated with decreased phospholipid exposure in platelets from a patient with a bleeding disorder. *Blood*, **65**:1557–1561.

Rosing, J., Tans, G., Govers-Riemslag, J.W.P., Zwaal, R.F.A. and Hemker, H.C. (1980). The role of phospholipids and factor Va in the prothrombinase complex. *J. Biol. Chem.*, **255**:274–283.

Rosing, J., van Rijn, J.L.M.L., Bevers, E.M., van Dieijen, G., Comfurius, P. and Zwaal, R.F.A. (1985b). The role of activated human platelets in prothrombin and factor X activation. *Blood*, **65**:319–332.

Ruf, W., Rehemtulla, A. and Edgington, T.S. (1991). Phospholipid-independent and -dependent interactions required for tissue factor receptor and cofactor function. *J. Biol. Chem.*, **266**:2158–2166.

Ryan, J., Brett, J., Tijburg, P., Bach, R.R., Kisiel, W. and Stern, D. (1992). Tumor necrosis factor-induced endothelial tissue factor is associated with subendothelial matrix vesicles but is not expressed on the apical surface. *Blood*, **80**:966–974.

Ryan, J., Wolitzky, B., Heimer, E., Lambrose, T., Felix, A., Tam, J.P., Huang, L.H., Nawroth, P., Wilner, G., Kisiel, W., Nelsestuen, G.L. and Stern, D.M. (1989). Structural determinants of the Factor IX molecule mediating interaction with the endothelial cell binding site are distinct from those involved in phospholipid binding. *J. Biol. Chem.*, **264**: 20283–20287.

Scarpati, E.M. and Sadler, J.E. (1989). Regulation of endothelial cell coagulant properties. *J. Biol. Chem.*, **264**:20705–20713.

Schoen, P., Reutelingsperger, C. and Lindhout, T. (1992). Activation of prothrombin in the presence of human umbilical-vein endothelial cells. *Biochem. J.*, **281**:661–664.

Schwager, I. and Jungi, T.W. (1994). Effect of human recombinant cytokines on the induction of macrophage procoagulant activity. *Blood*, **83**:152–160.

Shima, M., Scandella, D., Yoshioka, A., Nakai, H., Tanaka, I., Kamisue, S., Terada, S. and Fukui H. (1993). A factor VIII neutralizing monoclonal antibody and a human inhibitor alloantibody recognizing epitopes in the C2 domain inhibit factor VIII binding to von Willebrand factor and to phospholipids. *Thromb. Haemost.*, **69**:240–246

Sims, P.J., Wiedmer, T., Esmon, C.T., Weiss, H.J. and Shattil, S.J. (1989). Assembly of the platelet prothrombinase complex is linked to vesiculation of the platelet plasma membrane. *J. Biol. Chem.*, **264**:17049–17057.

Soriano-Garcia, M., Padmanabhan, K., de Vos, A.M. and Tulinsky, A. (1992). The Ca^{2+} ion and membrane binding structure of the gla domain of Ca-prothrombin fragment 1. *Biochemistry*, **31**:2554–2566.

Stern, D.M., Drillings, M., Nossel, H.L., Hurlet-Jensen, A., LaGamma, K.S. and Owen, J. (1983). Binding of factors IX and IXa to cultured vascular endothelial cells. *Proc. Natl. Acad. Sci. USA*, **80**:4119–4123.

Stern, D.M., Drillings, M., Kisiel, W., Nawroth, P., Nossel, H.L. and LaGamma, K.S. (1984a). Activation of factor IX bound to cultured bovine aortic endothelial cells. *Proc. Natl. Acad. Sci. USA*, **81**:913–917.

Stern, D.M., Knitter, G., Kisiel, W. and Nawroth, P.P. (1987). *In vivo* evidence of intravascular binding sites for coagulation factor IX. *Br. J. Hematol.*, **66**:227–232.

Stern, D.M., Nawroth, P.P., Kisiel, W., Handley, D., Drillings, M. and Bartos, J. (1984b). A coagulation pathway on bovine aortic segments leading to generation of factor Xa and thrombin. *J. Clin. Invest.*, **74**:1910–1921.

Stern, D.M., Nawroth, P.P., Kisiel, W., Vehar, G. and Esmon, C.T. (1985). The binding of factor IXa to cultured bovine aortic endothelial cells: Induction of a specific site in the presence of factors VIII and X. *J. Biol. Chem.*, **260**:6717–6722.

Tijburg, P.N.M., van Heerde, W.L., Leenhouts, H.M., Hessing, M., Bouma, B.N. and De Groot, P.G. (1991). Formation of meizothrombin as intermediate in factor Xa-catalysed prothrombin activation on endothelial cells. *J. Biol. Chem.*, **266**:4017–4022.

Toomey, J.R., Smith, K.J., Roberts, H.R. and Stafford, D.W. (1992). The endothelial cell binding determinant of human factor IX resides in the y-carboxyglutamic acid domain. *Biochemistry*, **31**:1806–1808.

Tracy, P.B., Eide, L.L. and Mann, K.G. (1985). Human prothrombinase complex assembly and function on isolated peripheral blood cell populations. *J. Biol. Chem.*, **260**:2119–2124.

Tracy, P.B., Nesheim, M.E. and Mann, K.G. (1981). Coordinate binding of factor Va and factor Xa to the unstimulated platelet. *J. Biol. Chem.*, **256**:743–751.

Van Dieijen, G., Tans, G., Rosing, J. and Hemker, H.C. (1981a). The role of phospholipid and factor VIIIa in the activation of bovine factor X. *J. Biol. Chem.*, **256**:3433–3442.

Van Dieijen, G., Tans, G., Van Rijn, J., Zwaal, R.F.A. and Rosing, J.(1981b). Simple and rapid method to determine the binding of blood clotting factor X to phospholipid vesicles. *Biochemistry*, **20**:7096–7101.

Van Heerde, W.L., Poort, S., Van 't Veer, C., Reutelingsperger, C.P.M., De Groot, P.G. (1994). Binding of recombinant annexin V to endothelial cells: effect of annexin V binding on endothelial-cell-mediated thrombin formation. *Biochem. J.*, **302**:305–312

Varadi, K. and Elodi, S. (1987). Formation and functioning of the factor IXa-VIII complex on the surface of endothelial cells. *Blood*, **69**:442–445.

Verweij, C.L. (1988). Biosynthesis of human von Willebrand Factor. *Haemostasis*, **18**:224–245.

Visser, M.R., Tracy, P.B., Vercellotti, G.M., Goodman, J.L., White, J.G. and Jacob, H.S. (1988). Enhanced thrombin generation and platelet binding on herpes simplex virus-infected endothelium. *Proc. Natl. Acad. Sci. USA*, **85**:8227–8230.

Wagner, D.D. (1993). The Weibel-Palade body: the storage granule for von Willebrand factor and P-selectin. *Thromb. Haemostas.*, **70**:105–110.

Wilcox, J.N., Smith, K.M., Schwartz, S.M. and Gordon, D. (1989). Localization of tissue factor in the normal vessel wall and in the atherosclerotic plaque. *Proc. Natl. Acad. Sci. USA*, **86**:2839–2843.

Wildgoose, P., Berkner, K.L. and Kisiel, W. (1990). Synthesis, purification and characterization of an agr152 → glu site-directed mutant of recombinant human blood clotting factor VII. *Biochemistry*, **29**:3413–3420.

Wildgoose, P., Jorgensen, T., Komiyama, Y., Nakagaki, T., Pedersen, A. and Kisiel, W. (1992). The role of phospholipids and the factor VII Gla-domain in the interaction of factor VII with tissue factor. *Thromb. Haemost.*, **67**:679–685.

Williams, E.B., Krishnaswamy, S. and Mann, K.G. (1989). Zymogen/enzyme discrimination using peptide chloromethyl ketones. *J. Biol. Chem.*, **264**:7536–7545.

6 Properties and Biosynthesis of von Willebrand Factor: A Critical Review

Caroline Hop and Hans Pannekoek

University of Amsterdam, Academic Medical Center, Department of Biochemistry, Amsterdam, The Netherlands

INTRODUCTION

Von Willebrand factor (vWF) is a glycoprotein that is synthesized in endothelial cells and megakaryocytes. Secretion from endothelial cells results in the appearance of vWF in plasma and in deposition in the subendothelium. vWF synthesized by megakaryocytes is ultimately encountered in the α-granules of platelets, shedded from mature megakaryocytes. Clinical investigations have shown that congenital deficiencies of vWF may lead to a mild, moderate or severe bleeding diathesis, denoted von Willebrand disease (vWD) (reviewed in: Ruggeri and Zimmerman, 1987). Extensive biochemical, molecular biological and cell biological studies have provided a rational basis for the clinical observations. The view, emerging from these studies, is that vWF is an essential protein for the formation of the hemostatic plug. It acts as a "molecular bridge" that connects the platelet to the subendothelium that is exposed upon injury of the vessel wall. In addition, vWF may promote platelet-platelet interaction, resulting in aggregation of platelets.

vWF, isolated from plasma, platelets or from the subendothelium, consists of a series of multimers, ranging from dimers to high molecular weight proteins composed of 50 to about 100 vWF monomers. It has now been well established that the extent of multimerization determines the ability of vWF to promote adhesion of platelets to the subendothelium. As outlined in this Chapter, the degree of multimerization is the resultant of intracellular trafficking of newly synthesized vWF.

Apart from its function in adhesion and aggregation, vWF is the obligatory carrier protein of Factor VIII (FVIII), an essential cofactor of the intrinsic coagulation cascade. It is generally assumed that vWF protects FVIII from proteolytic degradation. Hence, a complete deficiency of vWF results in uncontrolled degradation of FVIII and dysfunctioning of the coagulation cascade. The interaction between vWF and FVIII will be briefly discussed below.

Recently, comprehensive reviews have appeared on the properties and the biosynthesis of vWF (Wagner, 1990; Ruggeri and Ware, 1992, 1993). For that reason, we will briefly

107

summarize the major biochemical, molecular biological and cell biological aspects of the vWF protein and focus both on new developments in vWF biology, controversial issues and several of the questions that remain to be solved.

PROPERTIES OF vWF

vWF consists of repetitive domains

The molecular cloning of full-length vWF cDNA has been a milestone in vWF biology (Verweij *et al.*, 1986; Bonthron *et al.*, 1986). Initially, four groups independently reported on the cloning of a partial vWF cDNA (Ginsburg *et al.*, 1985; Lynch *et al.*, 1985; Sadler *et al.*, 1985; Verweij *et al.*, 1985). From those partial sequences it was predicted that vWF is a repetitive protein, composed of homologous domains (Sadler *et al.*, 1985). Full-length cDNA allowed the conclusion that about 90% of the precursor protein of vWF (pro-vWF) is contained within four repetitive domains, namely three A domains, three B domains, two C domains, four D domains and a partial duplication of a D domain (Verweij *et al.*, 1986; Bonthron *et al.*, 1986). Reading from the amino- to the carboxyl-terminus, these pro-vWF domains are arranged in the following order: D1-D2-D'-D3-A1-A2-A3-D4-B1-B2-B3-C1-C2. At this point, it should be noted that the region beyond the C2 domain till the carboxyl-terminus of mature vWF is not contained within a repetitive domain. The amino-terminus of mature vWF had been determined before by Edman degradation of plasma vWF (Titani *et al.*, 1986). The amino-terminus (serine-leucine-serine etc.) coincides with the designated amino-terminus of the D' domain and is preceded by an arginine residue as derived from the vWF nucleotide sequence. Consequently, pro-vWF is composed of a pro-polypeptide of 741 amino-acid residues (domains D1 and D2), followed by mature vWF of 2050 amino acids (domains D'-D3-A1-A2-A3-D4-B1-B2-B3-C1-C2) (Figure 6.1).

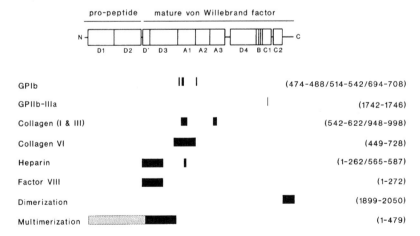

Figure 6.1   Schematic representation of pre-pro-vWF monomer and its ligand binding sites. The upper part represents pre-pro-vWF with its typical domain structure. Pre-pro-vWF (2813 amino acids) is composed of a signal peptide of 22 amino acids, the pro-polypeptide of 741 residues and, at the carboxyl-terminal end, mature vWF of 2050 amino acid residues. The lower part shows all known ligand binding sites for pro-vWF as well as the domains involved in dimerization and multimerization. The numbers at the right side indicate amino-acid residues of mature vWF (2050 amino acids).

The homology of the different repetitive domains varies between 29 and 43%. The distribution of cysteine residues is non-random: the B, C and D domains consist of 10 to 20% cysteine residues, whereas the A domains contain only a few cysteines. The atypical distribution of these residues constitutes the basis for the generation of dimers and multimers that are linked by disulphide bonds (Fretto *et al.*, 1986; Marti *et al.*, 1987). By transfecting heterologous cells with a set of vWF cDNA domain-deletion mutants, it was concluded that dimerization is mediated by cysteine residues located in the utmost 151 carboxyl-terminal amino-acid residues, present in a non-repetitive region (Voorberg *et al.*, 1991). By contrast, multimerization requires the participation of cysteine residues located in each of the domains D1, D2, D' and D3 (Voorberg *et al.*, 1990). In addition, it was shown that dimerization and multimerization are independent processes. The localization of the areas, that are involved in intermolecular disulphide bonding, agrees with electron microscopic observations that indicated the involvement of an extended area at the amino-terminus vWF in multimerization, while only a relatively small region at the carboxyl-terminus of vWF mediates dimerization (Fretto *et al.*, 1986).

Adhesive function of vWF

Exposure of the subendothelium to the circulation triggers the adhesion of platelets to the vessel wall. In this process the presence of vWF, deposited in the subendothelium and possibly supported by plasma vWF, is essential (Sakariassen *et al.*, 1979). To that end, vWF connects two different entities and, consequently, at least two different counterparts. The vWF receptor on the platelet surface for adhesion is a unique molecule, i.e. the glycoprotein Ib (GPIb) receptor (reviewed in: Ruggeri and Ware, 1992, 1993). By contrast, the vessel wall harbours a variety of candidates that are able to bind vWF. These includes a number of defined collagens, heparan sulphate-containing proteoglycans and sulphatides. Under selected flow conditions, vWF also promotes platelet aggregation. For that purpose, vWF binds to the glycoprotein IIB/IIIA (GPIIB/IIIA) receptor on platelets (Fressinaud *et al.*, 1986; Sakariassen *et al.*, 1986a,b; Weiss *et al.*, 1986). Furthermore, it has been suggested that platelet vWF, released from the α-granules upon activation, is particularly suited to bind to GPIIb/IIIa, whereas plasma vWF displays a higher affinity for GPIb than platelet vWF (Gralnick *et al.*, 1992). Both for GPIb and for GPIIb/IIIa specific binding sites have been determined on mature vWF monomers. The localization and characteristics of the different binding sites will be summarized below (Figure 6.1).

Interaction of vWF with GPIb

The platelet surface harbours approximately 28,000 GPIb receptors (Du *et al.*, 1987). GPIb is a heterodimeric protein, composed of the integral membrane proteins GPIbα and GPIbβ. GPIbα (145 kDa) is disulphide-linked to GPIbβ (24 kDa), each being the product of different genes (López *et al.*, 1988). The extracellular segment of the GPIbα chain contains the vWF binding site (Vicente *et al.*, 1990). On the platelet surface, GPIb heterodimers are complexed with glycoprotein IX (GPIX; 22 kDa) and, possibly, with glycoprotein V (GPV) (82 kDa) (Berndt *et al.*, 1985; Modderman *et al.*, 1992).

Recent studies have indicated that exposure of the GPIb receptor on the platelet surface is subject to regulation. Evidence has been presented showing that the GPIb complex is translocated from the surface of the platelets to the surface connected canicular system after activation of platelets with thrombin (Hourdille *et al.*, 1992). Interestingly, when vWF is bound to the GPIb receptor during thrombin activation, then most of the vWF is also translocated to the surface connected canicular system. Hence, during activation of platelets with thrombin the adhesiveness is regulated by translocation-mediated surface clearance of vWF.

It is assumed that the interaction between vWF and GPIb requires prior binding of vWF to the subendothelium (Sakariassen *et al.*, 1979). This binding would cause a conformational change of the vWF molecule that results in efficient interaction with GPIb. This process can be mimicked by the addition of certain modulators, i.e. the antibiotic ristocetin and the snake venom botrocetin, but also by desialation of vWF (Howard *et al.*, 1984; Berndt, 1992; Peng *et al.*, 1993). The interaction between vWF and the modulators ristocetin, botrocetin and with GPIb are localized in the A1 domain. Most of this domain is represented by a large "loop", held together by a single disulphide bond between the cysteine residues 509 and 695 of mature vWF (Marti *et al.*, 1987; Mohri *et al.*, 1988). Ristocetin and botrocetin occupy different binding sites on the vWF molecule. Amino-acid residues 702–704 are important for ristocetin-mediated interaction between vWF and GPIb, but are not essential for the GPIb binding site on vWF (Azuma *et al.*, 1993). The botrocetin-dependent binding site on vWF is localized within the A1 loop between residues 539 and 643 (Girma *et al.*, 1990; Sugimoto *et al.*, 1991).

The binding site on vWF for GPIb is constituted of at least three discontinuous regions of vWF, i.e. the region between the amino-acid residues 474 and 488 (at the boundary of the domains D3 and A1) and the region between the residues 694 and 708 (within the A1 domain) (Mohri *et al.*, 1988). In addition, it has been shown that the region between residues 514 and 542, located within the A1 loop, is also involved in binding to the GPIb receptor (Berndt *et al.*, 1991) (Figure 6.1). It is evident that the binding of vWF to GPIb requires an intact disulphide bond between the cysteines at 509 and 695 (Cruz *et al.*, 1993). Asparagine-linked glycosylation, and subsequent sialation, of the loop structure is thought to increase the solubility of vWF, but to reduce the affinity of vWF for GPIb (Ruggeri and Ware, 1992).

It is becoming increasingly apparent that the interaction between GPIb and vWF leads to signal transduction and activation of the platelet (Kroll *et al.*, 1991). The mechanism involves an arachidonic acid metabolite-dependent activation of phospholipase C after vWF binding to platelet membrane GPIb. Subsequently, protein kinase C is activated, followed by an increase of the intracellular calcium concentration that ultimately promotes platelet secretion and aggregation. Furthermore, it has been demonstrated that shear stress induces the binding of vWF multimers to GPIb, leading to an increase in intracellular calcium concentration and aggregation, due to the binding of vWF to the exposed GPIIB/IIIA complex (Chow *et al.*, 1992).

Interaction of vWF with GPIIb/IIIa

The receptor on the platelet surface that mediates aggregation is the GPIIb/IIIa (integrin α_{IIb}/β_3) complex (reviewed in: Philips *et al.*, 1991). This complex represents the most abundant platelet receptor exposing amounts of 40,000 to 80,000 molecules per platelet. GPIIb/IIIa is a heterodimer, composed of equimolar quantities of the integral membrane proteins GPIIb (145 kDa) and GPIIIa (95 kDa) (Kunicki *et al.*, 1981). The GPIIb part of the complex consists of a heavy chain (GPIIbα) that is disulphide-linked to a transmembrane light chain (GPIIbβ). The amino-terminal part of the GPIIIa polypeptide chain has been shown to contain the binding site for vWF (D'Souza *et al.*, 1988). The arginine-glycine-aspartate (RGD) tripeptide segment (Ruoslahti and Pierschbacher, 1985), present in the C1 domain of vWF, is probably important for the interaction of vWF and the GPIIb/IIIa complex although point mutations in the RGD sequence only lead to a partial reduction of vWF binding to GPIIb/IIIa (Beacham *et al.*, 1992; Ruggeri and Ware, 1992) (Figure 6.1). Under normal shear stress conditions, the GPIIb/IIIa receptor complex predominantly binds to fibrinogen. However, at high shear stress vWF is the preferred ligand, resulting in platelet aggregation and, ultimately, in thrombus formation (Ikeda *et al.*, 1991). It has been proposed that binding of vWF to GPIb on non-activated platelets/leads to a change in the ligand recognition specificity of GPIIb/IIIa (Savage *et al.*, 1992). Prior binding of vWF to GPIb induces the binding of vWF to GPIIb/IIIa, whereas this "activation" of GPIIb/IIIa could be prevented by inhibiting the protein kinase C-dependent signal transduction pathway. These newly delineated pathways for platelet activation would thus proceed in the absence of agonists and may substitute for or complement platelet activation by well-characterized agonists such as thrombin or collagen.

Interaction of vWF with the subendothelium

Numerous candidates have been proposed as counterpart of vWF in the vessel wall. Most of these suggestions originate from binding experiments, using purified proteins. For example, it has been shown that vWF binds to both monomeric and fibrillar collagen type III and to fibrillar collagen type I *in vitro* (Santoro, 1983; Morton *et al.*, 1983). Two collagen binding sites have been determined on the vWF monomer: one binding site is present in the A1 domain, whereas the other is contained within the A3 domain (reviewed by Ruggeri and Ware, 1992, 1993). Furthermore, vWF was shown to bind to immobilized heparin (Fujimura *et al.*, 1987). Heparin-binding is mediated by a high affinity site between residues 565 and 587 in the A1 domain and by a low affinity binding site in domains D'-D3 (residues 1 till 262) (Fujimura *et al.*, 1987; Mohri *et al.*, 1988; Sobel *et al.*, 1992). However, Rand and colleagues recently isolated a vWF-binding protein (MW 150 kDa) from human vascular endothelium and identified this protein as collagen type VI (Rand *et al.*, 1991). Immunofluorescence and electron microscopic analyses of the subendothelium of human umbilical veins revealed that vWF and collagen VI colocalize, whereas no colocalization was observed of vWF and collagen type I or type III (Rand *et al.*, 1993). It is concluded that collagen type VI constitutes the actual vWF binding site in the vessel wall (Figure 6.1).

There is no evident consensus on the localization of the binding site on vWF for the vessel wall and/or to collagen type VI. First, the binding of vWF to the endothelial cell matrix (ECM) could be completely abolished by a proteolytic fragment of vWF, consisting of amino-acid residues from 449 to 728, corresponding to the A1 domain (Denis *et al.*, 1993). Second, an anti-vWF monoclonal antibody prevented the interaction between vWF and the ECM: the corresponding epitope of this antibody is located, however, in the carboxyl-terminal part of vWF (de Groot *et al.*, 1988). Third, both the proteolytic vWF fragment 449–728 and a fragment derived from the carboxyl-terminus

(1366–2050) could block the binding of vWF to collagen type VI. Apparently, purification and subsequent immobilization of collagen type VI leads to the appearance of a binding site that is not revealed within the subendothelium. Significantly, a proteolytic fragment of vWF, harbouring the heparin binding site, did not displace vWF bound to the ECM, indicating that heparan sulphate-containing proteoglycans do not play a key role in binding of vWF to the subendothelium (Denis *et al.*, 1993). Hence, evidence has been presented on the involvement of collagen type VI in binding vWF to the vessel wall, whereas the participation of other subendothelial components *in vivo* requires further experimentation.

The view that emerges from the data presented in the previous paragraphs can be summarized as follows. First, vWF bound to the injured vessel wall (presumably to collagen type VI) undergoes a conformational change that enables the protein to bind to GPIb (Sakariassen *et al.*, 1979). Second, binding of vWF to GPIb activates the platelet (Kroll *et al.*, 1991; Savage *et al.*, 1992), leading to exposure of the GPIIb/IIIa complex. Third, preferably platelet vWF binds to the GPIIb/IIIa complex, an event that supports platelet-platelet interaction (Fressinaud *et al.*, 1986; Sakariassen *et al.*, 1986a, b; Weiss *et al.*, 1986; Gralnick *et al.*, 1992). Fourth, binding of high multimers of vWF to GPIIb/IIIa results in platelet aggregation, secretion of the contents of platelet granules, subsequent platelet spreading and, ultimately, to the formation of a thrombus (Sakariassen *et al.*, 1979; Weiss *et al.*, 1989).

Interaction of vWF with the basolateral endothelial cell surface

The endothelial cell displays polar growth properties and secretes a distinct spectrum of proteins to the apical and to the basolateral side, respectively (see section Biosynthesis). vWF routed to the basolateral side, and deposited in the ECM, is thought to be involved in anchoring of the cells to the subendothelium. Evidence has been presented that indicates an essential interaction between vWF and the vitronectin receptor (integrin $\alpha_v\beta_3$; Hynes, 1987) since antibodies, directed against this receptor cause detachment of cultured endothelial cells from the extracellular matrix (Cheresh, 1987; Charo *et al.*, 1987; Dejana *et al.*, 1989). An crucial role has been attributed to the RGD sequence in the C1 domain of the molecule with regard to the interaction with the basolateral endothelial cell surface (Hynes, 1987). It has been suggested that an important "housekeeping" function of vWF bound to the vitronectin receptor would be to fortify endothelial cell adhesion to the vessel wall (Wagner, 1990). Consequently, it is speculated that high shear stress may promote basolateral secretion of adhesive-competent vWF molecules (Sporn *et al.*, 1989).

Interaction of vWF with the apical endothelial cell surface?

A new option for yet another function of vWF has been recently offered by the results reported by Konkle and colleagues (Konkle *et al.*, 1990). These investigators demonstrated that cultured endothelial cells, preferentially treated simultaneously with tumor necrosis factor α (TNF-α) and IL-1, synthesize the glycoprotein GPIbα chain. In addition, it was shown that the GPIbα protein is expressed *in vivo* by high venule endothelium of tonsils. Although, no formal proof has been reported that endothelial GPIbα is actually exposed at the apical surface, the observations potentially support the view that (multimeric) vWF could be bound to the apical endothelial cell surface. Subsequently, multimeric vWF bound to the surface of the intact endothelial cell might interact with GPIb on the platelet surface and constitute a "molecular bridge" between the endothelium and the platelet. Since expression of endothelial GPIbα is only observed in the presence of inflammatory cytokines, it is speculated that these interactions may occur as a response of platelets to inflammation.

Interaction of vWF with FVIII

vWF is encountered in plasma as a complex with the glycoprotein FVIII. FVIII is an obligatory cofactor of activated Factor IX (FIX$_a$), a serine protease that is essential in the intrinsic coagulation pathway (Weiss *et al.*, 1977; Tuddenham *et al.*, 1982; Brinkhous *et al.*, 1985). In contrast to vWF, FVIII is synthesized by hepatocytes (Zelechowska *et al.*, 1985), and a number of other tissues (Wion *et al.*, 1985), and associates with vWF in a non-covalent manner (White and Shoemaker, 1989). The molar ratio of vWF and FVIII in vWF/FVIII complexes is approximately 50:1 (Counts *et al.*, 1977; Leyte *et al.*, 1990). The degree of multimerization of vWF is apparently not relevant for the ability to bind FVIII (Counts *et al.*, 1977). *In vitro*, the complex can be dissociated under conditions of high ionic strength (Cooper *et al.*, 1973). It is thought that dissociation of vWF and FVIII is a prerequisite for the cofactor function of FVIII *in vivo* (Hill-Eubanks *et al.*, 1989). Complex formation, however, protects FVIII from proteolytic degradation as has been deduced from observations with patients who completely lack vWF and, consequently, are deficient of FVIII (Tuddenham *et al.*, 1982).

The FVIII binding site on mature vWF is located within the amino-terminal region of mature vWF, spanning the region between residues 1 and 272 (Foster *et al.*, 1987; Bahou *et al.*, 1991; Pietu *et al.*, 1989) (Figure 6.1). Residues 78 to 96 probably are particularly important, since the corresponding epitope of anti-vWF monoclonal antibodies, that block the interaction between vWF and FVIII, is located in this area (Bahou *et al.*, 1991). It is conceivable that the ternary structure of the FVIII binding area is essential, since mutations that disturb the formation of disulphide bonds prevent binding to FVIII (Foster *et al.*, 1987). A potential (indirect) involvement of the pro-polypeptide of pro-vWF has been proposed, based on the properties of a deletion mutant, lacking the pro-polypeptide, which is unable to multimerize beyond the stage of dimers (Leyte *et al.*, 1991). However, this conclusion is in apparent contradiction with the data of others who have reported that similar vWF deletion mutants were able to bind FVIII (Wise *et al.*, 1991).

BIOSYNTHESIS OF vWF

Platelet vWF

The biosynthesis of vWF is restricted to two cell types, i.e. the endothelial cell and the megakaryocyte (reviewed by Wagner, 1990). At present, cell-specific transcriptional regulation of the vWF genes is still poorly understood. Most of our knowledge on vWF biosynthesis has been derived from studies using cultured vascular endothelial cells, mostly isolated from veins of human umbilical cords (Jaffe *et al.*, 1973). In this paragraph, however, we will discuss data on platelet vWF that originates from biosynthesis in megakaryocytes. Although there is formally little proof, it is assumed that the biosynthesis of vWF in megakaryocytes is similar to that in endothelial cells. An exception might be that megakaryocytes apparently do not secrete vWF in a constitutive manner (see next paragraph), but only store the protein in α-granules (mentioned in: Ruggeri and Ware, 1993). After shedding of platelets from the megakaryocyte, vWF remains within the α-granules of non-activated platelets together with a number of other proteins that are vital to hemostasis (e.g. fibrinogen, fibronectin, thrombospondin, α_2-antiplasmin and multimerin (Hayward *et al.*, 1991)). It should be mentioned that some of these proteins originate from the megakaryocyte, whereas others are endocytosed from plasma. The pool of vWF in the α-granules of platelets represents about 20% of the vWF that is present in blood. Electron microscopic inspection of vWF, stored in the α-granules, reveals striped structures due to condensed vWF molecules. These structures predominantly cover the periphery of the α-granules (Cramer *et al.*, 1985). When platelets are activated by agonists (e.g. by thrombin) then the contents of these organelles are released in plasma. In a previous paragraph, we discussed the function of platelet vWF and indicated that preliminary evidence has been presented, suggesting that platelet vWF may preferentially interact with the GPIIb/IIIa complex and promote platelet-platelet interaction.

Endothelial vWF

The vWF gene is situated on chromosome 12 (Verweij *et al.*, 1985; Ginsburg *et al.*, 1985) and spans approximately 200,000 basepairs (Mancuso *et al.*, 1989). Transcription of the gene yields a mature vWF mRNA of about 8,800 nucleotides that is translated into a polypeptide chain (pre-pro-vWF) of 2813 amino-acid residues (Verweij *et al.*, 1986; Bonthron *et al.*, 1986). Pre-pro-vWF is composed of a signal peptide (22 amino acids), an unusually long pro-polypeptide of 741 residues and, located carboxyl-terminally, mature vWF spanning 2050 amino-acid residues. Pre-pro-vWF is transported to the rough endoplasmatic reticulum (RER) (Figure 6.2). During translocation over the RER membrane to the lumen of the organelle, 12 asparagine-linked high mannose oligosaccharide chains are added (Titani *et al.*, 1989). Subsequently, the precursor protein undergoes proteolytic processing to remove the signal peptide, yielding pro-vWF. In the RER dimerization between two pro-vWF monomers occurs, mediated by intermolecular disulphide bond formation by cysteine residues located at the carboxyl-terminal region of the proteins (Fretto *et al.*, 1986; Marti *et al.*, 1987). Specifically, the utmost region of 151 amino-acid residues, that is not comprised in a repetitive domain, is responsible for dimerization (Voorberg *et al.*, 1991). This process is catalyzed by an RER-resident enzyme, presumably protein disulphide isomerase (PDI). Incorrect assembly of pro-vWF dimers elicits the formation of autophagosomes, containing pro-vWF, that are destined to degrade the protein (Voorberg *et al.*, 1991). Correctly assembled pro-vWF dimers are translocated to the Golgi apparatus where further processing steps take place. In this compartment, the high mannose oligosaccharides are processed to the complex form and, in addition 10 O-linked high mannose residues are added to threonyl and seryl residues (Titani *et al.*, 1986). Furthermore, it has been shown that the protein is sulphated in the trans-Golgi network (Vischer and Wagner, 1994).

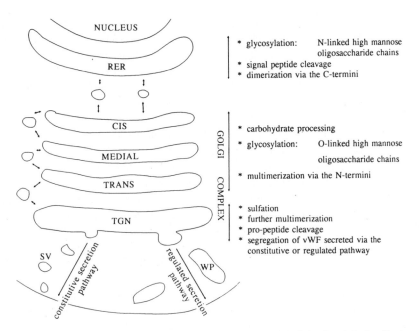

Figure 6.2 Schematic representation of the routing of vWF in the endothelial cell and the localization of the post-translational modification events. RER: rough endoplasmatic reticulum, TGN: trans-Golgi network, SV: secretory vescicle, WP: Weibel Palade body.

Multimerization is thought to be initiated in the Golgi apparatus and can proceed in a non-enzymatic manner (Mayadas and Wagner, 1989). It has been observed that cysteine residues in the amino-terminal region of vWF are involved in disulphide-mediated multimerization by "head-to-head" association of pro-vWF dimers (Fretto *et al.*, 1986; Marti *et al.*, 1987). Transfection studies with a set of vWF cDNA domain deletion mutants demonstrated that multimerization requires the presence of an extended area, consisting of the domains D1, D2, D′ and D3 (Voorberg *et al.*, 1990). Interestingly, it was shown that the *in-trans* action of the domains D1-D2 and the domains D′-D3 also yields vWF multimers (Wise *et al.*, 1988). After transport of vWF from the Golgi apparatus to the trans-Golgi network, the pro-peptide is proteolytically removed, yielding mature vWF and a pro-peptide that is also called vWF antigen II (vW AgII). The pro-peptide and mature vWF remain non-covalently associated and are simultaneously transported through the cell and ultimately secreted (Vischer and Wagner, 1994).

vWF secretion by the endothelial cell

In the endothelial cell, (partially) multimerized vWF that exits the trans-Golgi network is routed by two different pathways (reviewed in Wagner, 1990). In cultured endothelial cells, about 95% of the newly synthesized vWF is packaged in secretory vesicles that rapidly fuse with the plasma membrane, followed by secretion of the contents either at the apical or at the basolateral side ("constitutive secretory pathway") (Sporn *et al.*, 1989; Van Buul-Wortelboer *et al.*, 1989). Approximately 5% of vWF, synthesized in cultured endothelial cells, is stored in endothelial-cell specific organelles, namely the Weibel-Palade bodies (Weibel and Palade, 1964) ("regulated secretory pathway"). Important differences have been noted concerning the composition of the material routed by either one the indicated secretory pathways. Constitutively secreted vWF is not completely proteolytically processed and thus consists of a mixture of pro-vWF and mature vWF. Moreover, vWF routed by this pathway is only partially multimerized and lacks high molecular weight vWF multimers. By contrast, vWF secreted via the regulated pathway is fully processed, while a relatively large part of the material is composed of high molecular weight multimers (Sporn *et al.*, 1986; Ewenstein *et al.*, 1987; Reinders *et al.*, 1988). Apparently, routing of vWF to the Weibel-Palade bodies allows ongoing multimerization in this compartment that contains a high concentration of vWF and favourable conditions (i.e. low pH) for the generation of high molecular weight multimers (Mayadas and Wagner, 1989). At this point, it should be emphasized that the adhesive property of high molecular weight vWF greatly exceeds that of low molecular weight vWF. The affinity of high molecular weight vWF for GPIb is about 100 fold higher than that of low molecular weight vWF for this receptor of the platelet surface (Frederici *et al.*, 1989). This is probably due to the multiplicity of binding sites on high molecular weight material as compared to low molecular weight multimers. Hence, the adhesive properties of vWF are strongly determined by the destination of vWF to proceed into either one of the secretory pathways. No data are available on parameters that affect the destination of vWF into a particular secretory pathway. Results from studies on the routing of newly synthesized hormones in their cell of origin have suggested that constitutive secretion should be considered as a default pathway that is available when the regulated pathway has been "saturated" (Kelly, 1985).

vWF storage in Weibel-Palade bodies

Weibel-Palade bodies are endothelial-cell specific, electron-dense organelles (Weibel and Palade, 1964). These rod-shaped organelles have a length of approximately 4 μm long and a thickness of about 0.1 μm. Initially, it was believed that the lumen of Weibel-Palade bodies contained exclusively vWF and its pro-polypeptide (vW AgII) (Wagner *et al.*, 1982; McCarroll *et al.*, 1985, Ewenstein *et al.*, 1987). Recently, however, a number of other Weibel-Palade body resident proteins have been identified. First, a membrane-bound protein, denoted P-selectin (also called GMP-140 or PADGEM), has been described (Bonfanti *et al.*, 1989; McEver *et al.*, 1989). Release of the contents of the Weibel-Palade body, due to the presence of secretagogues, results in the exposure of P-selectin on the plasma membrane. In this configuration, P-selectin acts as a receptor for the adherence of leucocytes to the endothelial lining, an event that precedes transmigration to combat a focus of inflammation (reviewed in Ross, 1993). Subsequently, P-selectin is recycled to the Weibel-Palade bodies. Second, a protein, denoted CD63, has been found in the Weibel-Palade bodies (Metzelaar *et al.*, 1991; Vischer and Wagner, 1993). CD63 is a membrane glycoprotein that is also present in lysosomal membranes of platelets and other cell types. Third, it has been recently discovered that multimerin, a protein previously identified in the α-granules of platelets (Hayward *et al.*, 1991), is present in the lumen of the Weibel-Palade body (Kelton, personal communication). Like vWF, multimerin (MW of the monomer is 150 kDa) is encountered as a series of multimers. At present, the function of (multimerized) multimerin has not yet been reported.

Weibel-Palade bodies release their contents by exocytosis in the presence of an agonist that stimulates the protein kinase C-dependent signal transduction pathway. *In vitro*, release of vWF can be achieved by treatment of cultured endothelial cells with the calcium ionophore A231187 or with phorbol myristate acetate (PMA) (Loesberg *et al.*, 1983, de Groot *et al.*, 1984). Likely agonists *in vivo* are elevated levels of thrombin (Levine *et al.*, 1982, Loesberg *et al.*, 1983), histamine (Hamilton and Simms, 1987), fibrin (Ribes *et al.*, 1987) and complement proteins C5b-9 (Hattori *et al.*, 1989).

Routing of vWF to the Weibel-Palade bodies

The requirements for routing of (partially) multimerized vWF from the trans-Golgi network to the Weibel-Palade bodies is subject to discussion. At present, there is no consensus on such requirements, possibly due to use of the different cell types that have been employed for transfection experiments with vWF cDNA or variants thereof. Initially, it was proposed that storage of vWF in Weibel-Palade body-like organelles could only be achieved in transfected cells that harbour a regulated pathway, such as the adreno-corticotropic hormone (ACTH)- producing, murine pituitary cell line AtT-20 and the insulin-producing cell line RIN-5 (Wagner *et al.*, 1991). However, it has now been demonstrated that Monkey kidney CV-1 cells, that are not known to store proteins, exhibit vWF-containing Weibel-Palade body-like organelles, upon transfection with vWF cDNA (Voorberg *et al.*, 1993). Furthermore, it was claimed that proteolytic processing of pro-vWF is obligatory for storage in AtT-20 and RIN-5 cells, transfected with cDNA containing a mutation at the cleavage site (pro-vWF arg741gly) (Journet *et al.*, 1993). Nevertheless, transfection of CV-1 cells with vWF arg741gly cDNA showed storage of vWF protein in Weibel-Palade-like organelles (Voorberg *et al.*, 1993). Finally, intriguing discrepancies have been reported on structural requirements for routing of vWF to the Weibel-Palade bodies. The data reported sofar can be interpreted both in terms of a specific sorting signal required for routing the Weibel-Palade bodies and in terms of condensation (i.e. multimerization) as the "trigger" for the biogenesis of these organelles. First, stable transfectants of the regulated cell lines (AtT-20, RIN-5) with vWF cDNA, truncated at the carboxyl-terminus and, conceivably, not able to dimerize and multimerize, were found to generate Weibel-Palade-like organelles (Wagner *et al.*, 1991). These findings prompted the investigators to propose that the pro-polypeptide of pro-vWF plays an important role ("sorting signal") in routing to the Weibel-Palade bodies. On the other hand, data have been reported on the transfection of CV-1 cells with a set of vWF cDNA deletion mutants, lacking successive domains of pro-vWF, that demonstrate a correlation between the ability of particular mutants to dimerize, and subsequently to multimerize, and the generation of Weibel-Palade body-like organelles (Voorberg *et al.*, 1993). Thus, in the latter case, storage of vWF could be detected provided the domains D1, D2, D', D3 and the utmost 151 amino-acid residues of mature vWF were present. In addition, it was found that domains D1 and D2 could act *in-trans*, since cotransfection of CV-1 cells with a plasmid containing the D1 and D2 cDNA and another plasmid with cDNA, encoding only mature vWF, generated vWF multimers (Wise *et al.*, 1988; Voorberg *et al.*, 1993), but also elicited the formation of Weibel-Palade-like organelles (Voorberg *et al.*, 1993). In conclusion, data have been reported that argue in favour of a specific sorting signal to direct vWF to the Weibel-Palade body, reminiscent to sorting of a specific set of proteins to other organelles, e.g. to the endoplasmatic reticulum (Pelham, 1990). On the other hand, results have been presented that agree with the view that condensation (or multimerization) of the protein is the triggering event for the formation of these organelles, similar to storage of the condensation of hormones before storage (Kelly, 1985).

Proteolytic processing of pro-VWF

Initial experiments with cultured endothelial cells, using pulse-chase labelling of newly synthesized proteins in combination with metabolic inhibitors, showed that proteolytic processing of pro-VWF occurs in the Golgi apparatus or in post-Golgi compartments, such as the Weibel-Palade bodies and secretory vesicles (Wagner and Marder, 1984). Subsequently, it was described, using sub-cellular fractionation, that Weibel-Palade bodies contain stoichiometric amounts of mature vWF and of the vWF pro-polypeptide (vW Ag II), indicative for proteolytic processing of pro-vWF within these organelles (Ewenstein *et al.*, 1987). Recently, however, new insight has been presented into the cellular compartment responsible for cleavage of pro-vWF in mature vWF and vW AgII (Vischer and Wagner, 1994). These authors provided conclusive evidence that proteolytic processing occurs in the trans-Golgi network. Interestingly, the two segments of pro-vWF remain associated and are routed together to the Weibel-Palade bodies, in agreement with the finding that stoichiometric amounts of these entities are encountered in the Weibel-Palade bodies (Ewenstein *et al.*, 1987). Non-covalent association of the pro-polypeptide with mature vWF is promoted by high calcium concentrations and an acidic environment, conditions that met by the trans-Golgi network. The ability of a non-covalent association had been demonstrated previously by co-transfection studies of Monkey kidney COS and CV-1 cells with cDNA, encoding separately for the pro-polypeptide and for mature vWF (Wise *et al.*, 1988). The experiments revealed that also under these conditions vWF multimers are generated.

From the observations, reported by Vischer and Wagner (1994), it can be speculated that a single proteolytic enzyme, present in the trans-Golgi network, is responsible for the processing of both constitutively secreted vWF and for vWF routed by the regulated pathway. According to this view, proteolytic processing occurs prior to "sorting" into either one of the two secretory pathways. If the constitutive route is considered as a default pathway then the observation that only part of constitutively secreted vWF is proteolytically processed might be explained by saturation of the processing system. Recently, a potential processing enzyme has been independently identified by two groups, employing the same approach (Van de Ven *et al.*, 1990; Wise *et al.*, 1990). Co-transfection of COS cells with cDNA, encoding pro-vWF, and full-length human furin cDNA demonstrated complete processing of pro-vWF in the pro-polypeptide and mature vWF. In the absence of furin cDNA, pro-vWF is only partially proteolytically processed in transfected COS cells. The substrate specificity of furin, a di-basic endopeptidase, agrees with the amino-acid sequence that precedes the amino-terminus of mature vWF, namely arginine (-4), serine (-3), lysine (-2), arginine (-1). Replacement of arginine (-1) by glycine prevents cleavage by furin, underscoring the substrate specificity of the enzyme (Van de Ven *et al.*, 1990; Wise *et al.*, 1990). Since furin is a member of a family of enzymes with similar activities (di-basic endopeptidases), further experiments are required to demonstrate that this particular enzyme is responsible for pro-vWF processing in the endothelial cell.

Polar secretion of vWF by endothelial cells

Independent observations, using different systems to allow polar growth of cultured endothelial cells, have demonstrated that constitutive release of vWF is equally distributed to the apical- and the basolateral side of the cell (Sporn *et al.*, 1989; Van Buul-Wortelboer *et al.*, 1989). However, by using these different systems, dissimilar observations have been reported on the regulated secretion after stimulation of cultured endothelial cells with a secretagogue. Both preferential apical secretion (Van Buul-Wortelboer *et al.*, 1989) and predominantly basolateral deposition have been claimed (Sporn *et al.*, 1989). Studies with *in vivo* specimens support the view of a regulated apical secretion. Electron microscopic observations of rat aorta vascular endothelial cells, treated with the agonist thrombin, revealed large vWF-containing vacuoles, presumably due to fusion of Weibel-Palade bodies, that were located near the plasma membrane (Richardson *et al.*, 1994). Moreover, confocal scanning electron microscopy of Madin-Darby Canine Kidney cells (MDCK), stably transfected with vWF DNA, also revealed that most of the Weibel-Palade-like organelles are situated at the apical side of the cells (Hop and Pannekoek, unpublished observations). Hence, the data reported sofar suggest that release of vWF via the regulated secretory pathway predominantly occurs at the apical side of the cell. However, on a conceptional basis the opposite conclusion would have been anticipated for reasons discussed before. First, the regulated pathway delivers high molecular vWF multimers that are particularly suited for the interaction with the GPIb receptor on platelets. Apparently, this material is secreted at the apical side and will appear in plasma. Second, it is generally believed that vWF deposited in the subendothelial matrix undergoes a conformational change and is the principal source of vWF that interacts with GPIb, whereas plasma vWF only has a supportive role in this process. To reconcile these observations, we speculate that binding of constitutively secreted, low and intermediate vWF multimers to the subendothelium induces a conformational change that compensates for the lack of adhesive properties that are attributed to high molecular weight plasma vWF. The function of vWF, secreted at the apical side through the constitutive pathway and composed of dimers and intermediately multimerized vWF, would be to support FVIII binding and protect the cofactor from proteolytic degradation in plasma (Counts *et al.*, 1977; Tuddenham *et al.*, 1982).

Final remarks on remaining issues

Clearly, the construction and expression of full-length vWF cDNA has initiated a new era for studies on the biology of vWF (Verweij *et al.*, 1986; Bonthron *et al.*, 1986). This and other extensive reviews (Wagner, 1990; Ruggeri and Ware, 1992, 1993) illustrate the wealth of new information on the properties and the biosynthesis of this complex protein. Undoubtedly, much of the interest in vWF stems from clinical issues, related to the frequent occurrence of mutations in the vWF alleles that constitute the genetic background for a bleeding diathesis. We have restricted this review to biochemical, cell biological and molecular biological aspects of vWF and refer to other reviews for a discussion on the clinical issues (e.g. Ruggeri and Zimmerman, 1987). In this review, we have briefly recapitulated the most prominent recent developments and emphasized some unsolved topics. Finally, we will present a selection of other remaining unsolved issues on the properties and the biosynthesis of vWF:

- A full inventory of transcriptional regulatory elements and of the corresponding trans-acting transcriptional regulatory proteins is required to explain the restricted expression of vWF in endothelial cells and megakaryocytes.

- Although it is assumed that the biosynthesis and processing of vWF in megakaryocytes is similar to that in endothelial cells, experimental evidence is lacking. Obviously, such studies are hampered by the laborious manipulations to isolate primary megakaryocytes.

- A longstanding enigma is the cellular or extracellular association of vWF and FVIII to form vWF/FVIII complexes. Clearly, these entities originate from different cell types: FVIII is synthesized in hepatocytes and other cell types, whereas vWF is made in endothelial cells lining the vessel wall.

- Many of the questions related to the requirements on the vWF molecule for routing either to the regulated or to the constitutive pathway have been discussed in this review. Since, vWF is the major soluble protein of the Weibel-Palade body it is possible that the biogenesis of Weibel-Palade bodies is "driven" by the biosynthesis and assembly of (multimeric) vWF. Definite proof for this option or, conversely, for independent biosynthesis of vWF and biogenesis of these organelles await further experimentation.

- An intriguing issue concerns the proposed conformational change of vWF that is deposited in the subendothelium. The conformational change is assumed to yield an adhesive competent protein able to directly interact with the GPIb receptor on the platelet surface. However, the nature of the proposed conformational change of the molecule has not been established.

- Conceivably due to divergent endothelial cell culturing conditions, confusing data have been reported on the level of vWF biosynthesis after activation with cytokines (de Groot *et al.*, 1987, Zavoico *et al.*, 1989, Paleolog *et al.*, 1990; Giddings and Shall, 1987). Hence, the eminent question remains as to whether differences in the level of vWF synthesis would have consequences for the partition of the protein in the regulated and the constitutive pathway.

- Crystallization of vWF or of specific domains of the protein, preferably followed by co-crystallization with its biological counterparts, in order to elucidate the three-dimensional structure would obviously greatly deepen our insight into the diverse interaction of this adhesive protein that plays an essential role in hemostasis.

- Most of the data on the properties and biosynthesis of vWF described in this Chapter have been derived from *in vitro* experiments, predominantly by using cultured vascular endothelial cells. One should be cautious to extrapolate those data to the properties and biosynthesis of vWF, synthesized in non-vascular endothelial cells. Finally, a major future challenge will undoubtedly be the "translation" of the data, obtained with cultured vascular endothelial cells, to the strucure, function and biosynthesis of vWF *in vivo* under pathological and non-pathological conditions.

Acknowledgements

This work was supported by grant no. 91–126 from the Netherlands Heart Foundation (NHS). We are grateful to Dr. Jan A. van Mourik for critical reading of the manuscript.

References

Azuma, H., Sugimoto, M., Ruggeri, Z.M. and Ware, J. (1993). A role for von Willebrand factor proline residues 702–704 in ristocetin-mediated binding to platelet glycoprotein Ib. *Thromb. Haemostas.*, **69**:192–196.

Bahou, W.F., Ginsburg, D., Sikkink, R., Litwiller, R. and Fass, D.N. (1991). A monoclonal antibody to von Willebrand factor (vWF) inhibits factor VIII binding. Localization of its antigenic determinant to a non-adecapeptide at the amino terminus of the mature vWF polypeptide. *J. Clin. Invest.*, **84**:56–61.

Beacham, D.A., Wise, R.J., Turci, S.M. and Handin, R.I. (1992). Selective inactivation of the Arg-Gly-Asp-Ser (RGDS) binding site in von Willebrand factor by site-directed mutagenesis. *J. Biol. Chem.*, **267**:3409–3415.

Berndt, M.C., Gregory, C., Kabral, A., Zola, H., Fournier, D. and Castaldi, P.A. (1985). Purification and preliminary characterization of the glycoprotein Ib complex in the human platelet membrane. *Eur. J. Biochem.*, **151**:637–649.

Berndt, M.C., Booth, W.J., Andrews, R.K. and Castaldi, P.A. (1991). Definition of von Willebrand factor (vWF) GPIb-IX complex interaction using vWF-based peptides. *Thromb. Haemostas.*, **65**:748 (abstr.).

Berndt, M.C., Ward, C.M., Booth, W.J., Castaldi, P.A., Mazurov, A.V. and Andrews, R.K. (1992). Identification of aspartic acid 514 through glutamic acid 542 as a glycoprotein Ib-IX complex receptor recognition sequence in von Willebrand factor. Mechanism of modulation of von Willebrand factor by ristocetin and botrocetin. *Biochemistry*, **31**:11144–11151.

Bonfanti, R., Furie, B.C., Furie, B. and Wagner, D.D. (1989). PADGEM (GMP-140) is a component of Weibel Palade bodies of human endothelial cells. *Blood*, **73**:1109–1112.

Bonthron, D.T., Handin, R.I., Kaufman, R.J., Wasley, L.C., Orr, E.C., Mitsock, L.M., Ewenstein, B., Loscalzo, J., Ginsburg, D. and Orkin, S.H. (1986). Structure of pre-pro-von Willebrand factor and its expression in heterologous cells. *Nature*, **324**:270–273.

Brinkhous, K.M., Sandberg, H., Garris, J.R., Mattron, C., Palm, M., Griggs, T. and Read, M.S. (1985). Purified factor VIII procoagulant protein: comparative hemostatic response after infusions into hemophilic and von Willebrand disease dogs. *Proc. Natl. Acad. Sci. USA*, **82**:8752–8756.

Buul-Wortelboer, M. van, Brinkman, H.J., Reinders, J.H., van Aken, W.G. and van Mourik, J.A. (1989). Polar secretion of von Willebrand factor by endothelial cells. *Biochim. Biophys. Acta*, **1011**:129–133.

Charo, I.F., Bekeart, L.S. and Phillips, D.R. (1987). Platelet glycoprotein IIb-IIIa-like proteins mediate endothelial cell attachment to adhesive protein and extracellular matrix. *J. Biol. Chem.*, **262**:9935–9938.

Cheresh, D. (1987). Human endothelial cells synthesize and express an Arg-Gly-Asp-directed adhesion receptor involved in attachment to fibrinogen and von Willebrand factor. *Proc. Natl. Acad. Sci. USA*, **84**:6471–6475.

Chow, T.W., Hellums, J.D., Moake, J.L. and Kroll, M.H. (1992). Shear stress-induced von Willebrand factor binding to platelet glycoprotein Ib initiates calcium influx associated with aggregation. *Blood*, **80**:113–120.

Cooper, H.A., Griggs, T.R. and Wagner, R.H. (1973). Factor VIII recombination after dissociation by CaCl2. *Proc. Natl. Acad. Sci. USA*, **70**:2326–2329.

Counts, R.B., Paskell, S.L. and Elgee, S.K. (1977). Disulfide bonds and quarternary structure of factor VIII/von Willebrand factor. *J. Clin. Invest.*, **62**:702–709.

Cramer, E.M., Meyer, D., Le Menn, R. and Breton-Gorius, J. (1985). Excentric localization of von Willebrand factor in an internal structure of platelet alpha granule resembling that of Weibel Palade bodies. *Blood*, **66**:710–713.

Cruz, M.A., Handin, R.I. and Wise, R.J. (1993). The interaction of the von Willebrand factor A1 domain with platelet glycoprotein Ib/IX. *J. Biol. Chem.*, **268**:21238–21245.

Dejana, E., Lampugnani, M.G., Giorgi, M., Gaboli, M., Federici, A.B., Ruggeri, Z.M. and Marchiso, P.C. (1989). Von Willebrand factor promotes endothelial cell adhesion via an arg-gly-asp-dependent mechanism. *J. Cell Biol.*, **109**:367–375.

De Marco, L., Girolami, A., Russell, S. and Ruggeri, Z.M. (1985). Interaction of asialo von Willebrand factor with glycoprotein Ib induces fibrinogen binding to the glycoprotein IIb/IIIa complex and mediates platelet aggregation. *J. Clin. Invest.*, **75**:1198–1203.

Denis, C., Baruch, D., Kielty, C.M., Ajzenberg, N., Christophe, O. and Meyer, D. (1993). Localization of von Willebrand factor binding domains to endothelial extracellular matrix and to type VI collagen. Arterioscler. *Thromb.*, **13**:398–406.

D'Souza, S.E., Ginsberg, M.H., Burke, T.A., Lam, S.C.-.T. and Plow, E.F. (1988). Localization of an Arg-Gly-Asp recognition site within an integrin adhesion receptor. *Science*, **242**:91–93.

Du, X., Beutler, L., Ruan, C., Castaldi, P.A. and Berndt, M.C. (1987). Glycoprotein Ib and Glycoprotein IX are fully complexed in the intact platelet membrane. *Blood*, **69**:1524–1527.

Ewenstein, B.M., Warhol, M.J., Handin, R.I. and Pober, J.S. (1987). Composition of von Willebrand factor storage organelle (Weibel-Palade body) isolated from cultured umbilical vein endothelial cells. *J. Cell Biol.*, **104**:1423–1433.

Foster, P.A., Fulcher, C.A., Marti, T., Titani, K. and Zimmerman, T.S. (1987). A major factor VIII binding domain resides within the amino terminal 272 amino acid residues of von Willebrand factor. *J. Biol. Chem.*, **262**:8443–8446.

Frederici, A.B., Bader, R., Coliberti, M.L., de Marco, L. and Mannucci, P.M. (1989). Binding of von Willebrand factor to glycoproteins Ib and IIb/IIIa complex: affinity is related to multimer size. *Brit. J. Haematol.*, **73**:93–99.

Fressinaud, E., Sakariassen, K.S., Girma, J.P., Meyer, D. and Baumgarten, H.R. (1986). Role of GPIIb/IIIa as well as GPIb in von Willebrand factor-mediated platelet adhesion to collagen. *Thromb. Res.*, **suppl. 6**, 138 (abstr.).

Fretto, L.J., Fowler, W.E., McCaslin, D.R., Erickson, H.P. and McKee, P.A. (1986). Substructure of human von Willebrand factor. *J. Biol. Chem.*, **261**:15679–15689

Fujimura, Y., Titani, K., Holland, L.Z., Roberts, J.R., Kostel, P., Ruggeri, Z.M. and Zimmerman, T.S. (1987). A heparin-binding domain of human von Willebrand factor. *J. Biol. Chem.*, **267**:8857–8862.

Giddings, J.C. and Shall, L. (1987). Enhanced release of von Willebrand factor by human endothelial cells in culture in the presence of phorbol myristate acetate and interleukin 1. *Thromb. Res.*, **47** 259–267.

Ginsburg, D., Handin, R.I., Bonthron, D.T., Donlon, T.A., Bruns, G.A.P., Latt, S.A. and Orkin, S.H. (1985). Human von Willebrand factor (vWF): Isolation of complementary DNA (cDNA) clones and chromosomal localization. *Science*, **228**:1401–1406.

Girma, J.P., Takahashi, Y., Yoshioka, A., Diaz, J. and Meyer, D. (1990). Ristocetin and botrocetin involve two distinct domains of von Willebrand factor for binding to platelet membrane glycoprotein Ib. *Thromb. Haemostas.*, **64**:326–332.

Gralnick, H.R., Williams, S., McKeown, L. and Krutzsch, H. (1992). Purification and partial characterization of platelet von Willebrand factor. In: 3rd Bari Intern. Conf. on Factor VIII/von Willebrand factor: Biological and Clinical Advances (Eds. N. Ciavarella, P.M. Mannucci, Z.M. Ruggeri, M. Schiavoni), pp. 31.

Groot, Ph.G. de, Gonsalves, M.D., Loesberg, C., van Buul-Wortelboer, M.F., van Aken, W.G. and van Mourik, J.A. (1984). Thrombin-induced release of von Willebrand factor from endothelial cells is mediated by phospholipid methylation. *J. Biol. Chem.*, **259**:13329–13333.

Groot, Ph.G. de, Verweij, C.L., Nawroth, P.P., de Boer, H.H., Stern, D.M. and Sixma, J.J. (1987). Interleukin 1 inhibits the synthesis of von Willebrand factor in endothelial cells which results in a decreased reactivity of their matrix towards platelets. *Arteriosclerosis*, **7**:605–611.

Groot, P.G. de, Ottenhof-Rovers, M., van Mourik, J.A. and Sixma, J.J. (1988). Evidence that the primary binding site of von Willebrand factor that mediates platelet adhesion on subendothelium is not collagen. *J. Clin. Invest.*, **82**:65–73.

Hattori, R., Hamilton, K.K., McEver, R.P. and Sims, P.J. (1989). Complement proteins C5b-9 induce secretion of high molecular weight multimers of endothelial von Willebrand factor and translocation of granule membrane protein GMP-140 to the cell surface. *J. Biol. Chem.*, **264**:9053–9060.

Hamilton, K.K. and Sims, P.J. (1987). Changes in cytosolic Ca^{2+} associated with von Willebrand factor release in human endothelial cells exposed to histamine. *J. Clin. Invest.*, **79**:600–608.

Hayward, C.P., Warkentin, T.E., Horsewood, P. and Kelton, J.G. (1991). Multimerin: a series of large disulfide-linked multimeric proteins within platelets. *Blood*, **77**:(12), 2556–2560.

Hill-Eubanks, D.C., Parker, C.G. and Lollar, P. (1989). Differential proteolytic activation of factor VIII-von Willebrand factor complex by thrombin. *Proc. Natl. Acad. Sci. USA*, **86**:6508–6512.

Howard, M.A., Perkin, J., Salem, H.H. and Firkin, B. (1984). The agglutination of human platelets by botrocetin: evidence that botrocetin and ristocetin act at different sites on the factor VIII molecule and platelet membrane. *Brit. J. Haematol.*, **57**:25–35.

Hynes, R.O. (1987). Integrins: A family of cell surface receptors. *Cell*, **48**:549–554.

Ikeda, Y., Handa, M., Kawano, K., Kamata, T., Murata, M., Araki, Y., Anbo, H., Kawai, Y., Watanabe, K., Itagaki, I., Sakai, K. and Ruggeri, Z.M. (1991). The role of von Willebrand factor and fibrinogen in platelet aggregation under varying shear stress. *J. Clin. Invest.*, **87**:1234–1240.

Jaffe, E.A., Hoyer, L.W. and Nachmann, R.L. (1973). Synthesis of anti-haemophilic factor antigen by cultured human endothelial cells. *J. Clin. Invest.*, **52**:2757–2764.

Kelly, R.B. (1985). Pathways of protein secretion in eukaryocytes. *Science*, **230**:25–32.

Konkle, B.A., Shapiro, S.S., Asch, A.S. and Nachman, R.L. (1990). Cytokine-enhanced expression of glycoprotein Ibα in human endothelium. *J. Biol. Chem.*, **265**:19833–19838.

Kroll, M.H., Harris, T.S., Moake, J.L., Handin, R.I. and Schafer, A.I. (1991). Von Willebrand factor binding to platelet GPIb initiates signals for platelet activation. *J. Clin. Invest.*, **88**:1568–1573.

Kunicki, T.J., Pidard, D., Rosa, J.P. and Nurden, A.T. (1981). The formation of calcium-dependent complexes of platelet membrane glycoproteins IIb and IIIa in solution as determined by crossed immuno-electrophoresis. *Blood*, **58**:268–278.

Leyte, A., Verbeet, M.Ph., Brodniewicz-Proba, T., van Mourik, J.A. and Mertens, K. (1990). The interaction between human blood-coagulation factor VIII and von Willebrand factor: characterization of a high-affinity binding site on factor VIII. *Biochem. J.*, **257**:679–683.

Leyte, A., Voorberg, J., van Schijndel, H.B., Duim, B., Pannekoek, H. and van Mourik, J.A. (1991). The propolypeptide of von Willebrand factor is required for the formation of a functional Factor VIII-binding site on mature von Willebrand factor. *Biochem. J.*, **274**:257–261.

Levine, J.D., Harlan, J.M., Harker L.A., Joseph M.L. and Counts, R.B. (1982). Thrombin-mediated release of factor VIII antigen from human umbilical vein endothelial cells in culture. *Blood*, **60**:531–533.

Loesberg, C., Gonsalves, M.D., Zandbergen, J., Willems, C., van Aken, W.G., Stel, H.V., van Mourik, J.A. and de Groot Ph.G. (1983). The effect of calcium on the secretion of factor VIII-related antigen by cultured endothelial cells. *Biochim. Biophys. Acta*, **763**:160–168.

López, J.A., Chung, D.W., Fujikawa, K., Hagen, F.S., Davie, E.W. and Roth, G.J. (1988). The alpha and beta chains of human platelet glycoprotein Ib are both transmembrane proteins containing a leucine-rich alpha$_2$ glycoprotein. *Proc. Natl. Acad. Sci. USA*, **85**:2135–2139.

Lynch, D.C., Zimmerman, T.S., Collins, C.J., Brown, M., Morin, M.J., Ling, E.H. and Livingstone, D.M. (1985). Molecular cloning of cDNA for human von Willebrand factor: authentication by a new method. *Cell*, **41**:49–56.

Mancuso, D.J., Tuley, E.A., Westfield, L.A., Worrall, N.K., Shelton-Inloes, B.B., Sorace, J.M., Alevy, Y.G. and Sadler, J.E. (1989). The structure of the gene for von Willebrand factor. *J. Biol. Chem.*, **264**:19514–19527.

Marti, T., Rosselet, S.J., Titani, K. and Walsh, K.A. (1987). Identification of disulfide-bridged Substructures within human von Willebrand Factor. *Biochemistry*, **26**:8099–8109.

Mayadas, T. and Wagner, D.D. (1989). *In vitro* multimerization of von Willebrand factor is triggered by low pH: importance of the pro-polypeptide and free sulfhydryls groups. *J. Biol. Chem.*, **264**:13947–13503.

McCarroll, D.R., Levin, E.G. and Montgomery, R.R. (1985). Endothelial cell synthesis of von Willebrand antigen II, von Willebrand factor and von Willebrand factor/von Willebrand antigen II complex. *J. Clin. Invest.*, **75**:1089–1095.

McEver, R.P., Beckstead, J.H., Moore, K.L., Marshall-Carlson, L. and Bainton, D.F. (1989). GMP-140, a platelet alpha granule membrane protein, is also synthesized by vascular endothelial cells and is localized in Weibel-Palade bodies. *J. Clin. Invest.*, **84**:92–99.

Metzelaar, M.J., Wijngaard, P.L.J., Peters, P.J., Sixma, J.J., Nieuwenhuis, H.K. and Clevers, H.C. (1991). CD63 antigen: a novel lysosomal membrane glycoprotein, cloned by a screening procedure for intracellular antigens in eucaryotic cells. *J. Biol. Chem.*, **266**:3239–3245.

Moake, J.L., Olson, J.D., Troll, J.H., Tang, S.S., Funicella T. and Peterson D.M. (1980). Binding of radioiodinated human von Willebrand factor to Bernard Soulier, thrombasthenic and von Willebrand's disease platelets. *Thromb. Res.*, **19**:21–27.

Modderman, P.W., Admiraal, L.G., Sonnenberg, A. and von dem Borne, A.E.G.Kr. (1992). Glycoproteins V and Ib-IX form a noncovalent complex in the platelet membrane. *J. Biol. Chem.*, **267**:364–369.

Mohri, H., Fujimura, Y., Shima, M., Yoshioka, A., Houghton, R.A., Ruggeri, Z.M. and Zimmerman, T.S. (1988). Structure of the von Willebrand factor domain interacting with glycoprotein Ib. *J. Biol. Chem.*, **263**:17901–17904.

Morton, L.F., Griffin, B., Pepper, D.S. and Barnes, M.J. (1983). The interaction between collagens and factor VIII/von Willebrand factor: investigations of the structural requirements for interaction. *Thromb. Res.*, **32**:545–556.

Pelham, H.R.B. (1990). The retention signal for soluble proteins of the endoplasmic reticulum. Trends Biochem. *Sci.*, **15**:483–486.

Philips, D.R., Charo, I.F. and Scarborough, R.M. (1991). GPIIb-IIIa: The responsive integrin. *Cell*, **65**:359–362.

Pietu, G., Ribba, A.S., Meulien, P. and Meyer, D. (1989). Localization within the 106 N-terminal amino acids of von Willebrand factor (vWF) of the epitope corresponding to a monoclonal antibody which inhibits vWF binding to factor VIII. *Biochem. Biophys. Res. Comm.*, **163**:618–626.

Rand, J.H., Patel, N.D., Schwartz, E., Zhou, S.L. and Potter, B.J. (1991). 150 kD von Willebrand factor binding protein extracted from human vascular subendothelium is type VI collagen. *J. Clin. Invest.*, **88**:253–259.

Rand, J.H., Xiao-Xuan, W., Potter, B.J., Uson, R.R. and Gordon, R.E. (1993). Co-localization of von Willebrand factor and type VI collagen in human vascular subendothelium. *Amer. J. Pathol.*, **142**:843–850.

Reinders, J.H., de Groot, P.G., Sixma, J.J. and van Mourik, J.A. (1988). Storage and secretion of von Willebrand factor by endothelial cells. *Haemostasis,* **18**:246–261.

Ribes, J.A., Francis, C.W. and Wagner, D.D. (1987). Fibrin induces release of von Willebrand factor from endothelial cells. *J. Clin. Invest.,* **79**:117–123.

Richardson, M., Tinlin, S., Senis, Y. and Giles, A.R. (1994). Morphological alterations in endothelial cells associated with the release of von Willebrand factor following thrombin generation *in vivo*. Arterioscler. Thromb., **14**:990–999.

Ross, R. (1993). The pathogenesis of atherosclerosis: a perspective for the 1990s. *Nature*, **362**:801–809.

Ruggeri, Z.M. and Zimmerman, T.S. (1987). Von Willebrand factor and von Willebrand disease. *Blood*, **70**:895–904.

Ruggeri, Z.M. and Ware, J. (1992). The structure and function of von Willebrand factor. *Thromb. Haemostas.,* **67**:594–599.

Ruggeri, Z.M. and Ware, J. (1993). Von Willebrand factor. *FASEB. J.,* **7**:308–316.

Ruoslahti, E. and Pierschbacher, M.D. (1985). Arg/Gly/Asp: a versatile cell's recognition signal. *Cell,* **44**:517–518.

Sadler, J.E., Shelton-Inloes, B.B., Sorace, J.M., Harlan, J.M., Titani, K. and Davie, E.W. (1985). Cloning and characterization of two cDNAs coding for human von Willebrand factor. *Proc. Natl. Acad. Sci. USA*, **82**:6394–6398.

Sakariassen, K.S., Bolhuis, P.A. and Sixma, J.J. (1979). Human blood platelet adhesion to artery subendothelium is mediated by factor VIII/von Willebrand factor bound to the subendothelium. *Nature*, **279**:636–638.

Sakariassen, K.S., Fressinaud, E., Girma, J.P., Baumgarten, H.R. and Meyer, D. (1986a). Mediation of platelet adhesion to fibrillar collagen in flowing blood by a proteolytic fragment of human von Willebrand factor. *Blood*, **67**:1515–1518.

Sakariassen, K.S., Nievelstein, P.F.E.M., Coller, B.S. and Sixma, J.J. (1986b). The role of platelet membrane glycoprotein Ib and IIb/IIIa in platelet adherence to human artery subendothelium. *Brit. J. Haematol.,* **63**:681–691.

Santoro, S. (1983). Preferential binding of high molecular weight form of von Willebrand factor to fibrillar collagen. *Biochim. Biophys. Acta*, **756**:123–126.

Savage, B., Shattil, S.J. and Ruggeri, Z.M. (1992). Modulation of platelet function through adhesion receptors. A dual role for glycoprotein IIb-IIIa (integrin alpha IIb beta 3) mediated by fibrinogen and glycoprotein Ib-von Willebrand factor. *J. Biol. Chem.,* **267**:11300–11306.

Sobel, M., Soler, D.F., Kermode, J.C. and Harris, R.B. (1992). Localization and characterization of a heparin binding domain peptide of human von Willebrand factor. *J. Biol. Chem.,* **267**:8857–8862.

Sporn, L.A., Marder, V.J. and Wagner, D.D. (1986). Inducible secretion of large biologically potent von Willebrand factor multimers. *Cell,* **46**:185–190.

Sporn, L.A., Marder, V.J. and Wagner, D.D. (1987). Von Willebrand factor released from Weibel-Palade bodies binds more avidly to extracellular matrix than secreted constitutively. *Blood*, **69**:1531–1534.

Sporn, L.A., Marder, V.J. and Wagner, D.D. (1989). Differing polarity of the constitutive and regulated secretory pathways for von Willebrand factor in endothelial cells. *J. Cell. Biol.,* **108**:1283–1289.

Sugimoto, M., Mohri, H., McClintock, R.A. and Ruggeri, Z.M. (1991). Identification of discontinuous von Willebrand factor sequences involved in complex formation with botrocetin: a model for the regulation of von Willebrand factor binding to platelet glycoprotein Ib. *J. Biol. Chem.,* **266**:18172–18178.

Titani, K., Kumar, S., Takio, K., Ericksson, L.H., Wade, R.D., Ashida, K., Walsh, K.A., Chopek, M.W., Sadler, J.E. and Fujikawa, K. (1986). Amino-acid sequence of human von Willebrand factor. *Biochemistry*, **25**:3171–3184.

Titani, K., Marti, T., Takio, K. and Walsh, K.A. (1989). Primary structure of von Willebrand factor. In: Coagulation and Bleeding disorders; the role of Factor VIII and von Willebrand factor. (Eds. T.S. Zimmerman and Z. Ruggeri). Dekker, New York/Basel, vol. 9, pp. 99–116.

Tuddenham, E.G.D., Lane, R.S., Rothblat, F., Johnson, A.J., Snape, T.J., Middleton, S. and Kernoff, P.B.A. (1982). Response to infusions of electrolyte-fractionated human factor-VIII concentrate in human haemophilia A and von Willebrand's disease. *Brit. J. Haematol.,* **52**:259–267.

Ven, W.J.M. van de, Voorberg, J., Fontijn, R., Pannekoek, H., van den Ouwehand, A.M.W., van Duijnhoven, H.L.P., Roebroek, A.J.M. and Siezen, R.J. (1990). Furin is a subtilisin-like proprotein processing enzyme in higher eukaryotes. *Mol. Biol. Rep.,* **14**:265–275.

Verweij, C.L., de Vries, C.J.M., Distel, B., van Zonneveld, A.J., Geurts van Kessel, A., van Mourik, J.A. and Pannekoek, H. (1985). Construction of cDNA coding for human von Willebrand factor using antibody probes for colony-screening and mapping of the chromosomal gene. *Nucl. Acids Res.,* **13**:4699–4717.

Verweij, C.L., Diergaarde, P.J., Hart, M. and Pannekoek, H. (1986). Full-length von Willebrand factor (vWF) cDNA encodes a highly repetitive protein considerably larger than the mature vWF subunit. *EMBO J.,* **5**:1839–1847.

Vicente, V., Houghten, R.A. and Ruggeri, Z.M. (1990). Identification of a site in the α chain of platelet glycoprotein Ib that participates in von Willebrand factor binding. *J. Biol. Chem.,* **265**:274–280.

Voorberg, J., Fontijn, R., van Mourik, J.A. and Pannekoek, H. (1990). Domains involved in multimer assembly of von Willebrand factor (vWF): multimerization is independent of dimerization. *EMBO J.*, **9**:797–803.

Voorberg, J., Fontijn, R., Calafat, J., Janssen, H., van Mourik, J.A. and Pannekoek, H. (1991). Assembly and routing of von Willebrand factor variants: the requirements for disulfide-linked dimerization reside within the carboxyl-terminal 151 amino acids. *J. Cell Biol.*, **113**:195–205.

Voorberg, J., Fontijn, R., Calafat, J., Janssen, H., van Mourik, J.A., Pannekoek, H. (1993). Biogenesis of von Willebrand factor-containing organelles in heterologous transfected CV-1 cells. *EMBO J.*, **12**:749–758.

Wagner, D.D., Olmsted, J.B. and Marder, V.J. (1982). Immunolocalization of von Willebrand protein in Weibel Palade bodies of human endothelial cells. *J. Cell Biol.*, **95**:355–360.

Wagner, D.D. (1990). Cell biology of von Willebrand factor. *Ann. Rev. Cell Biol.*, **6**:217–246.

Wagner, D.D., Saffaripour, S., Bonfanti, R., Sadler J.W., Cramer, E.M., Chapman, B. and Mayadas, T.M. (1991). Induction of specific storage organelles by von Willebrand factor propolypeptide. *Cell*, **46**:403–413.

Weibel, E.R. and Palade, G.E. (1964). New cytoplasmic components in arterial endothelia. *J. Cell Biol.*, **23**:101–112.

Weiss, H.J., Sussman, I.I. and Hoyer, L.W. (1977). Stabilization of factor VIII in plasma by the von Willebrand factor. *J. Clin. Invest.*, **60**:390–404.

Weiss, H.J., Turitto, V.T. and Baumgarten, H.R. (1986). Platelet adhesion and thrombus formation on suben-dothelium in platelet deficient in glycoproteins IIb/IIIa and Ib and storage in alpha-granules. *Blood*, **67**:322–330.

Weiss, H.J., Hawiger, J., Ruggeri, Z.M., Turitto, V.I., Thiagarajan, P. and Hoffmann, T. (1989). Fibrinogen-independent platelet adhesion and thrombus formation on subendothelium mediated by glycoprotein IIb/IIIa complex at high shear rate. *J. Clin. Invest.*, **83**:288–297.

White, G.C. and Schoemaker, C.B. (1989). Factor VIII gene and haemophilia A. *Blood*, **73**:1–12.

Wion, K.L., Kelly, D., Summerfield, J.A., Tuddenham, E.G.D. and Lawn, R.M. (1985). Distribution of factor VIII mRNA and antigen in human liver and other tissues. *Nature*, **317**:726–728.

Wise, R.J., Pitmann, D.D., Handin, R.I., Kaufman, R.J. and Orkin, S.H. (1988). The propolypeptide of von Willebrand factor independently mediates the assembly of von Willebrand multimers. *Cell*, **52**:229–236.

Wise, R.J., Barr, P.J., Wong, P.A., Kiefer, M.C., Brake, A.J. and Kaufman, R.J. (1990). Expression of a human proprotein processing enzyme: correct cleavage of the von Willebrand factor precursor at a paired basic amino acid site. *Proc. Natl. Acad. Sci. USA*, **87**:9378–9382.

Wise, R.J., Dorner, A.J., Krane, M., Pittman, D.D. and Kaufman, R.J. (1991). The role of von Willebrand factors multimers and propeptide cleavage in binding and stabilization of Factor VIII. *J. Biol. Chem.*, **266**:21948–21955.

Zelechowska, M.G., van Mourik, J.A. and Brodniewicz-Proba, T. (1985). Ultrastructural localization of factor VIII procoagulant antigen in human liver hepatocytes. *Nature*, **317**:729–730.

7 Regulation of Platelet-Rich Thrombus Formation by the Endothelium

Philip G. de Groot and Jan J. Sixma

University Hospital Utrecht, Department of Haematology (G03.647), P.O. Box 85.500, 3508 GA UTRECHT, The Netherlands, Tel.: #31-30-250.72.30, Fax: #31-30-251.18.93, E-mail: ph.g.degroot@lab.azu.nl/jsixma@lab.azu.nl

INTRODUCTION

Platelets in the circulation are not activated as long as the endothelium remains biochemically and physically intact. When a vessel is transected, the normal hemostatic response starts immediately to prevent loss of blood. The first step in the hemostatic response is the adhesion of platelets. Platelets immediately adhere to exposed collagen and to von Willebrand factor present in the subendothelial structures (de Groot and Sixma, 1990). After activation of the platelets, vasoconstriction takes place and the injury is sealed by a platelet plug (Sixma and Wester, 1977). The hemostatic plug is subsequently strengthened by the formation of a fibrin network. Thrombosis can be considered as an abnormal consequence of the normal hemostatic process (Ratnoff, 1994). Thrombosis occurs after a superficial injury of the lumen of an intact vessel. It starts with a small rupture in the intact endothelial layer. Normally, the endothelial cells in the vicinity of the injury respond to limit the activation of the platelets and to downregulate thrombin formation. Only when the endothelial cells have lost (a part of) their normal function due to pathological conditions a thrombus can develop. The development of thrombi can thus be regarded as the consequence of a combination of the loss of endothelial cell integrity and an inadequate functioning of the metabolic activity of the endothelial cells covering the vessel wall.

One of the major functions of the endothelium is to separate the circulating platelets and clotting factors from the reactive deeper layers of the vessel wall. The endothelial cell is a cell with two faces. The plasma membrane on the luminal side of the endothelial cell has a completely different composition compared to the basolateral side (Muller and Gimbrone, 1986). The hemocompatibility of the luminal side of the endothelium is due to heparan sulphate-like structures which prevent platelets to interact with the endothelium, and the absence of surface molecules that can initiate coagulation or interact with platelets. On the basolateral side an extracellular matrix is formed which contains a large number of adhesive proteins, such as von Willebrand factor, laminin, fibronectin and

Table 7.1   Endothelial cell metabolites that regulate Hemostatic functions

Metabolite	Properties
Expression not known to be influenced in response to stimuli:	
Ectonucleotidases	Breakdown of platelet active nucleotides
Heparan sulphates	Prevent platelet-endothelial cell interaction
	Increase activity of antithrombin III
Binding sites for clotting factors	Support coagulation
TFPI I & II	Inhibition of tissue factor activity
Protein S	Member of protein C anticoagulant pathway
Factor V	Clotting factor
Production/release rapidly influenced in response to stimuli	
Prostacyclin	Inhibitor of platelet adhesion and aggregation Vasodilator
Nitric Oxide	Inhibitor of platelet adhesion and aggregation Vasodilator
Platelet Activating Factor	Cell surface associated platelet activator
von Willebrand factor	Main adhesive protein for platelets
Expression slowly influenced in response to stimuli	
Thrombomodulin	Cell surface expressed anticoagulant
Von Willebrand Factor	Main adhesive protein for platelets
Tissue factor	Activator of coagulation, only expressed on activated endothelium
Prostacyclin	Inhibitor of platelet adhesion and aggregation Vasodilator
Nitric oxide	Inhibitor of platelet adhesion and aggregation Vasodilator

collagen type IV, which are all able to support platelet adhesion. In addition, an intact endothelial cell layer expresses a large range of metabolic activities that prevent the activation of platelets and the coagulation cascade (Table 7.1). The endothelial cell surface contains a number of compounds such as heparan sulphates and ecto-nucleotidases which support the inactivation of platelet agonists (Borin and Lindahl, 1993, Marcus and Safier, 1993). When platelets are activated as the consequence of e.g. a superficial injury, the endothelial cells respond in a way that is directed towards the limitation of the activation of the platelets or even suppress platelet activation. The endothelial cells react on signals from their surrounding by releasing low molecular weight secretion product designed to inhibit platelet function. The most important products secreted by the endothelium which influence platelet function include prostacyclin (PGI_2) and nitric oxide (NO) (Lüscher, 1993).

The regulation of the hemostatic response by endothelial cells depends on their interaction with signals from the surroundings (Gimbrone, 1986, Pober and Cotran, 1990). A number of stimuli, in particular those which also stimulate a platelet response such as ADP and thrombin, induce a rapid and short lasting increase of antithrombotic functions (Table 7.1). Other stimuli, such as intermediates of immunological responses such as interleukin-1 (IL-1) and tumor necrosis factor (TNF) or endotoxins (LPS) induce a slow and long-lasting response that modulates endothelial cell properties to a more prothrombotic state (Table 7.1). In this chapter a review will be given of the control of platelet function and coagulation by endothelial cells.

ANTITHROMBOTIC ACTIVITIES OF ENDOTHELIAL CELLS

Prostacyclin

Almost every cell in the body is able to metabolize arachidonic acid to a large number of biological active oxidation products. Probably the major metabolic pathway is the synthesis of eicosanoids (Maclouf, 1993). Eicosanoids such as prostacyclin and thromboxane

A2 are autocoids which exert their biological effects in a microenvironment; only cells in the proximity of the producing cells are influenced. The major eicosanoid produced by endothelial cells is prostacyclin whereas the major product produced by platelets is thromboxane A_2 (TXA2) (Hamberg *et al.*, 1975, Moncada *et al.*, 1976). The biological effects of PGI2 and TXA2 on platelets are completely opposite. PGI2 is one of the most potent inhibitors of platelet function known while TXA2 is one of the most potent inducers of platelet aggregation. It has been postulated that the balance between PGI2 and TXA2 determines whether a platelet will aggregate (Moncada and Vane, 1979). Although much is learned about new mechanisms in the regulation of platelet aggregation since 1979, a contribution of the PGI2/TXA2 balance in the determination of a platelet response is undisputed. As long as the production of PGI2 dominates, the responses of platelets on agonists is suppressed. Only in those situation where the PGI2 production is limited (e.g. outside the lumen of a vessel) platelets can respond to agonists with TXA2 synthesis to support their aggregation.

Although levels of circulating PGI2 are detectable in perfused vessels, the levels are too low to influence platelet function (Blair *et al.*, 1982). The production of PGI2 is rapidly and transiently stimulated locally up to at least 100-fold by a variety of agonists such as thrombin, ADP, histamine and bradykinin, but also by variations in shear stress (Weksler *et al.*, 1977, Baenziger *et al.*, 1979, Frangos *et al.*, 1985). A number of agonists are secreted by activated platelets, which thus initiate a negative feed-back for their inhibition. The eicosanoid pathway of the endothelial cell is initiated via the liberation of arachidonic acid from phospholipids. This process is triggered by a rise in intracellular Ca^{2+} which results in an activation of phospholipase A2 (De Nucci *et al.*, 1988). The arachidonic acid liberated from the phospholipids is converted into endoperoxides by the enzyme prostaglandin endoperoxide synthase (PHS). The major product in endothelial cells formed from the endoperoxides is prostacyclin. PGI2 is not only a strong inhibitor of platelet aggregation, it also inhibits platelet adhesion (Weiss and Turitto, 1979) and it is a potent vasodilator. Released PGI2 can react with a specific receptor on the platelet, coupled to a stimulatory G-protein (Gs). This Gs-protein is linked to a signal transduction pathway which in turn activates adenylate cyclase (Gorman *et al.*, 1977, Moncada, 1982). The latter enzyme induces the formation of the second messenger cAMP from ATP. Probably all the prostacyclin-induced platelet responses are mediated via a rise in cAMP which results in the activation of a cAMP-dependent protein kinase (PKA) (Walter *et al.*, 1993). PKA stimulates the phosphorylation of the low molecular weight GTP-binding protein rap1B (Torti and Lapetina, 1993). This phosphorylation induces the dissociation of rap1B from the membranes and prevents binding of phospholipase C to the membranes, thereby inhibiting the hydrolysis of inositol phospholipids, an essential intermediate in the response to all platelet stimuli.

PHS is an important pharmacological target for nonsteroidal anti-inflammatory drugs such as aspirin (Roth and Calverley, 1994). Clinical studies have identified low doses of aspirin as effective in preventing myocardial infarction, transient ischemic attacks and angina pectoris. The protective effect of acetyl salicylic acid, the active compound in aspirin is due to inactivation of platelet PHS. Platelets are uniquely sensitive to oral administration of small doses of the drug. Apparently, after absorption from the upper tract, aspirin enters the portal blood circulation with the same rate as platelets from the preportal circulation and the direct contact between the newly absorbed aspirin and platelets facilitates the rapid inactivation of PHS (Roth and Calverley, 1994). Moreover, since platelets do not synthesize proteins, PHS is inactivated for the rest of the platelet life span and TXA2 production is inhibited. Endothelial cell PHS escapes from continuous suppression because the endothelial cells have the capacity to synthesize new PHS.

Prostacyclin production by endothelial cells is regulated at different levels. The production of prostacyclin is induced within seconds by agents such as thrombin, ADP and histamine and is complete within 5 minutes, even in the continuous presence of the agonists (Botherton and Hoak, 1983, Dejana *et al.*, 1983). A ten-fold elevation of intracellular Ca^{2+} above resting cytosolic levels (about 0.1 $\mu mol/L$) is needed to activate phospholipase A2 (Hallam *et al.*, 1988a, Hallam 1988b). Phospholipase A2 is the rate limiting enzyme in the formation of prostaglandins but is not responsible for the desensitization of prostaglandin formation. The rapid-down regulation of PGI2 synthesis is not fully understood but since the desensitization is agonist specific, it is thought to be related to the inactivation or uncoupling of the agonist-specific receptors. The production of prostacyclin is also regulated at the level of PHS, the first enzyme in the formation of eicosanoids. Components such as IL-1, TNF, the phorbol ester PMA and endotoxins (LPS) induce the transcription and translation of PHS, which results in an increased capacity to convert arachidonic acid into eicosanoids (Maier *et al.*, 1990). Recently, it has been shown that there are two enzymes with PHS activity present in endothelial cells, PHS-I and PHS-II (Jones *et al.*, 1993). The proteins share 61% identity and are located on different chromosomes. The expression of both enzymes is upregulated by LPS, IL-1 and PMA and they characteristically behave as immediate-early genes. It is not clear at the moment why endothelial cells have two almost similarly behaving enzymes.

A third mechanism by which endothelial cells can increase their PGI2 production is through transcellular transfer of substrates. This can only take place when other cells in the proximity of the endothelium produce these substrates. Stimulated platelets produce eicosanoids. The intermediates of the platelet eicosanoid synthesis, such as arachidonic acid and endoperoxides can be used by endothelial cells to form PGI2, thereby increasing their own PGI2 production and decreasing the platelet thromboxane production (Schafer *et al.*, 1984, Marcus *et al.*, 1980). This mechanism, also called the "stealing hypothesis", is an elegant way to reduce the platelet response. It is only relevant when platelets are activated and is an example of cellular cooperation or cellular cross-talk.

PGI2 not only inhibits platelet aggregation, but also inhibits platelet adhesion (Weiss and Turitto, 1979). It prevents adhesion via the inhibition of the spreading of the adhered platelet over the surface. Spreading of a platelet after adhesion is necessary to increase the affinity of the platelet for the surface. The affinity of platelets for the surface must be high because there is a continuous shear stress exerted on the platelet by the flowing blood. In the presence of PGI2 only contact platelets are seen and these platelets are easier washed away by the flowing blood. PGI2 inhibits platelet adhesion much better at higher shear stress.

Nitric oxide

Nitric oxide was first recognized as an endothelial cell secretion product when it was demonstrated that NO could account for the activity of Endothelial Cell Relaxing Factor (EDRF) (Palmer *et al.*, 1987). EDRF is an important endothelial cell metabolite involved in the regulation of the vascular tone and blood pressure (Furchgott and Zawadski, 1980).

NO is not only involved in relaxation of smooth muscle cells, it also expresses an important antithrombotic activity (Radomski *et al.*, 1987a). Just like PGI2, NO is a strong inhibitor of platelet activation and it is even a better inhibitor of platelet adhesion (Radomski *et al.*, 1987b, de Graaf *et al.*, 1992). NO is a simple diatomic molecule which has a half life of a few seconds and can therefore only exert its functional activity locally (Moncada *et al.*, 1991). Pure NO is a gas which easily dissolves in water. It can be inactivated by a large number of other compounds but *in vivo* the most important inhibitor of NO is hemoglobin (Martin *et al.*, 1985). It has been suggested that NO forms more stable S-nitrosothiol compounds when it is secreted and transported to function in the communication between cells (Myers *et al.*, 1990, Scharfstein *et al.*, 1994). However, there is also evidence that the main effector of the observed responses is NO itself (Feelisch *et al.*, 1994). NO increases cGMP-levels in the target cells (Hogan *et al.*, 1988, Moncada *et al.*, 1991). The precise mechanism of this process is not known but there are indications that NO directly interacts with the heme moiety of guanylate cyclase, the enzyme responsible for the formation of cGMP. Increase of the cGMP content in platelets results in activation of specific cGMP dependent serine/threonine protein kinases and causes a decrease of intracellular Ca^{2+} which leads to a down regulation of platelet activation (Moncada *et al.*, 1991).

NO is synthesized from the precursors L-arginine and O_2 by the enzyme NO synthase (NOS) (Palmer *et al.*, 1988). This enzyme converts L-arginine and O_2 to NO and L-citrulline. The last compound can be recycled to L-arginine via the urea cycle. Nitric oxidases are unique among eukaryotic enzymes in being dimeric, calmodulin-dependent or calmodulin-containing cytochrome P450-like hemeproteins that combine reductase and oxygenase catalytic domains in one monomer, bear both FAD and FMN, and carry out a 5-electron oxidation of a non aromatic amino acid with the aid of tetrahydrobiopterin (Marletta, 1993, Nathan and Xie, 1994). Four constitutive NOSs (cNOS) have been described, of which two are apparently present in endothelium (Smith *et al.*, 1994). One endothelial cNOS is recovered from the cytosol, the other type is membrane bound. Endothelial cells secrete NO constitutively but after stimulation of the cells the production is strongly increased. The NO production is stimulated by the same range of agonists as PGI2 synthesis (Cooke *et al.*, 1991). cNOS is probably already active at basal cytosolic Ca^{2+} concentrations, since only a Ca^{2+} concentration of 0.4 μM is required for its full activity (Mulsch *et al.*, 1989, Parsaee *et al.*, 1992). The mechanism by which agonists such as bradykinin transiently activate NO synthesis is not only because of a rise in intracellular Ca^{2+}-levels but also via a transient increase of arginine uptake by the cells (Bogle *et al.*, 1991). Besides the constitutive form (cNOS) an inducible form (iNOS) exists. The expression of iNOS, a calmodulin independent enzyme, needs de-novo protein synthesis. It is only expressed after activation of the cells by cytokines or endotoxins. iNOS is also present in endothelial cells but its contribution to NO production in e.g. septic shock seems to be much less than NO from other sources.

Despite the short half life of NO *in vivo* and its rapid inactivation by hemoglobin, there are numerous indications that endogenous NO synthesis continuously regulates platelet function *in vivo*. In contrast to PGI2, NO synthesis *in vivo* occurs at sufficient basal levels to influence vascular tone, since infusion of inhibitors of NO-synthase elevates blood pressure (Vallance *et al.*, 1989). The resting cytosolic Ca^{2+}-concentrations are high enough to allow NO synthesis and after an agonist induced activation, NO production continues when PGI2 synthesis has already stopped. This indicates that NO synthesis is not desensitized and the NO production lasts longer than PGI2 production. There is now substantial evidence that the NO production is impaired in atherosclerosis and diabetes mellitus (Lüscher, 1993) and these functional alterations in platelet-vessel wall interactions may play an important role in the pathogenesis of these cardiovascular diseases.

The release of NO and PGI2 is often induced by the same agonists (De Nucci *et al.*, 1988). The simultaneous release of PGI2 and NO may be a powerful mechanism by which endothelial cells inhibit platelet response (Figure 7.1). It has been shown that NO and PGI2 act synergistically. Activation of subthreshold concentrations of NO and PGI2 are able to effectively inhibit platelet aggregation (Radomsky *et al.*, 1987a). The increase of both cAMP and cGMP in the platelet is probably more effective to suppress Ca^{2+}-dependent platelet responses. It has been shown that the cAMP-dependent protein kinase and the cGMP dependent protein kinase have a common substrate, a 46/50 kDa protein VASP, whose phosphorylation correlates very well with platelet inhibition (Walter *et al.*, 1993). Another mechanism to explain the synergistic effect is the presence of a cGMP inhibited cAMP-phosphodiesterase. Elevation of cGMP levels delay the half life of cAMP in the platelets (Maurice and Haslam, 1990).

Platelets produce NO themselves (Radomski *et al.*, 1990). Addition of inhibitors of NO-synthase increases the aggregability of platelets to various agonists. However, it is most likely that endothelial cells are the main source of NO production. Aggregating platelets secrete ADP and serotonin which stimulate NO production by endothelial cells. Thus, like PGI2, NO production by endothelial cells forms a part of a feedback mechanism in which platelet-inhibiting factors are produced at sites where platelets aggregate.

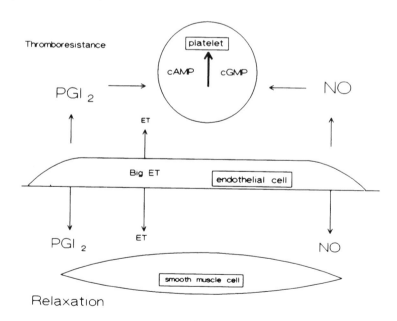

Figure 7.1   Synergistic inhibition of platelet function by endothelial cell derived NO and PGI2.

The continuous production of NO and PGI2 is not the major cause for the non-thrombogenicity of an intact endothelial cell surface. When endothelial cell PGI2 and NO synthesis is inhibited by acetylsalicylic acid and L-N-monomethyl arginine, respectively, platelets do not adhere to intact endothelial cells (de Graaf *et al.*, 1992). The locally produced NO and PGI2 may reduce platelet deposition on endothelial cell injuries in close proximity to the endothelial cells. The nonthrombogenicity of the intact endothelial cell is caused by other mechanisms. However, when the endothelial cell lost its non-thrombogenicity, as happens after viral infection, PGI2 and NO can reduce platelet deposition on the intact cell.

Other endothelial cell low molecular weight compounds claimed to influence platelet function

Endothelins are potent vasoconstrictor peptides produced by endothelial cells but also by other cell types (Yanagisawa *et al.*, 1988, Yanagisawa and Masaki, 1989). Three endothelins have been identified until now. Endothelin-1, a 21 amino acid peptide, is the only form synthesized by endothelial cells. The synthesis of endothelin-1 is induced by a large number of agonists, such as shear stress and the releasate of activated platelets (Yanagisawa and Masaki, 1989, Rubanyi, 1992). The endothelial cells possess an enzyme on their surface able to convert an inactive precursor present in the circulation, big endothelin, into active endothelin (Kimura *et al.*, 1989). Endothelin-1 has been postulated as an inhibitor of platelet aggregation (Thiemermann *et al.*, 1988). However, the influence of endothelin is probably indirect. It has been shown that endothelin induces the production of PGI2 and NO by endothelial cells (Edlund and Wennmalm, 1990). A direct influence of endothelin on platelet function has not been demonstrated.

Endothelial cells can convert linoleic acid to 13-hydroxyoctadienoic acid (13-HODE). It has been suggested that 13-HODE has non-thrombogenic properties (Buchanan *et al.*, 1987). However, studies with purified 13-HODE have shown that it has no influence on platelet adhesion (de Graaf *et al.*, 1989) and is only a very weak inhibitor of platelet aggregation (Coene *et al.*, 1986).

Surface characteristics of the luminal endothelial membrane

Platelets do not stick to endothelial cells in contrast to fibroblasts and smooth muscle cells and there is evidence that this is caused by the proteoglycan composition of the endothelial cell surface (Born and Palinski, 1985). Proteoglycans are macromolecules composed of glycosaminoglycan chains linked to a core protein (Kjellen and Lindahl, 1991). The glycosaminoglycans consist of hexosamine and either hexuronic acid or galactose units. These structural subunits are arranged in an altering unbranched sequence and they carry sulphate substitutions in various positions. The most common glycosaminoglycans are chondroitin sulphate, dermatan sulphate, heparin, heparan sulphate and keratan sulphate. Enormous variation exists in the structure of proteoglycans because of the inherent heterogeneity in glycosaminoglycan structure, caused by variation in length and degree of sulphation. The following proteoglycans have been characterized in endothelial cells: syndecan, ryudocan/amphiglycan, glypican, fibroglycan and perlecan (Kojima *et al.*, 1992, David *et al.*, 1992, Mertens *et al.*, 1992). The first four are membrane bound proteoglycans, while perlecan is a matrix component. Recent studies in our laboratory demonstrated platelet adhesion to endothelial cells treated with heparinitase, indicating that the heparan sulphate proteoglycans on the endothelial cell membrane are responsible for lack of adhesion of platelets to endothelial cells. Virus transformed endothelial cells have a changed glycosaminoglycan composition together with a lost thromboresistence (Curwen *et al.*, 1980)

Ectonucleotidase activity

Activation of platelets results in release of additional agonists such as ADP from their α-granula. Secretion of ADP leads to recruitment and activation of other platelets, thereby facilitating the formation of a haemostatic plug. Leakage of ADP from red blood cells during haemolysis or from injured tissue can induce platelet activation in an intact vessel. Adenosine nucleotides are relatively stable in plasma and to prevent platelet activation removal of ATP and ADP is needed. Endothelial cells can regulate this unwanted platelet activation via the presence of ectonucleotidases on their luminal surface that metabolize ATP and ADP to AMP and adenosine (Pearson and Gordon, 1985, Marcus *et al.*, 1991). Adenosine itself inhibits platelet aggregation. As red blood cells also contain strong ectonucleotidase activity on their surface, the *in vivo* relevance of endothelial cell ectonucleotidase activity is not yet established.

Inactivation of thrombin activity

Thrombin is the final enzyme of the coagulation cascade and responsible for the conversion of soluble fibrinogen into insoluble fibrin. In addition, it is one of the most potent agonists of platelets. Endothelial cells are the major physiological site of thrombin inactivation. Endothelial cells express heparan sulphates as side chains of proteoglycans and endothelial cells can bind heparin with high affinity. Both heparin and heparan sulphate can bind antithrombin III and dramatically increase the inactivation of thrombin by antithrombin III (Marcum *et al.*, 1984, Mertens *et al.*, 1992). A second and even more important anticoagulant function of the endothelium is the synthesis and expression of thrombomodulin (Esmon and Owen, 1981, Stern *et al.*, 1985a). Thrombomodulin binds thrombin and alters its substrate specificity. The affinity of thrombin for platelets and fibrinogen is lost but it now accelerates the activation of protein C. Activated protein C inactivates factors Va and VIIIa thereby downregulating further thrombin formation (Esmon, 1992). The catalytic action of protein C is enhanced by protein S, also synthesized by the endothelium (Fair *et al.*, 1986, Stern *et al.*, 1986). Thrombin bound to thrombomodulin is also faster inactivated by antithrombin III (Preissner *et al.*, 1987). Thrombomodulin expression is downregulated by IL-1, TNF and endotoxins (Nawroth and Stern, 1986). The downregulation of thrombomodulin is counteracted by interleukin-4 (IL-4) (Kapiotis *et al.*, 1991).

Recently, an activated protein C independent function of protein S was reported (Mitchell *et al.*, 1988). Protein S can directly inhibit the prothrombinase complex by interacting with factor Xa and factor Va (Heeb *et al.*, 1993). Protein S probably binds to negatively charged phospholipids, thereby shielding off binding sites for the coagulation factors. A comparable mechanism takes place on endothelial cells. When protein S binds

Table 7.2   Alteration of endothelial cell hemostatic Properties after activation

Product	Activation	Effect
Prostacyclin	Thr, ADP, BK	Increased production due to liberation of substrates
	Cytokines, LPS	Upregulation of producing enzymes
Nitric oxide	Thr, ADP, BK	Increased production due to increased supply of substrates
	Cytokines, LPS	Upregulation of producing enzymes
Von Willebrand factor	Thr	Release from storage organelles
	cytokines	Decreased deposition in the subendothelium
Platelet activating factor	Thr, ADP, BK	Increased production due to liberation substrates
Tissue factor	Cytokines, LPS	Induction of synthesis
Thrombomodulin	Cytokines, LPS	Downregulation of synthesis

Abbreviations: Thr: thrombin, BK: bradykinin, LPS: endotoxin

to endothelial cells, it interacts with factor Va and factor Xa and inhibits the formation of an active prothrombinase complex on the cells (Hackeng *et al.*, 1993, 1994)

UPREGULATION OF PROTHROMBOTIC ACTIVITIES

An important feature of endothelial cell functioning is that endothelial cell responses are modulated in response to stimuli (Table 7.2). Endothelial cells participate in a number of physiological processes such as inflammation, hemostasis and immunology in a different way when they are activated with cytokines (Nawroth and Stern, 1986, Pearson, 1994). As already described, endothelial cell PGI2 and NO synthesis increases when the cells are activated with IL-1 and TNF. But not only the anticoagulant properties of the cells are stimulated, also a number of prothrombotic activities are induced, such as the synthesis of tissue factor (Lyberg *et al.*, 1983, Colucci *et al.*, 1983, Bevilacqua *et al.*, 1984) and the down-regulation of thrombomodulin (Moore *et al.*, 1987). These changes in the hemo-compatibility of the endothelial cells may be important in the regulation of local inflammation and hemostatic processes. When these changes take place systematically, it may have a dramatic effect. Atherosclerotic disease has been thought to be the result of a slow change in the endothelial cell phenotype, resulting in a cell that is less capable to prevent platelet activation and to suppress smooth muscle cell migration and proliferation (Ross, 1986).

Platelet adhesion to the endothelium is an early event in animal models of inflammation and atherosclerosis. Platelets normally do not stick to an intact viable endothelial cell layer. *In vitro* studies have shown that when the phenotypic expression of endothelial cells is changed due to changes in their surroundings, the surface of endothelial cells becomes adhesive for platelets. The first studies on a direct interaction between platelets and endothelial cells have been performed in the presence of relatively high concentrations of thrombin (Czervionke *et al.*, 1979, Kaplan *et al.*, 1989). Thrombin strongly influences the expression of adhesive receptors on both platelets and endothelial cells. Interesting results were obtained in experiments with virus infected endothelial cells. Herpes simplex infected endothelial cells have been shown to become prothrombotic and to support enhanced platelet adherence to the endothelial cells (Visser *et al.*, 1988). Also the presence of endotoxins and cytokines can induce a comparable shift in endothelial cell phenotype. Infected endothelial cells start to synthesize and express tissue factor on their surface. Tissue factor is the physiological initiator of the coagulation cascade and the presence of tissue factor on the surface of endothelial cells enables the formation of thrombin. The locally generated thrombin can activate platelets and thus induce the expression of glycoprotein IIb:IIIa, a major adhesive receptor for both platelet-surface interactions and platelet-platelet interactions. Thrombin also enables the formation of a fibrin network on the endothelium and fibrin is a perfect adhesive surface for platelets (Hantgan *et al.*, 1990). Moreover, thrombin can also activate the endothelial cells themselves, resulting in release of prothrombotic substances such as von Willebrand factor (Loesberg *et al.*, 1983), and platelet activating factor (PAF) (Zimmerman *et al.*, 1990).

Von Willebrand factor

Von Willebrand factor has a dual function in hemostasis. First, it is the most important adhesive protein for platelets and second, von Willebrand factor acts as carrier for clotting factor VIII (Sadler, 1991, Ruggeri and Ware, 1993). At lower shear rates of the blood, platelets can adhere to different adhesive proteins but with increasing shear rate, platelet adhesion is completely dependent on the interaction between von Willebrand factor and glycoprotein Ib on the surface of platelets (Sixma and de Groot, 1994). Deficiencies of von Willebrand factor result in a bleeding disorder (Sadler, 1994). In several disease states, such as diabetes mellitus, vasculitis and the antiphospholipid syndrome, von Willebrand factor levels in the circulation are chronically elevated (Pearson, 1994). The reason for this elevation is not known. Probably it reflects endothelial cell perturbation or injury. There are no indications that elevated levels of von Willebrand factor result in an increased thrombotic tendency.

Von Willebrand factor is a highly multimerized protein build up from dimers with a mol weight of 500.000. The multimerization enables multiple interaction between a von Willebrand molecule and a platelet which results in a much higher affinity for platelets than a single interaction. Von Willebrand factor is synthesized by endothelial cells and megakaryocytes (Wagner, 1990). The source of von Willebrand factor in plasma and subendothelium is the endothelial cells, because during bone marrow transplantation, when megakaryocytes are absent, no drop in von Willebrand factor plasma levels is seen (Bowie *et al.*, 1986). Megakaryocytes are the most likely source of the von Willebrand factor present in the α-granules of the platelets. Von Willebrand factor synthesized by the endothelial cells is constitutively secreted from the cells, deposited in the extracellular matrix or stored inside the cell in the Weibel-Palade bodies. The content of the Weibel-Palade bodies is released upon stimuli such as thrombin (de Groot *et al.*, 1984). The secreted von Willebrand factor from the Weibel-Palade bodies is predominantly in the form of the highly reactive high molecular weight multimers. The ability to form multimers is due to the presence of an N-terminal extension in the pro-von Willebrand factor polypeptide chain (Verwey *et al.*, 1987). This propeptide is cleaved off during incorporation in the Weibel-Palade bodies and both the propeptide (also called von Willebrand factor antigen II) and the mature protein are stored in the Weibel-Palade bodies.

Only a limited range of agonists induces the instantaneous release of von Willebrand factor from endothelial cells. Compounds such as ATP and bradykinin which stimulate PGI2 synthesis do not increase the release of von Willebrand factor, indicating that another intracellular signalling pathway is involved (Carew *et al.*, 1992). Also inhibitors of protein kinase C do not influence the release of von Willebrand factor. There are indications that the stimulated release of von Willebrand factor is mediated via a Ca^{2+}-calmodulin pathway (Birch *et al.*, 1992). It must be noted that agents such as DDAVP (1-deamino-8-D-arginine vasopressin) which induce acute release of von Willebrand factor *in vivo*, are not active when used in *in vitro* cell culture. DDAVP acts indirectly on the release of von Willebrand factor from endothelial cells, probably via an enhanced secretion of PAF from DDAVP-triggered monocytes (Hashemi *et al.*, 1993).

IL-1 and TNF have little effect on the total level of synthesis of von Willebrand factor by the endothelial cells. However, the routing of the newly synthesized von Willebrand factor is altered. After activation hardly any von Willebrand factor is deposited in the extracellular matrix (de Groot *et al.*, 1987). This makes the subendothelium less reactive for platelets. Also the endothelial cells seem to become more sensitive for agonists such as thrombin, which induce an instantaneous release of von Willebrand factor (Paleolog *et al.*, 1990).

There is some debate whether the stimulated von Willebrand factor release is predominantly directed towards the luminal side of the cells or towards the basolateral side of the cells (van Buul-Wortelboer, 1989, Mayadas *et al.*, 1989). The released von Willebrand factor binds very well to subendothelial structures, while binding to the luminal surface of endothelial cells is normally not seen. However, when the endothelial cell is phenotypically changed, as happens after viral infection or in the presence of endotoxins, the released von Willebrand factor from the Weibel-Palade bodies stays associated with the surface and is involved in the adhesion of platelet to an intact endothelial cell monolayer (Etingin *et al.*, 1993).

Platelet activating factor

Platelet activating factor (1-O-alkyl-2-acetyl-sn-glycero-3-phosphocholine) is a very potent platelet activator (Benveniste *et al.*, 1972). It activates platelets at concentrations as low as 2.10^{-8} mol/L. Endothelial cells synthesize significant amounts of PAF in response to agonists such as thrombin, bradykinin, histamine, IL-1 and ATP (Camussi *et al.*, 1983, McIntyre *et al.*, 1985). PAF is synthesized from 1-O-alkyl-2-arachidonyl-sn-glycero-3-phosphocholine via a combined action of phospholipase A2 and acetyl CoA:1-alkyl-2-hydroxy-sn-glycero-3-phosphocholine acetyltransferase. Virtually all of the PAF synthesized by endothelial cells has been found associated with the cells (Zimmerman *et al.*, 1990), although there are also publications that about 25% of the PAF is released. In *ex-vivo* studies with segments of pulmonary arteries the synthesized PAF is also not released. There is no convincing evidence that the synthesis of PAF by endothelial cells influences platelet function, although the production of PAF is linked to the synthesis of prostacyclin. In contrast PAF synthesis is tightly linked with augmented binding of PMNs to endothelial cells. A role of endothelial cell PAF synthesis in endothelial cell-PMN interaction has been suggested (Zimmerman *et al.*, 1990).

Activation of the coagulation cascade

After activation by IL-1, TNF or endotoxins, endothelial cells synthesize and express tissue factor (Lyberg *et al.*, 1983, Colucci *et al.*, 1983). IL-4 inhibits IL-1, TNF and endotoxin induced expression of tissue factor by endothelial cells (Herbert *et al.*, 1992, Martin *et al.*, 1993). Tissue factor is the main physiological initiator of the coagulation cascade (Nemerson, 1992). It is a single chain membrane protein able to bind factor VIIa and this complex activates factors X and IX. Both clotting factors are able to bind to endothelial cells and since endothelial cells bind factor VIII and synthesize factor V, thrombin formation can take place (Stern *et al.*, 1985b, Cerveny *et al.*, 1984, Koppelman *et al.*, 1994). In an *in vitro* thrombosis model with noncoagulated whole blood it is shown that endothelial cell formed thrombin is able to form a fibrin layer over the endothelial cells and on this fibrin layer platelet thrombi are formed (Kirchhofer, 1994). When thrombin formation was inhibited, no fibrin formation and no deposition of platelets was found. Under these conditions fibrin is the adhesive surface for platelets and the presence of fibrin is required for the adhesion of platelets.

Endothelial cells express binding sites for all clotting factors of the extrinsic pathway of coagulation (Stern *et al.*, 1985b). Although there are indications that some clotting factors have specific protein receptors on the surface of endothelial cells (Stern *et al.*, 1985c), expression of negatively charged phospholipids on the surface of endothelial cells is, at least partly, responsible for the support of the procoagulant activity, because endothelial cell mediated prothrombinase and tenase activity could be completely inhibited by annexin V, a protein whose only known function is to bind to negatively charged phospholipids with high affinity (van Heerde *et al.*, 1994). In contrast to platelets, activation of the endothelial cells does not influence the number of binding sites for clotting factors (van Heerde *et al.*, 1994, Brinkman *et al.*, 1994)

The coagulation cascade can not only be initiated via tissue factor but also via the intrinsic pathway (Kaplan and Silverberg, 1987). Four plasma proteins are required for this surface mediated process, high molecular weight kininogen (HMWK), prekallikrein, factor XII and factor XI. Endothelial cells contain a binding site for both factor HMWK and factor XII (van Iwaarden *et al.*, 1988, Reddigari *et al.*, 1993). Factor XI can bind to HMWK on the endothelial cell surface (Berrettini *et al.*, 1992). Endothelial cells express an activator of factor XII (Wiggins *et al.*, 1980). There is some evidence that factor XII undergoes slow activation to factor XIIa after binding to endothelial cells (Reddigari *et al.*, 1993). Factor XIIa formed on the surface of endothelial cells can activate factor XI to factor XIa and since factors IX and X are present on the endothelial cell surface, the whole coagulation cascade can be activated via the contact system. Whether this system really functions *in vivo* and how it is regulated remains to be investigated.

The last step of the coagulation cascade is the conversion of prothrombin to the active serine protease thrombin. Activation of prothrombin to thrombin results from the proteolytic cleavage of Arg271-Thr272 and Arg320-Ile 321 by the prothrombinase complex. Depending upon the order of peptide bond cleavage, two intermediate products, meizothrombin and prethrombin-2, can be formed (Figure 7.2) (Rosing *et al.*, 1986). Meizothrombin has about 5% of the activity of thrombin towards fibrinogen but the kinetics of the thrombomodulin-meizothrombin complex are identical to that of the thrombomodulin-thrombin complex (Doyle and Mann, 1990). This suggests that meizothrombin predominantly has an antithrombotic activity. On endothelial cells, meizothrombin was formed as an intermediate in prothrombin activation and considerable amounts of meizothrombin desfragment-1 are accumulated (Tijburg *et al.*, 1991) indicating that prothrombin activated on endothelial cells may have a more anticoagulant nature than thrombin formed on negatively charged phospholipids.

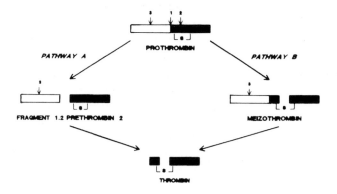

Figure 7.2   Activation pathway of prothrombin.

When α-thrombin is generated on the surface of endothelial cells, it is questionable whether the relatively low concentrations of thrombin formed are prothrombotic. Interesting experiments were performed by Hanson *et al.*, (1993). They infused 2 U/kg/min thrombin into baboons who were connected with an *ex-vivo* thrombosis model. The low doses thrombin infused strongly reduced the incorporation of fibrin and platelets in the *ex-vivo* thrombus without depleting platelets and fibrinogen in the circulation of the primates. Circulating levels of activated protein C increased significantly and addition of an antibody that inhibit the activation of protein C blocked the antithrombotic effects of the infused thrombin. This suggests that low doses of thrombin predominantly activate protein C. It is very well conceivable that thrombin formed on the surface of endothelial cells predominantly binds to thrombomodulin thereby functioning as a antithrombotic agent.

Endothelial cells in culture only express tissue factor when they are stimulated with cytokines or endotoxins. It is not really known whether endothelial cells *in vivo* express tissue factor activity when they are activated. The induction of tissue factor probably needs a combination of stimuli. When TNF is infused in a mouse model fibrin deposition is only found in tumor vasculature (Nawroth *et al.*, 1988). Cultured endothelial cells are already partly activated due to the *in vitro* proliferation and are therefore probably more sensitive for induction of tissue factor synthesis. It has been suggested that tissue factor synthesized by endothelial cells is deposited only in the extracellular matrix, however, others have shown that tissue factor is predominantly cell associated (Ryan *et al.*, 1992, Mulder *et al.*, 1994). The differences in tissue factor expression are probably induced by different culture media and/or different substrates on which the cells are cultured. This indicates that one should be careful with the results of *in vitro* experiments. Small changes in the culture conditions may strongly influence the results, which make translation to the *in vivo* situation hazardous (Almus *et al.*, 1991). Interesting observations were made in studies in which tissue factor induction by TNF was studied in cells grown in the presence of known risk factor of thrombosis, such as antiphospholipid antibodies or advanced glycosylated proteins (Hasselaar *et al.*, 1989, Esposito *et al.*, 1990, Oosting *et al.*, 1992). Under these conditions, much lower concentrations of TNF were needed to induce tissue factor response. This supports the hypothesis that multiple stimuli are necessary to activate endothelial cells. Risk factors for thrombosis which individually have little effect on endothelial cell function make the endothelial cells more susceptible to a change of their functional activity.

The expression of tissue factor by endothelial cells is balanced by the concomitant synthesis of TFPI (tissue factor pathway inhibitor) (Bajaj *et al.*, 1990). Endothelial cells synthesize and secrete the major inhibitor of tissue factor, TFPI. TFPI is also bound to the endothelial cell surface. TFPI binds to factor Xa and this combination forms a stable quaternary complex with tissue factor/factor VIIa, thereby removing factor Xa and inhibiting tissue factor. Recently, a second TFPI has been cloned and isolated (Sprecher *et al.*, 1994). TFPI-2 is also an endothelial cell product and it probably can inactivate tissue factor/factor VIIa without a first interaction with factor X_a. There is not much known about the regulation of the secretion of TFPI's by endothelial cells. Heparin stimulates the release of TFPI-1 but whether heparin really stimulates the release of TFPI from internal stores or it only releases TFPI which is bound to the cellular surface needs further studies (Novotny *et al.*, 1991).

CONCLUDING REMARKS

The endothelium is strongly involved in the regulation of thrombus growth, primarily via the synthesis of compounds able to suppress adhesion and aggregation of platelets and via proteins able to down-regulate the activation of coagulation cascade. Under normal, healthy conditions endothelial cells form an antithrombotic surface due to the composition of the luminal surface. In addition, a large range of metabolic activities is expressed to maintain the hemocompatibility. An important feature of endothelial cells is that they change their metabolic activity in response to changes in the environment. Especially after exposure to cytokines, a series of alterations in endothelial cell function takes place which changes the metabolic activity of the endothelial cell towards a more prothrombotic state. This shift in functioning is believed to be a major factor in the development of vascular diseases. It is of utmost importance to analyze the regulation of endothelial cell function at the molecular level. Until now, almost all studies were performed with cultured endothelial cells *in vitro*. Cultured endothelial cells are already partly activated due to the culture conditions. Moreover, *in vitro* cultured endothelial cells are proliferating cells while *in vivo* endothelial cells hardly proliferate. Increasing our knowledge about the *in vivo* endothelial cell function is crucial to understand the role of endothelial cells in hemostatic responses. In experiments in which low doses of TNF were perfused in human volunteers, a substantial procoagulant response was found (Bauer *et al.*, 1989, van der Poll *et al.*, 1990) Comparable results were found when LPS was infused into baboons (Taylor *et al.*, 1991). It is not known whether the endothelium was responsible for the increased hemostatic response. Interactions between different cells types take place *in vivo* and additional messenger molecules released from other cells may mediate possible effects on endothelial cells (Hashemi *et al.*, 1993). This assumption is supported by the observation that the *in vivo* effects seen on the hemostatic response when chimpanzees were treated with LPS seems to be mediated by monocytes (Levi *et al.*, 1994). It is now generally accepted that endothelial cells play an active role in many aspects of hemostasis, but studies with animal models and in patients are needed to understand the significance of all the *in vitro* observations. The development of sensitive tests for the detection of endothelial cell function in combination with sensitive tests for platelet activation and coagulation markers will help us to understand the role of endothelial cells in hemostatic responses.

References

Almus, F.E., Rao, L.V.M., Pendurthi, U.R., Quattrochi, L. and Rapaport, S.I. (1991). Mechanism for diminished tissue factor expression by endothelial cells cultured with heparin binding growth factor-1 and heparin. *Blood*, **77**:1256–1262.

Baenziger, N.L., Becherer, P.R. and Majerus, P.W. (1979). Characterization of prostaglandin synthesis in cultured human arterial smooth muscle cells, venous endothelial cells and skin fibroblasts. *Cell*, **16**:967–974.

Bajaj, M.S., Kuppuswamy, M.N., Saito, H., Spitzer, S.G. and Bajaj, S.P. (1990). Cultured normal human hepatocytes do not synthesize lipoprotein-associated coagulation inhibitor: Evidence that endothelium is the principal site of its synthesis. *Proceedings of the National Academy of Sciences USA*, **87**:8869–8873.

Bauer, K.A., ten Cate, H., Barzegar, S., Spriggs, D.R., Sherman, M.L. and Rosenberg, R.D. (1989). Tumor necrosis factor infusions have a procoagulant effect on the hemostatic mechanism of humans. *Blood*, **74**:165–172.

Bevilacqua, M.P., Pober, J.S., Majeau, G.R., Cotran, R.S. and Gimbrone, M.A.Jr. (1984). Interleukin-1 biosynthesis and cell surface expression of procoagulant activity in human vascular endothelial cells. *Journal of Experimental Medicine*, **60**:618–623.

Birch, K.A., Pober, J.S., Zavoico, G.B., Means, A.R. and Ewenstein, B.M. (1992). Calcium/calmodulin transduces thrombin stimulated secretion: Studies in intact and minimally-permeabilized human umbilical vein endothelial cells. *Journal of Cell Biology*, **118**:1501–1510.

Blair, I.A., Barrow, S.F. and Waddell, K.A. (1982). Prostacyclin is not a circulating hormone in man. *Prostagalandins*, **23**:577–589.

Bogle, R.G., Coade, S.B., Moncada, S., Pearson, J.D. and Mann, G.E. (1991). Bradykinin and ATP stimulate L-arginine uptake and nitric oxide release in vascular endothelial cells. *Biochemical Biophysical Research Communications*, **180**:926–932.

Born, G.V.R. and Palinsky, W. (1985). Unusually high concentrations of sialic acids on the surface of vascular endothelia. *British Journal of Experimental Pathology*, **66**:543–549.

Botherton, A.F.A. and Hoak, J.C. (1983). Prostacyclin biosynthesis in cultured vascular endothelium is limited by deactivation of cyclooxygenase. *Journal of Clinical Investigation*, **72**:1255–1261.

Bourin, M.C. and Lindahl, U. (1993). Glycosaminoglycans and the regulation of blood coagulation. *Biochemical Journal*, **289**:313–330.

Bowie, E.J.W., Solberg, L.A., Fass, D.N., Johnson, C.M., Knutsen, G.J., Steward, M.L. and Zoechlein, L.J. (1986). Transplantation of normal bone marrow into a pig with severe von Willebrand's disease. *Journal of Clinical Investigation*, **78**:26–30.

Brinkman, H.M., Mertens, K., Holthuis, J., Zwart-Huinink, L.A. and Grijm, K. (1994). The activation of human blood coagulation factor X on the surface of endothelial cells: a comparison with various vascular cells, platelets and monocytes. *British Journal of Haematology*, **87**:332–342.

Buchanan, M.R., Richardson, M., Haas, T.A. and Madri, J.A. (1986). The membrane underlying the vascular endothelium is not thrombogenic: *In vivo* and *in-vitro* studies with rabbit and human tissue. *Thrombosis and Haemostasis*, **58**:698–704.

Camussi, G., Anglietta, M., Malavasti, F., Tetta, C., Sanavio, F., Piacibello, W. and Bussolino, F. (1983). The release of platelet activating factor from human endothelial cells in culture. *The Journal of Immunology*, **131**:2397–2403.

Carew, M.A., Paleolog, E.M. and Pearson, J.D. (1992). The roles of protein kinase C and intracellular Ca^{++} in the secretion of von Willebrand factor from human vascular endothelial cells. *Biochemical Journal*, **286**:631–635.

Ceverny, J.T., Fass, D.N. and Mann K.G. (1985). Synthesis of coagulation factor V by cultured aortic endothelium. *Blood*, **63**:1467–1474.

Coene, M.C., Bult, H., Claeys, M., Laekman, G.M. and Herman, A.G. (1986). Inhibition of rabbit platelet activation by lipoxygenase products of arachidonic and linoleic acid. *Thrombosis Research*, **42**:205–214.

Colucci, M., Balconi, R., Lorenzet, A., Pietza, A., Locati, D., Donati, M.B. and Semeraro, N. (1983). Cultured endothelial cells generate tissue factor in response to endotoxin. *Journal of Clinical Investigation*, **71**:1893–1896.

Cooke, J.P., Rossitch, E., Andon, N.A., Loscalzo, J. and Dzau, V.J. (1991). Flow activates an endothelial cell potassium channel to release endogenous nitrovasodilator. *Journal of Clinical Investigation*, **88**:1663–1671.

Curwen, K., Gimbrone, M.A.Jr. and Handin, R.I. (1980). *In vitro* studies of thromboresistance: the role of prostacyclin (PGI2) in platelet adhesion to cultured normal and virus transformed human vascular endothelial cells. *Laboratory Investigation*, **42**:366–374.

Czervionke, R.L., Hoak, J.C. and Fry, G.L. (1978). Effect of aspirin on thrombin-induced adherence of platelets to cultured cells from the blood vessel wall. *Journal of Clinical Investigation*, **62**:847–856.

David, G., van der Schueren, B., Marynen, P., Cassiman, J.J. and van den Berghe, H. (1992). Molecular cloning of amphiglycan, a novel integral membrane heparan sulphate proteoglycan expressed in epithelial and fibroblastic cells. *Journal of Cell Biology*, **118**:961–969.

Dejana, E., Balconi, G., DeCastellarnau, C., Barbieri, B., Vergara-Dauden, M. and De Gaetano, G. (1983). Prostacyclin production by human endothelial and bovine smooth muscle cells in culture. Effect of repeated stimulation with arachidonic acid, thrombin and ionophore A23187. *Biochimica Biophysica Acta,* **750**:261–267.

De Graaf, J.C., Bult, H., De Meyer, G.R.Y., Sixma, J.J. and de Groot, Ph.G. (1989). Platelet adhesion to subendothelial structures under flow conditions: no effect of the lipoxygenase product 13-HODE. *Thrombosis and Haemostasis,* **62**:802–806.

De Graaf, J.C., Banga, J.D., Moncada, S., Palmer, R.M.J., de Groot, Ph.G. and Sixma, J.J. (1992). Nitric oxide functions as an inhibitor of platelet adhesion under flow conditions. *Circulation,* **85**:2284–2290.

De Groot, Ph.G., Gonsalves, M.D., Loesberg, C., van Buul-Wortelboer, M.F., van Aken, W.G. and van Mourik, J.A. (1984). Thrombin-induced release of von Willebrand factor is mediated by phospholipid methylation: prostacylin synthesis is independent of phospholipid methylation. *Journal of Biological Chemistry,* **259**:13329–13333.

De Groot, Ph.G., Reinders, J.H. and Sixma, J.J. (1987). Perturbation of human endothelial cells by thrombin or PMA changes the reactivity of their extracelluar matrices towards platelets. *Journal of Cell Biology,* **104**:697–704.

De Groot, Ph.G. and Sixma, J.J. (1990). Annotation: Platelet adhesion. *British Journal of Haematology,* **75**:308–312.

De Nucci, G., Gryglewski, R., Warner, T.D. and Vane, J.R. (1988). Receptor mediated release of endothelium-derived relaxing factor and prostacyclin from bovine endothelial cells is coupled. *Proceedings of the National Academy of Sciences USA,* **85**:2334–2338.

Doyle, M.F. and Mann, K.G. (1990). Multiple active forms of thrombin. IV Relative activities of meizothrombins. *Journal of Biological Chemistry,* **265**:10693–10701.

Edlung, A. and Wennmalm, A. (1990). Endothelin does not affect aggregation of human platelets. *Clinical Physiology,* **10**:585–590.

Esmon, C.T. and Owen, W.G. (1981). Identification of an endothelial cell cofactor for thrombin catalyzed activation of protein C. *Proceedings of the National Academy of Sciences USA,* **78**:2249–2252.

Esmon, C.T. The protein C anticoagulant pathway. *Arteriosclerosis and Thrombosis,* **12**:135–145.

Esposito, C., Gerlach, H., Brett, J., Stern, D. and Vlassara, H. (1990). Endothelial receptor-mediated binding of glucose-modified albumin is associated with increased monolayer permeability and modulation of cell surface coagulant properties. *Journal of Experimental Medicine,* **170**:1387–1407.

Etingin, O.R., Silverstein, R.L. and Hajjar, D.P. (1993). Von Willebrand factor mediates platelet adhesion to virally infected endothelial cells. *Proceedings of the National Academy of Sciences USA,* **90**:5153–5156.

Fair, D.S., Marler, R.A. and Levin, E.G. (1986). Human endothelial cells synthesize protein S. *Blood,* **67**:1168–1171.

Frangos, J.A., Eskin, S.G., McIntyre, L.V. and Ives, C.L. (1985). Flow effects on prostacyclin production by cultured human endothelial cells. *Science,* **277**:1477–1479.

Freelisch, M., De Poel, M., Zamora, R., Deussen, A. and Moncada, S. (1994). Understanding the controversy over the identity of EDRF. *Nature,* **368**:62–65.

Furchgott, R.F. and Zawadzki, J.V. (1980). The obligatory role of endothelial cells in the relaxation of arterial smooth muscle cells by acetylcholine. *Nature,* **299**:373–376.

Gimbrone, M.A. (1986). Vascular endothelium: nature's blood container. *In: Vascular endothelium in Haemostasis and Thrombosis,* M.A.Gimbrone (ed) pp. 1–13. Edinburgh: Churchill Livingstone

Gorman, R.R., Bunting, S. and Miller, O.V. (1977). Modulation of human platelet adenylate cyclase by prostaglandin. *Prostaglandins,* **13**:337–388.

Hackeng, T.M., Hessing, M., van't Veer, C., Meijer-Huizinga, F., Meijers, J.C.M., de Groot, Ph.G., van Mourik, J.A. and Bouma, B.N. (1993). Protein S binding to human endothelial cells is required for expression of cofactor activity for activated protein C. *Journal of Biological Chemistry,* **268**:3993–4000.

Hackeng, T.M., van't Veer, C., Meijers, J.C.M. and Bouma, B.N. (1994). Human protein S inhibits prothrombinase complex activity on endothelial cells and platelets via a direct interaction with factors Va and Xa. *Journal of Biological Chemistry,* **269**:21051–21058.

Hallam, T.J., Pearson, J.D. and Needham, L.A. (1988a). Thrombin stimulated elevation of endothelial cell cytoplasmic free calcium concentration causes prostacyclin production. *Biochemical Journal,* **251**: 243–249.

Hallam, T.J., Jacob, R. and Merrit, J.E. (1988b) Evidence that agonists stimulate bivalent cation influx into endothelial cells. *Biochemical Journal,* **255**:179–184.

Hamberg, M., Svensson, J. and Samuelsson, B. (1975). Thromboxanes: a new group of biologically active compounds derived from prostaglandin endoperoxides. *Proceedings of the National Academy of Sciences USA,* **72**:2994–

Hanson, S.R., Griffith, H.J., Harker, L.A., Kelly, A.B., Esmon, C.T. and Gruber, A. (1993). Antithrombotic effects of thrombin-induced activation of endogenous protein C in primates. *Journal of Clinical Investigation,* **92**:2003–2012.

Hantgan, R.R., Hindriks, G., Tayler, R.G., Sixma, J.J. and de Groot, Ph.G. (1990). Glycoprotein Ib, von Willebrand factor and glycoprotein IIb:IIIa are all involved in platelet adhesion to fibrin in flowing whole blood. *Blood,* **76**:345–353.

Hashemi, S., Palmer, D.S., Aye, M.T. and Ganz, P.R. (1993). Platelet activating factor secreted by DDAVP-treated monocytes mediates von Willebrand release from endothelial cells. *Journal of Cellular Physiology,* **154**:496–505.

Hasselaar, P., Derksen, R.H.W.M., Oosting, J.D., Blokzijl, L. and de Groot, Ph.G. (1989). Synergistic effect of low doses of tumor necrosis factor and sera of patients with systemic lupus erythematosus on the expression of procoagulant activity by cultured endothelial cells. *Thrombosis and Haemostasis,* **62**:654–660.

Heeb, M.J., Mesters, R.M., Tans, G., Rosing, J., and Griffin, J.H. (1993). Binding of protein S to factor Va associated with inhibition of prothrombinase that is independent of activated protein C. *Journal of Biological Chemistry,* **268**:2872–2877.

Herbert, J.M., Savi, P., Laplace, M.C. and Lale, A. (1992). IL-4 inhibits LPS, IL-1β and TNFα induced expression of tissue factor in endothelial cells and monocytes. *FEBS-letters,* **310**:31–33.

Hogan, J.C., Lewis, M.J. and Henderson, A.H. (1988). *In vivo* EDRF production influences platelet function. *British Journal of Pharmacology,* **94**:1020–1022.

Jones, D.A., Carlton, D.P., McIntyre, T.M., Zimmerman, G.A. and Prescott, S.M. (1993). Molecular cloning of human prostaglandin endoperoxide synthase type II and demonstration of expression in response to cytokines. *The Journal of Biological Chemistry,* **268**:9049–9054.

Kapiotis, S., Besemer, J., Bevec, D., Valent, P., Bettelheim, P., Lechner, K. and Speiser, W. (1991). Interleukin-4 counteracts pyrogen-induced downregulation of thrombomodulin in cultured human vascular endothelial cells. *Blood,* **78**:410–415.

Kaplan, A.P. and Silverberg, M. (1987). The coagulation-kinin pathway of human plasma. *Blood* **70**:1–15

Kaplan, J.E., Moon, D.G., Weston, L.K., Minnear, F.L., Del Vecchio, P.J., Shepard, J.M. and Fenton II, J.W. (1989). Platelets adhere to thrombin-treated endothelial cells *in vitro. American Journal Physiology,* **257**:H423–H433.

Kimura, S., Kasuya, Y., Sawamura, T. (1989). Conversion of big endothelin to 21-residue endothelin-1 is essential for the expression of full vasoconstrictor activity: Structure-activity relationship of big endothelin-1. *Journal of Cardiovascular Pharmacology,* **13**:S5–S7.

Kirchhofer, D., Tschopp, T.B., Hadvary, P. and Baumgartner, H.R. (1994). Endothelial cells stimulated with tumor necrosis factor-α express varying amounts of tissue factor resulting in inhomogeneous fibrin deposition in a native blood flow system. *Journal of Clinical Investigation,* **93**:2073–2083.

Kjellen, L. and Lindahl, U. (1991). Proteoglycans: structures and interactions. *Annual Review of Biochemistry,* **60**:443–475.

Kojima, T., Shworak, N.M. and Rosenberg, R.D. (1992). Molecular cloning and expression of two distinct cDNA-encoding heparan sulphate proteoglycan core proteins from a rat endothelial cell line. *Journal of Biological Chemistry,* **267**:4870–4877.

Koppelman, S.J., Koedam, J.A., van Wijnen, M., Stern, D.M., Nawroth, P.P., Sixma, J.J. and Bouma, B.N. (1994). Von Willebrand factor as a regulator of intrinsic factor X activation. *Journal of laboratory and Clinical Medicine,* **123**:585–593.

Levi, M., ten Cate, H., Bauer, K.A., van der Poll, T., Edgington, T.S., Büller, H.R., van Deventer, S.J.H., Hack, E., ten Cate, J.W. and Rosenberg, R.D. (1994). Inhibition of endotoxin-induced activation of coagulation and fibrinolysis by pentoxifylline or by a monoclonal anti-tissue factor antibody in chimpanzees. *Journal of Clinical Investigations,* **93**:114–120.

Loesberg, C., Gonsalvez, M.D., Zandbergen, J ., Willems, Ch., van Aken, W.G., Stel, H.V., van Mourik, J.A. and de Groot, Ph.G. (1985). The effect of calcium on the secretion of factor VIII-related antigen by cultured human endothelial cells. *Biochimica Biophysica Acta,* **763**:160–168.

Lüscher, T.F. (1993). Nitric oxide, prostaglandins and endothelins. *Ballière's Clinical Haematology,* **6**:609–627.

Lyberg, T., Galdal, S.A., Evensen, S.A. and Prydz, H. (1983). Cellular cooperation in endothelial cell thrombomodulin synthesis. *British Journal of Haematology,* **53**:89–95.

Maclouf, J. (1993). Transcellular biosynthesis of arachidonic acid metabolites: from *in vitro* investigations to the *in vivo* reality. In *Ballière's Clinical Haematology,* **6**:593–608.

Maier, J.A.M., Hla, T. and Maciag, T. (1990). Cyclooxygenase is an immediate early gene induced by interleukin-1 in human endothelial cells. *The Journal of Biological Chemistry,* **265**:10805–10808.

Marcum, J.A., Kenny, J.B. and Rosenberg, R.D. (1984). Acceleration of thrombin-antithrombin complex formation in rat hindquarters via heparin-like molecules bound to the endothelium. *Journal of Clinical Investigation,* **74**:341–350.

Marcus A.J., Weksler, B.B., Jaffe, E.A. and Broekman, M.J. (1980). Synthesis of prostacyclin from platelet-derived endoperoxides by cultured human endothelial cells. *Journal of Clinical Investigation,* **66**:979–986.

Marcus, A.J., Safier, L.B., Hajjar, K., Ullman, H.L., Islam, N., Broekman, M.J. and Eiroa, A.M. (1991). Inhibition of platelet function by an aspirin-insensitive endothelial cell ADPase. *Journal of Clinical Investigation,* **88**:1690–1696.

Marcus, A.J. and Safier, L. (1993). Thromboregulation: multicellular modulation of platelet reactivity in hemostasis and thrombosis. *FASEB Journal,* **7**:516–522.

Marletta, M.A. (1993). Nitric oxide synthase structure and mechanism. *Journal Biological Chemistry,* **268**:12231–12234.

Martin, W., Villiani, G.M., Jothianandan, D. and Furgchott, R.F. (1985). Selective blockade of endothelium dependent and glyceryl trinitrate-induced relaxation by hemoglobin and by methylene blue in the rabbit aorta. *Journal of Pharmacology and Experimental Ther,* **232**:708–716.

Martin, N.B., Jamieson, A. and Tuffin, D.P. (1993). The effect of interleukin-4 on tumor necrosis factor-alpha induced expression of tissue factor and plasminogen activator inhibitor-1 in human umbilical vein endothelial cells. *Thrombosis and Haemostasis,* **70**:1037–1042.

Maurice, D.H. and Haslam, R.J. (1990). Molecular basis of the synergistic inhibition of platelet function by nitrovasodilators and activators of adenylate cyclase: Inhibition of cAMP breakdown by cGMP. *Molecular Pharmacology,* **37**:671–691.

Mayadas, T.N., Wagner, D.D. and Simpson, P.J. (1989). Von Willebrand factor biosynthesis and partitioning between constitutive and regulated pathway of secretion after thrombin stimulation. *Blood,* **57**:2745–2756.

McIntyre, T.M., Zimmerman, G.A., Satoh, K. and Prescott, S.M. (1985). Human endothelial cells synthesize both platelet activating factor and prostacyclin in response to histamine, bradykinin and adenosine triphosphate. *Journal of Clinical Investigation,* **76**:275–280.

Mertens, G., Cassiman, J.J., van den Berghe, H., Vermylen, J and David, G. (1992). Cell surface heparin sulphate proteoglycans from human vascular endothelial cells: Core protein characterization and antithrombin III binding properties, *Journal of Biological Chemistry,* **267**:20435–20443.

Mitchell, C.A., Keleman, S.M. and Salem, H.H. (1988). The anticoagulant properties of a modified form of protein S. *Thrombosis and Haemostasis,* **60**:298–304.

Moncada, S., Gryglewski, R., Bunting, S. and Vane, J.R. (1976). An enzyme isolated from arteries transforms prostaglandin endoperoxides to an unstable substance that inhibits platelet aggregation. *Nature,* **263**:663–665.

Moncada, S. and Vane, J.R. (1979). Arachidonic acid metabolites and the interaction between platelets and blood vessel walls. *New England Journal of Medicine,* **300**:1141–0000.

Moncada, S. (1982). The biological importance of prostacyclin. *British Journal of Pharmacology,* **76**:3–31.

Moncada, S., Palmer, R.M.J. and Higgs, E.A. (1991). Nitric oxide: physiology, pathophysiology and pharmacology. *Pharmacological Reviews,* **43**:109–142.

Moore, K.L., Andreoli, S.P., Esmon, N.L., Esmon, C.T. and Bang, N.U, (1987). Endotoxin enhances tissue factor and suppresses thrombomodulin expression of human vascular endothelial cells *in vitro. Journal of Clinical Investigation,* **79**:124–130.

Mulder, A.B., Hegge-Paping, K.S.M., Magielse, C.P.E., Blom, N.R., Smit, J.W., van der Meer, J., Halie, M.R. and Blom, V.J.J. (1994). Tumor necrosis factor-induced endothelial cell tissue factor is located on the cell surface rather than in the subendothelial matrix. *Blood,* **84**:1559–1566.

Muller, W.A. and Gimbrone, M.A. (1986). Plasmalemmal proteins of cultured vascular endothelial cells exhibit apical-basal polarity: analysis by surface-selective iodonation. *Journal of Cell Biology,* **103**:2389–2402.

Mulsch, A., Busse, R. and Bassenge, E. (1989). Nitric oxide synthesis in endothelial cytosol: evidence for a calcium dependent and a calcium independent mechanism. *Archives of Pharmacology,* **340**:767–770.

Myers, P.R., Minor, R.L., Guerra, R., Bates, J.N. and Harrison, D.G. (1990). Vasorelaxant properties of the endothelium-derived relaxing factor more closely resembles S-nitrosocysteine than nitric oxide. *Nature,* **345**:161–163.

Nawroth, P.P. and Stern D.M. (1986). Modulation of endothelial cell hemostatic properties by tumor necrosis factor. *Journal of Experimental Medicine,* **163**:740–745.

Nawroth, P.P., Handley, D., Matsueda, M., de Waal, R., Gerlach, H., Blohm, D. and Stern, D.M. (1988). Tumor necrosis factor/cachetin induced intravascular fibrin formation in metA fibrosarcoma. *Journal of Experimental Medicine,* **168**:637–645.

Nathan, C. and Xie, Q.W. (1994). Regulation of biosynthesis of nitric oxide. *Journal of Biological Chemistry,* **269**:13725–13728.

Nemerson, Y. (1992). The tissue factor pathway of coagulation. *Seminars in Haematology,* **29**:170–176

Novotny, W.F., Palmier, M., Wun, T.C., Broze, G.J. and Miletich, J.P. (1991). Purification and properties of heparin-releasable lipoprotein-associated coagulation inhibitor. *Blood,* **78**:394–400.

Oosting, J.D., Derksen, R.H.W.M., Blokzijl, L., Sixma, J.J. and de Groot, Ph.G. (1992). Antiphospholipid antibodies positive sera enhance endothelial cell procoagulant activity. Studies in a thrombosis model. *Thrombosis and Haemostasis,* **68**:278–284.

Paleolog, E.M., Crossman, D.C., McVey, J.H. and Pearson, J.D. (1990). Differential regulation by cytokines of constitutive and stimulated secretion of vWf from endothelial cells. *Blood,* **75**:688–695.

Palmer, R.M.J., Ferrige, A.G. and Moncada, S. (1987). Nitric oxide release accounts for the biological activity of endothelium derived relaxing factor. *Nature, 327*:524–526.

Palmer, R.M.J., Ashton, D.S. and Moncada, S. (1988). Vascular endothelial cells synthesize nitric oxide from L-arginine. *Nature, 333*:664–666.

Parsaee, H., McEwan, J.R., Joseph, S. and MacDermot, J. (1992). Differential sensitivities of the prostacyclin and nitric oxide pathways to cytosolic calcium in bovine aortic endothelial cells. *British Journal of Pharmacology, 107*:1013–1019.

Pearson, J.D. and Gordon, J.L. (1985). Nucleotide metabolism by endothelium. *Annual Review of Physiology, 47*:617–627.

Pearson, J.D. (1994). Endothelial cell biology. In: *Haemostasis and Thrombosis 3rd edition* A.L. Bloom, C.D. Forbes, D.P. Thomas and E.G.D. Tuddenham (eds) pp. 219–232 Edinburgh: Churchill Livingstone

Preissner, K.T., Delvos, U. and Muller-Berghaus, G. (1987). Binding of thrombin to thrombomodulin accelerates inhibition of the enzyme by antithrombin III. Evidence for a heparin independent mechanism. *Biochemistry, 26*:2521–2528.

Pober, J.S. and Cotran, R.S. (1990). Cytokines and endothelial cell biology. *Physiological Reviews, 70*:427–451.

Radomski, M.W., Palmer, R.M.J. and Moncada, S. (1987a). The anti-aggregating properties of vascular endothelium: Interaction between prostacyclin and nitric oxide. *British Journal of Pharmacology, 92*:639–646.

Radomski, M.J., Palmer, R.M.J. and Moncada, S. (1987b). The role of nitric oxide and cGMP in platelet adhesion to vascular endothelium. *Biochemical and Biophysical Research Communications, 148*:1482–1489.

Radomski, M.W., Palmer, R.M.J. and Moncada, S. (1990). A L-arginine/nitric oxide pathway present in human platelets regulates aggregation. *Proceedings of the National Academy of Sciences USA, 87*:5193–5197.

Ratnoff, O.D. (1994). The development of knowledge about hemostasis and thrombosis. in: *Haemostasis and Thrombosis 3rd edition* A.L. Bloom, C.D. Forbes, D.P. Thomas and E.G.D. Tuddenham (eds). pp. 3–28 Edinburgh: Churchill Livingstone.

Reddigari, S.R., Shibayama, Y., Brunnee, T. and Kaplan, A.P. (1993). Human factor XI (Hageman factor) and high molecular weight kininogen compete for the same binding site on human umbilical vein endothelial cells. *Journal of Biological Chemistry, 268*:11982–11987.

Rosing, J., Zwaal, R.F.A. and Tans, G. (1986). Formation of meizothrombin as an intermediate in factor Xa-catalyzed prothrombin activation. *Journal of Biological Chemistry, 261*:4224–4228.

Ross, R. (1986). The pathogenesis of atherosclerose - An update. *New England Journal of Medicine, 314*:488–500.

Roth, G.J. and Calverley, D. (1994). Aspirin, platelets and thrombosis: Theory and practice. *Blood. 83*:885–898.

Ruggeri, Z.M. and Ware, J. (1993). von Willebrand factor. *FASEB Journal, 7*:308–316.

Rubanyi, G.M. (1992). Potential physiological and pathological significance of endothelins. *Drugs of the Future, 17*:915–936.

Ryan, J., Brett, J., Tijburg, P.N.M., Bach, R.R., Kisiel, W. and Stern, D.M. (1992). Tumor necrosis factor induced endothelial cell tissue factor is associated with subendothelial matrix vesicles but is not expressed on the apical surface. *Blood, 80*:966–974.

Sadler, J.E. (1991). Von Willebrand Factor. *Journal of Biological Chemistry, 266*:2277–2288.

Sadler, J.E. (1994). Von Willebrand disease In: *Haemostasis and Thrombosis 3rd edition* A.L. Bloom, C.D.Forbes, D.P.Thomas and E.G.D.Tuddenham (eds) pp. 859–887 Edinburgh: Churchill Livingstone

Schafer, A.I., Crawford, D.D. and Gimbrone, M.A.Jr. (1984). Unidirectional transfer of prostaglandin endoperoxides between platelets and endothelial cells. *Journal of Clinical Investigation, 73*:1105–1112.

Scharfstein, J.S., Keaney, J., Slivka, A., Welch, G.N., Vita, J.A., Stamler, J.S. and Loscalzo, J. (1994). *In vivo* transfer of nitric oxide between a plasma protein bound resevoir and low molecular weight thiols. *Journal of Clinical Investigation, 94*:1432–1439.

Sixma, J.J. and Wester, J. (1977). The hemostatic plug. *Seminars in Haematology, 14*:265–299.

Sixma, J.J. and de Groot, Ph.G. (1994). Regulation of platelet adhesion to the vessel wall. Annals of the New York *Academy of Sciences, 714*:190–199.

Smith, J.A., Henderson, A.H. and Randall, M.D. (1994). Endothelium derived relaxing factors, prostanoids and endothelins. In: *Haemostasis and Thrombosis 3rd edition* A.L. Bloom, C.D. Forbes, D.P. Thomas and E.G.D. Tuddenham (eds) pp. 183–197 Edinburgh: Churchill Livingstone

Sprecher, C.A., Kisiel, W., Mathewes, S. and Foster, D.C. (1994). Molecular cloning, expression, and partial characterization of a second human tissue factor pathway inhibitor. *Proceedings of the National Academy of Sciences USA, 91*:3353–3357.

Stern, D.M., Nawroth, P.P., Marcum, J., Kisiel, W., Rosenberg, R. and Stern, K. (1985). Interaction of antithrombin III with bovine aortic segments: role of heparin in the binding and enhanced anticoagulant activity. *Journal of Clinical Investigation, 75*:272–279.

Stern, D.M., Nawroth, P.P., Kisiel, W., Vehar, G. and Esmon, C.T. (1985a). The binding of factor IXa to cultured bovine endothelial cells: induction of a specific binding site in the presence of factors VIII and X. *Journal of Biological Chemistry, 260*:6717–6722.

Stern, D.M., Nawroth, P.P., Handley, D. and Kisiel, W. (1985b). An endothelial cell-dependent pathway of coagulation. *Proceedings of the National Academy of Sciences USA, 82*:2523–2527.

Stern, D.M., Brett, J., Harris, K. and Nawroth, P.P. (1986). Participation of endothelial cells in the protein C-protein S anticoagulant pathway: the synthesis and release of protein S. *Journal of Cell Biology,* **102**:1971–1978.

Stern, D.M., Nawroth, P.P., Kisiel, W., Vehar, G. and Esmon, C. (1985c). The binding of factor IXa to cultured bovine endothelial cells: Induction of a specific site in the presence of factors VIII and X. *Journal of Clinical Investigation,* **264**:3244–3251.

Taylor, F.B., Chang, A., Ruf, W., Morrissey, J.H., Hinshaw, L., Catlett, R., Blick, K. and Edgington, T.S. (1991). Lethal E.coli septic shock is prevented by blocking tissue factor with monoclonal antibody. *Circulatory Shock,* **33**:127–134.

Thiemermann, C., Lidbury, P.S., Thomas, G.R. and Vane, J.R. (1988). Endothelin-1 inhibits *ex-vivo* platelet aggregation in the rabbit. *European Journal of Pharmacology,* **158**:182–186.

Tijburg, P.M.N., van Heerde, W.L., Leenhouts, H.M., Hessing, M., Bouma, B.N. and de Groot, Ph.G. (1991). Formation of meizothrombin as intermediate in factor Xa-catalyzed activation of prothrombin on endothelial cells. *Journal of Biological Chemistry,* **266**:4071–4022.

Torti, M. and Lapertina, E.G. (1993). Prostacyclin and platelets: a novel signal transduction mechanism. in: *Prostacyclin: new perspectives for basic research and novel therapeutic indications.* Rubanyi, G.M. and Vane, J. (eds) pp. 25–35, Elsevier Scientific Publications, Amsterdam.

Vallance, P., Collier, J. and Moncada, S. (1989). Effect of endothelium derived nitric oxide on peripheral arteriolar tone in man. *Lancet,* **ii**:997–1000.

Van Buul-Wortelboer, M.F., Brinkman, H.M., Reinders, J.H., van Aken, W.G. and van Mourik, J.A. (1990). Polar secretion of von Willebrand factor by endothelial cells. *Biochimica Biophysica Acta,* **1011**:129–133.

Van der Poll, T, Büller, H.R., ten Cate, H., Wortel, C.H., Bauer, K.A., van Deventer, S.J.H., Hack, C.E., Sauerwein, H.P., Rosenberg, R.D. and ten Cate, J.W. (1990). Activation of coagulation after administration of tumor necrosis factor to normal subjects. *New England Journal of Medicine,* **322**:1622–1627.

Van Heerde, W.L, Poort, S., van't Veer, C., Reutelingsperger, C.P.M. and de Groot, Ph.G. (1994). Binding of recombinant annexin V to endothelial cells: effect of annexin V binding on endothelial cell mediated thrombin formation. *Biochemical Journal,* **302**:305–312.

Van Iwaarden, F., de Groot, Ph.G. and Bouma, B.N. (1988). The binding of high molecular weight kininogen to cultured human endothelial cells. *Journal of Biological Chemistry,* **263**:4698–4703.

Verweij, C.L., Hart, M. and Pannekoek, H. (1987). Expression of variant von Willebrand factor cDNA in heterologous cells: requirement of the propolypeptide in vWF multimer formation. *EMBO Journal,* **6**:2885–2890.

Visser, M.R., Tracy, P.B., Vercelotti, G.M., Goodman, J.L., White, J.G. and Jacob, H.S. (1988). Enhanced thrombin generation and platelet binding on herpes simplex virus infected endothelium. *Proceedings of the National Academy of Sciences,* **85**:8227–8230.

Walter, U., Eigenthaler, M., Geiger, J. and Reinhart, M. (1993). Role of cyclic nucleotide-dependent protein kinases and their common substrate VASP in the regulation of human platelets. in: Mechanisms of platelet Activation and Control, Authi, K.S. (ed) pp. 237–249, Plenum press, New York.

Wagner, D.D. (1990). Cell Biology of von Willebrand factor. *Annual Review of Cell Biology,* **6**:217–246.

Weksler, B.B., Marcus, A.J. and Jaffe, E.A. (1977). Synthesis of prostaglandin I2 (prostacyclin) by cultured human and bovine endothelial cells. *Proceedings of the National Academy of Sciences of the USA,* **74**:3922–3926.

Weiss, H.J and Turitto, V.T. (1979). Prostacyclin inhibits platelet adhesion and thrombus formation on subendothelium. *Blood,* **53**:244–250.

Wiggins, R.C., Loskutoff, D.J., Cochrane, C.G., Griffin, J.H. and Edgington, T.S. (1980). Activation of rabbit Hageman factor by homogenates of cultured rabbit endothelial cells. *Journal of Clinical Investigation,* **65**:197–206.

Yanagisawa, M., Kuhihara, H., Kimura, S., Tomobe., Kobayashi M., Mitsui, Y., Yazaki, Y., Goto, K. and Masaki, T. (1988). A novel potent vasoconstrictor peptide produced by vascular endothelial cells. *Nature,* **332**:411–415.

Yanagisawa, M. and Masaki, T. (1989). Endothelin, a novel endothelium-dependent peptide. *Biochemical Pharmacology,* **38**:1877–1883.

Zimmerman, G.A., McIntyre, T.M., Mehra, M. and Prescott, S.M. (1990). Endothelial cell associated platelet activating factor: a novel mechanism for signalling intracellular adhesion. *Journal of Cell Biology,* **110**:529–540.

8 Platelet Adhesion

Jan J. Sixma and Philip G. de Groot

Department of Haematology, University Utrecht, The Netherlands, University Hospital
Department of Haematology (G03.647), P.O. Box 85.500, 3508 GA UTRECHT,
The Netherlands, Tel.: #31-30-250.72.30, Fax: #31-30-251.18.93,
E-mail: ph.g.degroot@lab.azu.nl/jsixma@lab.azu.nl

INTRODUCTION

Cell adhesion is usually studied under static conditions. In the classic set-up, ELISA tray wells are coated with an adhesive protein. The adhesion is then measured by counting the cells which bind to the wells. This set-up is not optimal for the adhesion of blood cells, blood platelets in particular. Adhesion for these cells occurs physiologically under flow conditions and the shear stress induced by flow may cause qualitative and quantitative differences in adhesion (Baumgartner, 1973). The study of blood platelet adhesion under flow conditions also has other advantages. Blood platelets are of relative low density and do not settle well under gravity. Consequently static adhesion experiments need to be of long duration, and are strongly influenced by the viscosity of the suspending medium. Washed platelets in buffer or platelet rich plasma are used and the required centrifugation steps cause platelet activation. This is usually prevented by addition of inhibitors during the centrifugation step, but such inhibitors may also influence the actual adhesion process. In flowing blood, platelets are transported to the vessel wall and considerable adhesion occurs within short time spans. Most of the studies that will be reported in this review concern studies on platelet adhesion under flow conditions. Such studies were first performed by Baumgartner *et al.*, using an annual perfusion chamber in which a vessel wall segment was exposed to flowing blood (Baumgartner *et al.*, 1976). Later on, other flow chambers were developed and the results have been reviewed in several exhaustive review papers and chapters (Roth, 1991; Sixma *et al.*, 1995; Sixma, 1994; Sixma and De Groot, 1994; Sixma and De Groot, 1990). In the current chapter we will highlight recent data from ourselves and others, regarding platelet adhesion to isolated proteins, and the role of platelet activation. Recent data on thrombogenicity of atherosclerotic lesions will also be reviewed.

COLLAGEN

When a vessel is injured blood platelets adhere to the perivascular connective tissue. Already in 1963, Hovig demonstrated that collagen is an important reactive substance (Hovig, 1963). He showed that addition of fibrillar collagen to platelet rich plasma causes platelet aggregation. Electron microscopic observations of hemostatic plugs confirmed this by showing direct interaction between blood platelets and collagen fibrils (Hovig *et al.*, 1967). Many studies have been performed to distinguish between actual adhesion process, subsequent platelet secretion and platelet aggregation (Sakariassen *et al.*, 1990; Zijenah and Barnes, 1990; Zijenah *et al.*, 1990). More recently perfusion studies with flowing blood have been performed in which the adhesion of blood platelets to different types of collagen has been studied (Parsons *et al.*, 1986). In this chapter we will mainly concentrate on the results of such studies.

Eighteen different types of collagen have been recognized. Of these type I, III, IV, V, VI, and VIII and, sometimes, XI occur in the vessel wall. Platelet adhesion studies have been performed with collagens I through VIII (Saelman *et al.*, 1994). Such studies showed that the collagens could be broadly distinguished into three groups: reactive collagens: type I, II, III and IV, collagens with low reactivity: type VI, VII and VIII, and collagen type V which showed no adhesion under flow conditions, but which caused adhesion under static conditions, and aggregate formation in platelet rich plasma. Among the reactive collagens, adhesion to collagens type I, II and III goes up with the shear rate without a clear optimum up to a shear rate of 1500 s^{-1}. For collagen type III we recently found no optimum up to shear rates of 4000 s^{-1}. For collagen type IV some decrease of adhesion was seen at and above shear rates of 1500 s^{-1} (van Zanten *et al.*, 1995b). Collagen type VI had an optimum at a shear rate of 300 s^{-1}. Among the less reactive collagens, collagen type VII and VIII showed maximal adhesion at the lowest shear rate studied of 100 s^{-1} and almost no adhesion at a shear rate of 1000 s^{-1}. Platelet adhesion to the reactive collagens type I through IV caused aggregate formation whereas adhesion of dendritic platelets was seen on collagens type VII and VIII and of contact and dendritic platelets on type VI (Saelman *et al.*, 1994). Time course studies were done on collagen type I and III (Houdijk *et al.*, 1985). They showed almost linear increase of platelet deposition with time at a shear rate 800 s^{-1}. Studies with collagen type III in which aggregation was avoided by the use of platelets reconstituted in human albumin solution instead of plasma showed a linear increase of platelet adhesion at 300 s^{-1} over 15 minutes and initial faster adhesion for the first three minutes at 1600 s^{-1} (Wu *et al.*, 1994). Platelet adhesion to collagen type IV was also linear with time both at 300 and 1600 s^{-1} (Wu *et al.*, 1994).

The effect of divalent cations on platelet adhesion to collagen type I, III and IV was studied with reconstituted blood in which the concentrations of the calcium and magnesium were varied by dialysis of the plasma. These studies showed a clear cut magnesium dependence which was most pronounced for collagen type IV and more strongly expressed at higher shear rates. No adhesion of blood platelets to collagen type IV could be observed in the absence of Mg^{2+} (van Zanten *et al.*, 1995b). The observed effects of the magnesium concentration may have physiological relevance. Pronounced increase in adhesion was found between 0.6-1 mM free magnesium and concentrations in this range are encountered in normal individuals. Normal donors vary very strongly in their reaction to collagens and this has been attributed to strong variations in $\alpha 2\beta 1$ (glycoprotein Ia-IIa), the main receptor for collagen (Kunicki *et al.*, 1993). The observed variations in magnesium concentration in plasma may clearly also contribute, particularly in adhesion to collagen type IV and type III at high shear rates.

Platelet adhesion under static conditions has been distinguished in cation dependent and independent adhesion (Staatz *et al.*, 1989; Zijenah *et al.*, 1990). The cation dependent adhesion was attributed to mediation by glycoprotein Ia-IIa (GP Ia-IIa). This integrin forms an heterodimeric complex in the presence of magnesium and is then functional (Staatz *et al.*, 1989). Cation independent adhesion was thought not to be mediated by GP Ia-IIa. Studies with blood of a patient with deficiency of GP Ia-IIa (Nieuwenhuis *et al.*, 1985) and with the use of a monoclonal antibody against GP Ia showed, however, that adhesion of all collagens both under static and flow conditions require interaction of GP Ia-IIa with collagen (Saelman *et al.*, 1994).

GP Ia-IIa is an adhesion receptor belonging to the integrins. These are heterodimeric transmembrane receptors consisting of an α and a β chain. To date 7 different types of β chains have been identified (Hynes, 1992). GP Ia-IIa is a member of the $\beta 1$ family which consists mostly of integrins that are involved in the interaction of cells with connective tissue molecules (Hemler, 1990). GP Ia-IIa consists of an $\alpha 2$ chain of 140 kD and a $\beta 1$ chain of 105 kD (Takada and Hemler, 1989). $\alpha 2\beta 1$ (VLA-2) is present on many different cells and serves in general as a collagen receptor (Zutter and Santoro, 1990). In many cells, $\alpha 2\beta 1$ is also a laminin receptor. For platelets this is not the case (Elices and Hemler, 1989). The best demonstration that $\alpha 2\beta 1$ is important for platelet adhesion came from a patient with a livelong bleeding history in which the GP Ia was reduced to 200 molecules per platelet (normally > 1000) in whom all interactions with collagen were completely abolished (Nieuwenhuis *et al.*, 1985; Nieuwenhuis *et al.*, 1986; Beer *et al.*, 1988). A second patient with a similar disorder with also a decreased thrombospondin content of the α granules was described as transient disorder (Kehrel *et al.*, 1988) and auto-antibodies to GP Ia-IIa have been found to induce reduced interaction of platelets with collagen and a prolonged bleeding time (Deckmyn *et al.*, 1990). There is no doubt, however, that other receptors are also involved in interaction with collagen. A 61 kD membrane GP (GP VI) was found absent in Japanese individuals whose platelets did not react with collagen (Moroi *et al.*, 1989). An auto-antibody against a 80 kD GP also caused disturbed interaction of platelets with collagen (Deckmyn *et al.*, 1992) and also GP IV was quoted as potential collagen receptor (Tandon *et al.*, 1989). A 68 kD protein which may be identical to the C1q receptor has also been quoted as platelet receptor (Peerschke and Ghebrehiwet, 1990b; Peerschke and Ghebrehiwet, 1990a) and the possible involvement of GP IIb-IIIa has been pointed out (Kotite and Cunningham, 1986). Recent studies on normal Japanese volunteers who were found to lack GP IV on the platelet membranes (Yamamoto *et al.*, 1990) have shed some light on the potential role of GP IV. Studies under static conditions showed some decrease in initial adhesion (Tandon *et al.*, 1991) and absence of adhesion to collagen type V (Saelman *et al.*, 1993b; Kehrel *et al.*, 1993). Studies under flow conditions showed no abnormality at all (Saelman *et al.*, 1993b), although this is disputed (Diaz-Ricart *et al.*, 1993). It is difficult to reconcile all the data from various sources. Primary collagen induced adhesion and subsequent platelet activation should probably be seen as a series of steps in which different membrane molecules are involved. Some evidence for this is found by the action of moubatin isolated from the saliva of the leech Haementeria Officinalis (Keller *et al.*, 1993) and pallidipin from the tick Triatoma Pallidipennis (Noeske-Jungblut *et al.*, 1994). These components specifically inhibit collagen induced aggregation without affecting adhesion of blood platelets to collagen. They also have no effect on the aggregation induced by ADP and thrombin and by other platelet reactive agents. A similar effect was caused by C1q and antibodies to the C1q receptor which are able to block secretion and aggregation induced by collagen, but have no effect on adhesion (Peerschke and Ghebrehiwet, 1990b). The 68 kD protein which was thought to be a collagen receptor is in fact the receptor for C1q (Peerschke and Ghebrehiwet, 1990a; Peerschke and Ghebrehiwet, 1990b). It should be mentioned that a large part of C1q has a triple-helical structure similar to collagen.

This separation between primary adhesion and platelet activation would suggest that GP Ia-IIa by itself is not involved in platelet activation. There is one piece of evidence, however, that militates against this. The snake venom protein aggretin was found to activate platelets directly and to cause aggregation. There is strong evidence that these venoms work via GP Ia-IIa (Liu *et al.*, 1994). One speculation may be that clustering of GP Ia-IIa is required for platelet activation. The spacing of binding sites in collagen does not allow this clustering of the receptor. In that case another route may be followed in which other membrane proteins interact with GP Ia-IIa to cause activation of the different signalling pathways which leads to platelet activation. These other membrane proteins do not need to be receptors for collagen in their own right. Aggretin may cause the clustering of GP Ia-IIa directly.

Platelet adhesion to collagen under flow conditions differs from adhesion under static conditions particularly in that it has an absolute requirement for von Willebrand Factor (Houdijk *et al.*, 1985). Von Willebrand Factor has two collagen binding sites, one located in the A1 repeat and one in the A3 repeat. This latter is essential for collagen binding (Sixma *et al.*, 1991; Lankhof *et al.*, 1994; Dong and Sadler, 1994). Absence of von Willebrand Factor in the blood of a patient with severe von Willebrand's Disease or inhibition of the function of von Willebrand Factor with a monoclonal antibody completely inhibits adhesion to collagen type I and III (De Groot *et al.*, 1988; Fressinaud *et al.*, 1987; Fressinaud *et al.*, 1992). Collagen can be preincubated with von Willebrand Factor or von Willebrand Factor can be present in plasma in order to obtain normal adhesion (Houdijk *et al.*, 1985). Binding studies showed correlation between the number of platelets adhering to vessel wall and the number of von Willebrand Factor molecules binding to it (Sakariassen *et al.*, 1979), and von Willebrand Factor binding was found to precede platelet adhesion in a time sequence study (Bolhuis *et al.*, 1981). Platelet adhesion to collagen type I and III may be mediated by platelet von Willebrand Factor, but this is dependent on the reactivity of the collagen. Reactive collagens cause more platelet secretion and make more von Willebrand Factor available (D'Alessio *et al.*, 1990; Fressinaud *et al.*, 1987). Recent studies showed that also adhesion to collagen type IV is mediated by von Willebrand Factor-GP Ib interaction particularly at high shear rates, however, no binding is observed of von Willebrand Factor to collagen type IV (van Zanten *et al.*, 1995b). This situation is reminiscent of adhesion to fibronectin and fibrinogen/fibrin, which we will describe later. Von Willebrand Factor does not bind to these proteins, when they are coated on a coverslip, but adhesion of platelets, particularly at high shear rates, requires the support of von Willebrand Factor molecules. Localization studies have shown von Willebrand Factor to be localized only in the direct vicinity of the adhering platelet but not elsewhere on the surface and the same is true for adhesion to collagen type IV (van Zanten *et al.*, 1995b).

Studies with monoclonal antibodies directed against von Willebrand Factor have indicated that binding of von Willebrand Factor to the extracellular matrix of fibroblasts and endothelial cells is different from that to collagen type I and III. A monoclonal antibody which inhibited binding of von Willebrand Factor to collagen type I and III had no effect on binding to extracellular matrix (De Groot *et al.*, 1988). Conversely, another monoclonal antibody which inhibited binding of von Willebrand Factor to extracellular matrix had no effect on binding of von Willebrand Factor to collagen. Recently it has been suggested that collagen type VI is responsible for von Willebrand Factor binding to the extracellular matrix (Rand *et al.*, 1991; Rand *et al.*, 1993). Studies with a anti-platelet protein from the saliva of the leech Haementeria Officinalis expressed as recombinant product in yeast (rLAPP) showed that this protein inhibited platelet adhesion to collagen type I, III, and IV, but not to endothelial cell matrix and only weakly to collagen type VI (van Zanten *et al.*, 1995a). Further studies of its mechanism of action showed that rLAPP binds directly to collagen type I and III and competes with von Willebrand Factor binding. Inhibition of platelet adhesion to collagen type IV is not easy to understand in view of the inability of von Willebrand Factor to bind to collagen type IV.

Platelet adhesion to subendothelium and the matrix of endothelial cells is inhibited by antibodies to fibronectin. Studies of adhesion to collagen showed that fibronectin was also required for adhesion to monomeric collagen type I and III (Houdijk *et al.*, 1985). No fibronectin dependence was found for fibrillar collagen type III and only at a high shear rate for fibrillar collagen type I (Nievelstein *et al.*, 1988). The most likely explanation is that reactive collagen will release fibronectin from the platelet α granules, but this has not been proven.

Reactive sites on collagen have only been analyzed to a limited degree making use of cyanogen bromide (CB) fragments for the $\alpha 1$(I) chain. Adhesion under static conditions was observed with CB3, CB6, CB7 and CB8 (Zijenah *et al.*, 1990). Under flow conditions adhesion was only seen to CB3, CB7 and CB8 and not to CB6 (Saelman *et al.*, 1993a). Adhesion to CB3 was the strongest and was accompanied by aggregate formation, whereas adhesion to CB7 involved contact and dendritic platelets and adhesion to CB8 only contact platelets. Monoclonal antibodies against GP Ia-IIa inhibited adhesion under flow to all three CB fragments and so did antibodies to GP Ib. Previous studies had shown binding of von Willebrand Factor to various CB fragments of collagen type I (Morton *et al.*, 1983). These results indicate that these are at least three different functional binding sites for von Willebrand Factor on the $\alpha 1$(I) chain. No information is available about the $\alpha 2$(I) chain, but the current data show that a single monomeric triple-helical collagen type I molecule has at least six different interaction sites for GP Ia and for von Willebrand Factor binding. Peptide analysis of $\alpha 1$(I)CB3 showed that a DGEA sequence was involved in rat platelet adhesion (Staatz *et al.*, 1990; Staatz *et al.*, 1991). More recent studies, however, have not been able to confirm that DGEA derived peptides inhibit interaction of platelets with collagen (Morton *et al.*, 1994). The most reactive cyanogen bromide fragment of collagen type III is $\alpha 1$-(III)CB4 (Zijenah and Barnes, 1990). This fragment also causes $\alpha 2 \beta 1$ mediated adhesion of platelets under static conditions and a polymeric form causes platelet aggregation. More information is required about its reaction under flow conditions. Recently some information has been obtained from the work of Barnes and associates to distinguish between the effect of the GP Ia-IIa mediated adhesion on the one hand which involves specific sequences, and platelet activation on the other hand which may be caused by triple-helical fragments with the general repeated structure GPP (Morton *et al.,* 1995).

FIBRINOGEN AND FIBRIN

Platelet adhesion to fibrinogen has received much attention, because it was shown that platelet adhesion to biomaterials is caused by fibrinogen adsorption followed by platelet adhesion to this adsorbed fibrinogen (Lindon *et al.,* 1989). Most of the studies were performed under static conditions. They showed that this adhesion was strongly dependant on the surface induced denaturation of the fibrinogen molecule (Shiba *et al.,* 1991). More recently, more sophisticated and detailed studies of adhesion to fibrinogen have been performed under static (Kieffer *et al.,* 1991; Savage and Ruggeri, 1991; Savage *et al.,* 1992) and flow (Hantgan *et al.,* 1990) conditions. These studies show that platelets adhere to fibrinogen without preceding activation. This was first demonstrated with platelets washed in the presence of metabolic inhibitors (Savage and Ruggeri, 1991) and later in perfusions with whole blood, immediately after blood collection (Buchanan *et al.,* 1985). Platelet adhesion in flow is linear with time during the first ten minutes and then tends to level off because saturation of the surface is reached. In contrast to most other surfaces that will be discussed in this chapter there is very little effect of the shear rate and adhesion increases only up to 300 s^{-1} because of the improved transport of platelets towards the surface (Turitto and Baumgartner, 1974), but it then remains the same over a whole range of shear rates up to 2000 sec^{-1}. Platelets adhering to fibrinogen both under flow and under static conditions are strongly spread out in the form of thin pancakes. This spreading of the platelets is accompanied by a centripetal movement of the α-granules. Only a single layer of platelets is observed, platelet aggregation hardly occurs.

Studies with monoclonal antibodies directed against GP IIb-IIIa and with blood of Glanzmann's thrombasthenia disease patients show that GP IIb-IIIa is the receptor involved in adhesion at all shear rates (Hantgan *et al.,* 1990). Fibrinogen binding to GP IIb-IIIa on blood platelets in solution has been shown to be dependent on preceding platelet activation. However, there is ample evidence that such activation is not required when fibrinogen is adsorbed on the surface (Kieffer *et al.,* 1991; Savage and Ruggeri, 1991).

Fibrinogen has three potential reactive domains that are able to interact with GP IIb-IIIa (Hantgan *et al.,* 1994). These are the RGD S sequence between residue 572–575 on the Aα-chain, the RGD F sequence between residue 95–98 also on the Aα-chain and the last twelve carboxy-terminal amino acids of the γ-chain. Inhibition studies with an RGD containing peptide showed a pronounced inhibition at relatively low concentrations although adhesion to fibrinogen was less sensitive than platelet aggregation in a test tube (Hantgan *et al.,* 1992). Lower concentrations of the RGD peptide were required at high shear rates. The carboxy-terminal dodecapeptide of the γ-chain also caused inhibition of platelet adhesion, but the inhibition was much weaker and required large concentrations of the peptide (Hantgan *et al.,* 1992). These studies suggest that the RGD sequence is more important than the dodecapeptide for platelet adhesion, but this is in contrast to observations with recombinant fibrinogen (Farrell and Thiagarajan, 1994). The latter studies showed that the RGD sequences are not important for fibrinogen binding involved in platelet aggregation whereas the dodecapeptide is essential. More recently, monoclonal antibody studies have been performed both under static conditions and in flow and these studies show that the dodecapeptide is essential, whereas the RGDS sequence may contribute and the RGDF sequence is probably not very important (Hantgan *et al.*, 1995; Gartner *et al.*, 1993). It is surprising that the essential dodecapeptide sequence is a much weaker inhibitor of the function of GP IIb-IIIa than the RGD derived peptide. This may be in part due to the fact that more potent RGD peptides are now used than the original native sequence, but the same was also observed for platelet aggregation and fibrinogen binding to GP IIb-IIIa and it may be a native property of the RGD molecule.

Increased plasma fibrinogen levels have been shown to be a risk factor for cardiovascular disease. It is therefore of interest to study the effect of the circulating plasma fibrinogen in plasma on platelet adhesion to fibrinogen. Both in studies in which purified fibrinogen was added to plasma and in mixing experiments in which plasma from an afibrinogenemia patient was added in different proportions to normal plasma, increased platelet adhesion was found at low fibrinogen levels with a gradual decrease at higher levels. The highest platelet adhesion was found with whole blood of a patient with afibrinogenemia, and this may indicate that platelet granule fibrinogen plays a role (Endenburg *et al.*, 1995c). The results are in agreement with observations on platelet aggregation, which also showed inhibition of aggregation at higher fibrinogen levels (Landolfi *et al.*, 1991). However, the curve for aggregation is bell-shaped since fibrinogen is necessary to obtain aggregation at all and aggregation increases thus at low fibrinogen concentrations.

Adhesion to fibrinogen/fibrin at shear rates above 800 sec^{-1} has requirement for von Willebrand Factor (Buchanan *et al.*, 1985). This von Willebrand Factor interacts with GP Ib on the platelet membrane. This was demonstrated in studies with antibodies to GP Ib, antibodies to the GP Ib-binding domain on von Willebrand Factor, with blood of a patient with severe von Willebrand's Disease, and with blood of a Bernard Soulier Syndrome patient. Both plasma von Willebrand Factor or platelet von Willebrand Factor are able to provide this need. No direct binding of von Willebrand Factor to fibrinogen was observed in immune-electronmicroscopy studies which showed the presence of von Willebrand Factor only beneath and in the immediate vicinity of blood platelets (Endenburg *et al.*, 1995a). The actual mechanism is not resolved. One possibility would be the release of a substance from platelets which mediates interaction between fibrinogen and von Willebrand Factor.

Platelet adhesion to fibrin is in many respects similar to platelet adhesion to fibrinogen. Adhesion occurs linearly with time, but the adhesion rate is faster than on fibrinogen and lower concentrations of fibrin are required to obtain optimal adhesion (Hantgan *et al.*, 1992). Platelet adhesion to fibrin I is also not dependent on the shear rate. Platelets adhere as single spread platelets without platelet aggregation. Adhesion is mediated by GP IIb-IIIa, but there is also a dependence on von Willebrand Factor-GP Ib interaction at high shear rates (Buchanan *et al.*, 1985). Larger concentrations of RGD peptides and dodecapeptide are required to inhibit adhesion (Hantgan *et al.*, 1992). Unexpected and very interesting results were found when adhesion to preformed fibrin networks were studied (Endenburg *et al.*, 1995b). When such a network is formed under static conditions, platelets adhere to the fibrin fibres as single spread platelets and no aggregates are formed. When the fibrin network is formed under flow conditions a totally different picture emerges. Large aggregates are formed on the fibrin network. At high flow rates, the fibrin network aligns parallel with the flow direction. This alignment is not necessary for the thrombus generation. Even a flow of 10 sec^{-1} that did not cause alignment of the fibrin network induced aggregate formation. The formation of aggregates was not dependant on thrombin bound to the fibrin network as was shown by preincubation with the irreversible thrombin inhibitor PPACK. There is also no need for other adhesive molecules incorporated into the fibrin network, since a network formed from purified fibrinogen under flow conditions gives similar platelet aggregate formation. The exact nature of the changes in the fibrin network that are caused by flow is currently unknown.

FIBRONECTIN

Fibronectin is a heterodimeric protein consisting of two chains of 220 kD linked by two disulphide bonds near the carboxyterminus. The two chains in plasma are different due to alternative splicing in the so-called III connecting segment (IIICS). Plasma fibronectin differs from tissue fibronectin which has an extra type III domain also due to alternative splicing (Hynes, 1990). Fibronectin is present in plasma, in subendothelium of the vessel wall, and in α granules of platelets and is associated with all connective tissue. Fibronectin has been shown to support platelet adhesion and spreading under static condition (Grinnell *et al.*, 1979; Koteliansky *et al.*, 1981; Piotrowicz *et al.*, 1988). Activation of blood platelets by thrombin leads to binding of fibronectin to GP IIb-IIIa (Plow *et al.*, 1984; Plow *et al.*, 1985). Fibronectin has also been shown to be involved in platelet aggregation both in the aggregometer (Dixit *et al.*, 1985) and in a perfusion system (Bastida *et al.*, 1987). Evidence of the function of fibronectin as an adhesive protein under flow conditions was first obtained when it was demonstrated that platelet adhesion to subendothelium was inhibited by a polyclonal antibody directed against fibronectin. This effect was seen at shear rates of 500 s^{-1} and higher (Houdijk and Sixma, 1985; Houdijk *et al.*, 1986). A role of fibronectin was also found in adhesion to monomeric collagen type I and III (Houdijk *et al.*, 1985), but no fibronectin was required for adhesion to fibrillar collagen type I and III at 300 s^{-1} and to collagen type III at 1600 s^{-1}. More reactive collagens may have caused secretion of platelet α granules and this may have provided sufficient fibronectin to support platelet adhesion (Nievelstein P.F.E.M. *et al.*, 1988).

More recently platelet adhesion under flow conditions was studied to purified fibronectin coated to a glass coverslip (Beumer *et al.*, 1994). Fibronectin adsorption gave low adhesion which was irreproducible. Better adhesion was obtained by spraying a fibronectin solution as a fine mist of droplets with a retouching airbrush, a technique which is also used for application of collagen to a surface (Muggli *et al.*, 1980; Houdijk *et al.*, 1985). Optimal adhesion and platelet spreading was found at a concentration of 5 μg per cm^2. Higher concentrations of fibronectin gave less adhesion, but particularly less spreading. Adhesion was linear with time over the first 10 minutes and showed a optimum of about 20% coverage of the surface at a shear rate of 300 s^{-1}. At 1200 s^{-1} adhesion had dropped to a minimum of 4% surface coverage. Platelet spreading occurred over the whole range of shear rates.

Adhesion to surface coated fibronectin has no dependence on divalent cations. Pronounced inhibition was seen by heparin molecules. This inhibition was dependent on the size of the heparin chains. Molecules with a molecular weight of 21 kD showed the most pronounced inhibition (Beumer *et al.*, 1994).

Blood platelets have two integrin receptors for fibronectin. GP IIb-IIIa (αIIbβIII) which is absent in Glanzman's thrombasthenia, binds fibronectin when platelets are activated by thrombin (Plow *et al.*, 1985). GP Ic-IIa (very late antigen VLA-5, α5β1), is a receptor for fibronectin which is coated to a coverslip under static conditions (Piotrowicz *et al.*, 1988). Antibodies to α5 or β1 or both in combination inhibited adhesion to fibronectin in flow by 50%. They had no effect on platelet spreading. Antibodies to GP IIb-IIIa inhibited platelet adhesion by 90% and also inhibited platelet spreading (Beumer *et al.*, 1994). Low platelet adhesion was also seen with blood of a patient with Glanzman's thrombasthenia; spreading was absent with this blood. Both GP IIb-IIIa and VLA-5 interact with the RGD sequence of fibronectin. Platelet adhesion as well as platelet spreading were inhibited by a RGD peptide (Beumer *et al.*, 1994).

Studies with monoclonal antibodies directed against GP Ib or against the GP Ib-binding domain of von Willebrand Factor indicated that platelet adhesion to fibronectin was supported by a GP Ib-von Willebrand Factor interaction (Beumer *et al.*, 1995b). This was surprising because von Willebrand Factor does not bind to fibronectin. Immune electronmicroscopic studies after platelet adhesion showed that von Willebrand Factor was present beneath adhering platelets and linking platelets to the surface at the edges of the platelets, but no von Willebrand Factor was found bound to fibronectin where no platelets had adhered. This situation is similar as was found with collagen type IV and fibrinogen-fibrin, as described above. Von Willebrand Factor could be derived from plasma or from secretion from the platelet α granules. At present it is not known how von Willebrand Factor does interact with the fibronectin surface in the vicinity of adhering platelets. The possibility of a secreted substance from platelets that links fibronectin and von Willebrand Factor should be borne in mind.

There is an important difference in the role of fibronectin in supporting platelet adhesion to collagen and to subendothelium on the one hand or when fibronectin is coated to a surface on the other hand. In the latter case GP IIb-IIIa and VLA-5 are involved, both of which are RGD dependent integrins. In contrast, RGD peptides have little or no influence on platelet adhesion to subendothelium and collagen (Nievelstein and Sixma, 1988). At shear rates at which fibronectin is required for optimal adhesion, only a limited deficiency in platelet spreading was found in Glanzman's thrombasthenia. These data indicate that GP IIb-IIIa and VLA-5 may not be involved in the fibronectin mediated adhesion of platelets to the vessel wall (Nievelstein and Sixma, 1988).

Studies on reactive sites in fibronectin involved in cell adhesion have shown that the RGD sequence in repeat III-10 is involved in interaction with GP IIb-IIIa or the vitronectin receptor and in interaction with VLA-5. Different adhesive sequence have also been mapped to fibronectin repeat III-9. A stretch of five amino acids pro1376-asn1380 was found to competitively inhibit VLA-5 mediated cell spreading on fibronectin and it could support this cell spreading itself (Aota *et al.*, 1991; Aota *et al.*, 1994). Another sequence asp1373-pro1375 also contains some adhesive activity operating independently from the above mentioned sequence (Aota *et al.*, 1994). Bowditch *et al.*, (1991 and 1994) found that asp1373-thr1383 acted as recognition motif for purified GP IIb-IIIa. This sequence inhibited binding of repeat III-10 to GP IIb-IIIa which suggests that the RGD sequence and this sequence are two mutually exclusive adhesive sites of fibronectin. Adhesive sites were also found in the IIICS and in repeat III-14. These sites are involved in interaction with VLA-4 as integrin receptor which is not present on platelets. We studied the location of reactive sites using proteolytic fragments and recombinant peptides (Beumer *et al.,* 1995a). The essential information for platelet adhesion to surface coated fibronectin was found to be located in the III-10 repeat and the presence of the RGD site was absolutely essential. Essential information for the function of fibronectin in supporting platelet adhesion to endothelial cell matrix was found to be located in type III-9 and RGD-site had little effect. Further studies will be required to locate this domain more precisely and to find a putative receptor that is involved (Nievelstein and Sixma, 1988; Beumer *et al.,* 1995a).

VON WILLEBRAND FACTOR

That von Willebrand Factor might be involved in adhesion was first suggested by morphological studies of bleeding time wounds in patients with von Willebrand's Disease in which platelet aggregates were found to be present in the outflowing blood (Hovig and Stormorken, 1974). There was no hemostatic plug formed in the wound. Definitive proof of the involvement of von Willebrand Factor in adhesion was found when Tschopp *et al.,* demonstrated in perfusion studies that blood platelets from blood of a patient with von Willebrand's Disease did not adhere to subendothelium of rabbit aorta (Tschopp *et al.,* 1974). The role of von Willebrand Factor was subsequently confirmed in studies with monoclonal antibodies and in studies in which purified von Willebrand Factor was added to von Willebrand Factor deficient blood (Weiss *et al.,* 1978; Baumgartner *et al.,* 1980). Studies with radiolabeled von Willebrand Factor showed that von Willebrand Factor bound to the vessel wall and that this binding was correlated with the subsequent platelet adhesion (Sakariassen *et al.,* 1979). Binding was found to precede platelet adhesion (Bolhuis *et al.,* 1981). Studies at relatively high shear showed that von Willebrand Factor was also involved in platelet aggregate formation under flow conditions (Weiss *et al.,* 1989).

Relatively few studies have been performed regarding platelet adhesion to purified von Willebrand Factor coated on a surface (Olson *et al.,* 1989; Danton *et al.,* 1994; Wu *et al.,* 1994). Similar adhesion curves were found with von Willebrand Factor adsorbed to a surface or with spray coated von Willebrand Factor (Wu *et al.,* 1994). Optimal adhesion was found at an adsorption concentration of 10 μg/ml which deposited approximately 60 ng/cm^2 of von Willebrand Factor on the coverslip. Platelet adhesion to von Willebrand Factor showed a fast initial phase in the first minute following with a gradually decrease in adhesion rate over the following four minutes with a linear adhesion time up to 15 minutes. This pattern differed from that seen with fibrinogen-fibrin, collagen type III at low shear rates and collagen type IV which were linear with times, but was similar to that observed with endothelial cell matrix and collagen at high shear rates, both of which are strongly dependent on von Willebrand Factor. Adhesion to von Willebrand Factor was not dependent on the shear rate up to 4000 s^{-1}. There was a rapid increase which was due to increased platelet transport up to a shear rate of 1000 s^{-1} with a much more gradual increase above this value. Platelets adhered to von Willebrand

Factor were present as dendritic and spread platelets at all shear rates. No evidence of aggregate formation was observed.

The role of the multimeric composition of von Willebrand Factor was studied with different fractions of a gel filtration column. A linear decrease in adhesion was found with each subsequent fraction of low molecular weight reaching 50% reduction with the lowest molecular weight fraction. This was in contrast to observations on von Willebrand Factor mediated adhesion to collagen type III. On this surface adhesion only decreased with the last two fractions. The role of the multimeric composition was also studied with recombinant dimeric von Willebrand Factor. Adhesion was about 50% of that observed with native von Willebrand Factor and some decrease in adhesion was observed at shear rates above 1500 s^{-1} (Wu *et al.,* 1994).

Adhesion to surface coated von Willebrand Factor was not dependent on dimeric cations: adhesion in citrated blood was similar to adhesion from blood anticoagulated with hirudin. Heparin by itself caused inhibition of platelet adhesion to von Willebrand Factor. This effect was stronger with unfractionated heparin than with low molecular weight heparin (Wu *et al.,* 1994).

Platelets have two receptors for von Willebrand Factor, GP Ib and GP IIb-IIIa. Adhesion to von Willebrand Factor under static conditions appeared to be mediated by GP IB, although GP IIb-IIIa may be involved in spreading (Savage and Ruggeri, 1991; Savage *et al.,* 1992). Adhesion to von Willebrand Factor coated under flow conditions required both receptors. Adhesion to collagen incubated with von Willebrand Factor had an absolutely requirement for interaction of von Willebrand Factor with GP Ib whereas interaction with GP IIb-IIIa was relatively less important (Lankhof *et al.,* 1995; Wu *et al.,* 1994). The von Willebrand Factor-GPIIb-IIIa interaction was found to be involved in platelet spreading on collagen.

Von Willebrand Factor is a multimeric molecule consisting of a single subunit with a molecular weight of 270 kD. It is present in subendothelium, plasma, and platelet α granules and it is synthesized by endothelial cells and megakaryocytes (Wagner, 1990). A propeptide of 100 kD is cleaved off during synthesis although a small proportion of approximately 1% of plasma von Willebrand Factor still contains this propeptide (Wagner and Marder, 1984). An amino-terminal domain has been recognized for interaction of von Willebrand Factor with factor VIII (Foster *et al.,* 1987) of which von Willebrand Factor is the carrier protein and which it protects against degradation by protein C (Koedam *et al.,* 1988; Fay *et al.,* 1991). The domain interacting with GP Ib is located in the so-called A1 repeat. Collagen binding domains are present in the A1 and A3 repeat of which the A3 repeat is the essential one (Pareti *et al.,* 1986; Roth *et al.,* 1986; Sixma *et al.,* 1991; Lankhof *et al.,* 1994; Dong and Sadler, 1994). A heparin binding domain has been located in the A1 repeat (Sobel *et al.,* 1992) and the sulphatide binding domain is also present in the A1 repeat (Christophe *et al.,* 1991). A special domain is present in von Willebrand Factor involved in binding of von Willebrand Factor to subendothelium (De Groot *et al.,* 1988). Preliminary evidence indicated that this is located in the D4 domain (Vink *et al.,* 1991). Interaction of von Willebrand Factor with GP IIb-IIIa is mediated by the RGD sequence located between amino acids 1744–1747 (Nokes T.J.C. *et al.,* 1984; Beacham *et al.,* 1992; Lankhof *et al.,* 1995). A similar RGD sequence is present in the propeptide but it is not involved in binding to GP IIb-IIIa or the vitronectin receptor (Lankhof *et al.,* 1995). Collagen binding domains have also been recognized in the propeptide but these domains do not play a role in the interaction of multimeric plasma von Willebrand Factor with collagen (Fujisawa *et al.,* 1991; Usui *et al.,* 1992).

Studies under high shear stress in a cone-plate viscometer have shown that the von Willebrand Factor-GP Ib interaction may activate platelets and cause platelet aggregation (Ikeda *et al.,* 1991; Moake *et al.,* 1986; Aleviadou *et al.,* 1993). This platelet activation is associated with calcium influx into the platelets (Kroll *et al.,* 1991; Chow *et al.,* 1992). Studies with surface coated von Willebrand Factor, however, have failed to show aggregate formation at high shear rates. These results would indicate that platelet interaction with von Willebrand Factor present on a surface during adhesion is by itself not sufficient to cause platelet activation, but that von Willebrand Factor is able to do so when it is present on a platelet surface.

THROMBOSPONDIN AND LAMININ AND OTHER ADHESIVE PROTEINS

Platelet Adhesion to Thrombospondin

Thrombospondin can be present in two different forms, a calcium-repleted form and a calcium-depleted form with totally different adhesive functions. Platelets adhere to thrombospondin coated on a glass coverslip both under static and flow conditions. Optimal adhesion is achieved at shear rates of 1600 s^{-1} (Agbanyo *et al.,* 1993) with a rapid drop above this value. Platelets do not adhere to thrombospondin in the calcium-depleted form. Adhesion at low shear rates (300 s^{-1}) was characterised by a lack of platelet spreading. Studies with monoclonal antibodies against glycoprotein IV, glycoprotein Ia-IIa, glycoprotein IIb-IIIa $\alpha III \beta III$ which have been suggested as thrombospondin receptors had no clear-cut inhibitory effect. Further studies to identify the receptive thrombospondin are still required. When fibrinogen, fibronectin, or von Willebrand Factor were pre-coated with calcium-depleted thrombospondin a significant inhibition of platelet adhesion was seen. This inhibition was concentration dependent ranging from 40–70% and occurred both under static and flow conditions. On more thrombogenic surfaces the inhibition of thrombospondin was either donor dependent (on collagen type III) or modest (on fibrillar collagen type I).

Platelet adhesion to laminin and endothelial cell matrix was only inhibited by calcium-depleted thrombospondin under static conditions, but not under flow. Because of a lack of inhibitory antibodies against thrombospondin and because the thrombospondin receptor on platelets has not been identified, it has not yet been possible to delineate the contribution of thrombospondin to the total adhesion to the endothelial cell matrix. The fact that treatment of the endothelial cell matrix with EDTA did not have a pronounced effect on adhesion provided that sufficient calcium ions are present during the actual adhesion studies with flowing blood suggest that thrombospondin may not be an important contributor to the overall adhesion to the endothelial cell matrix or subendothelium. Further studies however are required to substantiate this.

Platelet Adhesion to Laminin

Platelet adhesion to surface coated laminin has been studied under static (Ill *et al.,* 1984) and flow conditions (Hindriks *et al.,* 1992). Here we will concentrate on the flow studies.

Purified laminin was coated for one hour onto glass coverslips by adsorption. Maximal coating was achieved at a concentration of 100 μg/ml of laminin corresponding to an adsorption of 350 ng/cm^2. Optimal adhesion at 5 minutes was seen corresponding to 40% coverage of the surface at this concentration. Platelets adhered in a strongly spread form with an occasional small aggregate. A study of the shear rate dependency showed a maximal adhesion at the shear rate of 1000 s^{-1} with a drop to 50% at 1300 s^{-1} and to 15% at 1800 s^{-1}. Adhesion was strongly affected by magnesium and calcium. The half-maximal effect of magnesium was found at 1 mM, the half-maximal effect of calcium was found at approximately 0.75 mM. This may mean that the plasma concentration of magnesium may affect adhesion to laminin under physiological conditions. The receptor for laminin was studied with use of monoclonal antibodies. GP Ic-IIa (VLA-6, $\alpha6\beta1$) was found to be the essential receptor. No role of VLA-5, VLA-2 or GP IIb-IIIa was found. Studies with deficient plasmas and antibodies showed no role of fibronectin or von Willebrand Factor in the adhesion to laminin. An antibody against the heparin binding E8-domain of laminin blocked adhesion completely. The importance of laminin adhesion to endothelial cell matrix was also studied. Antibodies against VLA-5 had a clear-cut effect at shear rates of 300 s^{-1} inhibiting for 40%, but has less effect at high shear rates.

CD 44/Hyaluronidate

Recently the presence of CD 44 on the platelet membrane has been demonstrated. CD 44 is a well known receptor for hyaluronidate. Some preliminary data suggesting adhesion of platelets to hyaluronidate under static conditions have been obtained (Koshiishi *et al.*, 1994).

Vitronectin

Vitronectin is an adhesive protein that is present in plasma and which may adsorb from plasma to the subendothelium. Studies with activated platelets under static conditions show considerable adhesion to glass coated vitronectin (Collins *et al.*, 1987; Thiagarajan and Kelly, 1988). Adhesion is absent if platelets are not pre-activated or when adhesion is studied from whole blood under flow conditions (HK Nieuwenhuis unpublished results). Vitronectin is involved in platelet aggregation (Asch and Podack, 1990) and interacts with GP IIb-IIIa on the platelet and also with the vitronectin receptor (Thiagarajan and Kelly, 1988; Lam *et al.*, 1989), but the total number of vitronectin receptor molecules is negligible (100–300) in comparison to the about 70.000 GP IIb-IIIa molecules per platelet (Lam *et al.*, 1989; Coller *et al.*, 1991).

COMPARISON OF ADHESION TO SINGLE PROTEINS AND TO THE VESSEL WALL

Studies of adhesion to single surface coated proteins were undertaken in order to better understand the action of every adhesive protein at the molecular level, but also in order to obtain more insight into the contribution of the various proteins to the total process. There is no doubt that the studies have been essential for the first topic. For von Willebrand Factor and fibronectin essential functional domains have been identified and such data are beginning to emerge for other proteins as well. It is important to consider, however, what has been learned about the role of various proteins in the total adhesion process. An important result of the studies is that they have underlines the importance of collagen(s) and von Willebrand Factor and to a lesser extent also fibronectin as adhesive proteins. Laminin and thrombospondin play only a contributory role.

Particularly von Willebrand Factor and its properties clearly dominated the overall adhesion process. Characteristics of adhesion to von Willebrand Factor found back in the total adhesion process are the fast initial adhesion and the resistance to high shear rate. This latter phenomenon was found back in the lack of detachment of platelets adhering to von Willebrand Factor when subjected to shear stress.

The relative importance of von Willebrand Factor was further supported by the finding that adhesion to fibronectin and to fibrinogen/fibrin at high shear rate required von Willebrand Factor for adhesion. This was somewhat unexpected since von Willebrand Factor did not bind to these adhesive proteins. Von Willebrand Factor was found to be located only near the adhesive platelet. The actual mechanism is not known yet but it is of great interest also in view of the fact that adhesion to collagen type IV may have features in common with this, with also low binding of von Willebrand Factor and presence of von Willebrand Factor only near adhering platelets. These studies also confirmed the importance of platelet von Willebrand Factor. Earlier studies in normal volunteers (Rodeghiero *et al.*, 1992) and patients with von Willebrand Disease (Fressinaud *et al.*, 1992) had shown a good correlation between platelet von Willebrand Factor and the bleeding time and our observations may partly explain this.

The studies on single adhesive proteins also point out that the adhesive process in general requires the interaction of the platelet with the adhesive surface via two receptors. Fibrinogen/fibrin at low shear rates and laminin may be exceptions, but these situations have not been studied in sufficient detail yet.

What has also come to light is that it is the adhesive interaction which determines whether there will be platelet thrombus formation. Two surfaces have been found that are able to induce platelet thrombus formation: reactive collagens (type I, III, and IV) and flow-formed fibrin. Both surfaces are characterized by the high local density of binding sites in either fibrils or a surface network (collagen type IV). Not much is known about the activation process of blood platelets under flow. Studies under resting conditions have recently been reviewed (Clark *et al.*, 1994). There is evidence that platelet adhesion under flow may follow different pathways of activation (Polanowska-Grabowska *et al.*, 1993). Whether these pathways are common to all adhesive proteins and only differ quantitatively for collagen and flow-formed fibrin or whether there are essential differences specific for each adhesive surface/receptor pair remains to be investigated.

The study of adhesion to single adhesive proteins has also provided tools to study the contribution of such proteins in various situations. A case in point is the adhesion of blood platelets to atherosclerotic lesions.

PLATELET ADHESION TO ATHEROSCLEROTIC LESIONS

Thrombus formation is closely related to the pathophysiology of atherosclerotic plaques. Advanced lesions often show defects in the endothelial cell lining on top of them which causes local formation of small platelet rich thrombi. There is ample evidence that growth factors released by platelets contribute to the proliferation of smooth muscle cells of the fibrous cap. Thrombus formation is particularly important when an atherosclerotic plaque ruptures and the thrombogenic deeper layer of the vessel wall are exposed to the blood. The ensuing thrombus may occlude the vessel and this may cause tissue ischemia and cell death as is the case in myocardial infarction. The thrombogenicity of the atherosclerotic lesions is partly explained by the tissue factor present in the lipid rich core of the lesion (Wilcox *et al.*, 1989). In order to study the reactivity for platelets, anticoagulated blood was circulated over cryostat frozen cross sections of coronary arteries. In normal vessels increased platelet deposition was found on subendothelium and adventitia. In vessels with atherosclerotic plaque, big platelet thrombi formed on the part of the connective tissue of the atherosclerotic lesion (van Zanten *et al.*, 1994). A immune-histochemical study showed that the area where platelet thrombi formed was rich in collagen type I and III. Using the insights obtained from studies with surface-coated isolated protein, we found that adhesion was indeed mediated by collagen and by von Willebrand Factor adsorbed from plasma. It is unclear why collagen type I and III in part of the lesion show this increased reactivity whereas collagen type I and III in the media and in other parts of the lesion is less reactive. Studies are under way to resolve this.

Conclusions

Platelet adhesion is a complex process in which many adhesive proteins, platelet receptors and perhaps also different activation pathways are involved. Adhesion studies under flow conditions have unravelled many of the different interactions that are involved. These studies have now come to the point that studies at the molecular level are required to precisely understand the nature of the ligand receptor interactions in terms of three-dimensional protein structure. As an offshoot of these studies amino acid sequences may be recognized that may act as competitive inhibitor of platelet adhesion. Peptidomimetics based on the structure of such peptides may have a role as antithrombotic drugs.

Also further studies are needed of the activation pathways involved in platelet activation when platelets adhere under flow. Such studies may provide also new avenues for therapeutic intervention in patients liable to have arterial thrombosis.

References

Agbanyo, F.R., Sixma, J.J., De Groot, P.G., Languino, L.R. and Plow, E.F. (1993). Thrombospondin-platelet interactions. Role of divalent cations, wall shear rate and platelet membrane glycoproteins. *J. Clin. Invest.*, **92**:288–296.

Aleviadou, B.R., Moake, J.L., Turner, N.A., Ruggeri, Z.M., Folie, B.J., Phillips, M.D., Schreiber, A.B., Hrinda, M.E. and McIntire, L.V. (1993). Real-time analysis of shear-dependent thrombus formation and its blockade by inhibitors of von Willebrand factor binding to platelets. *Blood,* **81**:1263–1276.

Aota, S., Nagai, T. and Yamada, K.M. (1991). Characterization of regions of fibronectin besides the arginine-glycine-aspartic acid sequence required for adhesive function of the cell-binding domain using site-directed mutagenesis. *J. Biol. Chem.,* **266**:15938–15943.

Aota, S., Nomizu, M. and Yamada, K.M. (1994). The short amino acid sequence Pro-His-Ser-Arg-Asn in human fibronectin enhances cell-adhesive function. *J. Biol. Chem.,* **269**:24756–24761.

Asch, E. and Podack, E. (1990). Vitronectin binds to activated human platelets and plays a role in platelet aggregation. *JCI,* **85**:1372–1378.

Bastida, E.B., Escolar, G., Ordinas, O. and Sixma, J.J. (1987). Fibronectin is required for platelet adhesion and for thrombus formation on subendothelium and collagen surfaces. *Blood,* **70**:1437–1442.

Baumgartner, H.R. (1973). The role of blood flow in platelet adhesion, fibrin deposition, and formation of mural thrombi. *Microvasc. Res.,* **5**:167–179.

Baumgartner, H.R., Muggli, R., Tschopp, T.B. and Turitto, V.T. (1976). Platelet adhesion, release and aggregation in flowing blood: Effects of surface properties and platelet function. *Thromb. Haemost.*, **35**:124–138.

Baumgartner, H.R., Tschopp, T.B. and Meyer, D. (1980). Shear rate dependent inhibition of platelet adhesion and aggregation on collagenous surfaces by antibodies to human factor VIII/von Willebrand Factor. *Brit. J. Haemat.*, **44**:127–139.

Beacham, D.A., Wise, R.J., Turci, S.M. and Handin, R.I. (1992). Selective inactivation of the Arg-Gly-Asp-Ser (RGDS) binding site in von Willebrand factor by site-directed mutagenesis. *J Biol. Chem.*, **267**:3409–3415.

Beer, J.H., Nieuwenhuis, H.K., Sixma, J.J. and Coller, B.S. (1988). Deficiency of antibody 6F1 binding to the platelets of a patient with an isolated defect in platelet-collagen interaction. *Circulation,* **78**: **suppl II**, 308 (abstract)

Beumer, S., IJsseldijk, M.J.W., De Groot, P.G. and Sixma, J.J. (1994). Platelet adhesion to fibronectin in flow: dependence on surface concentration and shear rate, role of membrane GP IIb/IIIa and VLA-5 and inhibition by heparin. *Blood,* **84**:3724–3733.

Beumer, S., Heijnen, G., IJsseldijk, M.J.W., De Groot, P.G. and Sixma, J.J. (1995a). Fibronectin in an extracellular matrix of cultured endothelial cells supports platelet adhesion via its ninth type III repeat. A comparison with platelet adhesion to isolated fibronectin. *Submitted*

Beumer, S., Heijnen, H.F.G., IJsseldijk, M.J.W., Orlando, E., De Groot, P.G. and Sixma, J.J. (1995b). Platelet adhesion to fibronectin in flow: the importance of von Willebrand Factor and GPIb. *Submitted*

Bolhuis, P.A., Sakariassen, K.S., Sander, H.J., Bouma, B.N. and Sixma, J.J. (1981). Binding of factor VIII-von Willebrand factor to human arterial subendothelium precedes increased platelet adherence and enhances platelet spreading. *J. Lab. Clin. Med.*, **97**:568–576.

Bowditch, R.D., Halloran, C.E., Aota, S., Obara, M., Plow, E.F., Yamada, K.M. and Ginsberg, M.H. (1991). Integrin $\alpha_{IIb}\beta_3$ (platelet GPIIb-IIIa) recognizes multiple sites in fibronectin. *J. Biol. Chem.*, **266**:23323–23328.

Bowditch. R.D., Hariharan. M., Tominna. E.F., Smith. J.W., Yamada. K.M., Getzoff. E.D. and Ginsberg. M.H. (1994) Identification of a novel integrin binding site in fibronectin. Differential utilization by $\beta3$ integrins. *J. Biol. Chem.,* **269**:10856–10663.

Buchanan, M.R., Blut,. R.W., Magaz, R.W., Van Rijn, J., Hirsch, J. and Nazir, D.J. (1985). Endothelial cells produce a lipoxygenase derived chemorepellant which influences platelet/endothelial cell interactions: effect of aspirin and salicylate. *Thromb. Haemostas.*, **53**:306–311.

Chow, T.W., Hellums, J.D., Moake, J.L. and Kroll, M.H. (1992). Shear stress-induced von Willebrand factor binding to platelet glycoprotein Ib initiates calcium influx associated with aggregation. *Blood,* **80**:113–120.

Christophe, O., Obert, B., Meyer, D. and Girma, J. (1991). The binding domain of von Willebrand factor to sulfatides is distinct from those interacting with glycoprotein Ib, heparin, and collagen and resides between residues Leu 512 and Lys 673. *Blood,* **78**:2310–2317.

Clark, E.A., Shattil, S.J. and Brugge, J.S. (1994). Regulation of protein tyrosine kinases in platelets. *Trends Biochem. Sci.*, **19**:464–469.

Coller, B.S., Cheresh, D.A., Asch, E. and Seligsohn, U. (1991). Platelet vitronectin receptor expression differentiates Iraqi-Jewish from Arab patients with Glanzmann thrombasthenia in Israel. *Blood,* **77**:75–83.

Collins, W.E., Mosher, D.F., Tomasini, B.R. and Cooper, S.L. (1987). A preliminary comparison of the thrombogenic activity of vitronectin and other RGD-containing proteins when bound to surfaces. *Ann. New York Acad. Sci.*, **516**:291–299.

D'Alessio, P., Zwaginga, J.J., de Boer, H.C., Federici, A.B., Rodeghiero, F., Castaman, G., Mariani, G., Mannucci, P.M., de Groot, P.G. and Sixma, J.J. (1990). Platelet adhesion to collagen in subtypes of type I von Willebrand's disease is dependent on platelet von Willebrand factor. *Thromb. Haemost.*, **64**:227–231.

Danton, M.C., Zaleski, A., Nichols, W.L. and Olson, J.D. (1994). Monoclonal antibodies to platelet glycoproteins Ib and IIb/IIIa inhibit adhesion of platelets to purified solid-phase von Willebrand factor. *J. Lab. Clin. Med.,* **124**:274–282.

De Groot, P.G., Ottenhof-Rovers, M., Van Mourik, J.A. and Sixma, J.J. (1988). Evidence that the primary binding site of von Willebrand factor that mediates platelet adhesion to subendothelium is not collagen. *J. Clin. Invest.*, **82**:65–73.

Deckmyn, H., Chews, S. L. and Vermylen, J. (1990). Lack of platelet response to collagen associated with an autoantibody against glycoprotein Ia. *Thromb. Haemost.*, **64**:74–79.

Deckmyn, H., Van Houtte, E. and Vermylen, J. (1992). Disturbed platelet aggregation to collagen associated with an antibody against an 85- to 90-Kd platelet glycoprotein in a patient with prolonged bleeding time. *Blood.*, **79**:1466–1471.

Diaz-Ricart, M., Tandon, N.N., Carretero, M., Ordinas, A., Bastida, E. and Jamieson, G.A. (1993). Platelets lacking functional CD36 (Glycoprotein IV) show reduced adhesion to collagen in flowing whole blood. *Blood,* **82**:491–496.

Dixit, V.M., Haverstick, D.M., O'Rourke, K., Hennessy, S.W., Broeklemann, T.J., McDonald, J.A., Grant, G.A., Santoro, S. A. and Frazier, W. A. (1985). Inhibition of platelet aggregation by a monoclonal antibody against human fibronectin. *Proc. Natl. Acad. Sci. USA*, **82**:3844–3848.

Dong, Z. and Sadler, J.E. (1994). Interactions of human von Willebrand Factor type A domains with collagen: heparin and extracellular matrix. *Blood*, **84**: **supplement**, 388a (Abstract)

Elices, M.J. and Hemler, M.E. (1989). The human integrin VLA-2 is a collagen receptor on some cells and a collagen/laminin receptor on others. *Proc. Natl. Acad. Sci. USA*, **86**:9906–9910.

Endenburg, S.C., Hantgan, R.R., Lindeboom-Blokzijl, L., Lankhof, H., Jerome, W.G., Lewis, J.C., Sixma, J.J. and De Groot, P.G. (1995a). On the role of vWF in promoting platelet adhesion to fibrin in flowing blood. *Submitted*

Endenburg, S.C., Lindeboom-Blokzijl, L., Sixma, J.J. and De Groot, P.G. (1995b). Thrombus formation in flowing whole blood on fibrin formed under flow conditions. *Submitted*

Endenburg, S.C., Lindeboom-Blokzijl, L., Zwaginga, J.J., Sixma, J.J. and De Groot, P.G. (1995c). Plasma fibrinogen inhibits platelet adhesion in flowing blood to immobilized fibrinogen. *Submitted*

Farrell, D.H. and Thiagarajan, P. (1994). Binding of recombinant fibrinogen mutants to platelets. *J. Biol. Chem.*, **269**:226–231.

Fay, P.J., Coumans, J.-V. and Walker, F.J. (1991). von Willebrand factor mediates protection of factor VIII from activated protein C-catalyzed inactivation. *J. Biol. Chem.*, **266**:2172–2177.

Foster, P.A., Fulcher, C.A., Marti, T., Titani, K. and Zimmerman, T.S. (1987). A major factor VIII binding domain resides within the amino-terminal 272 amino acid residues of von Willebrand factor. *J. Biol. Chem.*, **262**:8443–8446.

Fressinaud, E., Baruch, D., Rothschild, C., Baumgartner, H.R. and Meye, D. (1987). Platelet von Willebrand factor: evidence for its involvement in platelet adhesion to collagen. *Blood*, **70**:1214–1217.

Fressinaud, E., Sakariassen, K.S., Rothschild, C., Baumgartner, H.R. and Meyer, D. (1992). Shear rate-dependent impairment of thrombus growth on collagen in nonanticoagulated blood from patients with von Willebrand disease and hemophilia A. *Blood*, **80**:988–994.

Fujisawa, T., Takagi, J., Sekiya, F., Goto, A., Miake, F. and Saito, Y. (1991). Monoclonal antibodies that inhibit binding of propolypeptide of von Willebrand factor to collagen–Localization of epitopes. *Eur. J. Biochem.*, **196**:673–677.

Gartner, T.K., Amrani, D.L., Derrick, J.M., Kirschbaum, N.E., Matsueda, G.R. and Taylor, D.B. (1993). Characterization of adhesion of "resting" and stimulated platelets to fibrinogen and its fragments. *Thrombosis Research*, **71**:47–60.

Grinnell, F., Feld, M. and Snell, W. (1979). The influence of cold insoluble globulin on platelet morphological response to substrata. *Cell Biol. Intern. Rep.*, **3**:585–592.

Hantgan, R.R., Hindriks, G., Taylor, R., Sixma, J.J. and De Groot, P.G. (1990). Glycoprotein Ib, von Willebrand Factor, and glycoprotein IIb:IIIa are all involved in platelet adhesion to fibrin in flowing whole blood. *Blood*, **76**:345–353.

Hantgan, R.R., Endenburg, S.C., Cavero, I., Marguerie, G., Uzan, A., Sixma, J.J. and De Groot. P.G. (1992). Inhibition of platelet adhesion tofibrin(ogen) in flowing whole blood by Arg-Gly-Asp and fibrinogen gamma-chain carboxy-terminal peptides. *Thromb. Haemostasis*, **68**:694–700.

Hantgan, R.R., Francis, C.W. and Marder, V.J. (1994). Fibrinogen structure and physiology. In *Hemostasis and Thrombosis: Basic Principles and Clinical Practice* (Edited by Colman R.W., Hirsh J., Marder V.J. and Salzman E. W.), p. 277. JB Lippincott, Philadelphia.

Hantgan, R.R., Endenburg, S.C., Sixma, J.J. and De Groot, P.G. (1995). Evidence that fibrin α-chain RGDX sequences are not required for platelet adhesion in flowing blood. *Blood* in press

Hemler, M.E. (1990). VLA proteins in the integrin family: Structures, functions, and their role on leukocytes. *Annu. Rev. Immunol.*, **8**:365–400.

Hindriks, G.A., IJsseldijk, M.J.W., Sonnenberg, A., Sixma, J.J. and De Groot, P.G. (1992). Platelet adhesion to laminin: role of Ca^{2+} and Mg^{2+} ions, shear rate, and platelet membrane glycoproteins. *Blood*, **79**:928–935.

Houdijk, W.P.M., Sakariassen, K.S., Nievelstein, P.F.E.M. and Sixma, J.J. (1985). Role of factor VIII-von Willebrand factor and fibronectin in the interaction of platelets in flowing blood with monomeric and fibrillar collagen types I and III. *J. Clin. Invest.*, **75**:531–540.

Houdijk, W.P.M., De Groot, P.G., Nievelstein, P.F.E.M., Sakariassen, K.S. and Sixma, J.J. (1986). Subendothelial proteins and platelet adhesion: von Willebrand factor and fibronectin, not thrombospondin, are involved in platelet adhesion to extracellular matrix of human vascular endothelial cells. *Arteriosclerosis*, **6**:24–33.

Houdijk, W.P.M. and Sixma, J.J. (1985). Fibronectin in artery subendothelium is important for platelet adhesion. *Blood*, **65**:598–604.

Hovig, T. (1963). Release of a platelet aggregating substance (adenosine diphosphate) from rabbit blood platelets induced by saline extract of tendons. *Thromb. Diath. Haemorrh.*, **9**:264–278.

Hovig, T., Dodds, W.J., Rowsell, H.C., Joergensen, L. and Mustard, J.F. (1967). Experimental hemostasis in normal dogs and dogs with congenital disorders of blood coagulation. *Blood*, **40**:636–668.

Hovig, T. and Stormorken, H. (1974). Ultrastructural studies on the platelet plug formation in bleeding time wounds from normal individuals and patients with von Willebrand's disease. *Acta Pathol. Microbiol. Scand.*, **Suppl 248**:105–122.

Hynes, R.O. (1990). *Fibronectins*. Springer-Verlag, New York.

Hynes, R.O. (1992), Integrins: versatility, modulation, and signaling in cell adhesion. *Cell*, **69**:11–25.

Ikeda, Y., Handa, M., Kawano, K., Kamata,T., Murata, M., Araki, Y., Anbo, H., Kawai, Y., Watanabe, K., Itagaki, I., Sakai, K. and Ruggeri, Z. M. (1991). The role of von Willebrand Factor and fibrinogen in platelet aggregation under varying shear stress. *J. Clin. Invest.*, **87**:1234–1240.

Ill C.R., Engvall, E. and Ruohslahti, E. (1984). Adhesion of platelets to laminin in the absence of activation. *J. Cell Biol.*, **99**:2140–2145.

Kehrel, B., Balleisen, L., Kokott, R., Mester, R., Stenzinger, W., Clemetson, K.J. and van de Loo, J. (1988). Deficiency of intact thrombospondin and membrane glycoprotein Ia in platelets with defective collagen-induced aggregation and spontaneous loss of disorder. *Blood,* **71**:1074–1078.

Kehrel, B., Kronenberg, A., Rauterberg, J., Niesing-Bresch, D., Niehues, U., Kardoeus, J., Schwippert, B., Tschöpe, D., van de Loo, J. and Clemetson, K. J. (1993). Platelets deficient in glycoprotein IIIb aggregate normally to collagens type I and III but not to collagen type V. *Blood,* **82**:3364–3370.

Keller, P.M., Waxman, L., Arnold, B.A., Schultz, L.D., Condra, C. and Connolly, T.M. (1993). Cloning of the cDNA and expression of moubatin, an inhibitor of platelet aggregation. *J. Biol. Chem.,* **268**:5450–5456.

Kieffer, N., Fitzgerald, L.A., Wolf, D., Cheresh, D.A. and Phillips, D.R. (1991). Adhesive properties of the β_3 integrins: Comparison of GP IIb-IIIa and the vitronectin receptor individually expressed in human melanoma cells. *J. Cell Biol.,* **113**:451–461.

Koedam, J.A., Meijers, J.C.M., Sixma, J.J. and Bouma, B.N. (1988). Inactivation of human factor VIII by activated protein C. Cofactor activity of protein S and protective effect of von Willebrand factor. *J. Clin. Invest.,* **82**:1236–1243.

Koshiishi, I., Shizari, M. and Underhill, C.B. (1994). CD44 can mediate the adhesion of platelets to hyaluronan. *Blood,* **84**:390–396.

Koteliansky, V.E., Leytin, V.L., Sviridov, D.D., Repin, V.S. and Smirnov, V.N. (1981). Human plasma fibronectin promotes the adhesion and spreading of platelets on surfaces coated with collagen. *FEBS-letters,* **123**:59–62.

Kotite, N.J. and Cunningham, L.W. (1986). Specific adsorption of a platelet membrane glycoprotein by human insoluble collagen. *J. Biol. Chem.,* **261**:8342–8347.

Kroll, M.H., Harris, T.S., Moake, J.L., Handin, R.I. and Schafer, A.I. (1991). von Willebrand factor binding to platelet GpIb initiates signals for platelet activation. *J. Clin. Invest.,* **88**:1568–1573.

Kunicki, T.J., Orchekowski, R., Annis, D. and Honda, Y. (1993). Variability of integrin $\alpha 2\beta 1$ activity on human platelets. *Blood,* **82**:2693–2703.

Lam, S.C.-T., Plow, E.F., D'Souza, S.E., Cheresh, D.A., Frelinger, A.L., III and Ginsberg, M.H. (1989). Isolation and characterization of a platelet membrane protein related to the vitronectin receptor. *J. Biol. Chem.,* **264**:3742–3749.

Landolfi, R., De Cristofaro, R., De Candia, E., Rocca, B. and Bizzi, B. (1991). Effect of fibrinogen concentration on the velocity of platelet aggregation. *Blood,* **78**:377–381.

Lankhof, H., Schiphorst, M.E., Vink, T. and Sixma, J.J. (1994). Interaction of the A3 fragment of von Willebrand factor with collagen type III. *Brit. J. Haematol.,* **87**:79(Abstract)

Lankhof, H., Wu, Y.P., Vink, T., Schiphorst, M.E., Zerwes, H., De Groot, P.G. and Sixma, J.J. (1995). Role of the A1 domain and RGD-sequence in platelet adhesion to von Willebrand factor. *Blood,* **in press**

Lindon, J.N., Kushner, L. and Salzman, E.W. (1989). Platelet interaction with artificial surfaces: *In vitro* evaluation. *Methods Enzymol.,* **169**:104–116.

Liu, C.Z., Yang, S.H. and Huang, T.F. (1994). Action mechanism of a platelet aggregation inducer purified from calloselasma rhodostoma venom. *Thromb. Haemost.,* **69**:903(Abstract)

Moake, J.L., Turner, N.A., Stathopoulos, N.A., Nolasco, L.H. and Hellums, J.D. (1986). Involvement of large plasma von Willebrand Factor (vWF) multimers and unusually large vWF forms derived from endothelial cells in shear stress-induced platelet aggregation. *J. Clin. Invest.,* **78**:1456–1461.

Moroi, M., Jung, S.M., Okuma, M. and Shinmyozu, K. (1989). A patient with platelets deficient in glycoprotein VI that lack both collagen induced aggregation and adhesion. *J. Clin. Invest.,* **84**:1440

Morton, L.F., Griffin, B., Pepper, D.S. and Barnes, M.J. (1983). The interaction between collagens and factor VIII/von Willebrand factor: investigation of the structural requirements for interaction. *Thromb. Res.,* **32**:545–556.

Morton, L.F., Peachey, A.R., Zijenah, L.S., Goodall, A.H., Humphries, M.J. and Barnes, M.J. (1994). Conformation-dependent platelet adhesion to collagen involving integrin $\alpha 2\beta 1$-mediated and other mechanisms: Multiple $\alpha 2\beta 1$-recognition sites in collagen type I. *Biochem. J.,* **299**:791–797.

Morton, L.F., Hargreaves, P.G., Farndale, R.W., Young, R.D. and Barnes, M.J. (1995). Integrin α2β1-independent activation of platelets by simple collagen-like peptides: collagen tertiary (triple-helical) and quarternary (polymeric) structures are sufficient alone for α2β1-independent platelet reactivity. *Biochem. J.,* **in press**

Muggli, R., Baumgartner, H.R., Tschopp, T.B. and Keller, H. (1980). Automated microdensitometry and protein assay as a measure for platelet adhesion and aggregation on collagen-coated slides under controlled flow conditions. *J. Lab. Clin. Med.,* **95**:195–207.

Nieuwenhuis, H.K., Akkerman, J.W.N., Houdijk, W.P.M. and Sixma, J.J. (1985). Human blood platelets showing no response to collagen fail to express surface glycoprotein Ia. *Nature,* **318**:470–472.

Nieuwenhuis, H.K., Sakariassen, K.S., Houdijk, W.P.M., Nievelstein, P.F.E.M. and Sixma, J.J. (1986). Deficiency of platelet membrane glycoprotein Ia associated with a decreased platelet adhesion to subendothelium: a defect in platelet spreading. *Blood,* **68**:692–695.

Nievelstein, P.F.E.M., D'Alessio, P.A. and Sixma, J.J. (1988). Fibronectin in platelet adhesion to human collagen types I and III: Use of nonfibrillar and fibrillar collagen in flowing blood studies. *Arteriosclerosis,* **8**:200–206.

Nievelstein, P.F.E.M., D'Alessio, P.A. and Sixma, J.J. (1988). Fibronectin in platelet adhesion to human collagen types I and III. Use of nonfibrillar and fibrillar collagen in flowing blood studies. *Arteriosclerosis,* **8**:200–206.

Nievelstein, P.F.E.M. and Sixma, J.J. (1988). Glycoprotein IIB-IIIa and RGD(S) are not important for fibronectin-dependent platelet adhesion under flow conditions. *Blood,* **72**:82–88.

Noeske-Jungblut, C., Krätzschmar, J., Haendler, B., Alagon, A., Possani, L., Verhalle,n P., Donner, P. and Schleuning, W.-D. (1994). An inhibitor of collagen-induced platelet aggregation from the saliva of Triatoma pallidipennis. *J. Biol. Chem.,* **269**:5050–5053.

Nokes, T.J.C., Mahmoud, N.A., Savidge, G.F., Goodall, A.H., Meyer, D., Edgington, T.S. and Hardisty, R.M. (1984). Von Willebrand factor has more than one binding site for platelets. *Thromb. Res.,* **34**:361–366.

Olson, J.D., Zaleski, A., Herrmann, D. and Flood, P.A. (1989). Adhesion of platelets to purified solid-phase von Willebrand factor: Effects of wall shear rate, ADP, thrombin, and ristocetin. *J. Lab.Clin. Med.* **114**:6–18.

Pareti, F.I., Fujimura, Y., Dent, J.A., Holland, L.Z., Zimmerman, T.S. and Ruggeri, Z.M. (1986). Isolation and characterization of a collagen binding site in human von Willebrand factor. *J. Biol. Chem.,* **261**: 15310–15315.

Parsons, I.J., Haycraft, D.L., Hoak, J.C. and Sage, H. (1986). Interaction of platelets and purified collagens in a laminar flow model. *Thromb. Res.,* **43**:435–443.

Peerschke, E.I.B. and Ghebrehiwet, B. (1990a). Platelet C1Q receptor interactions with collagen- and C1Q-coated surfaces. *J. Immunol.,* **145**:2984–2988.

Peerschke, E.I.B. and Ghebrehiwet, B. (1990b). Modulation of platelet responses to collagen by C1q receptors. *J. Immunol.,* **144**:221–225.

Piotrowicz, R.S., Orchekowski, R.P., Nugent, D.J., Yamada, K.Y. and Kunicki, T.J. (1988). Glycoprotein Ic-IIa functions as an activation independent fibronectin receptor on human platelets. *J. Cell Biol.,* **106**:1359–1364.

Plow, E.F., Srouji, A.H., Meyer, D., Marguerie, G. and Ginsberg, M.H. (1984). Evidence that three adhesive proteins interact with a common recognition site on activated platelets. *J. Biol. Chem.,* **259**:5388

Plow, E.F., McEver, R.P., Coller, B.S., Woods, V.L., Marguerie, G.A. and Ginsberg, M.H. (1985). Related binding mechanisms for fibrinogen, fibronectin, von Willebrand Factor and thrombospondin on thrombin-stimulated platelets. *Blood,* **66**:724–727.

Polanowska-Grabowska, R., Geanacopoulos, M. and Gear, A.R.L. (1993). Platelet adhesion to collagen via the α2β1 integrin under arterial flow conditions causes rapid tyrosine phosphorylation of pp. 125[FAK]. *Biochem J.,* **296**:543–547.

Rand, J.H., Patel, N.D., Schwartz, E., Zhou, S.-L. and Potter, B.J. (1991). 150-kD von Willebrand factor binding protein extracted from human vascular subendothelium is type VI collagen. *J. Clin. Invest.,* **88**:253–259.

Rand, J.H., Wu, X.-X., Potter, B.J., Uson, R.R. and Gordon, R.E. (1993). Co-localization of von Willebrand factor and type VI collagen in human vascular subendothelium. *Am. J. Pathol.,* **142**:843–850.

Rodeghiero, F., Castaman, G., Ruggeri, M. and Tosetto, A. (1992). The bleeding time in normal subjects is mainly determined by platelet von Willebrand factor and is independent from blood group. *Thrombosis Research,* **65**:605–615.

Roth, G.J., Titani, K., Hoyer, L.W. and Hickey, M.J. (1986). Localization of binding sites within human von Willebrand factor for monomeric type III collagen. *Biochemistry,* **25**:8357–8361.

Roth, G.J. (1991). Developing relationships: Arterial platelet adhesion, glycoprotein Ib, and leucine-rich glycoproteins. *Blood,* **77**:5–19.

Saelman, E.U.M., Horton, L.F., Barnes, M.J., Gralnick, H.R., Hese, K.M., Nieuwenhuis, H K., de Groot, P.G. and Sixma, J.J. (1993a). Platelet adhesion to cyanogen-bromide fragments of collagen α1(I) under flow conditions. *Blood,* **82**:3029–3033.

Saelman, E.U.M., Kehrel, B., Hese, K.M., De Groot, P.G., Sixma, J.J. and Nieuwenhuis, H.K. (1993b). Platelet adhesion to collagen and endothelial cell matrix under flow conditions is not dependent on platelet glycoprotein IV. *Blood,* **in press**.

Saelman, E.U.M., Nieuwenhuis, H.K., Hese, K.M., de Groot, P.G., Heijnen, H.F.G., Sage, E.H., Williams, S., McKeown, L., Gralnick, H.R. and Sixma, J.J. (1994). Platelet adhesion to collagen types I through VIII under conditions of stasis and flow is mediated by GPIa/IIa ($\alpha_2\beta_1$-integrin). *Blood,* **83**:1244–1250.

Sakariassen, K.S., Bolhuis, P.A. and Sixma, J.J. (1979). Human blood platelet adhesion to artery subendothelium is mediated by factor VIII-von Willebrand factor bound to the subendothelium. *Nature,* **279**:635–638.

Sakariassen, K.S., Joss, R., Muggli, R., Kuhn, H., Tschopp, T.B., Sage, H. and Baumgartner, H.R. (1990). Collagen type III induced *ex vivo* thrombogenesis in humans. Role of platelets and leukocytes in deposition of fibrin. *Arteriosclerosis,* **10**:276–284.

Savage, B., Shattil, S.J. and Ruggeri, Z.M. (1992). Modulation of platelet function through adhesion receptors. A dual role for glycoprotein IIb-IIIa (integrin αIIbβ3) mediated by fibrinogen and glycoprotein Ib-von Willebrand factor. *J. Biol. Chem.,* **267**:11300–11306.

Savage, B. and Ruggeri, Z.M. (1991). Selective recognition of adhesive sites in surface-bound fibrinogen by glycoprotein IIb-IIIa on nonactivated platelets. *J. Biol. Chem.,* **266**:11227–11233.

Shiba, E., Lindon, J.N., Kushner, L., Matsueda, G.R., Hawiger, J., Kloczewiak, M., Kudryk, B. and Salzman, E.W. (1991). Antibody-detectable changes in fibrinogen adsorption affecting platelet activation on polymer surfaces. *Am. J. Physiol. Cell Physiol.,* **260**:C965–C974.

Sixma, J.J., Schiphorst, M.E., Verweij, C.L. and Pannekoek, H. (1991). Effect of deletion of the A1 domain of von Willebrand factor on its binding to heparin, collagen and platelets in the presence of ristocetin. *Eur. J. Biochem.,* **196**:369–375.

Sixma, J.J. (1994). Interaction of blood platelets with the vessel wall. In *Haemostasis and Thrombosis* (Edited by Bloom A.L., Forbes C.D., Thomas D.P. and Tuddenham E.G.D.), p. 259. Churchill Livingstone, Edinburgh.

Sixma, J.J., van Zanten, G.H., Banga, J.D., Nieuwenhuis, H.K. and De Groot, P.G. (1995). Platelet Adhesion. *Semin. Haemat.,* **32**:1–6.

Sixma, J.J. and De Groot, P.G. (1990). Platelet Adhesion. *Brit. J. Haemat.,* **75**:308–312.

Sixma, J.J. and De Groot, P.G. (1994). Regulation of platelet adhesion to the vessel wall. *Ann. New York Acad. Sci.,* **714**:190–199.

Sobel, M., Soler, D.F., Kermode, J.C. and Harris, R.B. (1992). Localization and characterization of a heparin binding domain peptide of human von Willebrand Factor. *J. Biol. Chem.,* **267**:8857–8862.

Staatz, W.D., Rajpara, S.M., Wayner, E.A., Carter, W.G. and Santoro, S.A. (1989). The membrane glycoprotein Ia-IIa (VLA-2) complex mediates the Mg^{++}-dependent adhesion of platelets to collagen. *J. Cell Biol.,* **108**:1917–1924.

Staatz, W.D., Walsh, J.J., Pexton, J. and Santoro, S.A. (1990). The $\alpha_2\beta_1$ integrin cell surface collagen receptor binds to the α1(I)-CB3 peptide of collagen. *J. Biol. Chem.,* **265**:4778–4781.

Staatz, W.D., Fok, K.F., Zutter, M.M., Adams, S.P., Rodriguez, B.A. and Santoro, S.A. (1991). Identification of a tetrapeptide recognition sequence for the $\alpha_2\beta_1$ integrin in collagen. *J. Biol. Chem.,* **266**:7363–7367.

Takada, Y. and Hemler, M.E. (1989). The primary structure of the VLA-2/collagen receptor α_2 subunit (platelet GPIa): homology to other integrins and the presence of a possible collagen-binding domain. *J. Cell Biol.,* **109**:397–407.

Tandon, N.N., Kralisz, U. and Jamieson, G.A. (1989). Identification of glycoprotein IV (CD36) as a primary receptor for platelet-collagen adhesion. *J. Biol. Chem.,* **264**:7576–7583.

Tandon, N.N., Ockenhouse, C.F., Greco, J. and Jamieson, G.A. (1991). Adhesive functions of platelets lacking glycoprotein IV (CD36). *Blood,* **78**:2809–2813.

Thiagarajan, P. and Kelly, K. (1988). Interaction of thrombin-stimulated platelets with vitronectin (S-protein of complement) substrate: Inhibition by a monoclonal antibody to glycoprotein IIb-IIIa complex. *Thromb. Hemostas.* **60**:514–517.

Thiagarajan, P. and Kelly, K.L. (1988). Exposure of binding sites for vitronectin on platelets following stimulation. *J. Biol Chem.,* **263**:3035–3038.

Tschopp T.B., Weiss H.J. and Baumgartner H.R. (1974) Decreased adhesion of platelets to subendothelium in von Willebrand's disease. *J. Lab. Clin. Med.,* **83**: 296–300.

Turitto, V.T. and Baumgartner, H.R. (1974). Effect of physical factors on platelet adhesion to subendothelium. *Thromb. Diath. Haemorrh.,* **Suppl. 60**:17–24.

Usui, T., Fujisawa, T., Takagi, J. and Saito, Y. (1992). Propolypeptide and mature portions of von Willebrand factor of bovine origin recognize different sites on type-I collagen obtained from bovine tendon. *Eur. J. Biochem.,* **205**:363–367.

van Zanten, G.H., De Graaf, S., Slootweg, P.J., Heijnen, H.F.G., Connolly, T.M., de Groot, P.G. and Sixma, J.J. (1994). Increased platelet deposition on atherosclerotic coronary arteries. *J. Clin. Invest.,* **93**:615–632.

van Zanten, G.H., Connolly, T.M., Schiphorst, M.E., De Graaf, S., Slootweg, P.J. and Sixma, J.J. (1995a). Recombinant leech anti platelet protein specifically blocks platelet deposition on collagen surfaces under flow conditions. *Submitted* van Zanten, G.H., Saelman, E.U.M., Schut-Heese, K.M., Wu, Y.P., Slootweg, P.J., Nieuwenhuis, H.K., De Groot, P. G. and Sixma, J. J. (1995b) Platelet adhesion to collagen type IV under flow conditions. *Submitted*

Vink, T., Kanters, D., Schiphorst, M., Van Mourik, J.A., De Groot, P.G. and Sixma, J.J. (1991) Localization of the epitope of a monoclonal antibody, which inhibits the binding of von Willebrand Factor (VWF) to subendothelium. *Thromb. Haemost.*, **65**: 798(Abstract)

Wagner, D.D. (1990) Cell biology of von Willebrand factor. *Annu. Rev. Cell Biol.*, **6**: 217–246.

Wagner, D.D. and Marder, V.J. (1984) Biosynthesis of von Willebrand protein in endothelial cells, processing steps and their intracellular localization. *J. Cell Biol.*, **99**: 2123–2130.

Weiss, H.J., Baumgartner, H.R., Tschopp, T.B., Turitto, V.T. and Cohen, D. (1978) Correction by factor VIII of the impaired platelet adhesion to subendothelium in von Willebrand's disease. *Blood*, **51**: 267–279.

Weiss, H.J., Hawiger, J., Ruggeri, Z.M., Turitto, V.T., Thiagarajan, R. and Hoffmann, T. (1989) Fibrinogen independent adhesion and thrombus formation on subendothelium mediated by GPIIb-IIIa complex at high shear rate. *J. Clin. Invest.*, **83**: 288–297.

Wilcox, J.N., Smith, K.M., Schwartz, S.M. and Gordon, D. (1989) Localization of tissue factor in the normal vessel wall and in the atherosclerotic plaque. *Proc. Natl. Acad. Sci. USA*, **86**: 2839–2843.

Wu, Y.P., van Breuge, H.F.I., Lankhof, H., Wise, R.J., Handin, R.I., de Groot, P.G. and Sixma, J.J. (1994) Platelet adhesion and von Willebrand Factor. Platelet adhesion to multimeric and dimeric von Willebrand factor and to Collagen type III preincubated with von Willebrand Factor. *Submitted*.

Yamamoto, N., Ikeda, H., Tandon, N.N., Herman, J., Tomiyama, Y., Mitani, T., Sekiguchi, S., Lipsky, R., Kralisz, U. and Jamieson, G. A. (1990) A platelet membrane glycoprotein (GP) deficiency in healthy blood donors: Nak^a- platelets lack detectable GPIV (CD36). *Blood,* **76**: 1698–1703.

Zijenah, L.S., Morton, L.F. and Barnes, M.J. (1990) Platelet adhesion to collagen. Factors affecting Mg^{2+}-dependent and bivalent-cation-independent adhesion. *Biochem. J.,* **268**: 481–486.

Zijenah, L.S. and Barnes, M.J. (1990) Platelet-reactive sites in human collagens I and III: Evidence for cell-recognition sites in collagen unrelated to RGD and like sequences. *Thromb. Res.*, **59**: 553–566.

Zutter, M.M. and Santoro, S.A. (1990) Widespread histologic distribution of the $\alpha_2\beta_1$ integrin cell-surface collagen receptor. *Am. J. Pathol.*, **137**: 113–120.

9 Vitronectin as Link between Protease Cascades and Cell Adhesion in Hemostasis

Klaus T. Preissner

Hemostasis Research Unit, Kerckhoff Klinik, Max-Planck-Institut, D-61231 Bad Nauheim, Germany

Abbreviations used: PAI-1, plasminogen activator inhibitor-1; SERPIN, serine protease inhibitor; tPA, tissue-type plasminogen activator

KEYWORDS: Cell adhesion, pericellular proteolysis, vitronectin, PAI-1, thrombin-SERPIN complexes

INTRODUCTION

The biological concept of protease cascades in the haemostasis and immune systems is essential for the fast, selective and localized operation of humoral defense in the organism and its control in the vascular system. An optimal response towards a given stimulus such as vascular injury or bacterial infection is achieved by specialized enzymatic functions of the contact, blood coagulation, fibrinolysis, and complement systems as well as by matrix metalloproteinases. As opposed to the conventional endopeptidases of the digestive tract, enzymes of the haemostatic cascade systems contain a large non-catalytic region with specific regulatory modules such as the epidermal growth factor precursor-domain, the finger and kringle domains or the hemopexin-like repeats of matrix metallo-proteinases, respectively. These elements allow interaction with specific cell surface receptors, with extracellular matrix and fibrin binding sites for proper juxtaposition towards macromolecular substrates or for the assembly of typical multicomponent enzyme complexes on negatively charged phospholipid surfaces (Rosing *et al.*, 1980). Finally, most proteolytic enzymes become inactivated through direct (covalent) linkage to protease inhibitors including serine protease inhibitors (SERPINs) and α_2-macroglobulin, and subsequent clearance is thereby initiated. Most of these inhibition reactions are modulated by exogeneous heparinoids and endogeneous heparin-like cell surface components of the endothelium, by basic proteins from platelet releasate or by components of the extracellular matrix (Preissner, 1990b).

At various stages of control in the protease cascade systems the multifunctional adhesive glycoprotein vitronectin appears to constitute a common factor for different

169

functions: Vitronectin is a major inhibitor of the terminal phase of the complement cascade and due to its heparin binding properties it may affect the kinetics of SERPIN-mediated reactions *in vivo*. Moreover, vitronectin is considered to be the major scavenger for thrombin-SERPIN complexes in the circulation, and may become translocated into the vessel wall where it serves adhesive functions and control of pericullar proteolysis through stabilization of SERPINs, in particular plasminogen activator inhibitor (PAI-1). Recent work also suggests a role for the adhesive protein in directing urokinase-receptor related processes. In the following, these properties of vitronectin as well as the functional consequences for the vascular regulation of hemostasis are discussed indicating that vitronectin can be considered as the molecular link between intra- and extravascular protease cascade systems.

STRUCTURE AND FUNCTION OF VITRONECTIN

Vitronectin belongs to the group of multifunctional adhesive glycoproteins which include fibronectin, fibrinogen and von Willebrand factor that all are present both in the blood plasma and found immobilized with extracellular matrix sites. Liver cells predominantly synthesize vitronectin (Barnes and Reing, 1985) which undergoes post-translational modification (including N-glycosylation, sulfation and possibly phosphorylation) but no alternative splicing mechanisms during processing (Jenne and Stanley, 1987). Although vitronectin mRNA is found in other organs in the mouse (Seiffert *et al.*, 1991), only a few non-hepatic cell types and transformed cell lines (Yasumitsu *et al.*, 1993) express vitronectin. Several histochemical studies have described the association of vitronectin at sites distant from actual biosynthesis with dermal elastic fibers in skin (Dahlbäck *et al.*, 1986) as well as with renal tissue (Falk *et al.*, 1987) and the media of the vascular wall (Niculescu *et al.*, 1987; Reilly and Nash, 1988; Guettier *et al.*, 1989). The accumulation at sites of fibrosis and necrosis and co-localization with the terminal complement complex in diseases such as glomerulonephritis (Falk *et al.*, 1987; Bariety *et al.*, 1989) and arteriosclerosis (Niculescu *et al.*, 1987; Guettier *et al.*, 1989; Sato *et al.*, 1990) suggests a role for vitronectin in preventing tissue damage in proximity to local complement activation. The mechanism of deposition of exogenous vitronectin alone or in association with other proteins *in vivo* remains unclear at present. The binding of vitronectin to glycosamino glycans/proteoglycans (Lane *et al.*, 1987) or to different types of native collagens (Gebb *et al.*, 1986) as well as crosslinking of vitronectin by transglutaminase/factor XIIIa (Sane *et al.*, 1988) are reactions that are likely to occur in order to stabilize interactions with the extracellular matrix.

The primary structures of human, rabbit and mouse vitronectins have been reported (Suzuki *et al.*, 1985; Jenne and Stanley, 1985; Sato *et al.*, 1990; Seiffert *et al.*, 1991) indicating more than 80% sequence homology within the mature proteins (Ehrlich *et al.*, 1993) derived from eight exons transcripts. Moreover, the amino-terminal portion encoded by exon 2 (Jenne and Stanley, 1987) shows appreciable homology with domains in other factors including "plasma cell protein 1", "megakaryocyte stimulating factor" or "placental protein 11" (Merberg *et al.*, 1993) which all contain four disulfide bridges at conserved positions. Except for this "somatomedin B" domain, the exon/intron organization of the human and mouse vitronectin gene (Jenne and Stanley, 1987; Seiffert *et al.*,

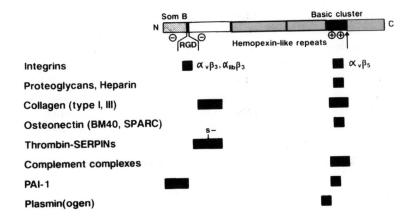

Figure 9.1 **Vitronectin structure and ligand binding domains. A** schematic representation of the domain organization of vitronectin is depicted showing the "somatomedin B" domain (Som B), the cell attachment site (RGD), hemopexin-like repeats and the heparin-binding site (basic cluster). The arrow indicates the position of an endogenous protease cleavage site which is adjacent to the protein kinase A-dependent phosphorylation site. Binding sites in vitronectin for macromolecular ligands (listed at the left margin) are highlighted by filled bars according to their position within the molecule. Note that these binding domains are concentrated around the acidic (– –) amino-terminus and the basic (++) carboxy-terminus.

1993) does not imply a typical mosaic arrangement of functional domains (Figure 9.1). Distant sequence homology between carboxy-terminal portions of vitronectin exist with the heme-binding plasma protein hemopexin (Jenne and Stanley, 1987) whose ligand-binding properties strongly depend on conformational flexibility (Smith *et al.*, 1988). Although the "hemopexin-type" protein family also includes matrix-metalloproteinases, their possible functional relation to vitronectin remains to be analyzed.

The predominant form of vitronectin in plasma (more than 98%) (Izumi *et al.*, 1989) appears to exist as an internally folded molecule that is stabilized by hetero-polar interactions between complementary charged regions (Preissner and Müller-Berghaus, 1987; Jenne *et al.*, 1989) and can undergo a transition into an "extended" form. This concept is supported by electron-microscopical analysis (Stockmann *et al.*, 1993), hydrodynamic data (Bittorf *et al.*, 1993) and ligand binding properties (Tomasini and Mosher, 1990; Preissner, 1991). The transition process which is central to the interaction of vitronectin with other proteins may be provoked by physiological ligands such as the thrombin-antithrombin III or the complement C5b-7 complex, or artificially by surface coating or with denaturants. Concomitant to unfolding, previously cryptic binding sites such as for heparin or protein ligands become exposed indicating that heparin binding forms of vitronectin are endowed with altered reactive properties.

Studies with conformational-type monoclonal antibodies that do not react with internally folded circulating plasma vitronectin but recognize different altered molecular isoforms including multimers, aggregates or ternary complexes (Tomasini and Mosher, 1988) indicated that platelet releasate as well as vessel wall extracellular matrix appears to be enriched in these forms of vitronectin (Stockmann *et al.*, 1993). In a number of histochemical studies and experiments with vitronectin receptor (integrin $\alpha V\beta 3$) bearing cells, the role of vitronectin in cell adhesion and migration particularly of non-differentiated cells during tumor metastasis (Felding-Habermann *et al.*, 1992) and angiogenesis has been suggested (Brooks *et al.*, 1994). Endothelial cell adhesion is promoted both by an integrin- and a proteoglycan-dependent mechanism (Preissner *et al.*, 1988) (H. de Boer *et al.*, unpublished observations), and the participation of vitronectin/αvβ3 in phagocytosis (Parker *et al.*, 1988) and apoptotic mechanisms (Savill *et al.*, 1990) has been proposed.

The localization of binding sites for macromolecular ligands as well as reactive sites for e.g. transglutaminase-mediated crosslinking (Skoorstengaard *et al.*, 1990) or protein kinase A-dependent phosphorylation (Korc-Grodzicki *et al.*, 1988) are concentrated around the acidic amino-terminal region and within or adjacent to the basic cluster at the carboxy-terminus, respectively (Figure 9.1). The characterization of interactions with PAI-1, thrombin-SERPIN complexes, integrins, collagen(s), heparinoids, complement components, perforin and plasminogen was established mostly by *in vitro* binding experiments and emphasizes the multifunctional role of this adhesive protein in defense mechanisms such as hemostasis and complement.

TERNARY VITRONECTIN COMPLEXES AND THEIR METABOLISM

Glycosaminoglycan Binding Proteins

Within the blood coagulation cascade antithrombin III appears to be the most efficient inhibitor for thrombin, and covalent, stoichiometric complex formation is accompanied by changes in the conformation of both, enzyme and inhibitor (Villanueva and Danishefsky, 1979), such that under non-denaturing conditions multimerization of the complex occurs (Binder, 1973; Marciniak and Gora-Maslak, 1983; Preissner, 1993). Various glycosaminoglycans are potent cofactors by drastically enhancing the rate of inhibition of thrombin and other coagulation enzymes (Damus *et al.*, 1973), and due to its unique structural features heparin has thus found wide application as an anticoagulant drug (Bourin and Lindahl, 1993). Due to their potent heparin-binding properties, several plasma proteins including vitronectin, platelet factor 4, histidine-rich glycoprotein or serum amyloid P component are believed to neutralize the acceleratory action of heparinoids also *in vivo* (Lane *et al.*, 1986; Preissner and Müller-Berghaus, 1987; Lane *et al.*, 1987; Zammit *et al.*, 1993). The quantitative effect of vitronectin to neutralize glycosaminoglycans in plasma and at the vascular endothelium appears to be comparable with the other factors, although only 2% of the adhesive protein in plasma is present in the heparin binding conformer (Izumi *et al.*, 1989). Vitronectin acts as non-competitive inhibitor for the heparin-accelerated reaction of thrombin or factor Xa with antithrombin III and thereby protects the enzymes against rapid inactivation (Preissner *et al.*, 1985; Podack *et al.*, 1986). Using overlapping synthetic peptides, a 15-mer linear sequence within the basic region of vitronectin was identified as moderate affinity (10^{-8} M) binding site for glycosaminoglycans which showed appreciable homology to heparin-binding consensus sequences in other basic proteins (Cardin and Weintraub, 1989) and directly competes with SERPINs for the essential binding site on the oligosaccharide chain (Lane *et al.*, 1987). Due to direct binding of vitronectin to the higher sulfated glycosaminoglycans heparin, fucoidan or dextran sulfate but not to dermatan, chondroitin, or keratan sulfates (Akama *et al.*, 1986; Preissner and Sie, 1988; Tomasini and Mosher, 1988), differential neutralization in enzyme inhibition reactions with antithrombin III or heparin cofactor II was found. Unlike histidine-rich glycoprotein, vitronectin and platelet factor 4 readily neutralize vessel wall-derived heparan sulfate (Lane *et al.*, 1987) and both display specific binding to endothelial cell monolayers inhibited by heparinoids (Hess *et al.*, 1993). These observations may be related to a modulation of the anticoagulant heparin-like activities proposed to be expressed at the luminal side of the endothelium *in vivo* (Preissner, 1990b).

Formation and Metabolism of Ternary Complexes

A unique feature of vitronectin relates to its association with different thrombin-SERPIN complexes in ternary product(s) (Podack and Müller-Eberhard, 1979), comprising an additional "modified" form of vitronectin during blood clotting (Ill and Ruoslahti, 1985; Jenne *et al.*, 1985; Podack *et al.*, 1986; Preissner *et al.*, 1987) and thereby regulating the distribution of thrombin-containing products. The majority of thrombin added to fibrino-gen-depleted plasma is found in complex with antithrombin III and subsequently enters a ternary product with vitronectin, whereas only 10% of thrombin is inhibited by α_2-macroglobulin (de Boer *et al.*, 1993a). The initial electrostatic interactions between thrombin-antithrombin-III and vitronectin result in alteration of its folded conformation with concomitant stabilization of a ternary complex by disulfide bridge(s) (Tomasini *et al.*, 1989) between thrombin and vitronectin (de Boer *et al.*, 1993b). High M_r associa-tion products were also documented when antithrombin III was replaced by other throm-bin-targeting SERPINs such as heparin cofactor II, protease nexin I (Preissner and Sie, 1988; Rovelli *et al.*, 1990) the Pittsburgh mutant of α_1-proteinase inhibitor (Tomasini *et al.*, 1989) or protein C inhibitor (H. de Boer *et al.*, unpublished results) implicating a general scavenger function of vitronectin (Figure 9.2). In thrombin-SERPIN complexes

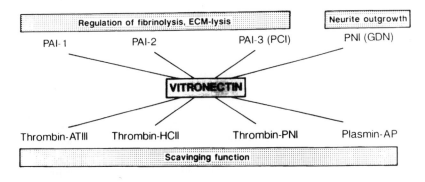

Figure 9.2   Incorporation of vitronectin into binary and ternary complexes of protease cascades. The for-mation of binary vitronectin — PAI complexes relates to the localization and stabilization of these SERPINs at extravascular matrix sites and are believed to efficiently control the function of plasminogen activators in peri-cellular proteolysis. In contrast, ternary complexes of vitronectin with thrombin-SERPINs constitute end-products of the blood coagulation cascade that acquire heparin-binding properties and become distributed into the extracellular matrix of blood vessels where they contribute to the regulation of extravascular thrombin; (PCI, protein C inhibitor; PNI = GDN, protease nexin = glia-derived nexin; AT III, antithrombin III; HC II, heparin cofactor II; AP, α_2-plasmin inhibitor; ECM, extracellular matrix).

the heparin-binding affinities of the single components, critical for the catalytic function of glycosaminoglycans during inhibition, are virtually lost. However, the exposure of the heparin-binding domain in vitronectin converts the ternary products into potent heparin scavengers, provided that sufficient quantities of complexes are formed *in vivo*. Thus, thrombin–SERPIN complexes are not only the major physiological inducers of conformational transition(s) in plasma vitronectin, but they also stabilize the nascent "multimeric" vitronectin conformer which otherwise would tend to self-associate with partial neutralization of complementary binding domains (Stockmann *et al.*, 1993).

Most enzyme-SERPIN complexes including the thrombin-antithrombin III have exposed a (formerly cryptic) region in the modified inhibitor that is responsible for binding to hepatocytes (or hepatoma cells) and monocytes (Perlmutter *et al.*, 1990). The responsible SERPIN-enzyme complex receptor (SEC-receptor) mediates moderate affinity binding and participates in *in vivo* clearance, respectively. These interactions have been best characterized for the prototype α_1-proteinase inhibitor-enzyme complex (Joslin *et al.*, 1991) which does not form ternary products with vitronectin. Since virtually all thrombin-antithrombin III in the circulation will enter a ternary complex with vitronectin (de Boer *et al.*, 1993a) which is particularly increased under conditions of septicemia and disseminated intravascular coagulation, it is questionable whether the uncomplexed thrombin-antithrombin III complex may ever reach the SEC-receptor. Moreover, all complexes appear to be catabolized very rapidly, a finding that is directly deduced from *in vivo* clearance studies of administered thrombin-antithrombin III complex and subsequent accumulation of a fraction thereof in the liver (Shifman and Pizzo, 1982). In addition, ternary complexes exhibit specific binding particularly to vascular endothelial cells mediated through ionic interactions of the altered vitronectin component (de Boer *et al.*, 1992). Although the ternary complex mediates cell attachment indistinguishable from isolated vitronectin through interaction with $\alpha v \beta 3$ integrin (Preissner *et al.*, 1988), competition experiments showed that binding to intact monolayers was mediated through the heparin-binding site of vitronectin possibly involving surface proteoglycan(s). While syndecan did not express affinity for vitronectin (Elenius *et al.*, 1990), fibroglycan, amphiglycan or other yet unidentified proteoglycans are candidates for ternary complex binding proteins (Mertens *et al.*, 1992).

Binding experiments at physiological temperature indicated a possible role for the vessel wall in the clearance of the ternary complexes, since metabolically active cells internalized and deposited these products into their extracellular matrix (de Boer *et al.*, 1992) mainly in undegraded form. Since the pathway of internalization did not involve lysosomal processing, it was proposed that transcytosis rather than endocytosis is involved in the translocation of the ternary complex from the luminal to the basolateral side of endothelial cells, although lateral diffusion or transport via cell junctions cannot totally be ruled out (de Boer *et al.*, 1993b). These findings are compatible with the afore mentioned distribution of vitronectin (-complexes) in the vessel wall of different organs. It remains, however, to be established in which way different vascular beds such as liver endothelium or the blood-brain barrier differ in their ability to recognize and translocate ternary complexes. In the extravascular compartments vitronectin will endow these complexes with potent cell adhesive properties, both through the RGD- and the heparin binding site, and the ternary complex was found to bind PAI-1 in an equivalent way as matrix-associated vitronectin does (de Boer *et al.*, 1993b). Recent experimental evidence also points to a possible counteracting effect of the ternary complex in the thrombin-induced proliferation of vascular smooth muscle cells (R. Bar-Shavit and K.T. Preissner, unpublished observations). Together, these activities of vitronectin provide a novel molecular link between clearance and extravasation of coagulation end-products and their regulatory functions important for the homeostasis of the vessel wall.

VITRONECTIN AND EXTRAVASCULAR PROTEASE INHIBITION

Pericellular Proteolysis

Different classes of extracellular proteolytic enzymes have a combined ability to degrade various macromolecules at the cell surface or in the connective tissue extracellular matrix (Chen, 1992). The plasminogen activation system as well as matrix metalloproteinases and their respective counteracting inhibitors are the major players in normal remodelling processes or in the accelerated tissue destruction occuring in many diseases including tumor metastasis (Vassalli *et al.*, 1991; Murphy and Docherty, 1992). The components of these proteolytic systems are synthesized and secreted by various cell types in the vessel wall and elsewhere, all of which appear to be in close proximity to sites of potential proteolytic modification. In general, the level of active protease is controlled and regulated by (a) the mode of gene expression and regulation of synthesis of (pro-)enzyme and of potential cell surface receptors and inhibitor(s) for these enzymes; (b) the rate of secretion and extracellular localization of (pro-)enzyme and inhibitor(s); (c) the rate of activation of latent (pro-)enzyme; (d) the accessibility of active enzyme towards respective inhibitor(s) and the rate of inhibition; (e) the mode of clerence of inactive enzyme-inhibitor complexes. Moreover, cell surface or extracellular matrix binding of plasminogen activators is a requirement for efficient plasmin generation and subsequent enzymatic modification of the pericellular environment (Saksela and Rifkin, 1988).

Direct binding of plasminogen activators to a reconstituted matrix/basement membrane (Korner *et al.*, 1993) and to isolated matrix molecules, such as laminin and fibronectin as well as to different types of collagen has been reported. Similarly, the local concentration of plasmin(ogen) is drastically increased by low affinity but high capacity binding to cell surface components such as α-enolase (Miles *et al.*, 1991) or matrix-associated proteins such as fibronectin (Salonen *et al.*, 1985), laminin (Salonen *et al.*, 1984), thrombospondin (Silverstein and Nachman, 1987), vitronectin (Preissner, 1990a) or others (Table 9.1). These plasminogen binding proteins share considerable homology within a consensus recognition site which is required for the interaction with lysine binding site(s) in the

Table 9.1   Binding of vitronectin to components of the plasminogen activation system

Component	Binding affinity (nM)
Glu-plasminogen	800–1000
Lys-plasminogen	85–100
DIP-plasmin	80
α_2-plasmin inhibitor	—
Plasmin-α_2-plasmin inhibitor	20–30
Plasmin-aprotinin	6–10
PAI-1	4 and 20

plasminogen kringle structures. The presence of liver-derived plasminogen in appreciable quantities in extracellular body fluids as well as in extravascular compartments is a prerequisite for its activation by both tissue plasminogen activator (t-PA) and urokinase.

Besides fibrin as an established example of a physiological surface which provides assembly of enzyme and substrate in the t-PA-mediated proteolysis of plasmin formation, other matrix components have a similar but weaker effect on the kinetics of plasminogen activation (Stack *et al.*, 1990). Vitronectin was found to inhibit plasmin formation in the presence of fibrin, possibly due to its more than 50-fold higher affinity for the proenzyme plasminogen (Preissner, 1990a). Although only minor quantities of plasma vitronectin become incorporated into a fibrin clot, multimeric vitronectin shows appreciable affinity for interaction with fibrin as deduced from direct binding studies and ultrastructural analysis (K.T. Preissner and E. Morgenstern, unpublished observations). Interestingly, while (extracellular) actin stimulates plasmin generation by t-PA appreciably (Lind and Smith, 1991a), actin as well as thrombospondin recruited from platelets inhibit the enzymatic activity of plasmin in a non-competitive manner (Lind and Smith, 1991b; Hogg *et al.*, 1992) in order to limit possible systemic effects of this protease during fibrinolysis.

Vitronectin-PAI-1 Interactions

At least five inhibitors in the plasminogen activation system, designated PAI-1, PAI-2, PAI-3, protease nexin I and α_2-plasmin inhibitor are known as distinct gene products with similar molecular mass which serve to limit plasmin formation and action, respectively. PAI-1 has the broadest tissue distribution among this group of arginine-specific serine proteinase inhibitors (Loskutoff *et al.*, 1989) and is produced by e.g. vascular cells, hepatocytes and haematopoietic progenitor cells as well as by a number of transformed or tumor cell lines. *In vitro*, gene expression of PAI-1 and urokinase has been studied in detail (Sawdey *et al.*, 1989; Andreasen *et al.*, 1990) indicating that growth factors and cytokines may sometimes have opposing effects on the transcription of inhibitor and activator in the same cell system.

The majority of PAI-1 deposited in the subendothelium appears to be stabilized in its active form (Levin and Santell, 1987; Mimuro *et al.*, 1987), whereas active PAI-1 found in the circulation (or culture medium) decays with a half-life of about two hours at 37°C into the conformationally altered latent form (Hekman and Loskutoff, 1988). Analysis of high molecular weight PAI-1 fractions in the circulation as well as of PAI-1 deposited in the vessel wall matrix revealed complex formation with vitronectin which thereby constitutes the major binding protein for the inhibitor (Declerck *et al.*, 1988; Wiman *et al.*, 1988; Mimuro and Loskutoff, 1989a; Preissner *et al.*, 1990). Polarized secretion and the quantities of deposited PAI-1 strongly correlate with available matrix-associated vitronectin (Grulich-Henn *et al.*, 1992). Moreover, following platelet stimulation by physiological agonists, a fraction of secreted PAI-1 is bound to platelet vitronectin in platelet releasate (Preissner *et al.*, 1989), and both components were co-localized also in areas of arteriosclerotic lesions (Lupu *et al.*, 1993). As a functional consequence, complex formation does not only increase the half-life of PAI-1 in the circulation by two-to four-fold (Declerck *et al.*, 1988; Lindahl *et al.*, 1989) but enables the active inhibitor to be stabilized at sites of vascular injury and initial platelet plug formation which are not necessarily reached by plasma-derived SERPINs. Thus, effective control of endothelial cell derived plasminogen activators during early hemostatic plaque formation is achieved through vessel wall- and platelet-derived vitronectin-stabilized PAI-1 which warrants initial thrombus formation and stabilization and prevents bleeding. Conversely, high level PAI-1 deposits in the vessel wall/thrombus are likely to postpone the necessary switch from blood clotting to fibrinolysis (Stringer *et al.*, 1994) such that restenosis may affect the vessel patency, whereas administration of antibodies to PAI-1 reduced thrombus extension and promoted low-dose t-PA-mediated thrombolysis (Levi *et al.*, 1992).

Based on the observations that the vitronectin-PAI-1 interactions are mainly of ionic nature, that polycations may disturb this interaction (Mimuro and Loskutoff, 1989b) that chaotropic agents such as guanidine (Hekman and Loskutoff, 1988) or arginine (Keijer *et al.*, 1990) as well as low pH (Lindahl *et al.*, 1989) may stabilize the PAI-1 molecule, it was concluded that latent and active PAI-1 differ in respective conformational states and that vitronectin serves to maintain PAI-1 in its strained form, the characteristic reactive conformation of SERPINs (Huber and Carrell, 1989). Hence, highly charged domains exposed in immobilized vitronectin may provide the structural motif for PAI-1 binding and stabilization, since the inhibitor was found to specifically bind to synthetic peptides adjacent to the heparin-binding domain of vitronectin (Preissner *et al.*, 1990). Alternatively, the amino-terminal portion of vitronectin was identified to interact with PAI-1 as well (Seiffert and Loskutoff, 1991) and a third site was also described (Mimuro *et al.*, 1993). Together, the idenfication of two major binding sites in vitronectin for PAI-1 supports previous kinetic data (Salonen *et al.*, 1989) and is compatible with the folding pattern of vitronectin which suggests cooperative complex formation (Stockmann *et al.*, 1993; Gechtman *et al.*, 1993). It appears plausible that complementary domain(s) of PAI-1 are involved in binding to vitronectin, and a highly charged region in PAI-1 (between residues 90 and 130) which overlaps with fibrin and heparin binding sites of the inhibitor (Keijer *et al.*, 1991) was localized as vitronectin binding domain using both mutagenesis and immunological approaches (Sane and Padmanabhan, 1993; Lawrence *et al.*, 1994; van Meijer *et al.*, 1994). Since the strained loop of PAI-1 containing the reactive site was not involved in binding to vitronectin (Lawrence *et al.*, 1990), a "hugging" mechanism between both proteins is proposed which is compatible with ultra-structural data of latent PAI-1 (Mottonen *et al.*, 1992) and which allows the inhibitor to retain its stressed conformation. Since PAI-1 neither modulates the function of vitronectin as attachment promoting factor (Salonen *et al.*, 1989) nor does the inhibitor affect the binding of vitronectin to heparin (Preissner *et al.*, 1990), and conversely, crosslinking of vitronectin does not change its PAI-1 binding properties (Sane *et al.*, 1990), vitronectin may simultaneously express several functions.

Upon reaction of vitronectin-associated PAI-1 with the respective target plasminogen activators, the binary complex dissociates with the concomitant appearance of inactive enzyme-PAI-1 products (Declerck *et al.*, 1988; Salonen *et al.*, 1989). PAI-1 has also been identified as "heparin cofactor" and kinetic data indicate that both, vitronectin and heparin, drastically change the specificity of PAI-1 for thrombin, such that this procoagulant enzyme becomes recognized and subsequently neutralized by PAI-1 (Ehrlich *et al.*, 1990; Ehrlich *et al.*, 1991a). Vitronectin thereby can be considered as a novel protein cofactor for SERPIN function. Although the overall rate of inhibition for the latter system is about 100-fold lower than for interaction of PAI-1 with plasminogen activators, thrombin inhibition by the PAI-1-vitronectin complex appears to be the major event *in vitro* when (pro-coagulant) thrombin interacts with the subendothelial cell matrix (Ehrlich *et al.*, 1991b). Since thrombin as well as PAI-1 are incorporated into the initial thrombus, their mutual neutralization promoted by the cofactor vitronectin appears to be beneficial for the dynamic switch from blood coagulation to fibrinolysis during the hemostatic process. Although transgenic mice lacking PAI-1 expression apparently develop normally (Carmeliet *et al.*, 1993), the cellular material found initially in totally occluded vessels following injury consists of vascularized neointima tissue. Not only the uncontrolled excess of plasminogen activators in these challenged animals was responsible for the observed cellular invasion, but due to the lack of PAI-1, extravascular thrombin inhibition could be hampered as well.

Modulation of vitronectin-PAI-1 interactions can occur by: (a) partial proteolysis of vitronectin (Chain *et al.*, 1991; Kost *et al.*, 1992), (b) competitive binding of vitronectin to other matrix-associated proteins such as osteonectin, and (c) non-enzymatic modification of critical residues in vitronectin by glucose metabolites (resulting in advanced glycosylation endproducts) (Preissner *et al.*, 1993). Initial plasmin-catalyzed limited proteolysis produces a vitronectin fragment which lacks both heparin and major PAI-1 binding sites leading to liberation and mobilization of the inhibitor within the vessel wall (Kost *et al.*, 1992; Gechtman *et al.*, 1993). Moreover, this intermediate fragment exhibits sequence homology in its carboxy-terminus with respective sites in α_2-plasmin inhibitor or α-enolase critical for plasminogen binding. In accordance with these *in vitro* data, in areas of skin inflammation associated with bullous pemphigoid the majority of blister-fluid derived vitronectin was present as the plasminogen-binding fragment and co-localized with plasmin(ogen) at sites of the dermal-epidermal junction (Kramer *et al.*, 1993). In Table 9.1 the interaction of vitronectin with components of the plasminogen activation system are summarized. Like for thrombin-containing complexes, vitronectin also shows appreciable affinity for plasmin-inhibitor complexes and may thus serve scavenging function as well (Figure 9.2) (C. Kost and K. T. Preissner, unpublished observations).

Interaction of vitronectin with other PAI-molecules has been observed as well which support the general role of the adhesive protein for localizing anti-proteolytic events (Figure 9.2). Direct binding of vitronectin to protease nexin I, a heparin-binding SERPIN which is found associated with platelet and endothelial cell surface and which exhibits inhibitory potential against both, urokinase and thrombin (Baker *et al.*, 1980), was noted (Rovelli *et al.*, 1990). Besides its potent neurite-outgrowth promoting activity, protease nexin I may thus become concentrated in extravascular compartments at vitronectin-rich sites where protease control is required. A possible disulfide-mediated association of vitronectin with PAI-2 extracted from placenta tissue was described (Radtke *et al.*, 1990), but it remains to be determined whether this interaction has consequences for the localized action or the function of monocyte/macrophage derived PAI-2 at sites of vascular injury or inflammation.

Taken together, the described examples indicate that intact matrix-associated vitronectin acts as adhesive anti-proteolytic cofactor not only for initial thrombus stabilization but also for control of thrombin that has escaped intravascular inhibition. Taken vitronectin as a constant denominator present in the extracellular environment, regulation of these inhibitory reactions can be envisaged to occur on the level of inhibitor expression and subsequent binding/stabilization by vitronectin.

VITRONECTIN-MEDIATED COORDINATION OF CELLULAR INTERACTIONS

The expression and modulation of adhesive functions in a given cell system is believed to determine cell morphology and motility as well as cellular metabolism relevant for proliferation and differentiation. Besides the firm association between cells and the extracellular matrix at sites of focal contacts that may prevent cells from apoptosis (Meredith *et al.*, 1993), integrins such as the $\alpha v \beta 3$ — vitronectin receptor have been implicated in the migration and differentiation of endothelial cells into capillary-like structures (Davis *et al.*, 1993) or during angiogenesis (Brooks *et al.*, 1994) and in the growth advantage of metastatic melanoma cells (Felding-Habermann *et al.*, 1992). The strength and duration of temporary or long-lasting interactions not only depend on the relative expression of different vitronectin-responsive integrins and the extent of receptor clustering (Felding-Habermann and Cheresh, 1993), but also on the composition of the extracellular matrix where anti-adhesive proteins such as osteonectin, thrombospondin and tenascin may serve as morpho-regulatory factors (Sage and Bornstein, 1991). Finally, proteolytic degradation predominantly of matrix material is believed to promote cell detachment important for migration and invasion to occur as mentioned earlier. Due to its broad distribution, the vitronectin PAI-1 complex appears to be of general importance for the control of pericellular proteolysis and for the stabilization of cell-matrix contacts (Ciambrone and McKeown-Longo, 1990), since vitronectin-containing focal adhesions associated with PAI-1-producing cells are much more protected against proteolysis than those containing predominantly fibronectin. Moreover, vitronectin-containing substrata may direct the localization of urokinase receptors into focal areas (Ciambrone and McKeown-Longo, 1992). The co-localization of urokinase receptors with integrins in focal contacts (Pöllänen *et al.*, 1988) which contrasts with a more scattered distribution of vitronectin-bound PAI-1 in extracellular matrices (Pöllänen *et al.*, 1987) could allow focal urokinase-mediated proteolysis to occur (Pöllänen *et al.*, 1991). While receptor-bound urokinase is not protected against inhibition by PAI-1, urokinase-PAI-1 complexes may remain in association with the receptor, and, through the cooperative action of low-density lipoprotein receptor-related protein/α_2-macroglobulin receptor, uptake and metabolism of the ligand is initiated (Orth *et al.*, 1992; Bu *et al.*, 1994). Another unusual way of regulation is achieved by urokinase-mediated proteolysis of its own receptor with subsequent release of the ligand-binding domain (Hoyer-Hansen *et al.*, 1992).

Besides the plasminogen activation-dependent modifications of the pericellular environment, additional observations support a role for the urokinase-receptor in cell adhesion and motility independent of plasmin formation: Increased urokinase-receptor expression has been described in migrating endothelial cells, and localization of the receptor to the leading edge of migrating monocytes appears to be essential for cell locomotion independent of urokinase activity (Gyetko *et al.*, 1994). Moreover, cellular migration of myeloid cells is dependent upon continued occupation of the urokinase receptor by its ligand, and vitronectin complexed PAI-1 apparently regulates adhesion by promoting urokinase/urokinase receptor turnover (Waltz *et al.*, 1993). Thus, urokinase receptor-related invasiveness or differentiation of tumor cells (Kook *et al.*, 1994; Howell *et al.*, 1994) may not be necessarily related to pericellular plasmin generation. Recently,

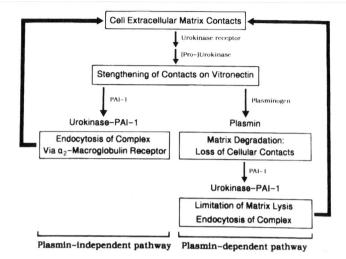

Figure 9.3 Communication between the urokinase receptor/urokinase and the vitronectin/PAI-1 system: Hypothetical reactions that modulate and regulate cell-matrix interactions. Cellular contacts with vitronectin-rich extracellular matrix may become strengthened and focalized by urokinase receptor and (pro-)urokinase expression. In the absence of plasminogen activation (plasmin-independent pathway), the addition of PAI-1 leads to inactivation of urokinase with subsequent induction of endocytosis via the $\alpha_2$macroglobulin-receptor pathway. The strength of cellular interactions may thus be modulated by the local concentrations of receptor-bound urokinase and vitronectin- stabilized PAI-1 without involving matrix lysis. In the presence of plasminogen activation (plasmin-dependent pathway) at PAI-1-depleted sites, efficient extracellular matrix lysis can occur necessary for cellular invasion before additional PAI-1 may limit this process by preventing further plasmin generation. Vitronectin appears to be the matrix-associated key element for linking these reactions.

vitronectin has been suggested to act as linking molecule between the extracellular matrix and some of the described urokinase-dependent mechanisms, since attachment of myeloid cells to immobilized vitronectin was observed (Waltz and Chapman, 1994), and direct binding of multimeric vitronectin to these cells as well as to urokinase receptor was augmented in the presence of urokinase (S. Kanse and K. T. Preissner, unpublished observations). Taken together, these findings suggest a novel communication between the urokinase receptor/urokinase and the vitronectin-PAI-1 system in the regulation of plasmin-dependent and plasmin-independent adhesive functions which control the variable strength of cell-matrix interactions (Figure 9.3). Although urokinase binding to its receptor may induce phosphorylation of an intracellular receptor-associated protein (Dumler *et al.*, 1993), it is unclear which signalling pathways are used.

Due to the translocation pathways of vitronectin between intra-and extra-vascular compartments as well as its association with vessel wall extracellular matrix, the redistribution of components of protease cascades is achieved. This trafficking together with unique protein-protein interactions described here allows the molecular link between control of protease cascades and adhesive functions in hemostasis. Moreover, the properties of vitronectin in this regard are of general importance not only for the homeostasis of the vascular system but are also relevant for the management of pathological processes related to thrombosis and atherosclerosis.

Acknowledgement:

Part of the author's work mentioned was supported by a grant (Pr 327/1–2) from the Deutsche Forschungsgemeinschaft, Bonn (Germany)

References

Akama, T., Yamada, K.M., Seno, N., Matsumoto, I., Kono, I., Kashiwagi, H., Funaki, T. and Hayashi, M. (1986). Immunological characterization of human vitronectin and its binding to glycosaminoglycans. *J. Biochem.*, **100**:1343–1351.

Andreasen, P.A., Georg, B., Lund, L.R., Riccio, A. and Stacey, S.N. (1990). Plasminogen activator inhibitors: hormonally regulated serpins. *Mol. Cell. Endocrinol.*, **68**:1–19.

Baker, J.B., Low, D.A., Simmer, R.L. and Cunningham, D.D. (1980). Protease nexin: a cellular component that links thrombin and plasminogen activator and mediates their binding to cells. *Cell*, **21**:37–45.

Bariety, J., Hinglais, N., Bhakdi, S., Mandet, C., Rouchon, M. and Kazatchkine, M.D. (1989). Immunohistochemical study of complement S protein (vitronectin) in normal and diseased human kidneys: Relationship to neoantigens of the C5b-9 terminal complex. *J. Clin. Exp. Immunol.*, **75**:76–81.

Barnes, D.W. and Reing, J. (1985). Human spreading factor: Synthesis and response by HepG2 hepatoma cells in culture. *J. Cell. Physiol.*, **125**:207–214.

Binder, B. (1973). On the complex formation of antithrombin III with thrombin. Gelfiltration studies on human plasma and serum. *Thrombos. Diathes. Haemorrh.*, **30**:280–283.

Bittorf, S.V., Williams, E.C. and Mosher, D.F. (1993). Alteration of vitronectin. Characterization of changes induced by treatment with urea. *J. Biol. Chem.*, **268**:24838–24846.

Bourin, M.C. and Lindahl, U. (1993). Glycosaminoglycans and the regulation of blood coagulation. *Biochem. J.*, **289**:313–330.

Brooks, P.C., Clark, R.A.F. and Cheresh, D.A. (1994). Requirement of vascular integrin $\alpha v \beta 3$ for angiogenesis. *Science*, **264**:569–571.

Bu, G., Warshawsky, I. and Schwartz, A.L. (1994). Cellular receptors for the plasminogen activators. *Blood*, **83**:3427–3436.

Cardin, A.D. and Weintraub, H.J.R. (1989). Molecular modeling of protein-glycosaminoglycan interactions. *Arteriosclerosis*, **9**:21–31.

Carmeliet, P., Stassen, J.M., Schoonjans, L., Ream, B., van den Oord, J.J., Demol, M., Mulligan, R.C. and Collen, D. (1993). Plasminogen activator inhibitor-1 gene-deficient mice. *J. Clin. Invest.*, **92**:2756–2760.

Chain, D., Kreizman, T., Shapira, H. and Shaltiel, S. (1991). Plasmin cleavage of vitronectin: Identification of the site and consequent attenuation in binding plasminogen activator inhibitor-1. *FEBS Lett.*, **285**:251–256.

Chen, W.T. (1992). Membrane proteases: roles in tissue remodeling and tumour invasion. *Curr. Opin. Cell Biol.*, **4**:802–809.

Ciambrone, G.J. and McKeown-Longo, P.J. (1990). Plasminogen activator inhibitor type I stabilizes vitronectin-dependent adhesions in HT-1080 cells. *J. Cell Biol.*, **111**:2183–2195.

Ciambrone, G.J. and McKeown-Longo, P.J. (1992). Vitronectin regulates the synthesis and localization of urokinase-type plasminogen activator in HT-1080 cells. *J. Biol. Chem.*, **267**:13617–13622.

Dahlbäck, K., Löfberg, H. and Dahlbäck, B. (1986). Localization of vitronectin (S-protein of complement) in normal human skin. *Acta Derm. Venereol.*, **66**:461–467.

Damus, P.S., Hicks, M. and Rosenberg, R.D. (1973). A generalized view of heparin's anticoagulant action. *Nature*, **246**:355–357.

Davis, C.M., Danehower, S.C., Laurenza, A. and Molony, J.L. (1993). Identification of a role of the vitronectin receptor and protein kinase C in the induction of endothelial cell vascular formation. *J. Cell. Biol.*, **51**:206–218.

de Boer, H.C., de Groot, P.G., Bouma, B.N. and Preissner, K.T. (1993a). Ternary vitronectin-thrombin-antithrombin III complexes in human plasma: detection and mode of association. *J. Biol. Chem.*, **268**:1279–1283.

de Boer, H.C., de Groot, P.G. and Preissner, K.T. (1993b). Metabolism of vitronectin complexes. In *Biology of Vitronectins and Their Receptors*, K.T. Preissner, S. Rosenblatt, C. Kost, J. Wegerhoff, D.F. Mosher (eds.), pp. 103–110. Amsterdam: Elsevier.

de Boer, H.C., Preissner, K.T., Bouma, B.N. and de Groot, P.G. (1992). Binding of vitronectin-thrombin-antithrombin III complex to human endothelial cells is mediated by the heparin binding site of vitronectin. *J. Biol. Chem.*, **267**:2264–2268.

Declerck, P.J., De Mol, M., Alessi, M.-C., Baudner, S., Paques, E.-P., Preissner, K.T., Müller-Berghaus, G. and Collen, D. (1988). Purification and characterization of a plasminogen activator inhibitor 1 binding protein from human plasma. Identification as a multimeric form of S protein (vitronectin). *J. Biol. Chem.*, **263**:15454–15461.

Dumler, I., Petri, T. and Schleuning, W.-D. (1993). Interaction of urokinase-type plasminogen activator (u-PA) with its cellular receptor (u-PAR) induces phosphorylation on tyrosine of a 38 kDA protein. *FEBS Lett.*, **322**:37–40.

Ehrlich, H.J., Keijer, J., Preissner, K.T., Klein Gebbink, R. and Pannekoek, H. (1991a). Functional interaction of plasminogen activator inhibitor type 1 (PAI-1) and heparin. *Biochemistry*, **30**:1021–1028.

Ehrlich, H.J., Klein Gebbink, R., Keijer, J., Linders, M., Preissner, K.T. and Pannekoek, H. (1990). Alteration of serpin specificity by a protein cofactor. Vitronectin endows plasminogen activator inhibitor 1 with thrombin inhibitory properties. *J. Biol. Chem.*, **265**:13029–13035.

Ehrlich, H.J., Klein Gebbink, R., Preissner, K.T., Keijer, J., Esmon, N.L., Mertens, K. and Pannekoek, H. (1991b). Thrombin neutralizes plasminogen activator inhibitor 1 (PAI-1) that is complexed with vitronectin in the endothelial cell matrix. *J. Cell Biol.*, **115**:1773–1781.

Ehrlich, H.J., Richter, B., von der Ahe, D. and Preissner, K.T. (1993). Primary structure of vitronectins and homology with other proteins. In *Biology of Vitronectins and Their Receptors*, K.T. Preissner, S. Rosenblatt, J. Wegerhoff, C. Kost, D.F. Mosher (eds.), pp. 59–66. Amsterdam: Elsevier.

Elenius, K., Salmivirta, M., Inki, P., Mali, M. and Jalkanen, M. (1990). Binding of human syndecan to extracellular-matrix proteins. *J. Biol. Chem.*, **265**:17837–17843.

Falk, R.J., Podack, E., Dalmasso, A.P. and Jennette, J.C. (1987). Localization of S protein and its relationship to the membrane attack complex of complement in renal tissue. *Am. J. Pathol.*, **127**:182–190.

Felding-Habermann, B. and Cheresh, D.A. (1993). Vitronectin and its receptors. *Curr. Opin. Cell Biol.*, **5**:864–868.

Felding-Habermann, B. and Mueller, B.M., Romerdahl, C.A. and Cheresh, D.A. (1992). Involvement of integrin αv gene expression in human melanoma tumorigenicity. *J. Clin. Invest.*, **89**:2018–2022.

Gebb, C., Hayman, E.G., Engvall, E. and Ruoslahti, E. (1986). Interaction of vitronectin with collagen. *J. Biol. Chem.*, **261**:16698–16703.

Gechtman, Z., Sharma, R., Kreizman, T., Fridkin, M. and Shaltiel, S. (1993). Synthetic peptides derived from the sequence around the plasma cleavage site in vitronectin. Use in mapping the PAI-1 binding site. *FEBS Lett.*, **315**:293–297.

Grulich-Henn, J., Müller-Berghaus, G. and Preissner, K.T. (1992). The influence of growth substratum and cell activation on the deposition of plasminogen activator inhibitor-1 in the extracellular matrix of human endothelial cells. *Fibrinolysis*, **6**:Suppl.4, 131–137.

Guettier, C., Hinglais, N., Bruneval, P., Kazatchkine, M., Bariety, J. and Camilleri, J.-P. (1989). Immunohistochemical localization of S protein/vitronectin in human atherosclerotic versus arteriosclerotic arteries. Virchows *Arch. A Pathol. Anat.*, **414**:309–313.

Gyetko, M.R., Todd III, R.F., Wilkinson, C.C. and Sitrin, R.G. (1994). The urokinase receptor is required for human monocyte chemotaxis *in vitro. J. Clin. Invest.*, **93**:1380–1387.

Hekman, C.M. and Loskutoff, D.J. (1988). Bovine plasminogen acitvator inhibitor 1: Specificity determinations and comparison of the active, latent, and guanidine-activated forms. *Biochemistry*, **27**:2911–2918.

Hess, S., Stockmann, A., Völker, W. and Preissner, K.T. (1993). Multimeric vitronectin: structure and function. In *Biology of Vitronectins and Their Receptors*, K.T. Preissner, S. Rosenblatt, J. Wegerhoff, C. Kost, D.F. Mosher (eds.), pp. 21–30. Amsterdam: Elsevier.

Hogg, P.J., Stenflo, J. and Mosher, D.F. (1992). Thrombospondin is a slow tight-binding inhibitor of plasmin. *Biochemistry*, **31**:265–269.

Howell, A.L., Hunt, J.A., James, T.W., Mazar, A., Henkin, J. and Zacharski, L.R. (1994). Urokinase inhibits HL-60 cell proliferation *in vitro. Blood Coagul. Fibrinol.*, **5**:445–453.

Hoyer-Hansen, G., Ronne, E., Solberg, H., Behrendt, N., Ploug, M., Lund, L.R., Ellis, V and Dano, K. (1992). Urokinase plasminogen activator cleaves its cell surface receptor releasing the ligand-binding domain. *J. Biol. Chem.*, **267**:18224–18229.

Huber, R. and Carrell, R.W. (1989). Implications of the three-dimensional structure of $\alpha 1$-antitrypsin for structure and function of serpins. *Biochemistry*, **28**:8951–8966.

Ill, C.R. and Ruoslahti, E. (1985). Association of thrombin-antithrombin III complex with vitronectin in serum. *J. Biol. Chem.*, **260**:15610–15615.

Izumi, M., Yamada, K.M. and Hayashi, M. (1989). Vitronectin exists in two structurally and functionally distinct forms in human plasma. *Biochim. Biophys. Acta*, **990**:101–108.

Jenne, D., Hille, A., Stanley, K.K. and Huttner, W.B. (1989). Sulfation of two tyrosine-residues in human complement S-protein (vitronectin). *Eur. J. Biochem.*, **185**:391–395.

Jenne, D., Hugo, F. and Bhakdi, S. (1985). Interaction of complement S-protein with thrombin-antithrombin complexes: A role for the S-protein in hemostasis. *Thromb. Res.*, **38**:401–412.

Jenne, D. and Stanley, K.K. (1985). Molecular cloning of S-protein, a link between complement, coagulation and cell-substrate adhesion. *EMBO J.*, **4**:3153–3157.

Jenne, D. and Stanley, K.K. (1987). Nucleotide sequence and organization of the human S-protein gene: repeating peptide motifs in the "pexin" family and a model for their evolution. *Biochemistry*, **26**:6735–6742.

Joslin, G., Fallon, R.J., Bullock, J., Adams, S.P. and Perlmutter, D.H. (1991). The SEC receptor recognizes a pentapeptide neodomain of α1-antitrypsin-protease complexes. *J. Biol. Chem.*, **266**:11282–11288.

Keijer, J., Linders, M, Ehrlich, H., Klein Gebbink, R. and Pannekoek, H. (1990). Stabilisation of plasminogen activator inhibitor type 1 (PAI-1) activity by arginine: possible implications for the interaction of PAI-1 with vitronectin. *Fibrinolysis*, **4**:153–159.

Keijer, J., Linders, M., van Zonneveld, A.-J., Ehrlich, H.J., de Boer, J.-P. and Pannekoek, H. (1991). The interaction of plasminogen activator inhibitor 1 with plasminogen activators (tissue-type and urokinase-type) and fibrin: Localization of interaction sites and physiologic relevance. *Blood*, **78**:401–409.

Kook, Y.H., Adamski, J., Zelent, A. and Ossowski, L. (1994). The effect of antisense inhibition of urokinase receptor in human squamous cell carcinoma on malignancy. *EMBO J.*, **13**:3983–3991.

Korc-Grodzicki, B., Tauber-Finkelstein, M., Chain, D. and Shaltiel, S. (1988). Vitronectin is phosphorylated by a cAMP-dependent protein kinase released by activation of human platelets with thrombin. *Biochem. Biophys. Res. Commun.*, **157**:1131–1138.

Korner, G., Bjornsson, T.D. and Vlodavsky, I. (1993). Extracellular matrix produced by cultured corneal and aortic endothelial cells contains active tissue-type and urokinase-type plaminogen activators. *J. Cell. Physiol.*, **154**:456–465.

Kost, C., Stüber, W., Ehrlich, H., Pannekoek, H. and Preissner, K.T. (1992). Mapping of binding sites for heparin, plasminogen activator inhibitor-1 and plasminogen to vitronectin's heparin binding region reveals a novel vitronectin-dependent feedback mechanism for the control of plasmin formation. *J. Biol. Chem.*, **267**:12098–12105.

Kramer, M.D., Gissler, H.M., Weidenthaler-Barth, B. and Preissner, K.T. (1993). Vitronectin and plasmin(ogen) in lesional skin of the bullous pemphigoid. In *Biology of Vitronectins and Their Receptors*, K.T. Preissner, S. Rosenblatt, C. Kost, J. Wegerhoff, D.F. Mosher (eds.), pp. 295–301. Amsterdam: Elsevier.

Lane, D.A., Flynn, A.M., Pejler, G., Lindahl, U., Choay, J. and Preissner, K.T. (1987). Structural requirements for the neutralization of heparin-like saccharides by complement S protein/vitronectin. *J. Biol. Chem.*, **262**:16343–16349.

Lane, D.A., Pejler, G., Flynn, A.M., Thompson, E.A. and Lindahl, U. (1986). Neutralization of heparin-related saccharides by histidine-rich glycoprotein and platelet factor 4. *J. Biol. Chem.*, **261**:3980–3986.

Lawrence, D.A., Berkenpas, M.B., Palaniappan, S. and Ginsburg, D. (1994). Localization of vitronectin binding domain in plasminogen activator inhibitor-1. *J. Biol. Chem.*, **269**:15223–15228.

Lawrence, D.A., Strandberg, K., Ericson, J. and Ny, T. (1990). Structure-function studies of the SERPIN plasminogen activator inhibitor type-1. Analysis of chimeric strained loop mutants. *J. Biol. Chem.*, **265**, 20293–20301.

Levi, M., Biemond, B.J., van Zonneveld, A.-J., Tencate, J.W and, Pannekoek, H. (1992). Inhibition of plasminogen activator inhibitor-1 activity results in promotion of endogenous thrombolysis and inhibition of thrombin extension in models of experimental thrombosis. *Circulation*, **85**:305–312.

Levin, E.G. and Santell, L. (1987). Association of a plasminogen activator inhibitor (PAI-1) with the growth substratum and membrane of human endothelial cells. *J. Cell Biol.*, **105**:2543–2549.

Lind, S.E. and Smith, C.J. (1991a). Actin accelerates plasmin generation by tissue plasminogen activator. *J. Biol. Chem.*, **266**:17673–17678.

Lind, S.E. and Smith, C.J. (1991b). Actin is a noncompetitive plasmin inhibitor. *J. Biol. Chem.*, **266**:5273–5278.

Lindahl, T.L., Sigurdardottir, O. and Wiman, B. (1989). Stability of plasminogen activator inhibitor 1 (PAI-1). *Thromb. Haemost.*, **62**:748–751.

Loskutoff, D.J., Sawdey, M. and Mimuro, J. (1989). Type-1 plasminogen-activator inhibitor. *Prog. Hemostas. Thromb.*, **9**:87–115.

Lupu, F., Bergonzelli, G.E., Heim, D.A., Cousin, E., Genton, C.Y., Bachmann, F. and Kruithof, E.K.O. (1993). Localization and production of plasminogen activator inhibitor-1 in human healthy and atherosclerotic arteries. *Arterioscl. Thromb.*, **13**:1090–1100.

Marciniak, E. and Gora-Maslak, G. (1983). High molecular weight forms of antithrombin III complexes in blood. *Thromb. Haemostas.*, **49**:32–36.

Merberg, D.M., Fitz, L.J., Temple, P., Giannotti, J., Murtha, P., Fitzgerald, M., Scaltreto, H., Kelleher, K., Preissner, K.T., Kriz, R., Jacobs, K. and Turner, K. (1993). A comparison of vitronectin and megakaryocyte stimulating factor. In *Biology of Vitronectins and Their Receptors*, K.T. Preissner, S. Rosenblatt, J. Wegerhoff, C. Kost, D.F. Mosher (eds.), pp. 45–53. Amsterdam: Elsevier.

Meredith, J.E., Fazeli, B. and Schwartz, M.A. (1993). The extracellular matrix as a cell survival factor. *Mol. Biol. Cell*, **4**:953–961.

Mertens, G., Cassiman, J.J., Van den Berghe, H., Vermylen, J. and David, G. (1992). Cell surface heparan sulfate proteoglycans from human vascular endothelial cells. Core protein characterization and antithrombin III binding properties. *J. Biol. Chem.*, **267**:20435–20443.

Miles, L.A., Dahlberg, C.M., Plescia, J., Felez, J., Kato, K. and Plow, E.F. (1991). Role of cell-surface lysines in plasminogen binding to cells: Identification of α-enolase as a candidate plasminogen receptor. *Biochemistry*, **30**:1682–1691.

Mimuro, J. and Loskutoff, D.J. (1989a). Purification of a protein from bovine plasma that binds to type-1 plasminogen-activator inhibitor and prevents its interaction with extracellular-matrix.evidence that the protein is vitronectin. *J. Biol. Chem.*, **264**:936–939.

Mimuro, J. and Loskutoff, D.J. (1989b). Binding of type 1 plasminogen activator inhibitor to the extracellular matrix of cultured bovine endothelial cells. *J. Biol. Chem.*, **264**:5058–5063.

Mimuro, J., Muramatsu, S., Kurano, Y., Uchida, Y., Ikadai, H., Watanabe, S. and Sakata, Y. (1993). Identification of the plasminogen activator inhibitor-1 binding heptapeptide in vitronectin. *Biochemistry*, **32**:2314–2320.

Mimuro, J., Schleef, R.R. and Loskutoff, D.J. (1987). Extracellular matrix of cultured bovine aortic endothelial cells contains functionally active type 1 plasminogen activator inhibitor. *Blood*, **70**:721–728.

Mottonen, J., Strand, A., Symersky, J., Sweet, R.M., Danley, D.E., Geoghegan, K.F., Gerard, R.D. and Goldsmith, E.J. (1992). Structural basis of latency in plasminogen activator inhibitor-1. *Nature*, **355**:270–273.

Murphy, G. and Docherty, A.J.P. (1992). The matrix metalloproteinase and their inhibitors. *Am. J. Respir. Cell Mol. Biol.*, **7**:120–125.

Niculescu, F., Rus, H.G. and Vlaicu, R. (1987). Immunohistochemical localization of C5b-9, S-protein, C3d and apolipoprotein B in human arterial tissues with atherosclerosis. *Atherosclerosis*, **65**:1–11.

Orth, K., Madison, L.E., Gething, M., Sambrook, J.F. and Herz, J. (1992). Complexes of tissue-type plasminogen activator with PAI-1 are internalized by means of the low density lipoprotein receptor-related protein/α2-macroglobulin receptor. *Proc. Natl. Acad. Sci. USA*, **89**:7422–7426.

Parker, C.J., Frame, R.N. and Elstad, M.R. (1988). Vitronectin (S protein) augments the functional activity of monocyte receptors for IgG and complement C3b. *Blood*, **71**:86–93.

Perlmutter, D.H., Glover, G.I., Rivetna, M., Schasteen, C.S. and Fallon, R.J. (1990). Identification of a serpin-enzyme complex receptor on human hepatoma cells and human monocytes. *Proc. Natl. Acad. Sci. USA*, **87**:3753–3757.

Podack, E.R., Dahlbäck, B. and Griffin, J.H. (1986). Interaction of S-protein of complement with thrombin and antithrombin III during coagulation. Protection of thrombin by S-protein from antithrombin III inactivation. *J. Biol. Chem.*, **261**:7387–7392.

Podack, E.R. and Müller-Eberhard, H.J. (1979). Isolation of human S-protein, an inhibitor of the membrane attack complex of complement. *J. Biol. Chem.*, **254**:9908–9914.

Pöllänen, J., Hedman, K., Nielsen, L.S., Dano, K. and Vaheri, A. (1988). Ultrastructural localization of plasma membrane-associated urokinase-type plasminogen activator at focal contacts. *J. Cell Biol.*, **106**:87–95.

Pöllänen, J., Saksela, O., Salonen, E.-M., Andreasen, P., Nielsen, L., Dano, K. and Vaheri, A. (1987). Distinct localizations of urokinase-type plasminogen activator and its type 1 inhibitor under cultured human fibroblasts and sarcoma cells. *J. Cell Biol.*, **104**:1085–1096.

Pöllänen, J., Stephens, R.W. and Vaheri, A. (1991). Directed plasminogen activation at the surface of normal and malignant cells. *Adv. Cancer Res.*, **57**:273–328.

Preissner, K.T. (1990a). Specific binding of plasminogen to vitronectin. Evidence for a modulatory role of vitronectin on fibrin(ogen)-induced plasmin formation by tissue plasminogen activator. *Biochem. Biophys. Res. Commun.*, **168**:966–971.

Preissner, K.T. (1990b). Physiological role of vessel wall related antithrombotic mechanisms: Contribution of endogenous and exogenous heparin-like components to the anticoagulant potential of the endothelium. *Haemostasis*, **20**:30–49.

Preissner, K.T. (1991). Structure and biological role of vitronectin. *Ann. Rev. Cell Biol.*, **7**:275–310.

Preissner, K.T. (1993). Self-association of antithrombin III relates to multimer formation of thrombin-antithrombin III complexes. *Thromb. Haemostas.*, **69**:422–429.

Preissner, K.T., Anders, E., Grulich-Henn, J. and Müller-Berghaus, G. (1988). Attachment of cultured human endothelial cells is promoted by specific association with S protein (vitronectin) as well as with the ternary S protein-thrombin-antithrombin III complex. *Blood*, **71**:1581–1589.

Preissner, K.T., Grulich-Henn, J., Ehrlich, H.J., Declerck, P., Justus, C., Collen, D., Pannekoek, H. and Müller-Berghaus, G. (1990). Structural requirements for the extracellular interaction of plasminogen activator inhibitor 1 with endothelial cell matrix-associated vitronectin. *J. Biol. Chem.*, **265**:18490–18498.

Preissner, K.T., Holzhüter, S., Justus, C. and Müller-Berghaus, G. (1989). Identification and partial characterization of platelet vitronectin: Evidence for complex formation with platelet-derived plasminogen activator inhibitor-1. *Blood*, **74**:1989–1996.

Preissner, K.T., Kost, C., Rosenblatt, S., de Boer.H., , Hammes, H.P. and Pannekoek, H. (1993). The role of fibrinolysis in the cross-talks among vessel wall components: the vitronectin-PAI-1 axis. *Fibrinolysis*, **7** (**Suppl. 1**), 18–19.

Preissner, K.T. and Müller-Berghaus, G. (1987). Neutralisation and binding of heparin by S protein/vitronectin in the inhibition of factor Xa by antithrombin III. Involvement of an inducible heparin binding domain of S protein/vitronectin. *J. Biol. Chem.*, **262**:12247–12253.

Preissner, K.T. and Sie, P. (1988). Modulation of heparin cofactor II function by S protein (vitronectin) and formation of a ternary S protein-thrombin-heparin cofactor II complex. *Thromb. Haemostas.*, **60**:399–406.

Preissner, K.T., Wassmuth, R. and Müller-Berghaus, G. (1985). Physicochemical characterization of human S-protein and its function in the blood coagulation system. *Biochem. J.*, **231**:349–355.

Preissner, K.T., Zwicker, L. and Müller-Berghaus, G. (1987). Formation, characterization and detection of a ternary complex between S protein, thrombin and antithrombin III in serum. *Biochem. J.*, **243**:105–111.

Radtke, K.-P., Wenz, K.H. and Heimburger, N. (1990). Isolation of plasminogen activator inhibitor-2 (PAI-2) from human placenta. Evidence for vitronectin/PAI-2 complexes in human placenta extract. *Biol. Chem. Hoppe-Seyler*, **371**:1119–1127.

Reilly, J.T. and Nash, J.R.G. (1988). Vitronectin (serum spreading factor): Its localisation in normal and fibrotic tissue. *J. Clin. Pathol.*, **41**:1269–1272.

Rosing, J., Tans, G., Govers-Riemslag, J.W.P., Zwaal, R.F.A. and Hemker, H.C. (1980). The role of phospholipids and factor Va in the prothrombinase complex. *J. Biol. Chem.*, **255**:274–283.

Rovelli, G., Stone, S.R., Preissner, K.T. and Monard, D. (1990). Specific interaction of vitronectin with the cell-secreted protease inhibitor glia-derived nexin (GDN) and the GDN-thrombin complex. *Eur. J. Biochem.*, **192**:797–803.

Sage, E.H. and Bornstein, P. (1991). Extracellular proteins that modulate cell-matrix interactions: sparc, tenascin, and thrombospondin. *J. Biol. Chem.*, **266**:14831–14834.

Saksela, O. and Rifkin, D.B. (1988). Cell-associated plasminogen activation: Regulation and physiological functions. *Ann. Rev. Cell Biol.*, **4**:93–126.

Salonen, E.-M., Saksela, O., Vartio, T., Vaheri, A., Nielsen, L.S. and Zeuthen, J. (1985). Plasminogen and tissue-type plasminogen activator bind to immobilized fibronectin. *J. Biol. Chem.*, **260**:12302–12307.

Salonen, E.-M., Vaheri, A., Pöllänen, J., Stephens, R., Andreasen, P., Mayer, M., Dano, K., Gailit, J. and Ruoslahti, E. (1989). Interaction of plasminogen activator inhibitor (PAI-1) with vitronectin. *J. Biol. Chem.*, **264**:6339–6343.

Salonen, E.-M., Zitting, A. and Vaheri, A. (1984). Laminin interacts with plasminogen and its tissue-type activator. *FEBS Lett.*, **172**:29–32.

Sane, D.C., Moser, T.L., Parker, C.J., Seiffert, D., Loskutoff, D.J. and Greenberg, C.S. (1990). Highly sulfated glycosaminoglycans augment the cross-linking of vitronectin by guinea pig liver transglutaminase. Functional studies of the crosslinked vitronectin multimers. *J. Biol. Chem.*, **265**:3543–3548.

Sane, D.C., Moser, T.L., Pippen, A.M.M., Parker, C.J., Achyuthan, K.E. and Greenberg, C.S. (1988). Vitronectin is a substrate for transglutaminases. *Biochem. Biophys. Res. Commun.*, **157**:115–120.

Sane, D.C. and Padmanabhan, J. (1993). A vitronectin binding region of plasminogen activator inhibitor-1. Analysis by ligand binding and construction of PAI-1/PAI-2 chimeras. *Thromb. Haemostas.*, **69**:783.

Sato, R., Komine, Y., Imanaka, T. and Takano, T.J. (1990). Monoclonal antibody EMR 1a/212D recognizing site of deposition of extracellular lipid in atherosclerosis. Isolation and characterization of a cDNA clone for the antigen. *J. Biol. Chem.*, **265**:21232–21236.

Savill, J., Dransfield, I., Hogg, N. and Haslett, C. (1990). Vitronectin receptor-mediated phagocytosis of cells undergoing apoptosis. *Nature*, **343**:180–183.

Sawdey, M., Podor, T.J. and Loskutoff, D.J. (1989). Regulation of type 1 plasminogen activator inhibitor gene expression in cultured bovine aortic endothelial cells. Induction by transforming growth factor-β, lipopolysaccharide, and tumor necrosis factor-α. *J. Biol. Chem.*, **264**:10396–10401.

Seiffert, D., Keeton, M., Eguchi, Y., Sawdey, M. and Loskutoff, D.J. (1991). Detection of vitronectin mRNA in tissues and cells of the mouse. *Proc. Natl. Acad. Sci. USA*, **88**:9402–9406.

Seiffert, D. and Loskutoff, D.J. (1991). Evidence that type-1 plasminogen activator inhibitor binds to the somatomedin-B domain of vitronectin. *J. Biol. Chem.*, **266**:2824–2830.

Seiffert, D., Poenninger, J. and Binder, B.R. (1993). Organization of the gene encoding mouse vitronectin. *Gene*, **134**:303–304.

Shifman, M.A. and Pizzo, S.V. (1982). The *in vivo* metabolism of antithrombin III and antithrombin III complexes. *J. Biol. Chem.*, **257**:3243–3248.

Silverstein, R.L. and Nachman, R.L. (1987). Thrombospondin-plasminogen interactions: Modulation of plasmin generation. *Semin. Thromb. Haemostas.*, **13**:335–340.

Skoorstengaard, K., Halkier, T., Hojrup, P. and Mosher, D. (1990). Sequence location of a putative transglutaminase cross-linking site in human vitronectin. *FEBS Lett.*, **262**:269–274.

Smith, A., Tatum, F.M., Muster, P., Burch, M.K. and Morgan, T. (1988). Importance of ligand-induced conformational changes in hemopexin for receptor-mediated heme transport. *J. Biol. Chem.*, **263**:5224–5229.

Stack, S., Gonzales-Gronow, M. and Pizzo, S.V. (1990). Regulation of plasminogen activation by components of the extracellular matrix. *Biochemistry*, **29**:4966–4970.

Stockmann, A., Hess, S., Declerck, P., Timpl, R. and Preissner, K.T. (1993). Multimeric vitronectin. Identification and characterization of conformation-dependent self-association of the adhesive protein. *J. Biol. Chem.*, **268**:22874–22882.

Stringer, H.A.R., van Swieten, P., Heijnen, H.F.G., Sixma, J.J. and Pannekoek, H. (1994). Plasminogen activator inhibitor-1 released from activated platelets plays a key role in thrombolytic resistance. Studies with thrombi generated in the Chandler loop. *Arterioscl. Thromb.*, **14**:1452–1458.

Suzuki, S., Oldberg, A., Hayman, E.G., Pierschbacher, M.D. and Ruoslahti, E. (1985). Complete amino acid sequence of human vitronectin deduced from cDNA. Similarity of cell attachment sites in vitronectin and fibronectin. *EMBO J.*, **4**:2519–2524.

Tomasini, B. and Mosher, D.F. (1988). Conformational states of vitronectin: Preferential expression of an antigenic epitope when vitronectin is covalently and noncovalently complexed with thrombin-antithrombin III or treated with urea. *Blood*, **72**:903–912.

Tomasini, B.R. and Mosher, D.F. (1990). Vitronectin. *Prog. Haemostas. Thromb.*, **10**:269–305.

Tomasini, B.R. Mosher, D.F., Owen, M.C. and Fenton, J.W. (1989). Conformational lability of vitronectin: Induction of an antigenic change by alpha-thrombin-serpin complexes and by proteolytically modified thrombin. *Biochemistry*, **28**:832–842.

van Meijer, M., Klein Gebbink, R., Preissner, K.T. and Pannekoek, H. (1994). Localization of the vitronectin binding region in plasminogen activator inhibitor-1. *FEBS Lett.* **352**:342–346.

Vassalli, J.D., Sappino, A.P. and Belin, D. (1991). The plasminogen activator/plasmin system. *J. Clin. Invest.*, **88**:1067–1072.

Villanueva, G.B. and Danishefsky, I. (1979). Conformational changes accompanying the binding of antithrombin III to thrombin. *Biochemistry*, **18**:810–817.

Waltz, D.A. and Chapman, H.A. (1994). Reversible cellular adhesion to vitronectin linked to urokinase receptor occupancy. *J. Biol. Chem.*, **269**:14746–14750.

Waltz, D.A., Sailor, L.Z. and Chapman, H.A. (1993). Cytokines induce urokinase-dependent adhesion of human myeloid cells. A regulatory role for plasminogen activator inhibitors. *J. Clin. Invest.*, **91**:1541–1552.

Wiman, B., Almquist, A., Sigurdardottir, O. and Lindahl, T. (1988). Plasminogen-activator inhibitor-1 (PAI) is bound to vitronectin in plasma. *FEBS Lett.*, **242**:125–128.

Yasumitsu, H., Seo, N., Misugi, E., Morita, H., Miyazaki, K. and Umeda, M. (1993). Vitronectin secretion by hepatic and non-hepatic human cancer cells. *In Vitro Cell. Dev. Biol.*, **29A**:403–407.

Zammit, A., Pepper, D.S. and Dawes, J. (1993). Interaction of immobilised unfractionated and low molecular weight heparins with proteins in whole human plasma. *Thromb. Haemostas.*, **70**:951–958.

10 Tissue-Type Plasminogen Activator and the Vessel Wall: Synthesis, Storage and Secretion

Jef J. Emeis, Yvonne van den Eijnden-Schrauwen and Teake Kooistra

Gaubius Laboratory TNO-PG, Leiden, the Netherlands

INTRODUCTION

Of the three layers of the vessel wall: intima, media and adventitia, the intimal layer — which contains the endothelial cells — has always attracted most attention in studies on plasminogen activation. Understandably so, since the vascular endothelial cell is thought to be the major source of tissue-type plasminogen activator (tPA) in plasma. However, during the last few years, and especially since it was proposed that plasminogen activation may be an essential component of local proteolytic processes, attention is increasingly being paid to the presence of plasminogen activators, including tPA, in vascular smooth muscle cells, and to the role of plasminogen activation in vascular smooth muscle cell biology, especially restenosis and vascular remodelling. In this chapter, we will try to summarize our present knowledge as regards the synthesis, storage and secretion of tPA in the vessel wall. We will emphasise the situation as it pertains *in vivo*, but attention will also be paid to data on the metabolism and regulation of tPA in cultured vascular cells. We will restrict ourselves mainly to data regarding human blood vessels, but from time to time animal data will be discussed as well, in case the relevant human data are not available. Attention will be paid only in passing to the presence in the vessel wall of plasminogen activator inhibitors (PAIs) and of urokinase-type plasminogen activator (uPA), as these proteins will be discussed in other chapters of this book (Loskutoff; Quax *et al.*).

INTIMAL ENDOTHELIAL CELLS

The Association of tPA with Endothelial Cells *in vivo*

The association of plasminogen activation with vascular endothelial cells was first functionally demonstrated by Todd (1958). In his histochemical fibrin autography technique, frozen tissue sections are overlaid with a plasminogen-rich fibrin layer, and then incubated at 37°C ("Todd-slide procedure"). Lysis of the overlaying fibrin indicates the presence of

187

plasminogen activator activity, the speed of lysis of the fibrin layer being an indication of the intensity of enzyme activity. The technique allows a fairly precise identification of those cells in the tissue section where the PA activity is located. In vessels, these cells are invariably the endothelial cells (Todd, 1964, 1969, 1972; Warren, 1964).

A serious disadvantage of the technique, and the main reason why it has gradually fallen into disuse, is that the activity measured is the resultant of the interaction between plasminogen activator(s) (PAs) on the one hand, and plasminogen activator inhibitor(s) (PAIs) on the other. If the latter are present in excess, the presence of PAs may even be completely masked. This drawback was later exploited by Noordhoek Hecht and Brakman (1974) to develop a histochemical slide assay for fibrinolysis inhibitory activity, the "fibrin slide sandwich procedure" (note that Todd's original principle is still actively employed in the so-called fibrin autography procedure, while Noordhoek Hecht and Brakman's principle is still in use in the reverse fibrin autography technique). A second limitation of Todd's original procedure is that it does not allow differentiation between the various types of PA, such as tPA and uPA. This problem was finally solved when antisera against tPA and uPA became available. Rijken *et al.* (1980) then demonstrated, using Todd's procedure, that the endothelial cell-related PA activity of vessel walls was fully quenched by anti-tPA antibodies, but not by anti-uPA antibodies. This observation showed for the first time that the plasminogen activator associated with vascular endothelial cells was tPA. Rijken's study was subsequently confirmed by Ljungner *et al.* (1983), and by Kirchheimer and Binder (1983).

Despite the limitations of Todd's procedure, the data it has generated are still of great value, as no other technique has been used so extensively in such a wide variety of vessel types and vascular pathologies (see e.g. Todd, 1964; Warren, 1964; Pandolfi *et al.*, 1967; Todd 1969; Fischer, 1970; Isacson, 1971; Todd 1972; Browse *et al.*, 1977; Donner *et al.*, 1977; Noordhoek Hecht, 1977a and b). A reappraisal of these data in the light of our present understanding of the biology of tPA and of PAI-1 may well prove a rewarding exercise.

The demonstration of the association of tPA *activity* with endothelial cells was soon followed by the immunohistochemical localization of tPA *antigen* in endothelial cells (Kristensen *et al.*, 1984; review by Kristensen, 1992). Immunohistochemical studies on the presence of tPA in vascular endothelial cells are summarized in Tables 10.1 and 10.2. From these tables it can be concluded that tPA antigen is present in a wide variety of human (and animal) vascular endothelial cells. Negative results have, however, also been reported. An interesting study in this regard is that of Levin and del Zoppo (1994), who reported in their study on baboons that the endothelial cells in the adventitia of vessels were always well stained immunohistochemically for tPA, while the intimal endothelial cells of the same vessels consistently did *not* stain. Also, in many parts of the brain only a small percentage of capillaries became stained. In situ hybridization with a probe for tPA mRNA agreed with these immunohistochemical observations (Levin and del Zoppo, 1994). A second study to be remarked upon is that of Labarrere *et al.* (1993, 1994). These authors described, in heart transplant biopsies, tPA immunoreactivity not in the arterial and arteriolar endothelial cells, but in the corresponding smooth muscle cells, both in pre-transplantation hearts and in clinically stable transplants. Often, however, especially during graft rejection, would the endothelial cells become positive for tPA immunoreactivity.

Table 10.1 Immunohistochemical localization of tissue-type plasminogen activator in vascular endothelial cells

Tissue	Human tissues Reference
Various veins and arteries	Kristensen *et al.* (1984)
Ovary: venules, capillaries and arteries	Angles-Cano *et al.* (1985a)
Glomerular capillaries	Angles-Cano *et al.* (1985b)
Colon tumours	Kohga *et al.* (1985)
Various vessels	Larsson and Åstedt (1985) *(uPA very faint)**
Breast tumour	Clavet *et al.* (1986)
Saphenous vein	Risberg *et al.*(1986) *(no uPA)*
Inferior mesenteric artery	Takada *et al.* (1986)
Skin	Grøndahl-Hansen *et al.* (1987) *(no uPA)*
Eye	Tripathi *et al.* (1987) *(also uPA: Tripathi et al. 1990)*
Kidney: veins and small arteries	Hasui *et al.* (1988)
Appendix	Grøndahl-Hansen *et al.* (1989) *(uPA in inflamed vessels)*
Glomerular capillaries and small arteries in kidney	Rondeau *et al.* (1990) *(no uPA)*
Breast	Costantini *et al.* (1991)
Colon tumours	Grøndahl-Hansen *et al.* (1991) *(uPA in tumour vessels)*
Eye	Lutty *et al.* (1991)
Glomerular capillaries	Aya *et al.* (1992) *(no uPA)*
Colon (inflamed)	Kurose *et al.* (1992)
Skin tumours	Miller *et al.* (1992) *(no uPA)*
Cardiac allografts (failing**)	Labarrere *et al.* (1993, 1994)
Skin and melanoma tissue	de Vries *et al.* (1994)

* Reactivity of vascular endothelial cells to anti-uPA antibodies is indicated only when specifically mentioned in the publication.
** See text.

Table 10.2 Immunohistochemical localization of tissue-type plasminogen activator in vascular endothelial cells

Species and tissue	Animal tissues Reference
Baboon	
Various vessels	Levin and del Zoppo (1994)
Rat	
Gastric mucosa	Kurose *et al.* (1991)
Carotid artery	Jackson *et al.* (1993)
Aorta	Padró *et al.* (1994)

The association of tPA activity and antigen with endothelial cells *in vivo* has thus been established, by functional and by immunohistochemical assay, for a great number of endothelial cell types in various locations. The studies by Levin and del Zoppo (1994) and by Labarrere *et al.* (1993, 1994) have made clear, though, that this association is not necessarily true for all vascular endothelial cells.

Proof that endothelial cells had actually synthetized the tPA that they contain is, remarkably, still scanty. Recently, however, Levin and del Zoppo (1994) reported co-localization of tPA antigen (by immunohistochemistry) and of tPA mRNA (by in situ hybridization) in baboon endothelial cells. Similar in situ hybridization data have been reported in abstract form by Gordon *et al.* (1989) for some vessels in rhesus monkeys. Finally, Clowes *et al.* (1990) showed that removal of the endothelium from rat carotid artery acutely reduced the tPA mRNA concentration in the vessel extract, thus indirectly showing association of the mRNA for tPA with the vascular endothelium. By in situ hybridization, mRNA for tPA has also been localized in kidney glomeruli, but whether endothelial cells or mesangial cells were involved remained undetermined (Sappino *et al.*, 1991; Moll *et al.*, 1994).

A point to be noted is that uPA has been observed only rarely in normal vascular endothelial cells, exceptions being the study of Tripathi *et al.* (1987) who found uPA in eye vessels, and that of Larsson and Åstedt (1985), who reported very faint uPA immunoreactivity in endothelia from various vessels. In two other reports, the presence of uPA immunoreactivity associated with endothelial cells coincided with an inflammatory condition: an inflamed appendix (Grøndahl-Hansen *et al.*, 1989), or colon tumour growth (Grøndahl-Hansen *et al.*, 1991). In the latter case, no uPA mRNA was detectable, however (Pyke *et al.*, 1991). Increased uPA immunoreactivity was also described in the glomeruli of dysfunctional renal allografts, although its precise localization within the glomerulus was unclear (Bukovsky *et al.*, 1992). It is of interest that uPA mRNA was recently shown to be induced in capillary endothelial cells during angiogenesis (Bacharach *et al.*, 1992). Together these observations suggest that the (immunohistochemical) presence of uPA in endothelial cells is associated with endothelial cell activation.

Synthesis of tPA by Endothelial Cells

As discussed in the previous paragraph, there is good evidence that tPA is associated with endothelial cells *in vivo*. Whether vascular endothelial cells also synthetize tPA is, however, not so well established. There are two main reasons for assuming that tPA is synthetized by endothelial cells *in vivo*. Firstly, all types of endothelial cells synthetize tPA when cultured *in vitro*. Secondly, the endothelial cell is so far the only cell from normal tissues (ovaries excepted) in which tPA mRNA has been localized *in vivo* (Gordon *et al.*, 1989; Clowes *et al.*, 1990; Levin and del Zoppo, 1994). In addition, it should be mentioned that the concentrations of tPA in tissue extracts on the one hand, and the amounts of tPA mRNA that are found in those extracts on the other, are strongly correlated (Quax *et al.*, 1990; and our unpublished data; compare also Rickles and Strickland, 1988). This suggests that tPA antigen and/or activity found in extracts from a given tissue had been synthetized locally. The fact that so many tissues contain tPA make it likely that tPA is synthetized by a widely distributed cell type (or cell types), supporting (but obviously not proving) an endothelial origin for tPA. This, of course, does not exclude the possibility that other cells, such as pituitary, adrenal, and pancreatic cells (Kristensen *et al.*, 1985, 1986, 1987) may also locally contribute to tPA synthesis.

In view of this putative contribution of endothelial cells to tPA synthesis, it is likely that factors which influence endothelial tPA synthesis will have a significant effect on tPA levels in tissues (and plasma: see discussion below). Because low plasma tPA activity is widely regarded as a risk factor for the development of cardiovascular disease (Chandler and Stratton, 1994; Hamsten and Eriksson, 1994), it would be attractive to increase plasma levels of tPA by increasing endothelial synthesis of tPA. To develop ways (drugs, procedures, changes in life-style) to do so, the most obvious line of approach is to study tPA synthesis in cultured human endothelial cells (see e.g. Kooistra, 1990). Various ways to increase human endothelial tPA synthesis have been successfully explored, as reviewed by Kooistra *et al.* (1994). These developments have, for experimental animals, resulted in procedures that will increase tPA synthesis (measured as an increase in tPA mRNA) and tissue and plasma concentrations of tPA. The objective of increasing plasma tPA levels by increasing endothelial tPA synthesis has not yet been accomplished in man, mainly because of limitations on the experimental use of drugs in man. Variables that modulate tPA synthesis in cultured human endothelial cells have recently been reviewed in depth by Kooistra *et al.* (1994). They include the following (compare Table 10.3).

Activators of protein kinase C. Vasoactive compounds such as α-thrombin (Levin *et al.*, 1984; Hanss and Collen, 1987; van Hinsbergh *et al.*, 1987) and histamine (Hanss and Collen, 1987) will induce tPA synthesis in cultured endothelial cells. Following interaction of these ligands with their endothelial receptor (always the seven transmembrane-domain type of receptor: in the case of histamine the H_1-receptor, and for thrombin the tethered thrombin receptor), their corresponding G-proteins are activated. This results, via activation of a phosphatidylinositol-diphosphate-specific phospholipase C (PI-PLC) in an increase of intracellular calcium (via inositoltriphosphate formed by PI-PLC from PI), and in activation of a protein kinase C (via diacylglycerol, also formed from PI by a PI-PLC). After a lag phase of a few hours, increased tPA synthesis then occurs. The activation of protein kinase C is probably responsible for this induction of tPA synthesis, since direct activation of endothelial protein kinase C by activators such as phorbol esters will also induce tPA synthesis (Levin and Santell, 1988; Levin *et al.*, 1989; Grülich-Henn and Müller-Berghaus, 1990; Kooistra *et al.*, 1991a; Medh *et al.*, 1992), while protein kinase C inhibitors will inhibit the thrombin- and histamine-induced up-regulation of tPA synthesis (Levin and Santell, 1988). Likely candidates as targets for this activation are the protein

Table 10.3 Compounds that modulate tPA Synthesis in human endothelial cells *in vitro**

Activators of protein kinase C (phorbol esters, thrombin, histamine)
cAMP elevating agents (in combination with activation of protein kinase C)
Retinoids
Triazolobenzodiazepines
Sodium butyrate, and similar short-chain fatty acids
Haemodynamic, oxidative, or hyperosmotic stress
Cytokines (microvascular endothelial cells)

* Adapted from Kooistra *et al.*, (1994)

kinase C subtypes C-α, C-βI, and C-βII, as these subtypes are calcium-and phorbol ester-sensitive, and have been detected in cultured human endothelial cells (Bussolino *et al.*, 1994; and our unpublished data). The increase in intracellular calcium level that also occurs during thrombin or histamine stimulation is, in itself, not sufficient to increase tPA synthesis, as treatment of endothelial cells with calcium ionophore A-23187 will not induce increased tPA synthesis (Kooistra *et al.*, 1991a).

Another second messenger, cyclic AMP, can further potentiate protein kinase C-induced tPA synthesis, but an increase in intracellular cyclic AMP is, in itself, not sufficient to increase tPA synthesis in human cells (Santell and Levin, 1988; Kooistra *et al.*, 1991a). Interestingly, a change, compared to the human promotor, in the rat tPA promoter at position–181 has resulted in the occurrence of a perfect cyclic AMP-responsive element (CRE) in rats (Feng *et al.*, 1990). Consequently, compounds that will increase intracellular cAMP levels in rat endothelial cells (for instance forskolin, or cholera toxin) will cause a very pronounced increase in tPA synthesis in cultured rat endothelial cells (Emeis *et al.*, 1994). This effect also occurred *in vivo*: forskolin and cholera toxin very effectively induced increased tPA mRNA levels following intravenous injection into rats. Moreover, the two compounds increased tissue and plasma levels of tPA antigen and activity in rats (Emeis *et al.*, 1994, and unpublished data). Finally, the increased synthesis of tPA in these animals also resulted in an enhancement of (bradykinin-induced) acute release of tPA (Schrauwen *et al.*, 1995).

Retinoids. These compounds are very effective inducers of tPA synthesis in cultured human endothelial cells (Kooistra *et al.*, 1991b; Thompson *et al.*, 1991; Bulens *et al.*, 1992a; for a recent review see Kooistra, 1995, 1995). The induction by retinoids involves the retinoic acid α-receptor, and at least one other protein (Lansink *et al.*, 1994). Of the many retinoids that are effective on human endothelial cells *in vitro*, three have been tested in rats *in vivo* (retinyl palmitate, retinoic acid, and isotretinoin). Isotretinoin did not influence tPA in rats (van Bennekum *et al.*, 1993), but retinyl palmitate and retinoic acid induced significant increases in plasma and tissue levels of tPA (Kooistra *et al.*, 1991b; van Bennekum *et al.*, 1993; van Giezen *et al.*, 1993). Repletion of vitamin A-deficient rats with retinyl palmitate also increased the (originally reduced) tPA concentration in plasma and tissues of these deficient rats (Bulens *et al.*, 1992b; van Bennekum *et al.*, 1993). In view of the inability of isotretinoin to influence tPA synthesis in rats, the minimal effects of isotretinoin (a clinically well tolerated retinoid) in humans, though disappointing, were not surprising (Declerck *et al.*, 1993; Wallnöfer *et al.*, 1993).

Other compounds that will increase tPA synthesis in cultured endothelial cells (see Table 3) include triazolobenzodiazepines (Kooistra *et al.*, 1992), and sodium butyrate and related short-chain fatty acids (Kooistra *et al.*, 1987). The effect of butyrate probably results from a change in histon H_4 acetylation (Arts *et al.*, 1995). These compounds have not yet been tested *in vivo*.

Mechanisms involved in the modulation of tPA by conditions such as flow and strain (Diamond *et al.*, 1989, 1990; Iba *et al.*, 1991; Iba and Sumpio, 1992) are unknown, but may involve a shear-stress responsive element (Resnick *et al.*, 1993) in the tPA promotor. Stress, whether osmotic stress (Levin *et al.*, 1993) or oxidative stress (Shatos *et al.*, 1992; Kugiyama *et al.*, 1993), may also cause changes in tPA synthesis in endothelial cells. Kugiyama *et al.*, (1993) reported that the component in oxidized low-density lipoproteins that reduced tPA synthesis (oxysterol) differed from the compound that induced increased PAI-1 synthesis (lysophosphatidylcholine).

In summary: significant progress has over the last years been made in the development of compounds that will increase tPA synthesis in cultured human endothelial cells. Some of these compounds have been tested in animals, and have been found to increase tPA synthesis *in vivo* as well, resulting in increased tissue and plasma levels of tPA, and in increased acute release of tPA. However, up-regulation of tPA synthesis has, in contrast to the situation in experimental animals, not yet been accomplished in man. Our increased understanding of the regulation of the human tPA gene (Kooistra *et al.*, 1994) makes it, however, likely that this goal may be reached in the not too distant future.

Storage of tPA in Endothelial Cells

Tissue extraction experiments have shown that appreciable amounts of PA (activity and antigen) can be found in vessels. The earlier studies, in which only overall PA activity could be determined, demonstrated large variations in PA activity between vessel walls from different parts of the body, and also between the three layers (intima, media and adventitia) of a given vessel. Astrup and collaborators demonstrated, for instance, that in the human aorta only the adventitial layer showed plasminogen activator activity, while the media and the intima were totally inactive in this respect (e.g. Astrup and Coccheri, 1962). Similar observations were later made in rat aorta by Padró *et al.* (1994), who found that the differences in tPA activity between the media and the adventitia could be explained by differences in inhibitor content. In contrast, all three vascular layers showed PA activity in other vessels such as human coronary arteries and pulmonary artery (Coccheri and Astrup, 1961). Similarly, large differences have been found between different human veins (e.g. Coccheri and Astrup, 1961; De Cossart and Marcuson, 1982, 1983). Such large differences may even occur between animal species for a single type of artery (Astrup and Buluk, 1963). And even within a single vessel, large differences in activity may exist between segments of that vessel, especially if pathological changes have occurred (see e.g. for arteriosclerotic vessel wall lesions: Smokovitis *et al.*, 1988; Padró *et al.*, 1993; Underwood and De Bono, 1993; Reilly *et al.*, 1994). Differences had also been noted in histochemical studies (for example: Kwaan and Astrup, 1967; Fischer, 1970), a good example being the difference in histochemical PA activity between arm veins (active) and leg veins (inactive) (Pandolfi *et al.*, 1967). Impressive differences between endothelial cells only a small distance apart in a vessel have been described for other endothelial cell characteristics as well (see for example the study on endothelial L-arginine metabolism by Abbott and Schachter, 1994).

As was the case in the fibrin autography studies discussed above, one should be aware that in most of the extraction studies just mentioned, the activities measured were net activities, and to a variable, but undoubtedly large, extent the resultant of the presence in the tissue extracts of both PA activity and of PA inhibitory activity (or activities; see Padró *et al.*, 1991). As early as 1969 Pugatch and Poole (Pugatch and Poole, 1969; Pugatch *et al.*, 1970) had described the co-existence of PA activity and PA inhibitory activity in extracts from endothelial cells purified by a "Häutchen" technique (see also Warren, 1964). Antigen assays have subsequently shown that extracts from vessels contain tPA antigen (Danglot *et al.*, 1986; Padró *et al.*, 1990), and that in some cases large amounts of tPA antigen can be present in extracts without any detectable PA activity (Padró *et al.*, 1994).

So far, little (Danglot *et al.*, 1986) or no (Padró *et al.*, 1990; Reilly *et al.*, 1994) uPA antigen or activity has been found in vessel wall extracts. It should, however, be noted that Northeast *et al.* (1990, 1992) caution that some extraction buffers may be poor buffers for uPA extraction. Recently, Padró *et al.* (1993) analysed in detail the antigen concentration of plasminogen activators and inhibitors in histologically-graded vascular lesions from human coronary arteries, and found significant differences between the various types of lesions as regards tPA and uPA (and PAI-1) antigen concentrations (for PAI-1, see also Schneiderman *et al.*, 1992; Lupu *et al.*, 1993).

The tPA that is found in tissue extracts can be either recently synthetized tPA, on the way to being secreted, or it can be tPA that is stored in the cell. Animal experiments have shown (Tranquille and Emeis, 1989) that the inhibition of protein synthesis (by cyclohex-imide) for up to five hours has only a slight, or even no, effect on the amount of tPA that can be extracted from (lung and skeletal) tissue. This observation shows that most of the tPA that can be extracted is present in a stable storage compartment. This store of tPA is large, compared to the daily turnover of tPA in the blood compartment: calculations show that tissue stores of tPA are sufficiently large to maintain plasma levels in the rat for about two days (Padró *et al.*, 1990), and the same may well be true in humans (Emeis, 1992; 1995). The site of tPA storage in the endothelial cell is not precisely known; recent density gradient fractionation data suggest that tPA is present in a small, dense particle (d > 1.12), and that this particle is not identical to the Weibel-Palade body, the endothelial storage particle for von Willebrand factor (Emeis *et al.*, 1993; and unpublished data).

Plasma tPA and Endothelial Cells: tPA Secretion

Having established that vascular endothelial cells can synthetize and store tPA, the question arises, to what purpose? Recent studies in transgenic tPA-deficient mice (Carmeliet *et al.*, 1994; review by Carmeliet and Collen, 1994) have confirmed the idea (Astrup, 1978; Bachmann, 1987; Wun and Capuano, 1985, 1987) that tPA is intimately involved in the process of intravascular fibrinolysis: tPA-deficient mice showed an increased throm-bogenic tendency, and a reduced thrombolytic potential (Carmeliet *et al.*, 1994). If one then assumes that the primary function of tPA is to maintain the fluidity of the blood and to prevent vascular obstruction, it should be possible to explain the main features of endothelial tPA metabolism from this perspective. Some aspects of tPA functioning should be kept in mind in doing so.

A. tPA is much more effective in inducing the lysis of fibrin (or of a thrombus) if present prior to fibrin formation, rather than after fibrin formation has occurred (Brommer, 1984; Zamarron *et al.*, 1984; Fox *et al.*, 1985).

B. tPA is present in tissues and blood as an active enzyme, not as a pro-enzyme. In this respect, tPA is an exception to the rule that proteases of the coagulation and the fibri-nolytic system circulate as inactive pro-enzymes. An explanation for this exceptional situation might be that tPA functions as the trigger of the fibrinolytic system. By being present in an active form, tPA ensures that the fibrinolytic cascade is triggered rapidly (just as tissue factor, being intrinsically active, makes a rapid initiation of coagulation possible).

C. tPA circulates in blood in the presence of a number of fast-acting inhibitors, each present in molar excess (possibly to prevent tPA from being harmful outside the circulation).

From these three considerations various characteristics of tPA metabolism can be derived. Since tPA circulates as an active protease, it must have a short half-life in the circulation, to minimize inactivation by inhibitors: the circulatory half-life of tPA in humans is 3–5 minutes. In order to maintain a stable plasma level, tPA must therefore continuously be supplied, preferably from a site close to the blood. The plasma level of tPA should, on the one hand, be low enough to ensure proper hemostasis, but should on the other also be amenable to rapid up-regulation in case of a major adverse event (e.g. thrombosis). The explosive formation of fibrin during thrombus formation might easily exhaust the normal supply of tPA, especially when blood flow has been interrupted as well. In that case, a rapid additional local supply of tPA is needed to make enough tPA available in the earliest stages of fibrin formation. As mentioned above, these early stages are critical for a proper functioning of the fibrinolytic system (Brommer, 1984; Zamarron *et al.*, 1984; Fox *et al.*, 1985). The endothelium is ideally situated to supply tPA, both systemically to maintain steady-state plasma levels, and locally to provide additional tPA when and where needed.

Most cells dispose of two pathways to secrete proteins: constitutive secretion and regulated secretion. During constitutive secretion, newly-synthetized protein is immediately secreted by the cell. This results in a steady rate of continuous secretion, since this rate depends only upon the rate of protein synthesis, which will in general change only slowly with time. The second pathway (regulated secretion) is normally dormant, and will only become active after the cell has been appropriately stimulated by an external stimulus. During regulated secretion (acute release), intracellular storage granules fuse with the plasma membrane and release their contents (proteins, polypeptides, autacoids, etc) into the extracellular space. Stimulation generally starts with the interaction of a stimulus with its plasma membrane receptor, generally of the "seven transmembrane-domain" type. This results in activation of receptor-linked trimeric G-protein(s), and is followed by activation of intracellular phospholipases and kinases, production of phosphoinositides, release of intracellular calcium and calcium influx, protein phosphorylation, etc, finally resulting in secretion.

In vascular endothelial cells both the constitutive secretory pathway and the regulated secretory pathway are present. Endothelial von Willebrand factor (vWf), for example, is constitutively secreted, but it is also stored intracellularly in storage granules — the Weibel-Palade bodies — from which it can be acutely released following stimulation of the endothelial cell by e.g. thrombin, bradykinin or histamine (Loesberg *et al.*, 1983; Reinders *et al.*, 1985; Sporn *et al.*, 1986; reviews by Reinders *et al.*, 1988; Wagner, 1990; Wagner and Bonfanti, 1991). Proteins like thrombospondin and fibronectin are, in contrast, only secreted in endothelial cells via the constitutive pathway (Reinders *et al.*, 1985). The way in which tPA is handled by endothelial cells appears very similar to the way the cell handles vWf. tPA is constitutively secreted by vascular endothelial cells, at least in culture (see e.g. reviews by van Hinsbergh, 1988; Schleef and Loskutoff, 1988; van Hinsbergh *et al.*, 1991; Kooistra *et al.*, 1994), but tPA is also stored intracellularly in dense storage particles (see above), from which tPA can be acutely released upon stimulation. Acute release of tPA from the endothelium has been demonstrated both *in vivo* and in perfused vascular beds (reviews by Emeis, 1988, 1992, 1995; Klöcking, 1991; Kooistra *et al.*, 1994), as well as, more recently, *in vitro* in cultured human endothelial cells (Booyse *et al.*, 1986; Schrauwen *et al.*, 1994a, 1994b, 1995). Concomitantly with tPA, vWf is released in most (Tranquille, 1991; Tranquille and Emeis, 1990; Schrauwen *et al.*, in press), though not in all circumstances (Smalley *et al.*, 1993). This suggests that the mechanisms involved in the acute release of tPA, and in the acute release of vWf, are very similar, but not identical. Release of intracellular calcium and influx of calcium, activation of protein kinases (including protein kinase C), actin depolymerization, and phospholipase A_2 activation and arachidonic acid metabolism are possibly all involved in the mechanisms of acute secretion (Tranquille, 1991; Tranquille and Emeis, 1992).

Whether the steady-state level of tPA in plasma is maintained by constitutive secretion or by stimulated secretion is still being debated (Emeis, 1988, 1992, 1995; Kooistra *et al.*, 1994). The stability of the tPA level in plasma may suggest a major role for the constitutive pathway of tPA secretion. The possibility that the regulated pathway, too, is responsible for maintaining steady-state levels of tPA cannot, however, at present be totally excluded. One could imagine that endothelial cells are continuously being stimulated to secrete tPA by shear stress, or by blood-born stimuli such as epinephrine (Chandler *et al.*, 1992 a and b), norepinephrine (C. Jern *et al.*, 1994, S. Jern *et al.*, 1994), vasopressin (Grant 1990; Grant and Medcalf, 1990), endothelin, histamine or bradykinin (Emeis, 1988). No definitive evidence is, however, available on this question yet (Kooistra *et al.*, 1994; Emeis, 1995). For reasons discussed in detail elsewhere (Emeis, 1988), it is, however, very likely that a sudden increase in the circulating plasma level of tPA is due to acute release (regulated secretion) of tPA from intracellular stores. This latter mechanism can, because of the large amounts of tPA stored in the endothelium *in vivo*, give rise to very high local tPA concentrations. This will occur especially in small-diameter vessels, which have more favourable surface-volume ratios than do larger vessels. Calculations (Emeis, 1992; Schrauwen *et al.*, 1994b) have shown that acute release of all tPA that is stored in the endothelium may result in local tPA concentrations of up to 12 µg/ml in capillaries, and up to 40 ng/ml in coronary artery-sized vessels. The thrombin formed during coagulation might be an important stimulus to induce the release of such large amounts of tPA during thrombus formation (Emeis, 1992). In this way, thrombin will not only act as a local trigger of thrombosis, but will also act as a local trigger of thrombus dissolution, even apart from its anticoagulant role as activator of protein C (see chapter by Esmon).

In a recently published kinetic model of the circulatory regulation of tPA, Chandler (1990; Chandler *et al.*, 1993) postulated a continuous secretion of tPA into the circulation. By fitting his experimental data to the model, this continuous secretion was determined to be 0.1–0.4 pmol.liter^{-1}.sec^{-1} (7–28 ng.l^{-1}.sec^{-1}) (Chandler, 1990; Chandler *et al.*, 1993). These values encompass the value determined by Keber *et al.* (1990) by a completely different method using venous occlusion of the arm (0.3 pmol.liter^{-1}.sec^{-1}). And these values were also in good agreement with the data from the elegant studies C. Jern *et al.* (1994) and

S. Jern *et al.* (1994), who continuously took blood samples across the vascular bed of the human forearm. It should be realised, however, that not all vascular beds behave similarly with regard to tPA release (Brommer *et al.*, 1988; Gough *et al.* 1992). Keber (1988; Keber *et al.*, 1990), for instance, found that tPA release from the arms was higher, and release from the legs was lower, than tPA release averaged over the whole body. Release from a leg amounted to only 40% of that measured in an arm (Keber 1988). These observations, once more, point to a heterogeneity of tPA metabolism in the various vascular beds.

MEDIAL SMOOTH MUSCLE CELLS

Compared to endothelial cells, we know very little about the presence and function of PAs in vascular medial smooth muscle cells (SMCs). In the earlier studies, it was demonstrated by fibrin autography that medial SMCs inhibited endothelial cell-induced lysis of fibrin. This inhibitory effect was ascribed by Noordhoek Hecht and Brakman (1974) to a vascular SMC-related diffusable plasmin inhibitor. This inhibitor would explain the absence of PA activity in the medial layer of the vessel wall. Immunohistochemical observations on the presence of PAs in the media have been remarkably few, if one takes into account that the presence of PAs in vascular endothelial cells has been studied extensively (Tables 1 and 2). Larsson and Åstedt (1985) reported tPA immunoreactivity in SMCs from a number of peripheral arteries and veins, including umbilical artery and veins. In contrast, Takada *et al.* (1986) did not observe tPA immunoreactive material in inferior mesenteric artery SMCs.

In the rat, Padró *et al.* (1994) found immunohistochemically tPA-immunoreactive material in aortic medial SMCs. Jackson *et al.* (1993), however, did not observe any tPA immunoreactivity in normal resting SMCs of rat carotid artery. Only after endothelial denudation did immunoreactivity for tPA become evident in medial, and possibly intimal, SMCs (Jackson *et al.*, 1993). In agreement with these immunohistochemical observations, Clowes *et al.* (1990) had found that all tPA activity had, immediately after deëndothelialisation, disappeared from rat carotid artery, suggesting that all tPA activity had been localized in endothelial cells, and none in the medial SMCs. Padró *et al.* (1994), however, found tPA in extract from the deëndothelialized media of rat aorta, i.e. in extract from pure medial SMCs. These latter authors also commented that extracts from the rat aortic media contained excess PAI-1 activity, and that consequently all medial tPA was present in the extracts as tPA:PAI-1 complexes. This was in contrast to the findings of Clowes *et al.* (1990), who could not demonstrate PAI-1 activity in their extracts from carotid artery. Both Clowes *et al.* (1990) and Padró *et al.* (1994) could confirm their functional and immunological data by mRNA analysis. The induction of tPA activity in the rat carotid artery SMCs, following endothelial damage, was inhibited by heparin (Clowes *et al.*, 1992), by thrombocytopenia and by an antiserum against platelet-derived growth factor (Jackson *et al.*, 1993), and was enhanced by basic fibroblast growth factor (Jackson and Reidy, 1993).

Since SMC migration into the intima is inhibited by a plasmin inhibitor, and tPA activity and SMC migration often go hand in hand (Jackson *et al.*, 1993; Jackson and Reidy, 1993), it was suggested (Clowes *et al.*, 1990) that tPA activity was involved in SMC migration. Cultured vascular SMCs synthetize tPA (van Leeuwen *et al.*, 1994), and the plasminogen-plasmin system has been shown to be involved in SMC migration *in vitro* (Sperti *et al.*, 1992).

It seems fair to conclude that our knowledge of the presence of plasminogen activators, and their inhibitors, in vascular smooth muscle cells is still very limited. What knowledge is available, however, suggests that the picture may prove at least as varied as the picture sketched above for the presence of PAs and PAIs in endothelial cells.

THE ADVENTITIA

The least-studied of the three layers of the vascular wall, the adventitia, is without doubt the one with the highest PA activity. This is true both for the fibrin autography procedure (e.g. Kwaan and Astrup, 1967; Donner *et al.*, 1977), for tissue extracts (e.g. Astrup and Coccheri, 1962; Padró *et al.*, 1994) and for immunohistochemistry (e.g. Levin and del Zoppo, 1994). The high PA activity is associated with the endothelium of small adventitial vessels, and is probably due to high tPA levels, in combination with low PAI activity.

Conclusion

The vessel wall (or, more precisely: the vascular endothelial cell) is the main source of tPA. Endothelial cells lining the lumen of large vessels, small vessel endothelium, and microvascular endothelium have been reported to synthetize and store tPA. This endothelial tPA is the main source of plasma tPA, as endothelial cells maintain the steady-state plasma concentration of tPA, likely by constitutive secretion of tPA. In addition, endothelial cells are able to acutely release large amounts of tPA from an intracellular storage compartment, which release will contribute to the local and systemic thrombolytic defense reaction. It should be added immediately, however, that the above is not necessarily true for *all* endothelial cells at *all* sites of the vasculature. In many studies, at least some endothelial cells did *not* contain detectable amounts of tPA immunoreactive material or tPA activity. Also, synthesis of tPA, as evidenced by the presence of tPA mRNA, was not always detected when looked for. Apart from these qualitative differences, pronounced quantitative differences in plasminogen activator were found between endothelial cells in different locations. This variation may to some extent be apparent only, being due to interference in the assays used (especially the activity-based assays) by plasminogen activator inhibitors. However, other types of variation (for instance in antigen concentrations, or in immunohistochemical staining intensity) cannot be so explained, and point to a real heterogeneity in tPA metabolism (synthesis, storage, secretion) between endothelial cells at different sites of the vascular tree. This heterogeneity may be even more pronounced for the other vascular cell known to (occasionally?) contain tPA, the smooth muscle cell. The available data on changes in vascular tPA content during the development of vascular lesions point to yet another source of variability. Now that at least some of the basic facts regarding endothelial tPA metabolism have been elucidated, the heterogeneity of tPA metabolism *in vivo* in vascular endothelial cells, and in vascular smooth muscle cells, may constitute a fruitful area for further research.

Notes

Recently, four papers have appeared, describing in great detail the qualitative and quantitative distribution of tPA, uPA and PAI-1 in the normal and atherosclerotic human vessel wall:

Lupu, F., Heim, D.A., Bachmann, F., Hurni, M., Kakkar, V.V. and Kruithof, E.K.O. (1995) Plasminogen activator expression in human atherosclerotic lesions. *Anteriosclerosis Thrombosis and Vascular Biology*, **15**:1444–1455.

Padró, T., Emesis, J.J., Stein, M., Schmid, K.W. and Kienast, J. (1995) Quantification of plasminogen activators and their inhibitors in aortic vessel wall in relation to the presence and severity of atherosclerotic disease. *Arteriosclerosis Thrombosis and Vascular Biology*, **15**:893–902.

Raghunath, P.N., Tomaszewski, J.E., Brady, S.T., Caron, R.J., Okada, S.S. and Barnathan, E.S. (1995) Plasminogen activator system in human coronary atherosclerosis. *Arteriosclerosis Thrombosis and Vascular Biology*, **15**:1432–1443.

Schneiderman, J., Bordin, G.M., Engelberg, I., *et al.* (1995) Expression of fibrinolytic genes in atheroscletrotic abdominal aortic aneurysm wall. *Journal of Clinical Investigation*, **96**:639–645.

Acknowledgement

This study was supported by grants from the Netherlands Heart Foundation (90.075 and 90.267).

References

Abbott, R.E. and Schachter, D. (1994). Regional differentiation in rat aorta: L-arginine metabolism and cGMP content *in vitro. American Journal of Physiology*, **266**:H2287–H2295.

Angles-Cano, E., Balaton, A., Le Bonniec, B., Genot, E., Elion, J. and Sultan, Y. (1985a). Production of mono-clonal antibodies to the high fibrin-affinity, tissue-type plasminogen activator of human plasma. Demonstration of its endothelial origin by immunolocalization. *Blood*, **66**:913–920.

Angles-Cano, E., Rondeau, E., Delarue, F., Hagege, J., Sultan, Y. and Sraer, J.D. (1985b). Identification and cellular localization of plasminogen activators from human glomeruli. *Thrombosis and Haemostasis*, **54**:688–692.

Arts, J., Lansink, M., Grimbergen, J., Toet, K.H. and Kooistra, T. (1995) Stimulation of tissue-type plasminogen activator gene expression by sodium butyrate and trichostain A in human endothelial cells involves histone acetylation. *Biochemical Journal*, **310**, 171–176.

Astrup, T.and Arts *et al.* (1978). Fibrinolysis: an overview. In: *Progress in Chemical Fibrinolysis and Thrombolysis*, J.F. Davidson, R.M. Rowan, M.M. Samama and P.C. Desnoyers (eds), volume 3, pp. 1–57. New York: Raven Press.

Astrup, T. and Coccheri, S. (1962). Thromboplastic and fibrinolytic activity of the arteriosclerotic human aorta. *Nature*, **193**:182–183.

Astrup, T. and Buluk, K. (1963). Thromboplastic and fibrinolytic activities in vessels of animals. *Circulation Research*, **13**:253–260.

Aya, N., Yoshioka, K., Murakami, K., Hino, S., Okada, K., Matsuo, O. and Maki, S. (1992). Tissue-type plas-minogen activator and its inhibitor in human glomerulonephritis. *Journal of Pathology*, **166**:289–295.

Bacharach, E., Itin, A. and Keshet, E. (1992). *In vivo* patterns of expression of urokinase and its inhibitor PAI-1 suggest a concerted role in regulating physiological angiogenesis. *Proceedings of the National Academy of Sciences USA*, **89**:10686–10690.

Bachman, F. (1987). Plasminogen activators. In: *Haemostasis and Thrombosis*, R.W. Colman, J. Hirsh, V.J. Marder and E.W. Salzman Jr (eds), 1st ed, pp. 318–339. Philadelphia: J.B. Lippincott.

Booyse, F.M., Bruce, R., Dolenak, D., Grover, M., and Casey, L.C. (1986). Rapid release and deactivation of plasminogen activators in human endothelial cell cultures in the presence of thrombin and ionophore A23187. *Seminars in Thrombosis and Haemostasis*, **12**:228–232.

Brommer, E.J.P. (1984). The level of extrinsic plasminogen activator (t-PA) during clotting as a determinant of the rate of fibrinolysis; inefficiency of activators added afterwards. *Thrombosis Research*, **34**:109–115.

Brommer, E.J.P., Derkx, F.H.M., Schalekamp, M.A.D.H., Dooijewaard, G. and van der Klaauw, M.M. (1988). Renal and hepatic handling of endogenous tissue-type plasminogen activator (t-PA) and its inhibitor in man. *Thrombosis and Haemostasis*, **59**:404–411.

Browse, N.L., Gray, L., Jarrett, P.E.M. and Morland, M. (1977). Blood and vein wall fibrinolytic activity in health and vascular disease. *British Medical Journal*, **i**:478–481.

Bukovsky, A., Labarrere, C.A., Carter, C., Haag, B. and Faulk, W.P. (1992). Novel immunohistochemical markers of human renal allograft dysfunction — antithrombin III, Thy-1, urokinase, and alpha-smooth muscle actin. *Transplantation*, **54**:1064–1071.

Bulens, F., Nelles, L., van den Panhuyzen, N. and Collen, D. (1992a). Stimulation by retinoids of tissue-type plasminogen activator secretion in cultured human endothelial cells: relations of structure to effect. *Journal of Cardiovascular Pharmacology*, **19**:508–514.

Bulens, F., Thompson, A.E., Stassen, J.M., Moreau, H., Declerck, P.J., Nelles, L. and Collen, D. (1992b). Induction of t-PA synthesis with intravenous bolus injections of vitamin A palmitate in vitamin A deficient rats. *Fibrinolysis*, **6**:243–249.

Camiolo, S.M., Siuta, M.R. and Madeja, J.M. (1982). Improved medium for the extraction of plasminogen activator from tissue. *Preparative Biochemistry*, **12**:297–305.

Carmeliet, P. and Collen, D. Evaluation of the plasminogen/plasmin system in transgenic mice. *Fibrinolysis*, **8**, supplement 1, 269–275.

Carmeliet, P., Schoonjans, L., Kieckens, L. *et al.* (1994). Physiological consequences of loss of plasminogen activator gene function in mice. *Nature*, **368**:419–424.

Chandler, W.L. (1990). A kinetic model of the circulatory regulation of tissue plasminogen activator. *Thrombosis and Haemostasis*, **66**:321–328.

Chandler, W.C., Veith, R.C., Fellingham, G.W., Levy, W.C., Schwartz, R.S., Cerqueira, M.D., Kahn, S.E., Larson, V.G., Cain, K.C., Beard, J.C., Abrass, I.B. and Stratton, J.R. (1992a). Fibrinolytic response during exercise and epinephrine infusion in the same subjects. *Journal of the American College of Cardiology*, **19**:1412–1420.

Chandler, W.L., Loo, S.C. and Mornin, D. (1992b). Adrenergic stimulation of regional plasminogen activator release in rabbits. *Thrombosis and Haemostasis*, **68**:545–551.

Chandler, W.L., Levy, W.C., Veith, R.C. and Stratton, J.R. (1993). A kinetic model of the circulatory regulation of tissue plasminogen activator during exercise, epinephrine infusion, and endurance training. *Blood*, **81**:3293–3302.

Chandler, W.L. and Stratton, J.R. (1994). Laboratory evaluation of fibrinolysis in patients with a history of myocardial infarction. *American Journal of Clinical Pathology*, **102**:248–252.

Clavel, C., Chavanel, G. and Birembaut, P. (1986). Detection of the plasmin system in human mammary pathology using immunofluorescence. *Cancer Research*, **46**:5743–5747.

Clowes, A.W., Clowes, M.M., Au, Y.T.P., Reidy, A.M. and Belin, D. (1990). Smooth muscle cells express urokinase during mitogenesis and tissue-type plasminogen activator during migration in injured rat carotid artery. *Circulation Research*, **67**:61–67.

Clowes, A.W., Clowes, M.M., Kirkman, T.R., Jackson, C.L., Au, Y.P.T. and Kenagy, R. (1992). Heparin inhibits the expression of tissue-type plasminogen activator by smooth muscle cells in injured rat carotid artery. *Circulation Research*, **70**:1128–1136.

Coccheri, S. and Astrup, T. (1961). Thromboplastic and fibrinolytic activities of large human vessels. *Proceedings of the Society for Experimental Biology and Medicine*, **108**:369–372.

Collen, D. and Lijnen, H.R. (1991). Basic and clinical aspects of fibrinolysis and thrombolysis. *Blood*, **78**:3114–3124.

Costantini, V., Zacharski, L.R., Memoli, V.A., Kudryk, B.J., Rousseau, S.M. and Stump, D.C. (1991). Occurrence of components of fibrinolysis pathways in situ in neoplastic and nonneoplastic human breast tissue. *Cancer Research*, **51**:354–358.

Danglot, G., Vinson, D. and Chapeville, F. (1986). Qualitative and quantitative distribution of plasminogen activators in organs from healthy adult mice. *Federation of European Biochemical Societies Letters*, **194**:96–100.

Declerck, P.J., Boden, G., Degreef, H. and Collen, D. (1993). Influence of oral intake of retinoids on the human plasma fibrinolytic system. *Fibrinolysis*, **7**:347–351.

De Cossart, L. and Marcuson, R.W. (1982). A simple quantitative assay of tissue plasminogen activator. *Journal of Clinical Pathology*, **35**:980–983.

De Cossart, L. and Marcuson, R.W. (1983). Vascular plasminogen activator and deep vein thrombosis. *British Journal of Surgery*, **70**:369–370.

De Vries, T.J., Quax, P.H.A., Denijn, M., Verrijp, K.N., Verheijen, J.H., Verspaget, H.W., Weidle, U.H., Ruiter, D.J. and van Muijen, G.N.P. (1994). Plasminogen activators, their inhibitors, and urokinase receptor emerge in late stages of melanocyte tumor progression. *American Journal of Pathology*, **144**:70–81.

Diamond, S.L., Eskin, S.G. and McIntyre, L.V. (1989). Fluid flow stimulates tissue plasminogen activator secretion by cultured human endothelial cells. *Science*, **243**:1483–5.

Diamond, S.L., Sharefkin, J.B., Dieffenbach, C., Frasier-Scott, K., McIntyre, L.V. and Eskin, S.G. (1990). Tissue plasminogen activator messenger RNA levels increase in cultured human endothelial cells exposed to laminar shear stress. *Journal of Cellular Physiology*, **143**:364–371

Donner, L., Klener, P. and Roth, Z. (1977). The plasminogen activator of the arterial wall. *Thrombosis and Haemostasis*, **37**:436–443.

Emeis, J.J. (1988). Mechanisms involved in short-term changes in blood levels of t-PA. In *Tissue-type plasminogen activator: physiological and clinical aspects*, C. Kluft (ed.), volume 2, pp. 21–35. Boca Raton: CRC Press.

Emeis, J.J. (1992). Regulation of the acute release of tissue-type plasminogen activator from the endothelium by coagulation activation products. *Annals of the New York Academy of Sciences*, **667**:249–258.

Emeis, J.J. (1995) Normal and abnormal endothelial release of tissue-type plasminogen activator. In *Fibrinolysis in disease*, P. Glas-Greenwalt (ed.); pp. 55–64. Boca Raton: CRC Press.

Emeis, J.J., van den Hoogen, C.M. and Schrauwen, Y. (1993). An endothelial storage granule for tissue-type plasminogen activator (abstract). *Thrombosis and Haemostasis*, **69**:609.

Emeis, J.J., de Vries, R.E.M., Schrauwen, Y. and Kooistra, T. (1994). Enhancement of endogenous rat plasma tissue-type plasminogen activator antigen and activity by cAMP-enhancing compounds (abstract). *Fibrinolysis*, **8**: supplement 1, 21.

Feng, P., Ohlsson, M. and Ny, T. (1990). The structure of the TATA-less rat tissue plasminogen activator gene. *Journal of Biological Chemistry*, **265**:2022–2027.

Fischer, S. (1970). Fibrinolytic activity in human coronary arteries. Review and quantitative studies. *Advances in Cardiology*, **4**:187–210.

Fox, K.A.A., Robison, A.K., Knabb, R.M., Rosamond, T.L., Sobel, B.E. and Bergmann, S.R. (1985). Prevention of coronary thrombosis with subthrombolytic doses of tissue-type plasminogen activator. *Circulation*, **72**:1346–1354.

Gordon, D., Augustine, A.J., Smith, K.M., Schwartz, S.M. and Wilcox, J.N. (1989). Localization of cells expressing t-PA, PAI-1, and urokinase by in situ hybridization in human atherosclerotic plaques and in the normal rhesus monkey (abstract). *Thrombosis and Haemostasis*, **62**:131.

Gough, S.C.L., Smyllie, J., Sheldon, T., Rice, P.J.S. and Grant, P.J. (1992). The anatomical distribution of plasma fibrinolytic activity in man during cardiac catheterisation. *Thrombosis and Haemostasis*, **68**:442–447.

Grant, P.J. (1990). Hormonal regulation of the acute hemostatic response to stress. *Blood Coagulation and Fibrinolysis*, **1**:299–

Grant, P.J. and Medcalf, R.L. (1990). Hormonal regulation of haemostasis and the molecular biology of the fibrinolytic system. *Clinical Science*, **78**:3–11.

Grøndahl-Hansen, J., Ralfkiaer, E., Nielsen L.S., Kristensen, P., Frentz, G. and Danø, K. (1987). Immunohistochemical localization of urokinase- and tissue-type plasminogen activators in psoriatic skin. *Journal of Investigative Dermatology*, **88**:28–32.

Grøndahl-Hansen, J., Kirkeby, L.T., Ralfkiaer, E., Kristensen, P., Lund, L.R. and Danø, K. (1989). Urokinase-type plasminogen activator in endothelial cells during acute inflammation of the appendix. *American Journal of Pathology*, **135**:631–636.

Grøndahl-Hansen, J., Ralfkiaer, E., Kirkeby, L.T., Kristensen, P., Lund, L.R. and Danø, K. (1991). Localization of urokinase-type plasminogen activator in stromal cells in adenocarcinomas of the colon in humans. *American Journal of Pathology*, **138**:111–117.

Grülich-Henn, J. and Müller-Berghaus, G. (1990). Regulation of endothelial tissue plasminogen activator and plasminogen activator inhibitor type 1 synthesis by diacylglycerol, phorbol ester, and thrombin. *Blut*, **61**:38–44.

Hamsten, A. and Eriksson, P. (1994). Fibrinolysis and atherosclerosis: an update. *Fibrinolysis*, **8**, supplement 1, 253–262.

Hanss, M. and Collen, D. (1987). Secretion of tissue-type plasminogen activator and plasminogen activator inhibitor by cultured human endothelial cells: modulation by thrombin, endotoxin and histamine. Journal of *Laboratory and Clinical Medicine*, **109**:97–104.

Hasui, Y., Suzumiya, J., Sumoyoshi, A., Hashida, S. and Ishikawa, E. (1988). Distribution of plasminogen activators in human kidney and male genital organs using a highly sensitive enzyme immunoassay. *Thrombosis Research*, **51**:453–459.

Iba, T., Shin, T., Sonoda, T., Rosales, O. and Sumpio, B.E. (1991). Stimulation of endothelial secretion of tissue-type plasminogen activator by repetitive stress. *Journal of Surgical Research*, **50**:457–60.

Iba, T. and Sumpio, B.E. (1992). Tissue plasminogen activator expression in endothelial cells exposed to cyclic strain *in vitro*. *Cell Transplantation*, **1**:43–50.

Isacson, S. (1971). Low fibrinolytic activity of blood and vein walls in venous thrombosis. *Scandinavian Journal of Haematology*, supplementum **16**.

Jackson, C.L., Raines, E.W., Ross, R. and Reidy, M.A. (1993). Role of endogenous platelet-derived growth factor in arterial smooth muscle cell migration after balloon catheter injury. *Arteriosclerosis and Thrombosis*, **13**:1218–1226.

Jackson, C.L. and Reidy, M.A. (1993). Basic fibroblast growth factor: its role in the control of smooth muscle cell migration. *American Journal of Pathology*, **143**:1024–1031.

Jansson, J.-H., Olofsson, B.-O. and Nilsson, T.K. (1993). Predictive value of tissue plasminogen activator mass concentration on long-term mortality in patients with coronary artery disease. A 7-year follow-up. *Circulation*, **88**:2030–2034.

Jern, C., Selin, L. and Jern, S. (1994). *In vivo* release of tissue-type plasminogen activator across the human forearm during mental stress. *Thrombosis and Haemostasis*, **72**:285–291.

Jern, S., Selin, L., Bergbrant, A. and Jern, C. (1994). Release of tissue-type plasminogen activator in response to muscarinic receptor stimulation in human forearm. *Thrombosis and Haemostasis*, **72**:588–594.

Keber, D. (1988). Mechanism of tissue plasminogen activator release during venous occlusion. *Fibrinolysis*, **2**, supplement 2, 96–103.

Keber, D., Blinc, A. and Fettich, J. (1990). Increase of tissue plasminogen activator in limbs during venous occlusion: a simple hemodynamic model. *Thrombosis and Haemostasis*, **64**:433–437.

Kirchheimer, J. and Binder, B.R. (1983). Localization and immunological characterization of plasminogen activators in human prostate tissue. *Haemostasis*, **13** 358–362.

Klöcking, H.-P. (1991). Pharmakologische Beëinflussung der Freisetzung von t-PA aus dem Gefässendothel. *Hämostaseologie*, **11**:76–88.

Kohga, S., Harvey, S.R., Weaver, R.M. and Markus, G. (1985). Localization of plasminogen activators in human colon cancer by immunoperoxidase staining. *Cancer Research*, **45**:1787–1796.

Kooistra, T. (1990). The use of cultured human endothelial cells and hepatocytes as an *in vitro* model to study modulation of endogenous fibrinolysis. *Fibrinolysis*, **4**, supplement 2, 33–39.

Kooistra, T. (1995) The potentials of retinoids as stimulators of endogenous tissue-type plasminogen activator. In *Fibrinolysis in disease*, P. Glas-Greenwalt (ed.); pp. 237–245. Boca Raton: CRC Press.

Kooistra, T., van den Berg, J., Töns, A., Platenburg, G., Rijken, D.C. and van den Berg, E. (1987). Butyrate stimulates tissue-type plasminogen activator synthesis in cultured human endothelial cells. *Biochemical Journal*, **247**:605–612.

Kooistra, T., Bosma, P.J., Toet, K., Cohen, L.H., Griffioen, M., van den Berg, E., Le Clercq, L. and van Hinsbergh, V.W.M. (1991a). Role of protein kinase C and cAMP in the regulation of tissue-type plasminogen activator, plasminogen activator inhibitor 1 and platelet-derived growth factor mRNA levels in human endothelial cells. Possible involvement of proto-oncogenes *c-jun* and *c-fos*. *Arteriosclerosis and Thrombosis*, **11**:1042–1052.

Kooistra, T., Opdenberg, J.P., Toet, K., Hendriks, H.F.J., van den Hoogen, C.M. and Emeis, J.J. (1991b). Stimulation of tissue-type plasminogen activator synthesis by retinoids in cultured human endothelial cells and rat tissues *in vivo*. *Thrombosis and Haemostasis*, **65**:565–572.

Kooistra, T., Toet, K., Kluft, C., VonVoigtländer, P.F., Ennis, M.D., Aiken, J.W., Boadt, J.A. and Erickson, L.A. (1992). Triazolobenzodiazepines: a new class of stimulators of tissue-type plasminogen activator synthesis in human endothelial cells. *Biochemical Pharmacology*, **46**:61–67.

Kooistra, T., Schrauwen, Y., Arts, J. and Emeis, J.J. (1994). Regulation of endothelial cell t-PA synthesis and release. *International Journal of Haematology*, **59**:233–255.

Kristensen, P. (1992). Localization of components from the plasminogen activation system in mammalian tissues. *Acta Pathologica, Microbiologica et Immunologica Scandinavica*, **100**, supplementum 29.

Kristensen, P., Larsson, L.-I., Nielsen, L.S., Grøndahl-Hansen, J., Andreasen, P.A. and Danø, K. (1984). Human endothelial cells contain one type of plasminogen activator. *Federation of European Biochemical Societies Letters*, **168**:33–37.

Kristensen, P., Nielsen, L.S., Grøndahl-Hansen, J., Andresen, P.B., Larsson, L.-I. and Danø, K. (1985). Immunocytochemical demonstration of tissue-type plasminogen activator in endocrine cells of the rat pituitary gland. *Journal of Cell Biology*, **101**:305–311.

Kristensen, P., Hougaard, D.M., Nielsen, L.S. and Danø, K. (1986). Tissue-type plasminogen activator in rat adrenal medulla. *Histochemistry*, **85**:431–436.

Kristensen, P., Høiriis Nielsen, J., Larsson, L.-I. and Danø, K. (1987). Tissue-type plasminogen activator in somatostatin cells of rat pancreas and hypothalamus. *Endocrinology*, **88**:2238–2244.

Kugiyama, K., Sakamoto, T., Misumi, I., Sugiyama, S., Ohgushi, M., Ogawa, H., Horiguchi, M. and Yasue, H. (1993). Transferable lipids in oxidized low-density lipoprotein stimulate plasminogen activator inhibitor-1 and inhibit tissue-type plasminogen activator release from endothelial cells. *Circulation Research*, **73**:335–343.

Kurose, I., Suematsu, M., Miura, S., Suzuki, M., Nagata, H., Morishita, T., Sekizuka, E. and Tsuchiya, M. (1991). Involvement of superoxide anion and platelet-activating factor in increased tissue-typeplasminogen activator during rat gastric microvascular damages. *Thrombosis Research*, **62**:241–248.

Kurose, I., Miura, S., Suematsu, M., Serizawa, H., Fukumura, D., Asako, H., Hibi, T. and Tsuchiya, M. (1992). Tissue-type plasminogen activator of colonic mucosa in ulcerative colitis. *Digestive Diseases and Sciences*, **37**:307–311.

Kwaan, H.C. and Astrup, T. (1967). Fibrinolyic activity in human atherosclerotic coronary arteries. *Circulation Research*, **21**:799–804.

Labarrere, C.A., Pitts, D., Halbrook, H. and Faulk, W.P. (1993). Tissue plasminogen activator in human cardiac allografts. *Transplantation*, **55**:1056–1060.

Labarrere, C.A., Pitts, D., Halbrook, H. and Faulk, W.P. (1994). Tissue plasminogen activator, plasminogen activator inhibitor-1, and fibrin as indexes of clinical course in cardiac allograft recipients. An immunocytochemical study. *Circulation*, **89**:1599–1608.

Lansink, M., Toet, K. and Kooistra, T. (1994). Retinoids stimulate t-PA synthesis in cultured human endothelial cells by a hitherto unknown two-stage mechanism (abstract). *Fibrinolysis*, **8**, supplement 1, 21.

Larsson, A. and Åstedt, B. (1985). Immunohistochemical localisation of tissue plasminogen activator and urokinase in the vessel wall. *Journal of Clinical Pathology*, **38**:140–145.

Larsson, L.-I., Skriver, L., Nielsen, L.S., Grøndahl-Hansen, J., Kristensen, P. and Danø, K. (1984). Distribution of urokinase-type plasminogen activator immunoreactivity in the mouse. *Journal of Cell Biology*, **98**:894–903.

Levin, E.G., Marzec, U., Anderson, J. and Harker, L.A. (1984). Thrombin stimulates tissue plasminogen activator release from cultured human endothelial cells. *Journal of Clinical Investigation*, **74**:1988–1995.

Levin, E.G. and Santell, L. (1988). Stimulation and desensitization of tissue plasminogen activator release from human endothelial cells. *Journal of Biological Chemistry*, **263**:9360–9365.

Levin, E.G., Marotti, K.R. and Santell, L. (1989). Protein kinase C and the stimulation of tissue plasminogen activator release from human endothelial cells. Dependence on the elevation of messenger RNA. *Journal of Biological Chemistry*, **264**:16030–16036.

Levin, E.G., Santell, L. and Saljooque, F. (1993). Hyperosmotic stress stimulates tissue plasminogen activator expression by a PKC-independent pathway. *American Journal of Physiology*, **265**:C387–C396.

Levin, E.G. and del Zoppo, G.J. (1994). Localization of tissue plasminogen activator in the endothelium of a limited number of vessels. *American Journal of Pathology*, **144** 855–861.

Ljungner, H., Holmberg, L., Kjeldgaard, A., Nilsson, I.M. and Åstedt, B. (1983). Immunological characterisation of plasminogen activators in the human vessel wall. *Journal of Clinical Pathology*, **36**:1046–1049.

Loesberg, C., Gonsalves, M.D., Zandbergen, J., Willems, C., van Aken, W.G., Stel, H.V., van Mourik, J.A. and de Groot, P.G. (1983). The effect of calcium on the secretion of factor VIII-related antigen by cultured human endothelial cells. *Biochimica Biophysica Acta*, **763**:160–168.

Lupu, F., Bergonzelli, G.E., Heim, D.A., Cousin, E., Genton, C.Y., Bachmann, F. and Kruithof, E.K.O. (1993). Localization and production of plasminogen activator inhibitor-1 in human healthy and atherosclerotic arteries. *Arteriosclerosis and Thrombosis*, **13**:1090–1100.

Lutty, G.A., Ikeda, K., Chandler, C. and McLeod, D.S. (1991). Immunolocalization of tissue plasminogen activator in the diabetic and nondiabetic retina and choroid. *Investigative Ophthalmology and Visual Science*, **32**:237–245.

Medh, R.D., Santell, L. and Levin, E.G. (1992). Stimulation of tissue plasminogen activator production by retinoic acid: synergistic effect on protein kinase C-mediated activation. *Blood*, **80**:981–987.

Miller, S.J., Jensen, P.J., Dzubow, L.M. and Lazarus, G.S. (1992). Urokinase plasminogen activator is immunocytochemically detectable in squamous cell but not in basal cell carcinomas. *Journal of Investigative Dermatology*, **98**:351–358.

Moll, S., Schifferli, J.A., Huarte, J., Lemoine, R., Vassalli, J.-D. and Sappino, A.-P. (1994). LPS induces major changes in the extracellular proteolytic balance in the murine kidney. *Kidney International*, **45** 500–508.

Nguyen, H., Berleau, L., Modi, N., Bennett, W.F. and Keyt, B.A. (1994). Formation of tPA:PAI1 complex does not mediate rapid clearance of physiologic levels of tPA *in vivo* (abstract). *Fibrinolysis*, **8**, supplement 1, 7.

Noordhoek Hecht, V. and Brakman, P. (1974). Histochemical study of an inhibitor of fibrinolysis in the human arterial wall. *Nature*, **248**:75–76.

Noordhoek Hecht, V. (1977a). Localization and distribution of fibrinolytic inhibition in the walls of human arteries and veins. *Thrombosis Research*, **10**:121–133.

Noordhoek Hecht, V. (1977b). Relations between activation and inhibition of fibrinolysis in the walls of human arteries and veins. *Thrombosis and Haemostasis*, **38**:407–419.

Northeast, A.D.R., Eastham, D., Gaffney, P.J. and Burnand, K.G. (1990). The anatomical distribution of fibrinolytic activity in normal rat blood vessels (abstract). *Fibrinolysis*, **4**, supplement 3, 140.

Northeast, A.D.R. and Burnand, K.G. (1992). The response of the vessel wall to thrombosis: the *in vivo* study of venous thrombolysis. *Annals of the New York Academy of Sciences*, **667**:127–140.

Padró, T., van den Hoogen, C.M. and Emeis, J.J. (1990). Distribution of tissue-type plasminogen activator (activity and antigen) in rat tissues. *Blood Coagulation and Fibrinolysis*, **1** 601–608.

Padró, T., van den Hoogen, C.M. and Emeis, J.J. (1991). Plasmin inhibitory effect of rat tissues: comparison with antiplasmin activity of plasma. *Scandinavian Journal of Clinical and Laboratory Investigation*, **51**:599–603.

Padró, T., Steins, M., Hammel, D. and Kienast, J. (1993). Atherosclerosis-related alterations of the plasminogen activator/plasmin system in the vascular wall: studies in human coronary arteries (abstract). *Thrombosis and Haemostasis*, **69**:971.

Padró, T., Quax, P.H.A., van den Hoogen, C.M., Roholl, P., Verheijen, J. and Emeis, J.J. (1994). Tissue-type plasminogen activator and its inhibitor in rat aorta. Effect of endotoxin. *Arteriosclerosis and Thrombosis*, **14**:1459–1465.

Pandolfi, M., Nilsson, I.M., Robertson, B. and Isacson, S. (1967). Fibrinolytic activity of human veins. *The Lancet*, **ii**:127–128.

Pugatch, E.M.J. and Poole, J.C.F. (1969). Studies on the fibrinolytic activity of an extract from vascular endothelium. *Quarterly Journal of experimental Physiology*, **54**:80–84.

Pugatch, E.M.J., Foster, E.A., Macfarlane, D.E. and Poole, J.C.F. (1970). The extraction and separation of activators and inhibitors of fibrinolysis from bovine endothelium and mesothelium. *British Journal of Haematology*, **18**:669–681.

Pyke, C., Kristensen, P., Ralfkiaer, E., Grøndahl-Hansen, J., Eriksen, J., Blasi, F. and Danø, K. Urokinase-type plasminogen activator is expressed in stromal cells and its receptor in cancer cells at invasive foci in human colon adenocarcinomas. *American Journal of Pathology*, **138**:1059–1067.

Quax, P.H.A., van den Hoogen, C.M., Verheijen, J.H., Padró, T., Zeheb, R., Gelehrter, T.D., van Berkel, T.J.C., Kuiper, J. and Emeis, J.J. (1990). Endotoxin induction of plasminogen activator type 1 mRNA in rat tissues *in vivo*. *Journal of Biological Chemistry*, **265**:15560–15563.

Reilly, J.M., Sicard, G.A. and Lucore, C.L. (1994). Abnormal expression of plasminogen activators in aortic aneurysmal and occlusive disease. *Journal of Vascular Surgery*, **19**:865–872.

Reinders, J.H., de Groot, P.G., Dawes, J., Hunter, N.R., van Heusten, H.A., Zandbergen, J., Gonsalves, M.D. and van Mourik, J.A. (1985). Comparison of secretion and subcellular localization of von Willebrand protein with that of thrombospondin and fibronectin in cultured human vascular endothelial cells. *Biochimica Biophysica Acta*, **844**:306–313.

Reinders, J.H., de Groot, P.G., Sixma, J.J. and van Mourik, J.A. (1988). Storage and secretion of von Willebrand factor by endothelial cells. *Haemostasis*, **18**:246–261.

Resnick, N., Collins, T., Atkinson, W., Bonthron, D.T., Dewey, C.F. and Gimbrone, M.A. (1993). Platelet-derived growth factor B chain promotor contains a cis-acting fluid shear-stress-responsive element. *Proceedings of the National Academy of Sciences USA*, **90**:4591–4595.

Rickles, R.J. and Strickland, S. (1988). Tissue plasminogen activator mRNA in murine tissues. Federation of European Biochemical Societies Letters, **229**:100–106.

Ridker, P.M., Vaughan, D.E., Stampfer, M.J., Manson, J.E. and Hennekens, C.H. (1993). Endogenous tissue-type plasminogen activator and risk of myocardial infarction. *Lancet*, **341**:1165–1168.

Risberg, B., Eriksson, E., Björk, S. and Hansson, G.K. (1986). Immunohistochemical localization of plasminogen activators in human saphenous veins. *Thrombosis Research*, **37**:301–308.

Rondeau, E., Mougenot, B., Lacave, R., Peraldi, M.N., Kruithof, E.K.O. and Sraer, J.D. (1990). Plasminogen activator inhibitor 1 in renal fibrin deposits of human nephropathies. *Clinical Nephrology*, **33** 55–60.

Rijken, D.C., Wijngaards, G. and Welbergen, J. (1980). Relationship between tissue plasminogen activator and the activator in blood and vascular wall. *Thrombosis Research*, **18**:815–830.

Santell, L. and Levin, E.G. (1988). Cyclic AMP potentiates phorbol ester stimulation of tissue plasminogen activator release and inhibis secretion of plasminogen activator inhibitor-1 from human endothelial cells. *Journal of Biological Chemistry*, **263**:16802–16808.

Santell, L., Marotti, K., Bartfeld, N.S., Baynham, P. and Levin, E.G. (1992). Disruption of microtubules inhibits the stimulation of tissue plasminogen activator expression and promotes plasminogen activator inhibitor type 1 expression in human endothelial cells. *Experimental Cell Research*, **201**:358–365.

Sappino, A.-P., Huarte, J., Vassalli, J.-D. and Belin, D. (1991). Sites of synthesis of urokinase and tissue-type plasminogen activators in the murine kidney. *Journal of Clinical Investigation*, **87**:962–970.

Schleef, R.R. and Loskutoff, D.J. (1988). Fibrinolytic system of vascular endothelial cells. *Haemostasis*, **18**:328–341.

Schneiderman, J., Sawdey, M.S., Keeton, M., Bordin, G.M., Bernstein, E.F., Dilley, R.B. and Loskutoff D.J. (1992). Increased type 1 plasminogen activator inhibitor gene expression in atherosclerotic human arteries. *Proceedings of the National Academy of Sciences USA*, **89**:6998–7002.

Schrauwen, Y., Emeis. J.J. and Kooistra, T. (1994a). A sensitive ELISA for human tissue-type plasminogen activator applicable to the study of acute release from cultured human endothelial cells. *Thrombosis and Haematostasis*, **71**:225–229.

Schrauwen, Y., de Vries, R.E.M., Kooistra, T. and Emeis, J.J. (1994b). Acute release of tissue-type plasminogen activator (tPA) from the endothelium: regulatory mechanisms and therapeutic target. *Fibrinolysis*, **8**, supplement 2, 8–12.

Schrauwen, Y., Kooistra, T., de Vries, R.E.M. and Emeis, J.J. (1995) Studies on the acute release of tissue-type plasminogen activator from human endothelial cells *in vitro* and in rats *in vivo*: evidence for a dynamic storage pool. *Blood*, **85**, 3510–3517.

Shatos, M.A., Doherty, J.M., Orfeo, T., Hoak, J.C., Collen, D. and Stump, D.C. (1992). Modulation of the fibrinolytic response of cultured human vascular endothelium by extracellularly generated oxygen radicals. *Journal of Biological Chemistry*, **267**:597–601.

Smalley, D.M., Fitzgerald, J.E. and O'Rourke, J. (1990). Adenosine diphosphate stimulates the endothelial release of tissue-type plasminogen activator but not von Willebrand factor from isolated-perfused rat hind limbs. *Thrombosis and Haemostasis*, **70**:1043–1046.

Smokovitis, A., Kokolis, N. and Alexaki-Tzivanidou, E. (1988). Fatty streaks and fibrous plaques in human aorta show increased plasminogen activator activity. *Haemostasis*, **18**:146–153.

Sperti, G., van Leeuwen, R.T.J., Quax, P.H.A., Maseri, A. and Kluft, C. (1992). Vascular smooth muscle cells digest naturally produced extracellular matrices. *Circulation Research*, **71**:385–392.

Sporn, L.A., Marder, V.J. and Wagner, D.D. (1986). Inducible secretion of large biologically potent von Willebrand factor multimers. *Cell*, **46**:185–190.

Takada, A., Shizume, K., Ozawa, T., Takahashi, S. and Takada, Y. (1986). Characterization of various antibodies against plasminogen activator using highly sensitive enzyme immunoassays. *Thrombosis Research*, **42**:63–72.

Thompson, E.A., Nelles, L. and Collen, D. (1991). Effect of retinoic acid on the synthesis of tissue-type plasminogen activator and plasminogen activator inhibitor-1 in human endothelial cells. *European Journal of Biochemistry*, **201**:627–632.

Todd, A.S. (1958). Fibrinolysis autographs. *Nature*, **181**:495–496.

Todd, A.S. (1964). Localization of fibrinolytic activity in tissues. *British Medical Bulletin*, **20**:210–212.

Todd, A.S. (1969). The blood vessel wall and fibrinolytic activity. In *Dynamics of thrombus formation and dissolution*, S.A. Johnson and M.M. Guest (eds), pp. 321–339. Philadelphia: J.B. Lippincott.

Todd, A.S. (1972). Endothelium and fibrinolysis. *Bibliotheca Anatomica*, **12**:98–105.

Tranquille, N. (1991). Pharmacological modulation of the release of tissue-type plasminogen activator and von Willebrand factor. *Thesis*, University of Leiden.

Tranquille, N. and Emeis, J.J. (1989). Protein synthesis inhibition by cycloheximide does not affect the acute release of tissue-type plasminogen activator. *Thrombosis and Haemostasis*, **61**:442–447.

Tranquille, N. and Emeis, J.J. (1990). The simultaneous acute release of tissue-type plasminogen activator and von Willebrand factor in the perfused rat hindleg region. *Thrombosis and Haemostasis*, **63**:454–458.

Tranquille, N. and Emeis, J.J. (1991). On the role of calcium in the acute release of tissue-type plasminogen activator and von Willebrand factor from the rat perfused hindleg region. *Thrombosis and Haemostasis*, **66**:479–483.

Tranquille, N. and Emeis, J.J. (1992). The involvement of products of the phospholipase pathway in the acute release of tissue-type plasminogen activator from perfused rat hindlegs. *European Journal of Pharmacology*, **213**:285–292.

Tripathi, B.J., Geanon, J.D. and Tripathi, R.C. (1987). Distribution of tissue plasminogen activator in human and monkey eyes: an immunohistochemical study. *Ophthalmology*, **94**:1434–1438.

Tripathi, R.C., Tripathi, B.J. and Park, J.K. (1990). Localization of urokinase-type plasminogen activator in human eyes: an immunocytochemical study. *Experimental Eye Research*, **51**:545–552.

Underwood, M.J. and De Bono, D.P. (1993). Increased fibrinolytic activity in the intima of atheromatous coronary arteries: protection at a price. *Cardiovascular Research*, **27**:882–885.

Van Bennekum, A.M., Emeis, J.J., Kooistra, T. and Hendriks, H.F.J. (1993). Modulation of tissue-type plasminogen activator by retinoids in rat plasma and tissues. *American Journal of Physiology*, **264**:R931–R937.

Van Giezen, J.J.J., Boon G.d.I.A., Jansen, J.W.C.M. and Bouma, B.N. (1993). Retinoic acid enhances fibrinolytic activity *in vivo* by enhancing tissue plasminogen activator (t-PA) activity and inhibits venous thrombosis. *Thrombosis and Haemostasis*, **69**:381–386.

Van Hinsbergh, V.W.M. (1988). Synthesis and secretion of plasminogen activators and plasminogen activator inhibitor by endothelial cells. In *Tissue-type plasminogen activator: physiological and clinical aspects*, C. Kluft (ed.), volume 2, pp. 3–20. Boca Raton: CRC Press.

Van Hinsbergh, V.W.M., Sprengers, E.D. and Kooistra, T. (1987). Effect of thrombin on the production of plasminogen activators and PA inhibitor-1 by human foreskin microvascular endothelial cells. *Thrombosis and Haemostasis*, **57** 148–153.

Van Hinsbergh, V.W.M., Kooistra, T., Emeis, J.J. and Koolwijk, P. (1991). Regulation of plasminogen activator production by endothelial cells: role in fibrinolysis and local proteolysis. *International Journal of Radiation Biology*, **60**:261–272.

Van Leeuwen, R.T.J., Kol, A., Andreotti, F., Kluft, C., Maseri, A. and Sperti, G. (1994). Angiotensin II increases plasminogen activator inhibitor type 1 and tissue-type plasminogen activator messenger RNA in cultured rat aortic smooth muscle cells. *Circulation*, **90**:362–368.

Verheijen, J.H., Rijken, D.C., Chang, G.T.G., Preston, F.E. and Kluft C. (1984). Modulation of rapid plasminogen activator inhibitor in plasma by Stanozolol. *Thrombosis and Haemostasis*, **51**:396–397.

Wagner, D.D. (1990). Cell biology of von Willebrand factor. *Annual Review of Cell Biology*, **6**:217–246.

Wagner, D.D. and Bonfanti, R. (1991). Von Willebrand factor and the endothelium. *Mayo Clinic Proceedings*, **66**:621–627.

Wallnö fer, A.E., van Griensven, J.M.T., Schoemaker, H.C., Cohen, A.F., Lambert, W., Kluft, C., Meijer, P. and Kooistra, T. (1993). Effect of isotretinoin on endogenous tissue-type plasminogen activator (t-PA) and plasminogen activator inhibitor 1 (PAI-1) in humans. *Thrombosis and Haemostasis*, **70**:1005–1008.

Warren, B.A. (1964). Fibrinolytic activity of vascular endothelium. *British Medical Bulletin*, **20**:213–216.

Wun, T.-C. and Capuano, A. (1985). Spontaneous fibrinolysis in whole human plasma. Identification of tissue activator-related protein as the major plasminogen activator causing spontaneous activity *in vitro*. *Journal of Biological Chemistry*, **260**:5061–5066.

Wun, T.-C. and Capuano, A. (1987). Initiation and regulation of fibrinolysis in human plasma at the plasminogen activator level. *Blood*, **69**:1354–1362.

Zamarron, C., Lijnen, H.R., and Collen, D. (1984). Influence of exogenous and endogenous tissue-type plasminogen activator on the lysability of clots in a plasma milieu *in vitro*. *Thrombosis Research*, **35**:335–345.

11 Synthesis and Localization of PAI-1 in the Vessel Wall

Colleen Fearns, Fahumiya Samad and David J. Loskutoff

Department of Vascular Biology VB-3, The Scripps Research Institute, 10666 North Torrey Pines Road, La Jolla, CA 92037, USA

The plasminogen activator (PA) system provides an important source of proteolytic activity for a variety of physiological and pathological processes such as vascular fibrinolysis (Astrup, 1978; Collen and Lijnen, 1991; Vassalli *et al.*, 1991), angiogenesis (Vassalli *et al.*, 1991; Bacharach *et al.*, 1993), embryo implantation (Strickland *et al.*, 1976; Lala and Graham, 1990; Vassalli *et al.*, 1991), ovulation (Tsafriri *et al.*, 1989; Ohlsson *et al.*, 1991; Vassalli *et al.*, 1991;), tissue remodelling and tumor metastasis (Hart and Rehemtulla, 1988; Blasi and Verde, 1990; Liotta *et al.*, 1991). The primary regulator of plasminogen activation *in vivo* is type 1 plasminogen activator inhibitor (PAI-1), a rapid and specific inhibitor of both tissue-type and urokinase-type plasminogen activators (t-PA and u-PA), respectively (reviewed in Sprengers and Kluft, 1987; Loskutoff, 1988a). Limited clinical data suggest that abnormalities in the regulation of PAI-1 itself *in vivo* may contribute to the development of thrombotic or bleeding disease (reviewed in Loskutoff, 1991; Dawson and Henney, 1992). Most studies on the regulation of PAI-1 have used cultured cells. While such studies provide insights into the nature of molecules that regulate PAI-1 in the isolated cell growing *in vitro* in serum, their relevance to the regulation of PAI-1 in normal and pathological conditions *in vivo* remains to be determined. In this review, we summarize current knowledge of PAI-1 gene expression *in vivo*, from the nature of molecules now known to regulate it, to the tissues and cells that actually produce it. Special emphasis is placed on localization and synthesis of PAI-1 in the vessel wall.

BACKGROUND

Properties of PAI-1. PAI-1 is a single-chain glycoprotein of approximate M_r 50,000 daltons and is a member of the serine protease inhibitor (serpin) superfamily (Sprengers and Kluft, 1987; Carrell and Boswell, 1986; Loskutoff, 1991). The mature secreted form of PAI-1 consists of 379 amino acids, and lacks cysteine residues but contains multiple methionine residues. The reactive center of the inhibitor has been identified (Arg_{346}-Met_{347}), and is contained in the 'strained loop' region at the carboxy terminus of the molecule where it acts as a pseudosubstrate for the target serine protease. The reaction between PAI-1 and PA is rapid with second order rate constants above 10^7 $M^{-1}s^{-1}$. The human (Loskutoff *et al.*, 1987; Bosma *et al.*, 1988; Strandberg *et al.*, 1988), rat (Bruzdzinski *et al.*, 1990), and mouse (Prendergast *et al.*, 1990) PAI-1 genes have been isolated and characterized. In humans, PAI-1 is encoded by a single gene located on chromosome 7. The gene is 12.2kb in length, is organized into 9 exons and 8 introns, and gives rise to 2 distinct mRNA species (3.2kb and 2.3kb), which may be regulated differentially (Klinger *et al.*, 1987; Mayer *et al.*, 1988; Schleef *et al.*, 1988; van den Berg *et al.*, 1988; Follo and Ginsburg, 1989; Georg *et al.*, 1989). Only the higher molecular weight form of PAI-1 mRNA (3kb) is observed in rodents (Follo and Ginsburg, 1989; Bruzdzinski *et al.*, 1990; Prendergast *et al.*, 1990).

PAI-1 is a trace protein in plasma, ranging in concentration from 0 to 60 ng/ml under normal conditions, with an average of about 20 ng/ml (Booth *et al.*, 1988; Declerck *et al.*, 1988). It is also present in platelets (Erickson *et al.*, 1985) but at a much higher concentration (290ng/ml of blood). In fact it has been estimated that more than 90% of the total PAI-1 antigen in the blood is in platelets (Booth *et al.*, 1990). The inhibitor has been detected in both an active and an inactive state. It is synthesized in the active form by cultured cells but is unstable in solution and rapidly decays into the inactive (latent) form. The binding of PAI-1 to the adhesive glycoprotenectin stabilizes the inhibitor in its active conformation, thus increasing the biological half-life of the molecule (Declerck *et al.*, 1988). The majority of PAI-1 in plasma is active and circulates in complex with vitronectin (Wiman *et al.*, 1988; Declerck *et al.*, 1988). In contrast, the majority of PAI-1 detected in platelet extracts is latent (Booth *et al.*, 1990).

PAI-1 Biosynthesis in Vitro. PAI-1 is produced constitutively by a large variety of cells in culture including endothelial cells, smooth muscle cells, hepatocytes, granulosa cells, epithelial cells, megakaryocytes, fibroblasts and several tumor cell lines (reviewed in Loskutoff *et al.*, 1988b). However, the range of cells that constitutively produce it *in vivo* appears to be considerably more restricted (see below).

PAI-1 biosynthesis by cultured cells can be regulated by a diverse group of cytokines, growth factors and hormones. For the purpose of this review, we will focus on regulation of PAI-1 biosynthesis in cells of the vasculature (endothelial and smooth muscle cells; summarized in Table 11.1). One molecule of particular interest in this regard is endotoxin or lipopolysaccharide (LPS). Elevated plasma PAI-1 levels are found in patients with gram-negative septicemia (Colucci *et al.*, 1985; Pralong *et al.*, 1989). Moreover, PAI-1 levels in plasma of rabbits (Colucci *et al.*, 1985), rats (Quax *et al.*, 1990), and man (Suffredini *et al.*, 1989) increase dramatically after injection of low doses of LPS. Analysis of the effects of LPS on PAI-1 gene expression by cultured cells indicates that PAI-1 synthesis by human (Colucci *et al.*, 1985; Emeis and Kooistra, 1986; Hanss and Collen, 1987) and bovine (Crutchley and Conanan, 1986; Medina *et al.*, 1989; Sawdey *et al.*, 1989) endothelial cells is stimulated by LPS. Surprisingly, LPS has been shown to downregulate PAI-1 synthesis in cultured human monocytes (Hamilton *et al.*, 1993).

Table 11.1   Agents modulating PAI-1 in vascular cells *in vitro*

Agonist	Cell type	Reference
I. *STIMULATORS:*		
LPS	Human umbilical vein EC[1]	Colucci *et al.*, 1985; Emeis *et al.*, 1986; Hanss *et al.*, 1987
	Bovine aortic EC	Medina *et al.*, 1989; Sawdey *et al.*, 1989
	Bovine pulmonary artery EC	Crutchley *et al.*, 1986
TNF-α	Human umbilical vein EC	Schleef *et al.*, 1988; van Hinsbergh *et al.*, 1988
	Human umbilical arterial EC	van den Berg *et al.*, 1988
	Human foreskin microvascular EC	van Hinsbergh *et al.*, 1988
	Bovine aortic EC	Sawdey *et al.*, 1989; Medina *et al.*, 1989
IL-1	Human umbilical vein EC	Bevilacqua *et al.*, 1986b; Emeis *et al.*, 1986; Nachman *et al.*, 1986; Schleef *et al.*, 1988
	Human umbilical arterial EC	van den Berg *et al.*, 1988
	Human adult saphenous vein ESC	Bevilacqua *et al.*, 1986b
	Bovine aortic EC	Medina *et al.*, 1989
TGF-β	Human monocytes	Hamilton *et al.*, 1993
	Bovine aortic EC	Sawdey *et al.*, 1989
	Bovine capillary EC	Saksela *et al.*, 1987 Pepper *et al.*, 1990, 1991a
	Bovine vascular SM[2]	McFall *et al.*, 1990
bFGF	Bovine capillary EC	Saksela *et al.*, 1987
	Pepper *et al.*, 1990	
	Bovine lymphatic EC	Pepper *et al.*, 1994
PDGF	Bovine aortic EC	Slivka *et al.*, 1991b
	Bovine vascular SM	McFall *et al.*, 1990
	Rat vascular SM	Sperti *et al.*, 1992
VEGF	Bovine capillary EC	Pepper *et al.*, 1991b
	Bovine lymphatic EC	Pepper *et al.*, 1994
Thrombin	Human umbilical vein EC	Gelehrter *et al.*, 1986; Dichek *et al.*, 1989; Hanss *et al.*, 1987
	Human foreskin microvascular EC	van Hinsbergh *et al.*, 1987
	Human vascular SM	Noda-Heiny *et al.*, 1993; Wojta *et al.*, 1993
Glucocorticosteroids	Human umbilical vein EC	Partridge *et al.*, 1990
	Rabbit coronary microvascular EC	Partridge *et al.*, 1990
Lipoprotein(a)	Human umbilical vein EC	Etingin *et al.*, 1991
t-PA	Human umbilical vein EC	Fujii, 1990a

Table 11.1   (*Continued*)

Agonist	Cell type	Reference
II. *INHIBITORS:*		
LPS	Human monocytes	Hamilton *et al.*, 1993
Gemfibrozil	Human umbilical vein EC	Fujii *et al.*, 1993
Genistein	Human umbilical vein EC	van Hinsbergh *et al.*, 1994
Forskolin/IBMX	Bovine aortic EC	Santell *et al.*, 1988
	Human umbilical vein EC	Slivka *et al.*, 1991a
Herpes simplex virus	Human umbilical vein EC	Bok *et al.*, 1993

[1] EC denotes endothelial cells.
[2] SM denotes smooth muscle cells.

Endotoxin activates monocytes (Michalek *et al.*, 1980; Nathan, 1987) and endothelial cells (Gerritsen and Bloor, 1993) and leads to the elaboration of a variety of inflammatory cytokines. Cytokines are another group of molecules that induce PAI-1 biosynthesis. Tumor necrosis factor-α (TNF-α) (Schleef *et al.*, 1988; van den Berg *et al.*, 1988; van Hinsbergh *et al.*, 1988; Medina *et al.*, 1989; Sawdey *et al.*, 1989; Kooistra, 1990) and interleukin-1 (IL-1) (Bevilacqua *et al.*, 1986b; Emeis and Kooistra, 1986; Nachman *et al.*, 1986; van den Berg *et al.*, 1988; Medina *et al.*, 1989; Kooistra, 1990) both stimulate PAI-1 synthesis by endothelial cells. Interestingly, both of these cytokines also induce tissue factor activity in endothelial cells (Bevilacqua *et al.*, 1986a; Nawroth and Stern, 1986). The induction of tissue factor by inflammatory mediators such as TNF-α and IL-1 leads to the generation of thrombin which increases PAI-1 activity in umbilical vein endothelial cells (Gelehrter and Sznycer-Laszuk, 1986; Hanss and Collen, 1987; van Hinsbergh *et al.*, 1987; Dichek and Quertermous, 1989) and human smooth muscle cells (Noda-Heiny *et al.*, 1993; Wojta *et al.*, 1993).

One of the most potent growth factors known to stimulate PAI-1 expression is transforming growth factor-β (TGF-β), a polypeptide growth modulator present in platelets and released from platelet α-granules upon activation by thrombin. Picomolar concentrations of TGF-β significantly increased PAl-1 mRNA in endothelial cells (Saksela *et al.*, 1987; Sawdey *et al.*, 1989; Pepper *et al.*, 1990, 1991a), smooth muscle cells (McFall and Reilly, 1990) and monocytes (Hamilton *et al.*, 1993). It has been suggested that release of TGF-β from platelets at sites of vascular injury, inflammation and thrombosis may induce PAI-1 synthesis in surrounding endothelial cells (Loskutoff, 1988a) and thus suppress the fibrinolytic system of the vessel wall. This hypothesis is supported by recent observations that TGF-β from platelet extracts stimulates PAI-1 synthesis by endothelial cells (Slivka and Loskutoff, 1991b). Other growth factors reported to stimulate PAI-1 biosynthesis in vascular cells include platelet derived growth factor (PDGF) (McFall and Reilly, 1990; Slivka and Loskutoff, 1991b; Sperti *et al.*, 1992), and basic fibroblast growth factor (bFGF) (Saksela *et al.*, 1987; Pepper *et al.*, 1990, 1994) and vascular endothelial growth factor (VEGF) (Pepper *et al.*, 1991b, 1994).

Hormones and a variety of other agents also regulate PAI-1 biosynthesis. For example, corticosteroids stimulate PAI-1 synthesis in human and rabbit endothelial cells (Partridge and Gerritsen, 1990). PAI-1 biosynthesis is also stimulated by lipoprotein (a) (Etingin *et al.*, 1991), linking this atherogenic molecule to suppression of the fibrinolytic system.

In addition, atheromatous plaque macrophages both synthesize PAI-1 and stimulate PAI-1 production by endothelial cells and vascular smooth muscle cells (Tipping *et al.*, 1993). Lastly, excess t-PA itself may also stimulate PAI-1 biosynthesis (Fujii *et al.*, 1990a), suggesting the existence of a feed-back mechanism of regulation for this system.

Thus, a variety of agents have been shown to upregulate PAI-1 biosynthesis by cultured vascular cells. In comparison, the number of agents now known to downregulate PAI-1 expression is relatively small. For example, both basal and stimulated PAI-1 expression in endothelial cells is decreased by pharmacological concentrations of gemfibrozil, a lipid lowering drug (Fujii *et al.*, 1993). In addition, Genistein, a dietary-derived inhibitor of *in vitro* angiogenesis inhibits PAI-1 production in vascular endothelial cells (van Hinsbergh *et al.*, 1994). Similarly, agents that increase intracellular cAMP, such as forskolin and isobutylmethylxanthine (IBMX), have been shown to decrease both basal expression of PAI-1 as well as induced PAI-1 expression (Santell and Levin, 1988; Slivka and Loskutoff, 1991a). Decreased PAI-1 was also observed after viral (Herpes simplex) infection of human umbilical vein endothelial cells (Bok *et al.*, 1993). Lastly, the combination of heparin and endothelial cell growth factor downregulates PAI-1 synthesis in endothelial cells (Konkle and Ginsburg, 1988).

The diversity of molecules that modulate PAI-1 biosynthesis implies that the regulatory region of the PAI-1 gene must be unusually complex, containing DNA sequences that are either directly, or indirectly, responsive to all of these molecules. DNA response elements within the first 800 bp of the 5' flanking region of the human PAI-1 gene that might be important for regulation by dexamethasone (van Zonneveld *et al.*, 1988) and TGF-β (Keeton *et al.*, 1991; Riccio *et al.*, 1992) have been identified.

In summary, most of the early data on PAI-1 regulation have been obtained from cells in culture. It is well known that cultured cells undergo phenotypic and genotypic changes after several passages *in vitro*, and although some insights can be gained by studying the regulation of gene expression in isolated cells in culture, such results must be interpreted with caution. For one thing, cultured cells have been removed from their normal milieu where interactions with other cells, other factors and extracellular matrix play such a vital role. For another, vascular cells are normally exposed to plasma, not serum. Therefore, data on biosynthesis and regulation obtained from *in vitro* systems needs to be validated *in vivo*.

PHYSIOLOGICAL ROLE OF PAI-1 *in vivo*

It is generally assumed that vascular homeostasis results from the regulated interaction of the coagulation and fibrinolytic systems, and that these two systems are in dynamic equilibrium. The net fibrinolytic activity of cells and of blood is the result of the balance between the PAs on the one hand and PAI-1 on the other. Thus, changes in either the PAs or PAI-1 may alter this balance and lead to thrombotic problems or to a tendency to develop a bleeding diathesis.

Several individuals have now been identified with little or no detectable functional PAI-1 in their blood and all have had lifelong bleeding problems (Francis *et al.*, 1986; Schleef *et al.*, 1989; Dieval *et al.*, 1991; Fay *et al.*, 1992; Lee *et al.*, 1993). Moreover, in mice, disruption of the PAI-1 gene was associated with a mild hyperfibrinolytic state and increased resistance to thrombosis (Carmeliet *et al.*, 1993).

In contrast, individuals with elevated levels of the inhibitor tend to be at risk to develop thrombotic problems. For example, PAI-1 increases during the second and third trimester of pregnancy, the same period when the risk for thrombosis increases (Kruithof *et al.*, 1987). Familial thrombosis has been associated with an inherited elevation of plasma PAI-1 activity in a number of families (Berdeaux and Marlar, 1991; Schved *et al.*, 1991). In addition, elevated levels of PAI-1 mRNA are associated with severely atherosclerotic human arteries (Schneiderman *et al.*, 1992; Lupu *et al.*, 1993) and myocardial infarction (Hamsten *et al.*, 1985; Keber and Keber, 1992). Large increases in circulating PAI-1 are observed during gram-negative infections (Colucci *et al.*, 1985), which are also frequently associated with disseminated intravascular coagulation (Wada *et al.*, 1993a). Elevations in plasma PAI-1 levels may also be present in individuals with metabolic disorders associated with the development of atherosclerosis (Juhan-Vague and Alessi, 1993). Significant correlations have been established between PAI-1 levels and obesity (Legnani *et al.*, 1988; Vague *et al.*, 1989; Potter van Loon *et al.*, 1993; McGill *et al.*, 1994), non-insulin-dependent diabetes (Takada *et al.*, 1993), hypercholesterolemia (Wada *et al.*, 1993b), hyperinsulinemia (Juhan-Vague *et al.*, 1984; Sundell *et al.*, 1989) and hypertriglyceridemia (Sundell *et al.*, 1989), all conditions associated with an increased risk for thrombosis. While these examples emphasize that elevations in the concentration of PAI-1 may be associated with the pathogenesis of thrombotic disease, they remain, at best, only correlative. More definitive proof of the critical role that PAI-1 may play in regulating fibrinolysis has been obtained from a number of animal models developed recently, which directly address this issue.

Transgenic mice carrying the human PAI-1 cDNA under the control of the murine metallothionine promoter were born with high levels of PAI-1 in their blood which peaked soon after birth and then subsided (Erickson *et al.*, 1990). These animals developed venous thrombi and lesions in the tail, hind quarters and feet within the first week after birth, which receded as PAI-1 expression diminished. These results suggest a link between the existence of venous occlusions and expression of the transgene. The role of elevated PAI-1 activity in promoting fibrin deposition has also been studied in rabbits. In this model, ancrod (a venom-derived enzyme that clots fibrinogen) did not induce fibrin deposition in normal rabbits. However, it did induce fibrin deposition in LPS-treated rabbits (which have high levels of PAI-1), and in rabbits administered recombinant PAI-1 (Krishnamurti *et al.*, 1993). These results demonstrate that inhibition of the fibrinolytic system by PAI-1 is necessary for pathological fibrin deposition in ancrod-treated rabbits. In other studies, fibrin degradation in rabbits was inhibited in a dose-dependent manner by infusion of rPAI-1 (Knabb *et al.*, 1990), and high levels of circulating and clot-bound PAI-1 significantly inhibited clot lysis in a rat model of pulmonary embolism (Reilly *et al.*, 1991). Lastly, inhibition of PAI-1 activity by a monoclonal anti-human PAI-1 antibody enhanced endogenous thrombolysis and partially prevented thrombus extension in a rabbit model for thrombosis (Levi *et al.*, 1992).

The above examples provide experimental evidence to support the notion that PAI-1 synthesis *in vivo* must be precisely regulated, and that abnormalities in this regulation may be associated with the pathogenesis of vascular disease. It follows from this that understanding the nature of signals that regulate PAI-1 synthesis *in vivo* and delineating their mechanism of action may provide new insights into the role of the fibrinolytic system in vascular disease.

PAI-1 BIOSYNTHESIS *in vivo*

The origin of plasma PAI-1 under normal and pathological conditions and the tissues/cells involved in the synthesis of PAI-1 *in vivo* in man are largely unknown. Although the majority of PAI-1 in blood is present in platelets, platelets themselves do not appear to constitute a major source of plasma PAI-1 under normal conditions (Booth *et al.*, 1990). Analysis of PAI-1 protein levels in normal human tissues showed relatively high levels in liver, spleen, kidney and lung (Simpson *et al.*, 1991). It is not clear whether these results reflect synthesis of PAI-1, clearance of PAI-1 from plasma or circulating platelets, or storage of PAI-1. These ambiguities can begin to be resolved by determining the level of PAI-1 gene expression *in vivo* (i.e., by determining the concentrations of mRNA) in the various tissues, and by comparing the human results with results obtained using more carefully controlled animal models.

Normal tissue distribution of PAI-1 mRNA. The normal tissue distribution of PAI-1 mRNA has been examined in humans as well as in rodent model systems (Lucore *et al.*, 1988; Quax *et al.*, 1990; Sawdey and Loskutoff, 1991) (Table 11.2). For example, Northern blot analysis revealed high levels of PAI-1 mRNA in a number of highly vascularized human tissues, including placenta, uterus, myocardium and liver (Lucore *et al.*, 1988). In the rat, PAI-1 mRNA was detected mainly in the lung, with low levels detected in the heart (Quax

Table 11.2 Normal tissue distribution of PAI-1 *in vivo*

	Mouse		Human		Rat	
Tissues	*mRNA[1]*	*Protein[2]*	*mRNA*	*Protein*	*mRNA*	*Protein*
Aorta	2.018±0.358					
Adipose	0.606±0.070					
Heart	0.583±0.149	0.8	+	30.1	+	
Lung	0.357±0.196	0.1		108.1	++	
Muscle	0.180±0.102		+		−	
Kidney	0.091±0.031	ND[3]		279.4	−	
Adrenal	0.079±0.020					+
Thymus	0.048±0.028					
Brain	0.026±0.009	0.1		9.8		
Testis	0.024±0.010					
Liver	0.021±0.007	6.1	++	804.3	−	
Spleen	0.019±0.007	ND		534.4		
GIT	ND		−			
Placenta			+++			
Uterus			+			
Ovary					+	
Appendix			+[4]			
Platelets				620 ng/10^9		

[1] In the mouse, mRNA levels are expressed as pg PAI-1 mRNA/μg total RNA (Sawdey *et al.*, 1991). Absolute values for human and rat tissues are not known. Thus these results are expressed as relative levels with high levels expressed as +++, moderate levels as ++, and low levels as +. Values are taken from Lucore *et al.*, 1988 and Whawell *et al.*, 1993 (human tissues), and Quax *et al.*, 1990 and Chun *et al.*, 1992 (rat tissues).
[2] Protein levels are expressed as ng PAI-1/g wet weight of tissue. Figures are taken from Erickson *et al.*, 1990 (mouse tissues) and Simpson *et al.*, 1991 (human tissues). Levels have not been quantitated in rat tissues. In the column for rat protein, + signifies PAI-1 antigen detected by immunohistochemistry (Eriksen *et al.*, 1989).
[3] ND, not determined.
[4] Inflamed appendix.

et al., 1990). Studies from our lab on the normal distribution of PAI-1 mRNA in the mouse demonstrated relatively high levels in the aorta, lung, adipose tissue and myocardium, with intermediate levels in skeletal muscle and thymus (Sawdey and Loskutoff, 1991). Low but significant levels were detected in the liver and kidney. The finding of detectable levels of PAI-1 mRNA in most tissues examined, raises the possibility that plasma PAI-1 may originate from a variety of tissues under normal conditions, and suggests that some ubiquitous cell type, possibly endothelial or smooth muscle cells of the vasculature, or smooth muscle cells/fibroblasts of connective tissue, may be responsible for its production.

The high level of PAI-1 production by virtually all cultured endothelial cells (reviewed in Loskutoff *et al.*, 1988b) suggested that these cells may constitutively produce PAI-1 *in vivo*. Unexpectedly, *in situ* hybridization studies to localize PAI-1 mRNA producing cells in tissues of control mice revealed that endothelial cells in the large vessels as well as in the microvasculature of most organs (liver, kidney, heart, lung, adipose) were negative for PAI-1 mRNA. Although no PAI-1 mRNA was detected in vascular endothelium in normal mouse tissues, a weak hybridization signal for PAI-1 mRNA was consistently detected in vascular as well as non-vascular smooth muscle cells. For example, smooth muscle cells in the aorta, as well as in the vasculature of kidney, heart, liver and adipose tissue showed weak positivity for PAI-1 mRNA. A representative example of PAI-1 expression in vascular cells is shown in Figure 11.1. A positive PAI-1 signal also was

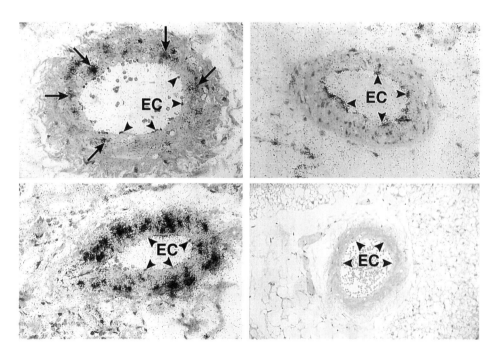

Figure 11.1 Cellular localization of PAI-1 mRNA in the vessel wall. Paraffine sections from mouse kidney were analyzed by *in situ* hybridization for PAI-1 mRNA as described in Keeton *et al.*, 1993. **Upper left**: Arteriole from kidney of an untreated mouse, showing PAI-1 mRNA in the smooth muscle cells of the tunica media (arrows). Note the endothelial cells (EC) are negative for PAI-1 mRNA. **Upper right**: Arteriole from kidney of an LPS-treated mouse, showing positive hybridization signal in EC. **Lower left**: Arteriole from kidney of a TGF-β-treated mouse, showing induction of PAI-1 mRNA in smooth muscle cells. **Lower right**: Arteriole from kidney of an untreated mouse hybridized with the sense riboprobe. No hybridization is seen.

detected in non-vascular smooth muscle cells underlying such structures as the bronchioles in lung and the bile duct in liver. These results suggest that smooth muscle cells from a variety of tissues may be involved in normal PAI-1 expression in the mouse. In addition to these results, a weak signal was observed in the myocardium and the renal papilla. The specific PAI-1 producing cells in these tissues remain to be determined.

In contrast to the results with murine vessels, PAI-1 immunoreactivity was detected in both endothelial cells and in the smooth muscle cell layer of human arteries and veins (Simpson *et al.*, 1991). PAI-1 mRNA was not measured in this study. In other studies, PAI-1 mRNA was detected in the smooth muscle cells of the tunica media and in luminal endothelial cells of normal human arteries (Schneiderman *et al.*, 1992; Lupu *et al.*, 1993). Data regarding the normal cellular distribution of PAI-1 in human tissues needs to be interpreted with caution, since most samples of human tissues are obtained from individuals undergoing surgery for various disease conditions. PAI-1 is an acute phase protein in humans (Aillaud *et al.*, 1985; Kluft *et al.*, 1985; Kruithof *et al.*, 1988), and its concentration in plasma increases during trauma, infection and surgery. Thus, the above results may not accurately reflect the normal *in vivo* cellular distribution of PAI-1.

In summary, it appears that both murine and human smooth muscle cells constitutively produce PAI-1 under normal conditions. In the human, in addition to the smooth muscle cells, the endothelial cells may also produce PAI-1.

PAI-1 expression after LPS, TNFα or TGF-β treatment. The concentration of plasma PAI-1 increases dramatically during endotoxemia (Colucci *et al.*, 1985). Moreover, LPS was shown to induce PAI-1 mRNA in the heart, lung, kidney and liver of the rat (Quax *et al.*, 1990) and in virtually all tissues of the mouse including liver, kidney, heart, lung, adipose, testes, brain, thymus, aorta, spleen, adrenals, gut, and muscle (Table 11.3) (Sawdey and Loskutoff, 1991). These observations suggest that plasma PAI-1 may originate from multiple tissues during sepsis. *In situ* hybridization performed to determine the cellular localization of PAI-1 mRNA in various mouse tissues after endotoxin treatment revealed a strong signal within endothelial cells at all levels of the vasculature, including larger arteries, veins and capillaries (Figure 11.1). For example, initial experiments focusing on the kidney from LPS-treated mice, showed a strong hybridization signal for PAI-1 in glomerular and peritubular cells in the cortex (Keeton *et al.*, 1993). These cells stained positively for von Willebrand factor antigen, an endothelial cell specific marker. The PAI-1 mRNA hybridization signal could further be observed in peritubular endothelial cells in the medulla and in the endothelial cells of veins and arteries throughout the kidney. Immunochemical analysis revealed that PAI-1 antigen co-localized to the cytoplasm of cells expressing PAI-1 mRNA. The cellular localization of PAI-1 mRNA after endotoxin treatment was also studied in the liver, heart, lung and adipose tissue (Fearns, Keeton and Loskutoff, submitted). In each of these organs, PAI-1 mRNA was induced in endothelial cells within the vessels, both within larger vessels (e.g., aorta and pulmonary vein) as well as within the capillary endothelium. Within the heart, the endocardium also showed a strong positive signal. Again, the endothelial cell origin of PAI-1 producing cells was confirmed by immunohistochemistry using an antibody to von Willebrand factor. Thus, the predominant cell type induced by LPS to produce PAI-1 mRNA in the mouse appears to be the endothelial cell in most organs (Eguchi *et al.*, 1991; Fearns *et al.*, 1992).

It should be noted that the response to LPS in the mouse was not restricted to the endothelium. Notable exceptions include the adipose tissue and liver. In the adipose

Table 11.3 Induction of PAI-1 gene expression *in vivo*

Tissues	LPS	TNF-α	TGF-β
MURINE:			
Aorta	+	ND	ND
Adipose	+	+	++
Heart	+	+	+
Lung	+++	++	+
Muscle	+	+	+
Kidney	+++	++	++
Adrenal	++	++	ND
Thymus	+	+	ND
Liver	++++	++	+
Spleen	+	+	+
RAT:			
Lung	+++		
Liver	++		
Kidney	+		
Heart	+		
Muscle	+		
RABBITS:[1]			
Aorta			+
Heart			++
Lung			−
Muscle			−
Kidney			−
Liver			++
Spleen			−

Results expressed as relative induction with very high induction expressed as ++++, high induction as +++, moderate induction as ++, and low induction as +. Values are taken from Sawdey *et al.*, 1991 (mouse tissues); Quax *et al.*, 1990 (rat tissues); and Fujii and Sobel, 1990 (rabbit tissues).
[1] Induction of PAI-1 mRNA in response to infusion of platelet lysates. Plasma PAI-1 increases were markedly attenuated by pretreatment of platelet lysate with a neutralizing anti-TGF-β antibody.

tissue, PAI-1 mRNA was induced in the endothelial cells and smooth muscle cells of the larger vessels and the microvasculature, and in cells that morphologically and biochemically resembled adipocytes (Samad *et al.*, 1994; Samad *et al.*, 1996). In the liver, in addition to induction within the sinusoidal endothelium, PAI-1 mRNA was also induced in hepatocytes (Fearns *et al.*, 1993). Similarly, analysis of isolated and fractionated rat liver cells showed that the marked increase in PAI-1 mRNA after endotoxin injection is mainly due to a strong increase of PAI-1 mRNA in the endothelial cell fraction. However, PAI-1 mRNA could also be detected within the hepatocyte and Kupffer cell fractions (Quax *et al.*, 1990; Podor *et al.*, 1993). In contrast to these results, dexamethasone transiently induced PAI-1 expression in rat hepatocytes without increasing PAI-1 expression in sinusoidal endothelial cells (Konkle *et al.*, 1992).

Many of the effects of endotoxin are mediated through the release of TNF-α and studies from our lab show that most of the same tissues of the mouse that produce PAI-1 in response to endotoxin (e.g.,liver, kidney, heart, lung) also produce it in response to TNF-α (Table 11.3). Again the major cell type within these tissues that responded to

TNF-α were the endothelial cells (Fearns, Keeton and Loskutoff, submitted). The adipose tissue was again an exception. While there was a weak induction of PAI-1 mRNA in the endothelial cells, there was also relatively strong induction in the smooth muscle cells, the adventitial cells, and in cells that morphologically resembled adipocytes (Samad *et al.*, 1994).

TGF-β induces plasma PAI-1 activity in rabbits (Fujii and Sobel, 1990b), and PAI-1 mRNA in the mouse (Table 11.3) (Sawdey and Loskutoff, 1991). In the mouse, in contrast to the results obtained after LPS and TNF-α treatment, induction of PAI-1 mRNA was not detected within the endothelium (Figure 11.1). In this case PAI-1 mRNA was induced in vascular and non-vascular smooth muscle cells. In addition, induction was also observed in the myocardium and the papilla region of the kidney. Thus TGF-β appeared to increase the rate of PAI-1 mRNA synthesis in the cells that make it constitutively (i.e., smooth muscle cells), without any apparent change in the cellular distribution (Fearns *et al.*, 1992).

The induction of PAI-1 expression by LPS and TNF-α *in vivo* occurred primarily in endothelial cells in most mouse tissues. These observations are in agreement with results obtained *in vitro*, since both agents induced PAI-1 expression in various bovine and human endothelial cells in culture. This is in contrast to the results obtained with TGF-β. In culture, TGF-β induced PAI-1 expression in both bovine smooth muscle cells and bovine endothelial cells (Sawdey *et al.*, 1989; Saksela *et al.*, 1987; McFall and Reilly, 1990) whereas, in the mouse, TGF-β induced PAI-1 expression only in smooth muscle cells. Whether this apparent inconsistency reflects differences between *in vitro* and *in vivo* systems or between species remains to be determined.

PAI-1 gene expression in atherosclerosis. Although the majority of patients with generalized arterial atherosclerosis exhibit normal plasma fibrinolytic profiles, the local fibrinolytic balance in these patients may be severely disturbed. Intravascular or mural thrombosis is a frequent histologic feature of atherosclerotic lesions and appears to play a role in the intimal thickening and fibrosis characteristic of advanced lesions (Juhan-Vague and Collen, 1992). To determine if localized alterations in fibrinolytic activity could influence this process, we evaluated PAI-1 mRNA expression in segments of 11 severely diseased and 5 relatively normal human arteries obtained from patients undergoing reconstructive surgery for aortic occlusive or aneurysmal disease (Schneiderman *et al.*, 1992). PAI-1 mRNA levels as analyzed by Northern blot analysis were significantly increased in severely atherosclerotic vessels compared with normal or mildly affected arteries. In most cases, the level of PAI-1 gene expression correlated with the degree of atherosclerosis. Analysis by *in situ* hybridization demonstrated an abundance of PAI-1 mRNA-positive cells within the thickened intima of atherosclerotic arteries, mainly around the base of the plaque, and in cells scattered within the necrotic material. In contrast to these results, PAI-1 mRNA was detected primarily within the luminal endothelial cells of normal-appearing aortic tissues (Schneiderman *et al.*, 1992). These observations have recently been confirmed and extended by Lupu *et al.*, (1993). These authors found that both endothelial cells and smooth muscle cells of normal arteries were positive for PAI-1 antigen and mRNA. In advanced atherosclerotic lesions, increased expression of PAI-1 was seen in the smooth muscle cells within the fibrous cap of the necrotic core. In addition, large quantities of PAI-1 were present in the extracellular matrix in close association with elastic laminae and collagen bundles. In another study, PAI-1 was localized to both cellular (endothelial and smooth muscle cells) and extracellular (intimal collagen fibers) components of human coronary atherosclerotic lesions (Yorimitsu *et al.*, 1993). In addition to these observations, a disturbance in local fibrinolytic balance also has been shown in a rabbit model. Induction of arterial thrombosis in rabbit carotid arteries increased expression of PAI-1 mRNA and antigen in the endothelium juxtaposed to the thrombi, in smooth muscle cells adjacent to the neointima and in macrophages (Sawa *et al.*, 1992). Qualitatively similar but much more marked increases in PAI-1 gene expression were seen when arterial injury was accompanied by hypercholesterolemia (Sawa *et al.*, 1993).

PAI-1 expression in other diseases. Many renal diseases are associated with fibrin deposition in the glomeruli (Holdsworth and Tipping, 1985; Takemura *et al.*, 1987; Kamitsuji *et al.*, 1988; Tomosugi *et al.*, 1990), and again may reflect abnormalities in the balance between coagulation and fibrinolysis. To investigate the possibility that overexpression of PAI-1 in the glomerulus may contribute to the pathology of renal disease, PAI-1 expression was studied in mice which develop early onset lupus glomerulonephritis (GN) (i.e., in female MRL/lpr mice) (Keeton *et al.*, 1995). Unlike the results with LPS, TNF-α and TGF-β (Table 11.3) where relatively specific expression was observed, a variety of cells were observed to produce PAI-1 in these GN mice. PAI-1 levels were expressed in relatively high levels in the kidneys of diseased mice, both within the glomeruli and in the tubules and vessels. PAI-1 expression was localized not only to endothelial cells, but also to parietal epithelial cells, tubular epithelial cells, and infiltrating mononuclear cells in the tubulointerstitium. The inappropriate expression of PAI-1 in the kidney of mice with lupus GN suggests that PAI-1 may play a role in the pathogenesis of this disease process. This possibility is supported by studies employing another murine model of autoimmune renal disease ((NZB x NZW) F_1). In this model, severe caloric restriction was found to delay the onset time and reduce the severity of disease. In a recent study, glomeruli of mice fed *ad libitum* showed much greater deposition of PAI-1 protein, increased expression of PAI-1 mRNA and more severe histological abnormalities than animals on a calorie restricted diet (Troyer *et al.*, 1995). These observations indicate that the known ameliorating effects of caloric restriction on disease include diminished PAI-1 gene expression as well as decreased localization of PAI-1 in the glomeruli.

PAI-1 also appears to be abnormally regulated in some cancers (Hart and Rehemtulla, 1988; Liotta *et al.*, 1991). These studies suggest that PAI-1 may play an important role in several malignant processes, such as tumorigenicity, invasion, metastasis, and neovascularization (Hart and Rehemtulla, 1988; Liotta *et al.*, 1991). In fact, high levels of PAI-1 are associated with a poor prognosis in several different tumors including gastric and breast carcinomas, as well as brain, ovarian and lung tumors (Janicke *et al.*, 1993; Pujade-Lauraine *et al.*, 1993; Bouchet *et al.*, 1994; Landau *et al.*, 1994; Nekarda *et al.*, 1994; Pedersen *et al.*, 1994). Few reports show the localization of PAI-1 within vessels in tumors. Studies in human colon carcinomas localized PAI-1 mRNA to vascular endothelial cells in the stroma immediately surrounding the invasive tumor glands, in granulation tissue and in some capillaries within the tumor (Pyke *et al.*, 1991). In human intracranial tumors, strong positivity for PAI-1 antigen was seen in proliferative vessels within high grade gliomas and metastatic tumors, as well as in blood vessels near necrotic foci (Kono *et al.*, 1994). In these studies, PAI-1 was localized in the vascular basement membrane and perivascular connective tissue, while endothelial cells themselves showed only weak reactivity. In contrast, an immunochemical study on Lewis lung carcinoma transplanted in mice showed PAI-1 protein in the tumor cells themselves (Kristensen *et al.*, 1990).

PAI-1 BINDING PROTEINS IN THE VESSEL WALL

The molecules to which PAI-1 binds in the vessel wall have been the subject of considerable attention. Vitronectin has been shown to localize and concentrate PAI-1 in the endothelial cell extracellular matrix (Preissner *et al.*, 1990; Seiffert *et al.*, 1990), and thus could be a potential PAI-1 binding protein in the vessel wall. In a recent study, vitronectin was found to co-localize with PAI-1 in extracellular areas of advanced atherosclerotic lesions (Lupu *et al.*, 1993). Preliminary results from our lab indicate that this is not always the case, that PAI-1 immunoreactivity frequently does not co-localize with vitronectin (van Aken and Loskutoff, unpublished observations). These observations suggest that other PAI-1 binding proteins must exist. It is known that PAI-1 binds to fibrin (Wagner *et al.*, 1989) and to negatively charged phospholipids (Lambers *et al.*, 1987), both of which are present in platelet-rich thrombi and can be incorporated as intramural thrombi into the atherosclerotic vessel wall (Woolf, 1981). PAI-1 also binds to vimentin-type intermediate filaments (Podor *et al.*, 1992), raising the possibility that the accumulation of this inhibitor at sites of cell damage and necrosis may promote the fibrin deposition frequently observed in such areas.

CONCLUSION

While much is known about regulation of PAI-1 biosynthesis *in vitro*, our knowledge of the tissue/cellular distribution and regulation of PAI-1 gene expression *in vivo* is still limited. What is apparent from these limited studies is that PAI-1 mRNA is widely distributed in most tissues under normal conditions. This suggests that many tissues may contribute to plasma PAI-1 and that some common cell/s is responsible for its production. From the mouse studies, it appears that PAI-1 mRNA is localized primarily to smooth muscle cells, both vascular and non-vascular. Human tissues on the other hand also contain PAI-1 in endothelial cells. Whether this represents true constitutive expression under basal conditions or is a reflection of a state of activation of these cells due to disease or trauma cannot be determined for reasons outlined above.

Induction of PAI-1 by agents such as LPS, TNF-α and TGF-β in the rat and mouse, and increases in PAI-1 in some pathological conditions such as atherosclerosis, appear to be relatively specific and are restricted to a limited number of cell types. For example, the endothelial cell from all levels of the vasculature is the LPS and TNF-α responsive cell in the mouse. In atherosclerosis, PAI-1 expression has been localized primarily to smooth muscle cells. However, in autoimmune diseases such as GN, a broad spectrum of cell types is observed to produce PAI-1, including endothelial cells, tubular epithelium and inflammatory cells. This observation may reflect the involvement of many different cell systems and cytokines in such diseases.

In conclusion, the inappropriate expression of PAI-1 *in vivo* may alter the fibrinolytic balance systemically, as seen in endotoxemia, or locally, as seen in atherosclerosis and glomerulonephritis. While the systemic increase in PAI-1 activity may result from its increased biosynthesis in endothelial cells throughout the vasculature, the local induction of PAI-1 activity may be a reflection of the action of mediators of inflammatory or repair processes on specific cells of the vessel wall. Continued investigation into the nature of signals that regulate PAI-1 synthesis *in vivo* and delineation of their mechanisms of action, will ultimately help to clarify the role of PAI-1 in vascular disease.

References

Aillaud, M.F., Juhan-Vague, I., Alessi, M.C., Marecal, M., Vinson, M.F., Arnaud, C., Vague, P.H. and Collen, D. (1985). Increased PA-inhibitor levels in the postoperative period: no cause-effect relation with increased cortisol. *Thromb. Haemost.*, **54**:466–468.

Astrup, T. (1978). Fibrinolysis: An overview. In: *Progress in Chemical Fibrinolysis and Thrombolysis*, Davidson, J.F., Rowan, R.M., Samama, M.M. and Desnoyers, P.C. (eds.), pp. 1–57. New York: Raven Press, Ltd.

Bacharach, E., Itin, A. and Keshet, E. (1993). *In vivo* patterns of expression of urokinase and its inhibitor PAI-1 suggest a concerted role in regulating physiological angiogenesis. *Proc. Natl. Acad. Sci. USA*, **89**:10686–10690.

Berdeaux, D. and Marlar, R. (1991). Report of an American family with elevated PAI as a cause of multiple thromboses response to prednisone. *Thromb. Haemost.*, **65**:1044 (Abstract).

Bevilacqua, M.P., Pober, J.S., Majeau, G.R., Fiers, W., Cotran, R.S. and Gimbrone, M.A., Jr. (1986a). Recombinant tumor necrosis factor induces procoagulant activity in cultured human vascular endothelium: Characterization and comparison with the actions of interleukin 1. *Proc. Natl. Acad. Sci. USA*, **83**:4533–4537.

Bevilacqua, M.P., Schleef, R.R., Gimbrone, M.A., Jr. and Loskutoff, D.J. (1986b). Regulation of the fibrinolytic system of cultured human vascular endothelium by interleukin 1. *J. Clin. Invest.*, **78**:587–591.

Blasi, F. and Verde, P. (1990). Urokinase-dependent cell surface proteolysis and cancer. *Semin. Cancer Biol.*, **1**:117–126.

Bok, R.A., Jacob, H.S., Balla, J., Juckett, M., Stella, T., Shatos, M.A. and Vercellotti, G.M. (1993). Herpes simplex virus decreases endothelial cell plasminogen activator inhibitor. *Thromb. Haemost.*, **69**:253–258.

Booth, N.A., Croll, A. and Bennett, B. (1990). The activity of plasminogen activator inhibitor-1 (PAI-1) of human platelet. *Fibrinolysis*, **4** (**Suppl 2**), 138–140.

Booth, N.A., Simpson, A.J., Croll, A., Bennett, B. and MacGregor, I.R. (1988). Plasminogen activator inhibitor (PAI-1) in plasma and platelets. *Br. J. Haematol.*, **70**:327–333.

Bosma, P.J., van den Berg, E.A., Kooistra, T., Siemieniak, D.R. and Slightom, J.L. (1988). Human plasminogen activator inhibitor-1 gene. *J. Biol. Chem.*, **263**:9129–9141.

Bouchet, C., Spyratos, F., Martin, P.M., Hacene, K., Gentile, A. and Oglobine, J. (1994). Prognostic value of urokinase-type plasminogen activator (uPA) and plasminogen activator inhibitors PAI-1 and PAI-2 in breast carcinomas. *Br. J. Cancer*, **69**:398–405.

Bruzdzinski, C.J., Riordan-Johnson, M., Nordby, E.C., Suter, S.M. and Gelehrter, T.D. (1990). Isolation and characterization of the rat plasminogen activator inhibitor-1 gene. *J. Biol. Chem.*, **265**:2078–2085.

Carmeliet, P., Stassen, J.M., Schoonjans, L., Ream, B., Van den Oord, J.J., De Mol, M., Mulligan, R.C. and Collen, D. (1993). Plasminogen activator inhibitor-1 gene-deficient mice. II. Effects on hemostasis, thrombosis, and thrombolysis. *J. Clin. Invest.*, **92**:2756–2760.

Carrell, R.W. and Boswell, D.R. (1986). Serpins: The superfamily of plasma serine proteinase inhibitors. In: Proteinase Inhibitors, Barrett, A.J. and Salvesen, G. (eds.), pp. 403–420. Amsterdam: Elsevier Science Publishers.

Chun, S.-Y., Popliker, M., Reich, R. and Tsafriri, A. (1992). Localization of preovulatory expression of plasminogen activator inhibitor type-1 and tissue inhibitor of metalloproteinase type-1 mRNAs in the rat ovary. *Biol. Reprod.*, **47**:245–253.

Collen, D. and Lijnen, H.R. (1991). Basic and clinical aspects of fibrinolysis and thrombolysis. *Blood*, **78**:3114–3124.

Colucci, M., Paramo, J.A. and Collen, D. (1985). Generation in plasma of a fast-acting inhibitor of plasminogen activator in response to endotoxin stimulation. *J. Clin. Invest.*, **75**:818–824.

Crutchley, D.J. and Conanan, L.B. (1986). Endotoxin induction of an inhibitor of plasminogen activator in bovine pulmonary artery endothelial cells. *J. Biol. Chem.*, **261**:154–159.

Dawson, S. and Henney, A. (1992). The status of PAI-1 as a risk factor for arterial and thrombotic disease: A review. *Atherosclerosis*, **95**:105–117.

Declerck, P.J., De Mol, M., Alessi, M-C., Baudner, S., Paques, E-P., Preissner, K.T., Muller-Berghaus, G. and Collen, D. (1988). Purification and characterization of a plasminogen activator inhibitor 1 binding protein from human plasma. *J. Biol. Chem.*, **263**:15454–15461.

Dichek, D. and Quertermous, T. (1989). Thrombin regulation of mRNA levels of tissue plasminogen activator and plasminogen activator inhibitor-1 in cultured human umbilical vein endothelial cells. *Blood*, **74**:222–228.

Dieval, J., Nguyen, G., Gross, S., Delobel, J. and Kruithof, E.K.O. (1991). A lifelong bleeding disorder associated with a deficiency of plasminogen activator inhibitor type 1. *Blood*, **77**:528–532.

Eguchi, Y., Keeton, M., Sawdey, M. and Loskutoff, D.J. (1991). Endotoxin induces the expression of type 1 plasminogen activator inhibitor (PAI-1) protein and mRNA by endothelial cells in mouse tissues *in vivo*. *Thromb. Haemost.*, **65**:652 (Abstract).

Emeis, J.J. and Kooistra, T. (1986). Interleukin 1 and lipopolysaccharide induce an inhibitor of tissue-type plasminogen activator *in vivo* and in cultured endothelial cells. *J. Exp. Med.*, **163**:1260–1266.

Erickson, L.A., Hekman, C.M. and Loskutoff, D.J. (1985). The primary plasminogen activator inhibitors in endothelial cells, platelets, serum, and plasma are immunologically related. *Proc. Natl. Acad. Sci. USA*, **82**:8710–8714.

Erickson, L.A., Fici, G.J., Lund, J.E., Boyle, T.P., Polites, H.G. and Marotti, K.R. (1990). Development of venous occlusions in mice transgenic for the plasminogen activator inhibitor-1 gene. *Nature*, **346**:74–76.

Eriksen, J., Kristensen, P., Pyke, C. and Dano, K. (1989). Plasminogen activator inhibitor (type-1) in rat adrenal medulla. *Histochemistry*, **92**:377–383.

Etingin, O.R., Hajjar, D.P., Hajjar, K.A., Harpel, P.C. and Nachman, R.L. (1991). Lipoprotein (a) regulates plasminogen activator inhibitor-1 expression in endothelial cells. *J. Biol. Chem.*, **266**:2459–2465.

Fay, W.P., Shapiro, A.D., Shih, J.L., Schleef, R.R. and Ginsburg, D. (1992). Complete deficiency of plasminogen-activator inhibitor type 1 due to a frameshift mutation. *N. Engl. J. Med.*, **327**:1729–1733.

Fearns, C., Keeton, M.R., Thinnes, T., Roegner, K. and Loskutoff, D.J. (1992). Induction of PAI-1 gene expression *in vivo* by TGF-β. *Fibrinolysis*, **6**:125 (Abstract).

Fearns, C., Thinnes, T., Roegner, K. and Loskutoff, D.J. (1993). Kinetics of induction of PAI-1 gene expression on liver endothelial cells and hepatocytes by lipopolysaccharide (LPS). *Thromb. Haemost.*, **69**:757 (Abstract).

Follo, M. and Ginsburg, D. (1989). Structure and expression of the human gene encoding plasminogen activator inhibitor, PAI-1. *Gene*, **84**:447–453.

Fotsis, T., Pepper, M., Adlercreutz, H., Fleischmann, G., Hase, T., Montesano, R. and Schweigerer, L. (1993). Genistein, a dietary-derived inhibitor of *in vitro* angiogenesis. *Proc. Natl. Acad. Sci. USA*, **90**:2690–2694.

Francis, R.B., Jr., Liebman, H., Koehler, S. and Feinstein, D.I. (1986). Accelerated fibrinolysis in amyloidosis. Specific binding of tissue plasminogen activator inhibitor by an amyloidogenic monoclonal IgG. *Blood*, **68**:333 (Abstract).

Fujii, S., Lucore, C.L., Hopkins, W.E., Billadello, J.J. and Sobel, B.E. (1990a). Induction of synthesis of plasminogen activator inhibitor type-1 by tissue-type plasminogen activator in human hepatic and endothelial cells. *Thromb. Haemost.*, **64**:412–419.

Fujii, S. and Sobel, B.E. (1990b). Induction of plasminogen activator inhibitor by products released from platelets. *Circulation*, **82**:1485–1493.

Fujii, S., Sawa, H. and Sobel, B.E. (1993). Inhibition of endothelial cell expression of plasminogen activator inhibitor type-1 by gemfibrozil. *Thromb. Haemost.*, **70**:642–647.

Gelehrter, T.D. and Sznycer-Laszuk, R. (1986). Thrombin induction of plasminogen activator-inhibitor in cultured human endothelial cells. *J. Clin. Invest.*, **77**:165–169.

Georg, B., Helseth, E., Lund, L.R., Skandsen, T., Riccio, A., Dano, K., Unsgaard, G. and Andreasen, P.A. (1989). Tumor necrosis factor-α regulates mRNA for urokinase-type plasminogen activator and type-1 plasminogen activator inhibitor in human neoplastic cell lines. *Mol. Cell. Endocrinol.*, **61** 87–96.

Gerritsen, M.E. and Bloor, C.M. (1993). Endothelial cell gene expression in response to injury. *FASEB J.*, **7**:523–532.

Hamilton, J.A., Whitty, G.A., Wojta, J., Gallichio, M., McGrath, K. and Ianches, G. (1993). Regulation of plasminogen activator inhibitor-1 levels in human monocytes. *Cell. Immunol.*, **152**:7–17.

Hamsten, A., Wiman, B., deFaire, U. and Blomback, M. (1985). Increased plasma levels of a rapid inhibitor of tissue plasminogen activator in young survivors of myocardial infarction. *N. Engl. J. Med.*, **313**:1557–1563.

Hanss, M. and Collen, D. (1987). Secretion of tissue type plasminogen activator and plasminogen activator inhibitor by cultured human endothelial cells, modulation by thrombin, endotoxin, and histamine. *J. Lab. Clin. Med.*, **109**:97–104.

Hart, D.A. and Rehemtulla, A. (1988). Plasminogen activators and their inhibitors: regulation of extracellular proteolysis and cell function. *Comp. Biochem. Physiol.*, **90B**:691–708.

Holdsworth, S.R. and Tipping, P.G. (1985). Macrophage-induced glomerular fibrin deposition in experimental glomerulonephritis in the rabbit. *J. Clin. Invest.*, **76**:1376–1374.

Janicke, F., Schmitt, M., Pache, L., Ulm, K., Harbeck, N., Hofler, H. and Graeff, H. (1993). Urokinase (uPA) and its inhibitor PAI-1 are strong and independent prognostic factors in node-negative breast cancer. *Breast Cancer Res. Treat.*, **24**:195–208.

Juhan-Vague, I., Moerman, B., De Cock, F., Aillaud, M.F. and Collen, D. (1984). Plasma levels of a specific inhibitor of tissue-type plasminogen activator (and urokinase) in normal and pathological conditions. *Thromb. Res.*, **33**:523–530.

Juhan-Vague, I. and Collen, D. (1992). On the role of coagulation and fibrinolysis in atherosclerosis. *Ann. Epidemiol.*, **2**:427–435.

Juhan-Vague, I. and Alessi, M.C. (1993). Plasminogen activator inhibitor 1 and atherothrombosis. *Thromb. Haemost.*, **70**:138–143.

Kamitsuji, H., Sakamoto, S., Matsunaga, T., Taira, K., Kawahara, S. and Nakajima, M. (1988). Intraglomerular deposition of fibrin/fibrinogen related antigen in children with various renal diseases. *Am. J. Pathol.*, **133**:61–72.

Keber, I. and Keber, D. (1992). Increased plasminogen activator inhibitor activity in survivors of myocardial infarction is associated with metabolic risk factors of atherosclerosis. *Haemostasis*, **22**:187–194.

Keeton, M., Curriden, S.A., van Zonneveld, A.J. and Loskutoff, D.J. (1991). Identification of regulatory sequences in the type 1 plasminogen activator inhibitor gene responsive to transforming growth factor β. *J. Biol. Chem.*, **266**:23048–23052.

Keeton, M., Eguchi, Y., Sawdey, M., Ahn, C. and Loskutoff, D.J. (1993). Cellular localization of type 1 plasminogen activator inhibitor mRNA and protein in murine renal tissue. *Am. J. Pathol.*, **142**:59–70.

Keeton, M., Ahn, C., Eguchi, Y., Burlingame, R. and Loskutoff, D.J. (1995). Expression of type 1 plasminogen activator inhibitor (PAI-1) in renal tissue in murine lupus. *Kidney Int.*, **47**:148–157.

Klinger, K.W., Winqvist, R., Riccio, A., Andreasen, P.A., Sartorio, R., Nielsen, L.S., Stuart, N., Stanislovitis, P., Watkins, P., Douglas, R., Grzeschik, K-H., Alitalo, K., Blasi, F. and Dano, K. (1987). Plasminogen activator inhibitor type 1 gene is located at region q21.3-q22 of chromosome 7 and genetically linked with cystic fibrosis. *Proc. Natl. Acad. Sci. USA*, **84**:8548–8552.

Kluft, C., Verheijen, J.H., Jie, A.F.H., Rijken, D.C., Preston, F.E., Sue-Ling, H.M., Jespersen, J. and Aasen, A.D. (1985). The postoperative fibrinolytic shutdown: a rapidly reverting acute phase pattern for the fast-acting inhibitor of tissue-type plasminogen activator after trauma. *Scand. J. Clin. Lab. Invest.*, **45**:605–610.

Knabb, R.M., Chiu, A.T. and Reilly, T.M. (1990). Effects of recombinant plasminogen activator inhibitor type 1 on fibrinolysis *in vitro* and *in vivo*. *Thromb. Res.*, **59**:309–317.

Konkle, B.A. and Ginsburg, D. (1988). The addition of endothelial cell growth factor and heparin to human umbilical vein endothelial cell cultures decreases plasminogen activator inhibitor-1 expression. *J. Clin. Invest.*, **82**:579–585.

Konkle, B.A., Schuster, S.J., Kelly, M.D., Harjes, K., Hassett, D.E., Bohrer, M. and Tavassoli, M. (1992). Plasminogen activator inhibitor-1 messenger RNA expression is induced in rat hepatocytes *in vivo* by dexamethasone. *Blood*, **79**:2636–2642.

Kono, S., Rao, J.S., Bruner, J.M. and Sawaya, R. (1994). Immunohistochemical localization of plasminogen activator inhibitor type 1 in human brain tumors. *J. Neuropath. Exp. Neurol.*, **53**:256–262.

Kooistra, T. (1990). The use of cultured human endothelial cells and hepatocytes as an *in vitro* model system to study modulation of endogenous fibrinolysis. *Fibrinolysis*, **4**:33–39.

Krishnamurti, C., Bolan, C., Colleton, C.A., Reilly, T.M. and Alving, B.M. (1993). Role of plasminogen activator inhibitor-1 in promoting fibrin deposition in rabbits infused with ancrod or thrombin. *Blood*, **82**:3631–3636.

Kristensen, P., Pyke, C., Lund, L.R., Andreasen, P.A. and Dano, K. (1990). Plasminogen activator inhibitor-type 1 in Lewis lung carcinoma. *Histochemistry*, **93**:559–566.

Kruithof, E.K.O., Tran-Thang, C., Gudinchet, A., Hauert, J., Nicoloso, G., Genton, C., Welti, H. and Bachmann, F.W. (1987). Fibrinolysis in pregnancy. A study of plasminogen activator inhibitors. *Blood*, **69**:460–466.

Kruithof, E.K.O., Gudinchet, A. and Bachmann, F. (1988). Plasminogen activator inhibitor 1 and plasminogen activator inhibitor 2 in various disease states. *Thromb. Haemost.*, **59**:7–12.

Lala, P.K. and Graham, C.H. (1990). Mechanisms of trophoblast invasiveness and their control: The role of proteases and protease inhibitors. *Cancer Metastasis Rev.*, **9**:369–379.

Lambers, J.W.J., Cammenga, M., Konig, B., Pannekoek, H. and van Mourik, J.A. (1987). Activation of human endothelial cell-type plasminogen activator inhibitor (PAI-1) by negatively charged phospholipids. *J. Biol. Chem.*, **262**:17492–17496.

Landau, B.J., Kwaan, H.C., Verrusio, E.N. and Brem, S.S. (1994). Elevated levels of urokinase-type plasminogen activator and plasminogen activator inhibitor type-1 in malignant human brain tumors. *Cancer Res.*, **54**:1105–1108.

Lee, M.H., Vosburgh, E., Anderson, K. and McDonagh, J. (1993). Deficiency of plasma plasminogen activator inhibitor 1 results in hyperfibrinolytic bleeding. *Blood*, **81**:2357–2362.

Legnani, C., Maccaferri, M., Tonini, P., Cassio, A., Cacciari, E. and Coccheri, S. (1988). Reduced fibrinolytic response in obese children: associations with high baseline activity of the fast acting plasminogen activator inhibitor (PAI-1). *Fibrinolysis*, **2**:211–214.

Levi, M., Biemond, B.J., van Zonneveld, A.-J., ten Cate, J.W. and Pannekoek, H. (1992). Inhibition of plasminogen activator inhibitor-1 activity results in promotion of endogenous thrombolysis and inhibition of thrombus extension in models of experimental thrombosis. *Circulation*, **85**:305–312.

Liotta, L.A., Steeg, P.S. and Stetler-Stevenson, W.G. (1991). Cancer metastasis and angiogenesis: an imbalance of positive and negative regulation. *Cell*, **64**:327–336.

Loskutoff, D.J., Linders, M., Keijer, J., Veerman, H., van Heerikhuizen, H. and Pannekoek, H. (1987). The structure of the human plasminogen activator inhibitor 1 gene: Non–random distribution of introns. *Biochemistry*, **26**:3763–3768.

Loskutoff, D.J. (1988a). Type 1 plasminogen activator inhibitor and its potential influence on thrombolytic therapy. *Sem. Thromb. Haemost.*, **14**:100–109.

Loskutoff, D.J., Sawdey, M. and Mimuro, J. (1988b). Type 1 plasminogen activator inhibitor. In: *Progress in Haemostasis and Thrombosis*, Coller, B. (ed.), pp. 87–115. Philadelphia: W.B.Saunders Company.

Loskutoff, D.J. (1991). Regulation of PAI-1 gene expression. *Fibrinolysis*, **5**:197–206.

Lucore, C.L., Fujii, S., Wun, T.C., Sobel, B.E. and Billadello, J.J. (1988). Regulation of the expression of type 1 plasminogen activator inhibitor in Hep G2 cells by epidermal growth factor. *J. Biol. Chem.*, **263**:15845–15848.

Lupu, F., Bergonzelli, G.E., Heim, D.A., Cousin, E., Genton, C.Y., Bachmann, F. and Kruithof, E.K.O. (1993). Localization and production of plasminogen activator inhibitor-1 in human healthy and atherosclerotic arteries. *Arterioscler. Thromb.*, **13**:1090–1100.

Mayer, M., Lund, L.R., Riccio, A., Skouv, J., Nielsen, L.S., Stacey, S.N., Dano, K. and Andreasen, P.A. (1988). Plasminogen activator inhibitor type-1 protein, mRNA and gene transcription are increased by phorbol esters in human rhabdomyosarcoma cells. *J. Biol. Chem.*, **263**:15688–15693.

McFall, B.C. and Reilly, C.F. (1990). TGFβ and PDGF induce plasminogen activator inhibitor release from vascular smooth muscle cells. *FASEB J.*,**4**:A892 (Abstract).

McGill, J.B., Schneider, D.J., Arfken, C.L., Lucore, C.L. and Sobel, B.E. (1994). Factors responsible for impaired fibrinolysis in obese subjects and NIDDM patients. *Diabetes*, **43**:104–109.

Medina, R., Socher, S.H., Han, J.H. and Friedman, P.A. (1989). Interleukin-1, endotoxin or tumor necrosis factor/cachectin enhance the level of plasminogen activator inhibitor messenger RNA in bovine aortic endothelial cells. *Thromb. Res.*, **54**:41–52.

Michalek, S.M., Moore, R.N., McGee, J.R., Rosenstreich, D.L. and Mergenhagen, S.E. (1980). The primary role of lymphoreticular cells in the mediation of host responses to bacterial endotoxin. *J. Infect. Dis.*, **141**:55–63.

Nachman, R.L., Hajjar, K.A., Silverstein, R.L. and Dinarello, C.A. (1986). Interleukin 1 induces endothelial cell synthesis of plasminogen activator inhibitor. *J. Exp. Med.*, **163**:1595–1600.

Nathan, C.F. (1987). Secretory products of macrophages. *J. Clin. Invest.*, **79**:319–326.

Nawroth, P.P. and Stern, D.M. (1986). Modulation of endothelial cell hemostatic properties by tumor necrosis factor. *J. Exp. Med.*, **163**:740–745.

Nekarda, H., Schmitt, M., Ulm, K., Wenninger, A., Vogelsang, H., Becker, K., Roder, J.D., Fink, U. and Siewert, J.R. (1994). Prognostic impact of urokinase-type plasminogen activator and its inhibitor PAI-1 in completely resected gastric cancer. *Cancer Res.*, **54**:2900–2907.

Noda-Heiny, H., Fujii, S. and Sobel, B.E. (1993). Induction of vascular smooth muscle cell expression of plasminogen activator inhibitor-1 by thrombin. *Circ. Res.*, **72**:36–43.

Ohlsson, M., Peng, X.R., Liu, Y.X., Jia, C., Hsueh, A.J.W. and Ny, T. (1991). Hormone regulation of tissue-type plasminogen activator gene expression and plasminogen activator-mediated proteolysis. *Semin. Thromb. Haemost.*, **17**:286–290.

Partridge, C.A. and Gerritsen, M.E. (1990). Dexamethasone increases the release of three 44 kD proteins immunologically related to plasminogen activator inhibitor-1 from human umbilical vein endothelial and rabbit coronary microvessel endothelial cells. *Thromb. Res.*, **57**:139–154.

Pedersen, H., Grondahl-Hansen, J., Francis, D., Osterlind, K., Hansen, H.H., Dano, K. and Brunner, N. (1994). Urokinase and plasminogen activator inhibitor type 1 in pulmonary adenocarcinoma. *Cancer Res.*, **54**:120–123.

Pepper, M.S., Belin, D., Montesano, R., Orci, L. and Vassalli, J.D. (1990). Transforming growth factor-beta 1 modulates basic fibroblast growth factor-induced proteolytic and angiogenic properties of endothelial cells *in vitro*. *J. Cell Biol.*, **111**:743–755.

Pepper, M.S., Montesano, R., Orci, L. and Vassalli, J.D. (1991a). Plasminogen activator inhibitor-1 is induced in microvascular endothelial cells by a chondrocyte-derived transforming growth factor-beta. *Biochem. Biophys. Res. Comm.*, **176**:633–638.

Pepper, M.S., Ferrara, N., Orci, L. and Montesano, R. (1991b). Vascular endothelial growth factor (VEGF) induces plasminogen activators and plasminogen activator inhibitor-1 in microvascular endothelial cells. *Biochem. Biophys. Res. Comm.*, **181**:902–906.

Pepper, M.S., Wasi, S., Ferrara, N., Orci, L. and Montesano, R. (1994). *In vitro* angiogenic and proteolytic properties of bovine lymphatic endothelial cells. *Exp. Cell Res.*, **210**:298–305.

Podor, T.J., Joshua, P., Butcher, M., Seiffert, D., Loskutoff, D. and Gauldie, J. (1992). Accumulation of type 1 plasminogen activator inhibitor and vitronectin at sites of cellular necrosis and inflammation. *Ann. N. Y. Acad. Sci.*, **667**:173–177.

Podor, T.J., Hirsh, J., Gelehrter, T.D., Zeheb, R., Torry, D., Guigoz, Y., Sierra, F. and Gauldie, J. (1993). Type 1 plasminogen activator inhibitor is not an acute phase reactant in rats: Lack of IL-6- and hepatocyte-dependent synthesis. *J. Immunol.*, **150**:225–235.

Potter van Loon, B.J., Kluft, C., Radder, J.K., Blankenstein, M.A. and Meinders, A.E. (1993). The cardiovascular risk factor plasminogen activator inhibitor type 1 is related to insulin resistance. *Metabolism*, **42**:945–949.

Pralong, G., Calandra, T., Glauser, M.P., Schellekens, J., Verhoef, J., Bachmann, F. and Kruithof, E.K.O. (1989). Plasminogen activator inhibitor 1: A new prognostic marker in septic shock. *Thromb. Haemost.*, **61**:459–462.

Preissner, K.T., Grulich-Henn, J., Ehrlich, H.J., Declerck, P., Justus, C., Collen, D., Pannekoek, H. and Muller-Berghaus, G. (1990). Structural requirements for the extracellular interaction of plasminogen activator inhibitor 1 with endothelial cell matrix-associated vitronectin. *J. Biol. Chem.*, **265**:18490–18498.

Prendergast, G.C., Diamond, L.E., Dahl, D. and Cole, M.D. (1990). The c-myc-regulated gene mr1 encodes plasminogen activator inhibitor 1. *Mol. Cell. Biol.*, **10**:1265–1269.

Pujade-Lauraine, E., Lu, H., Mirshahi, S., Soria, J., Soria, C., Bernadou, A., Kruithof, E.K.O., Lijnen, H.R. and Burtin, P. (1993). The plasminogen-activation system in ovarian tumors. *Int. J. Cancer*, **55**:27–31.

Pyke, C., Kristensen, P., Ralfkiaer, E., Eriksen, J. and Dano, K. (1991). The plasminogen activation system in human colon cancer: Messenger RNA for the inhibitor PAI-1 is located in endothelial cells of the tumor stroma. *Cancer Res.*, **51**:4067–4071.

Quax, P.H.A., van den Hoogen, C.M., Verheijen, J.H., Padro, T., Zeheb, R., Gelehrter, T.D., van Berkel, T.J.C., Kuiper, J. and Emeis, J.J. (1990). Endotoxin induction of plasminogen activator and plasminogen activator inhibitor type 1 mRNA in rat tissues *in vivo*. *J. Biol. Chem.*, **265**:15560–15563.

Reilly, C.F., Fujita, T., Mayer, E.J. and Siegfried, M.E. (1991). Both circulating and clot bound PAI-1 inhibit endogenous fibrinolysis in the rat. *Arterioscler. Thromb.*, **11**:1276–1286.

Riccio, A., Pedone, P.V., Lund, L.R., Olesen, T., Olsen, H.S. and Andreasen, P.A. (1992). Transforming growth factor β1-responsive element: Closely associated binding sites for USF and CCAAT- binding transcription factor-nuclear factor I in the type 1 plasminogen activator inhibitor gene. *Mol. Cell. Biol.*, **12**:1846–1855.

Saksela, O., Moscatelli, D. and Rifkin, D.B. (1987). The opposing effects of basic fibroblast growth factor and transforming growth factor β on the regulation of plasminogen activator activity in capillary endothelial cells. *J. Cell Biol.*, **105**:957–963.

Samad, F., Thinnes, T., Roegner, K. and Loskutoff, D.J. (1994). Regulation of plasminogen activator inhibitor-1 (PAI-1) gene expression in adipose tissue and in cultured adipocytes. *FASEB J.*, **8**, A268 (Abstract).

Samad, F., Yamaamoto, K. and Loskutoff, D.J. (1996). Distribution and regulation of plasminogen activator inhibitor-1 in murine adipose tissue *in vivo*: induction by tumor necrosis factor-α and lipopolysaccharide. *J. Clin. Invest.*, **In Press**.

Santell, L. and Levin, E.G. (1988). Cyclic AMP potentiates phorbol ester stimulation of tissue plasminogen activator release and inhibits secretion of plasminogen activator inhibitor-1 from human endothelial cells. *J. Biol. Chem.*, **263**:16802–16808.

Sawa, H., Fujii, S. and Sobel, B.E. (1992). Augmented arterial wall expression of type-1 plasminogen activator inhibitor induced by thrombosis. *Arterioscler. Thromb.*, **12**:1507–1515.

Sawa, H., Sobel, B.E. and Fujii, S. (1993). Potentiation by hypercholesterolemia of the induction of aortic intramural synthesis of plasminogen activator inhibitor type 1 by endothelial injury. *Circ. Res.*, **73**:671–680.

Sawdey, M., Podor, T.J. and Loskutoff, D.J. (1989). Regulation of type 1 plasminogen activator inhibitor gene expression in cultured bovine aortic endothelial cells: Induction by transforming growth factor-β, lipopolysaccharide, and tumor necrosis factor-α. *J. Biol. Chem.*, **264**:10396–10401.

Sawdey, M. and Loskutoff, D.J. (1991). Regulation of murine type 1 plasminogen activator inhibitor gene expression *in vivo*. Tissue specificity and induction by lipopolysaccharide, tumor necrosis factor-α, and transforming growth factor-β. *J. Clin. Invest.*, **88**:1346–1353.

Schleef, R.R., Bevilacqua, M.P., Sawdey, M., Gimbrone, M.A., Jr. and Loskutoff, D.J. (1988). Cytokine activation of vascular endothelium. Effects on tissue-type plasminogen activator and type 1 plasminogen activator inhibitor. *J. Biol. Chem.*, **263**:5797–5803.

Schleef, R.R., Higgins, D.L., Pillemer, E. and Levitt, J.J. (1989). Bleeding diathesis due to decreased functional activity of type 1 plasminogen activator inhibitor. *J. Clin. Invest.*, **83**:1747–1752.

Schneiderman, J., Sawdey, M.S., Keeton, M.R., Bordin, G.M., Bernstein, E.F., Dilley, R.B. and Loskutoff, D.J. (1992). Increased type 1 plasminogen activator inhibitor gene expression in atherosclerotic human arter-·ies. *Proc. Natl. Acad. Sci. USA*, **89**:6998–7002.

Schved, J.F., Gris, J.C., Martinez, P., Sarlat, C., Sanchez, N. and Arnaud, A. (1991). Familial thrombophilia associated with familial elevation of plasma histidin rich glycoprotein and type 1 PAI. *Thromb. Haemost.*, **65**: 1044 (Abstract).

Seiffert, D., Wagner, N.N. and Loskutoff, D.J. (1990). Serum-derived vitronectin influences the pericellular distribution of type 1 plasminogen activator inhibitor. *J. Cell Biol.*, **111**:1283–1291.

Simpson, A.J., Booth, N.A., Moore, N.R. and Bennett, B. (1991). Distribution of plasminogen activator inhibitor (PAI-1) in tissues. *J. Clin. Pathol.*, **44**:139–143.

Slivka, S.R. and Loskutoff, D.J. (1991a). Regulation of type 1 plasminogen activator inhibitor synthesis by protein kinase C and cAMP in bovine aortic endothelial cells. *Biochim. Biophys. Acta*, **1094**:317–322.

Slivka, S.R. and Loskutoff, D.J. (1991b). Platelets stimulate endothelial cells to synthesize type 1 plasminogen activator inhibitor. *Blood*, **77**:1013–1019.

Sperti, G., Van Leeuwen, R., Maseri, A. and Kluft, C. (1992). Platelet-derived growth factor increases plasminogen activator inhibitor-1 activity and mRNA in rat cultured vascular smooth muscle. *Ann. N. Y. Acad. Sci.*, **667**:178–180.

Sprengers, E.D. and Kluft, C. (1987). Plasminogen activator inhibitors. *Blood*, **69**:381–387.

Strandberg, L., Lawrence, D. and Ny, T. (1988). The organization of the human plasminogen activator inhibitor 1 gene. *Eur. J. Biochem.*, **176**:609–616.

Strickland, S., Reich, E. and Sherman, M.I. (1976). Plasminogen activator in early embryogenesis: enzyme production by trophoblast and parietal endoderm. *Cell*, **9**:231–240.

Suffredini, A.F., Harpel, P.C. and Parrillo, J.E. (1989). Promotion and subsequent inhibition of plasminogen activation after administration of intravenous endotoxin to normal subjects. *N. Engl. J. Med.*, **320**:1165–1172.

Sundell, I.B., Nilsson, T.K., Hallmans, G., Hellsten, G. and Dahlen, G.H. (1989). Interrelationship between plasma levels of plasminogen activator inhibitor, tissue plasminogen activator, lipoprotein (a), and established cardiovascular risk factors in a North Swedish population. *Atherosclerosis*, **80**:9–16.

Takada, Y., Urano, T., Watanabe, I., Taminato, A., Yoshimi, T. and Takada, A. (1993). Changes in fibrinolytic parameters in male patients with type 2 (non-insulin-dependent) diabetes mellitus. *Thromb. Res.*, **71**:405–415.

Takemura, T., Yoshioka, K. and Akano, N. (1987). Glomerular deposition of cross-linked fibrin in human kidney disease. *Kidney Int.*, **32**:102–111.

Tipping, P.G., Davenport, P., Gallicchio, M., Filonzi, E.L., Apostolopoulos, J. and Wojta, J. (1993). Atheromatous plaque macrophages produce plasminogen activator inhibitor type-1 and stimulate its production by endothelial cells and vascular smooth muscle cells. *Am. J. Pathol.*, **143** 875–885.

Tomosugi, N., Naito, T., Ikeda, K., Yokoyama, H., Kobayashi, K. and Kida, H. (1990). The role of plasminogen activator inhibitor (PAI) on anti-glomerular basement membrane antibody-mediated glomerular injury and its modulation by tumor necrosis factor (TNF). *Kidney Int.*, **37**:435 (Abstract).

Troyer, D.A., Chandrasekar, B., Thinnes, T., Stone, A., Loskutoff, D.J. and Fernandes, G. (1995). Effects of energy intake on type 1 plasminogen activator inhibitor levels in glomeruli of lupus prone B/W mice. *Am. J. Pathol.* **146**:111–120.

Tsafriri, A., Bicsak, T.A., Cajander, S.B., Ny, T. and Hsueh, A.J.W. (1989). Suppression of ovulation rate by antibodies to tissue-type plasminogen activator and α_2-antiplasmin. *Endocrinol.*, **124**:415–421.

Vague, P., Juhan-Vague, I., Chabert, V., Alessi, M.C. and Atlan, C. (1989). Fat distribution and plasminogen activator inhibitor activity in nondiabetic obese women. *Metabolism*, **38**:913–915.

van den Berg, E.A., Sprengers, E.D., Jaye, M., Burgess, W., Maciag, T. and van Hinsbergh, V.W.M. (1988). Regulation of plasminogen activator inhibitor-1 mRNA in human endothelial cells. *Thromb. Haemost.*, **60**:63–67.

van Hinsbergh, V.W.M., Sprengers, E.D. and Kooistra, T. (1987). Effect of thrombin on the production of plasminogen activators and PA inhibitor-1 by human foreskin microvascular endothelial cells. *Thromb. Haemost.*, **57**:148–153.

van Hinsbergh, V.W., Kooistra, T., van den Berg, E.A., Princen, H.M., Fiers, W. and Emeis, J.J. (1988). Tumor necrosis factor increases the production of plasminogen activator inhibitor in human endothelial cells *in vitro* and in rats *in vivo*. *Blood*, **72**:1467–1473.

van Hinsberg, V.W., Vermeer, M., Koolwijk, P., Grimbergen, J. and Kooistra, T. (1994). Genistein reduces tumor necrosis factor alpha-induced plasminogen activator inhibitor-1 transcription but not urokinase expression in human endothelial cells. *Blood*, 84:2984–2991.

van Zonneveld, A.J., Curriden, S.A. and Loskutoff, D.J. (1988). Type 1 plasminogen activator inhibitor gene: Functional analysis and glucocorticoid regulation of its promoter. *Proc. Natl. Acad. Sci. USA*, **85**:5525–5529.

Vassalli, J.D., Sappino, A.P. and Belin, D. (1991). The plasminogen activator/plasmin system. *J. Clin. Invest.*, **88**:1067–1072.

Wada, H., Minamikawa, K., Wakita, Y., Nakase, T., Kaneko, T., Ohiwa, M., Tamaki, S., Deguchi, K., Shirakawa, S., Hayashi, T. and Suzuki, K. (1993a). Increased vascular endothelial cell markers in patients with disseminated intravascular coagulation. *Am. J. Hematol.*, **44**:85–88.

Wada, H., Mori, Y., Kaneko, T., Wakita, Y., Nakase, T., Minamikawa, K., Ohiwa, M., Tamaki, S., Tanigawa, M., Kageyama, S. et al.., (1993b). Elevated plasma levels of vascular endothelial cell markers in patients with hypercholesterolemia. *Am. J. Hematol.*, **44**:112–116.

Wagner, O.F., de Vries, C., Hohmann, C., Veerman, H. and Pannekoek, H. (1989). Interaction between plasminogen activator inhibitor type 1 (PAI-1) bound to fibrin and either tissue-type plasminogen activator (t-PA) or urokinase-type plasminogen activator (u-PA): Binding of t-PA/PAI-1 complexes to fibrin mediated by both the finger and the kringle-2 domain of t-PA. *J. Clin. Invest.*, **84**:647–655.

Whawell, S.A., Wang, Y., Fleming, K.A., Thompson, E.M. and Thompson, J.N. (1993). Localization of plasminogen activator inhibitor-1 production in inflamed appendix by *in situ* mRNA hybridization. *J. Pathol.*, **169**:67–71.

Wiman, B., Almquist, A., Sigurdardottir, O. and Lindahl, T. (1988). Plasminogen activator inhibitor 1 (PAI) is bound to vitronectin in plasma. *FEBS Letters*, **242**:125–128.

Wojta, J., Gallicchio, M., Zoellner, H., Hufnagl, P., Last, K., Filonzi, E.L., Binder, B.R., Hamilton, J.A. and McGrath, K. (1993). Thrombin stimulates expression of tissue-type plasminogen activator and plasminogen activator inhibitor type 1 in cultured human vascular smooth muscle cells. *Thromb. Haemost.*, **70**:469–474.

Woolf, N. (1981). Thrombosis and atherosclerosis. In: *Haemostasis and Thrombosis*, Bloom, A.L. and Thomas, D.P. (eds.), pp. 527–553. Churchill Livingstone, Edinburgh.

Yorimitsu, K., Saito, T., Toyozaki, T., Ishide, T., Ohnuma, N. and Inagaki, Y. (1993). Immunohistochemical localization of plasminogen activator inhibitor-1 in human coronary atherosclerotic lesions involved in acute myocardial infarction. *Heart Vessels*, **8**:160–162

12 The Role of Plasminogen Activators in Vascular Pericellular Proteolysis

Paul H.A. Quax, Pieter Koolwijk, Jan H. Verheijen and Victor W.M. van Hinsbergh

Gaubius Laboratory, TNO-PG, Leiden, The Netherlands

INTRODUCTION

The repair matrix that the body uses after injury is fibrin. It is acutely deposited after wounding and slowly dissolves during tissue repair. This temporary repair matrix prevents blood loss and provides the scaffold for the invasion of cells during the subsequent healing process. Formation and removal of fibrin is regulated by two cascades-type systems of proteolytic activities: the coagulation and fibrinolysis system. Fibrin formation is initiated by the proteolytic conversion of fibrinogen into fibrin by thrombin, a serine protease formed by the coagulation pathway. Thrombin is not only a crucial factor in the prevention of blood loss by its abilities both to initiate fibrin formation and to activate platelets, but in addition it acts as a paracrine hormone at the vessel wall. On the endothelium, it interacts with two receptors, thrombomodulin and the G-protein-linked thrombin receptor, and thereby enhances anticoagulant properties of the endothelium, i.e. it induces the activation of protein C and the acute release of prostacyclin, nitric oxide and tissue-type plasminogen activator (t-PA). Thrombin also acts on smooth muscle cells, in particular in the thickened intima, via the thrombin receptor, and may stimulate the growth of smooth muscle cells. Thrombin thus not only initiates and regulates fibrin formation and platelet activation, but also is involved in the activation of the cells of the vessel wall.

The proteases that regulate the breakdown of fibrin, i.e. plasmin and plasminogen activators, also have a double function. Firstly, they are involved in the proteolytic degradation of fibrin (fibrinolysis). Secondly, plasminogen activators, in particular urokinase-type plasminogen activator (u-PA) and plasmin, are thought to function in pericellular proteolytic processes affecting matrix proteins and proteins involved in cell-matrix interactions. Pericellular proteolysis is required for matrix remodeling and cell migration, which occur in many pathophysiological processes, such as in tissue repair, outgrowth of neuronal extensions, leucocyte migration, tumor cell invasion, and (with respect to the vascular system) in angiogenesis and neointima formation. The activity of the u-PA/plasmin system is controlled by specific inhibitors and by specific cellular receptors,

227

which enable the cell to direct this activity. Because plasmin can activate stromelysin and other matrix-degrading metalloproteinases, the cell-bound u-PA/plasmin system may play an essential role in pericellular remodeling of matrix proteins, cell-matrix contacts and possibly cell-cell contacts. In addition to these functions, plasminogen activators are involved in the proteolytic activation of growth factors, in particular transforming growth factor-β (TGF-β).

By selected expression of different components of the fibrinolytic system vascular cells are able to remove fibrin before it obstructs a blood vessel and to respond in an adequate manner, i.e. by cell migration or angiogenesis, to local stimuli after tissue damage. Several proteases involved in hemostasis, including thrombin and plasminogen activators, have a dual role. On the one hand they contribute to the generation or dissolution of fibrin, on the other hand they contribute to the subsequent repair process by activation of tissue cells. Other chapters in this book (Carmeliet and Collen, 1995; Emeis *et al.*, 1995) focus on the role of the endothelium in fibrinolysis. In this chapter we shall discuss the role of the plasminogen activators in pericellular proteolysis of vascular cells.

COMPONENTS OF THE PLASMINOGEN ACTIVATION SYSTEM

The plasminogen activation system consists of several (pro-)enzymes, activators, inhibitors and receptors that regulate the activity and localization of the plasminogen activator/plasmin system. The main proteases and inhibitors are summarized in Figure 12.1.

Plasmin/Plasminogen

The key enzyme in this system is plasmin, which circulates as a zymogen: plasminogen. Plasminogen is synthesized by the liver as a single-chain glycoprotein of 92 kD and is

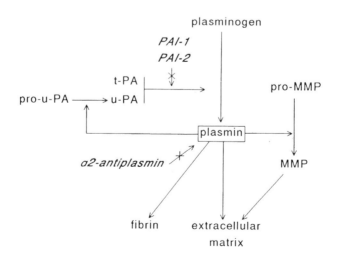

Figure 12.1   The plasminogen activation pathway.

secreted into the blood. It is also present in the interstitial fluid of tissues. Plasminogen can be converted into the active serine protease plasmin by specific plasminogen activators that cleave the Arg-560:Val-561 bond in the single chain plasminogen (Robbins *et al.*, 1967). Plasmin consists of a light chain and a heavy chain linked by a disulphide bond. The light chain contains a proteolytic domain which is similar to that of other serine proteases. The heavy chain, which consists of five kringle structures, mediates the binding to fibrin and related compounds (Bosma *et al.*, 1988; Castellino, 1988). Plasmin is a trypsin-like serine protease with a broad specificity. It can degrade many proteins including various extracellular matrix components and can activate other proteases, such as matrix-degrading metalloproteinases.

Plasminogen Activators

The conversion of plasminogen into active plasmin is catalyzed by specific plasminogen activators. Two types of plasminogen activators are presently known: tissue-type plasminogen activator (t-PA) and urokinase-type plasminogen activator (u-PA). These two enzymes, with a molecular weight of 68 kD and 55 kD, respectively are synthesized as single chain polypeptides and can be cleaved by plasmin. The resulting two chains remain connected by a disulphide bond. Single chain u-PA is a pro-enzyme whereas single chain t-PA is an active enzyme. t-PA binds to fibrin and its activity is enhanced by this binding (Hoylaerts *et al.*, 1982; Verheijen *et al.*, 1982; Nieuwenhuizen *et al.*, 1988). In contrast, u-PA does not bind to fibrin and its activity is not stimulated by fibrin.

Inhibitors

The activity of plasmin and the plasminogen activators is controlled by specific inhibitors. Plasmin is instantaneously inhibited by α_2-antiplasmin (Holmes *et al.*, 1987), which is present in blood, but this reaction is attenuated when plasmin is bound to fibrin or a cell surface receptor (Stephens *et al.*, 1989). The predominant inhibitors of t-PA and u-PA are plasminogen activator inhibitor type-1 (PAI-1) and type-2 (PAI-2). PAI-1 is a 50 kD glycoprotein present in plasma and blood platelets and is synthesized by endothelial cells, smooth muscle cells and many other cell types in culture (Fearns *et al.*, 1995). PAI-1 forms inactive complexes with single-chain and two-chain t-PA, as well as two- chain u-PA but not with single-chain u-PA. PAI activity in human plasma is normally exclusively PAI-1 (Sprengers and Kluft, 1987; Fearns *et al.*, 1995). PAI-2 is mainly produced by monocytes/macrophages and can be found as a glycosylated secreted molecule of 56 kD or as a non-glycosylated intracellular molecule of 46 kD. PAI-2 forms complexes with both t-PA and u-PA, similar to PAI-1. The reactivity of PAI-2 with the activators differs in the order two-chain u-PA > two-chain t-PA > single-chain t-PA. Similar to PAI-1, PAI-2 does not interact with single-chain u-PA (Kruithof, 1988).

Receptors

Cellular receptors are also involved in regulation of plasminogen activation. A number of these receptors concentrate and direct the action of plasminogen activators and plasmin to defined areas on the cell surface. High affinity binding sites for u-PA (Stoppelli *et al.*,

1985; Vassalli *et al.*, 1985), t-PA (Hajjar *et al.*, 1992, 1994) and plasminogen (Miles *et al.*, 1988; Stephens *et al.*, 1989) have been found on various types of cells including endothelial and smooth muscle cells. Other receptors are involved in the clearance of these proteases or their complexes with inhibitors.

A specific u-PA receptor (u-PAR) has been identified and cloned. This receptor binds both single-chain and two-chain u-PA via their growth factor domains (Blasi *et al.*, 1994; Danø *et al.*, 1994). Human u-PAR is synthesized as a 313 amino acid residue polypeptide (excluding a 22 residue signal peptide). It is a heavily glycosylated molecule of 55–60 kD. After proteolytic cleavage of the C-terminal part of the newly synthesized u-PAR molecule a glycosylphosphatidylinositol (GPI) -anchor is attached to the novel C-terminus which in human u-PAR is thought to be Gly-283 (Ploug *et al.*, 1991; Møller *et al.*, 1992). The mature u-PAR is anchored in the plasma membrane by its GPI-anchor. Binding of u-PA to its receptor not only concentrates u-PA activity on the cell surface, but also potentiates u-PA catalyzed plasminogen activation (Ellis *et al.*, 1991; Quax *et al.*, 1991).

The cellular binding of t-PA and plasminogen has been studied extensively, but the nature of the binding sites is less clear. A variety of proteins including α-enolase (as a plasminogen receptor) and annexin II (as a t-PA/plasminogen receptor) have been identified as cellular components which bind t-PA or plasmin(ogen) *in vitro* (Miles *et al.*, 1991; Hajjar *et al.*, 1992, 1994; Cesarman *et al.*, 1994).

Other types of receptors have been described that are involved in the clearance from the circulation by the liver of t-PA, u-PA and their PAI-1 complexes. They comprise the mannose receptor on liver endothelial cells and the α_2-macroglobulin receptor/LDL receptor-related protein (LRP) on hepatocytes and Kupffer cells. Whereas the mannose receptor on liver endothelial cells only binds t-PA, the LRP contributes to the internalization and degradation of both the proteases t-PA and u-PA and of their PA/PAI-1 complexes (Nykjaer *et al.*, 1992; Orth *et al.*, 1992, 1994; Kounnas *et al.*, 1993). The LRP consists of an 85 kD membrane-spanning β-chain and a 515 kD ligand binding α-chain (Herz *et al.*, 1988). The latter contains four clusters of cysteine-rich repeats that are also found in the LDL-receptor and the gp330 (Moestrup, 1994). The LRP has been demonstrated in the liver on hepatocytes and Kuppfer cells, in placenta and on many cell types including vascular smooth muscle cells, fibroblasts and monocytes (Moestrup *et al.*, 1992; Luoma *et al.*, 1994).

Recently, it has been recognized that the LRP and possibly two other members of the LDL receptor family, namely gp330 and the VLDL-receptor, are also involved in the regulation of the plasminogen activator activity on the cell surface since they can mediate the internalization and subsequent degradation of the u-PA/PAI-1 complex. This enables the cell to restore unoccupied u-PAR on its surface after dissociation of the ligand and receptor in the endosomes. The involvement of the LRP in u-PA/PAI-1 internalization has clearly been demonstrated in experiments with monocytic cells and smooth muscle cells. The u-PA/PAI-1 uptake can be inhibited by addition of receptor associated protein (RAP), a 39 kD protein that covers the protease binding sites of the LRP and related receptors. Although RAP can also reduce the uptake and degradation of u-PA/PAI-1 by endothelial cells by 25–30% (van Hinsbergh, unpublished), it is uncertain whether this occurs via the LRP or a related receptor, the VLDL receptor or gp330.

PRESENT MODEL OF THE INVOLVEMENT OF U-PA AND THE U-PA RECEPTOR IN LOCAL PERICELLULAR PROTEOLYSIS

An association between plasminogen activator activity and cell migration and invasion has been recognized for several decades (for review see: Danø *et al.*, 1985; Liotta *et al.*, 1992). In the last decade a number of studies have provided biochemical and genetic evidence regarding the involvement of plasminogen activators in cell migration. Most of the evidence is obtained for u-PA in man and mouse, but it is likely that t-PA may have a similar role in some species. The following model has emerged (Figure 12.2). Immediately after secretion u-PA binds to a specific receptor (u-PAR) and is converted from its single-chain pro-enzyme form into its active two-chain form. The u-PA/u-PAR complex has been localized at focal attachment sites and in areas of cell-cell contacts in fibrosarcoma cells (Pöllänen *et al.*, 1987, 1988) and endothelial cells (Conforti *et al.*, 1994). It is believed that active receptor-bound u-PA can convert cell-bound plasminogen into plasmin which causes proteolysis of matrix proteins. As a consequence cell-matrix contacts and possibly cell-cell contacts are disrupted. This, together with the formation of new cell-matrix contacts, is required for cell movement. Active u-PA is rapidly inhibited by PAI-1; on monocytes also by PAI-2. The receptor bound u-PA/PAI complex is subsequently internalized (Cubellis *et al.*, 1990; Estreicher *et al.*, 1990), eg. by the LRP or the VLDL receptor (Strickland *et al.*, 1994). During this process, the u-PA/PAI complex detaches from the u-PAR and is degraded, while the unoccupied u-PAR returns to the plasma membrane.

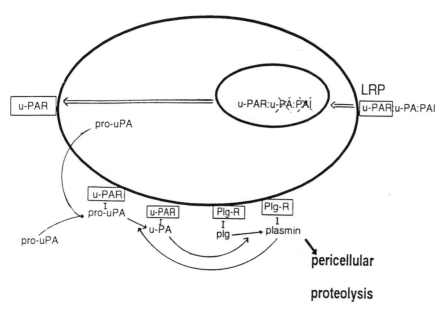

Figure 12.2   Pericellular plasminogen activation and the putative mechanisms of action of the various receptors and proteases. The mechanism is described in the text.

Next to their role in the proteolytic degradation of extracellular matrix components may plasminogen activators, in concert with plasminogen, play a role in the proteolytic activation of latent TGF-β and the liberation of b-FGF from the extracellular matrix (Sato and Rifkin, 1989; Flaumenhaft *et al.*, 1992a, 1992b) and may be involved in the activation of matrix metalloproteinases (He *et al.*, 1989; Murphy *et al.*, 1992).

ROLE OF PLASMINOGEN ACTIVATORS SYNTHESIZED BY VASCULAR CELLS

The plasminogen activation system is used by vascular cells to prevent fibrin deposition within the vessel lumen and in the vascular tissue, and to regulate pericellular proteolysis involved in cell migration and invasion into a fibrin matrix. This function is most pronounced in endothelial cells, which are the major if not only source of t-PA in the plasma. In addition to the synthesis and constitutive secretion of t-PA, endothelial cells are able to store t-PA and to release this stored t-PA acutely if they are stimulated by thrombi or other vasoactive substances (Emeis *et al.*, 1995). Plasma t-PA activity is modulated by circulating PAI-1, in particular in thrombi and in areas of stasis. However, the main function of PAI-1 synthesized by smooth muscle cells and endothelial cells may be to protect the cell environment against uncontrolled plasminogen activation. The relatively high concentration of PAI-1 in the vessel wall (Padro *et al.*, 1994) and the simultaneous induction of PAI-1 and u-PA by the inflammatory mediators tumor necrosis factor-α (TNFα) and interleukin-1 (IL-1) (van Hinsbergh *et al.*, 1990) support this suggestion. Induction of u-PA and its receptor occurs in tissue repair. It is generally assumed that this is related to cell migration and angiogenesis. In the following paragraphs the role of plasminogen activators in migration and angiogenesis by endothelial cells, and in smooth muscle cell migration will be discussed. Then, we will summarize the data on the expression of plasminogen activators and matrix degrading proteinases in intact and injured blood vessels *in vivo*.

INVOLVEMENT OF u-PA AND u-PAR IN ENDOTHELIAL CELL MIGRATION *IN VITRO*

During migration of endothelial cells and during formation of new blood vessels, existing cell-matrix contacts are disrupted by endothelial cells and new ones are generated. By this process endothelial cells can pull themselves over or into their basement membrane or the extracellular matrix. Local pericellular proteolysis is assumed to play a central role in the detachment of focal adhesion sites and possibly cell-cell contacts (Blasi, 1993). The fact that receptor-bound u-PA can be found at focal matrix contact sites and cell-cell contacts in a number of cells (Pollänen *et al.*, 1987, 1988; Hébert and Baker, 1988), including endothelial cells (Conforti *et al.*, 1994), supports this assumption. Cell-bound u-PA activity is induced in bovine microvascular endothelial cells, which migrate from the edges of a wounded monolayer *in vitro* (Pepper *et al.*, 1987, 1993; Sato and Rifkin, 1989). In these cells, u-PA synthesis is induced by basic fibroblast growth factor (b-FGF) which is liberated upon wounding of the monolayer (Tsuboi *et al.*, 1988; Odekon *et al.*,

1992). A b-FGF-dependent induction of PAI-1 and u-PAR expression was also observed in the endothelial cells in the migrating zone along a wound in a monolayer *in vitro*, suggesting tight control of u-PA activity (Pepper *et al.*, 1993). The involvement of u-PA activity in cell migration was further underscored by the fact that migration of endothelial cells in this model was inhibited by addition of antibodies against u-PA (Bell *et al.*, 1992; Odekon *et al.*, 1992) and by inhibition of the interaction of u-PA with its receptor (Pepper *et al.*, 1993). However, it remains uncertain whether the action of u-PA is due to direct interaction of u-PA with the cell, e.g. by signalling via the u-PA receptor (Busso *et al.*, 1994), or to the generation of plasmin. Several authors were unable to demonstrate that endothelial cell migration was plasmin(ogen)-dependent (Schleef and Birdwell, 1982; Odekon *et al.*, 1992). The recently reported interaction of vitronectin with the u-PAR (Waltz and Chapman, 1994) and the observed intracellular tyrosine phosphorylation after u-PA interaction with its receptor (Dumler *et al.*, 1994) add to the notion that the u-PA/u-PAR interaction may cause a plethora of effects on vascular cells.

PUTATIVE ROLE OF u-PA AND u-PAR IN ANGIOGENESIS

A similar mechanism involving cell-bound u-PA activity has been suggested as being involved in the formation of new microvessels (angiogenesis) in a fibrinous wound matrix (Pepper *et al.*, 1990; Montesano, 1992). A direct correlation between the expression of u-PA activity and the formation of capillary-like tubular structures in a three-dimensional fibrin matrix by bovine microvascular endothelial cells *in vitro* was demonstrated by Pepper *et al.*, (1990). The outgrowth of tubular structures was induced by b-FGF, which in bovine endothelial cells enhances cell-bound u-PA activity (Montesano *et al.*, 1986; Moscatelli *et al.*, 1986; Saksela *et al.*, 1987), and limited by TGF-β, which enhances predominantly PAI-1 synthesis and inhibits PA activity (Saksela *et al.*, 1987). These studies with fibrin matrices indicate that the extent of capillary sprout formation and the diameter of the newly formed tubuli depend on the interplay between u-PA and PAI-1. A similar co-localization of u-PA and PAI-1 expression was observed during *in vitro* "angiogenesis" of cultured aortic explants, where both u-PA and PAI-1 expression was detected in outgrowing capillary sprouts, but not in the underlying endothelial sheets (Bacharach *et al.*, 1992).

Using human microvascular endothelial cells, similar factors as mentioned above have been observed to induce the outgrowth of capillary-like tubular structures in a three-dimensional fibrin matrix (Figure 12.3) (Koolwijk *et al.*, 1994). In these cells, b-FGF enhances the number of u-PAR (Mignatti *et al.*, 1991), but does not induce u-PA. TNFα on the other hand, induces u-PA synthesis (van Hinsbergh *et al.*, 1990, 1994; Niedbala and Picarella, 1992). In addition to b-FGF and/or vascular endothelial growth factor (VEGF), TNFα appeared to be required to induce tubular structures (Koolwijk *et al.*, 1994). Inhibition of u-PA activity by blocking antibodies or competition of u-PA binding to its receptor by addition of soluble u-PAR largely prevented the outgrowth of tubular structures under these conditions. It is anticipated that in more complex matrices, which also contain collagen fibers, other proteases, such as matrix-degrading metalloproteinases, also contribute to the invasion of endothelial cells.

In early embryo development the production of u-PA and PAI-1 is found in cells involved and closely associated with angiogenesis and cell migration (Sappino *et al.*,

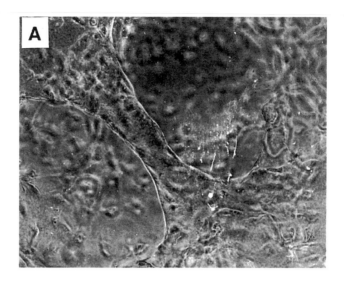

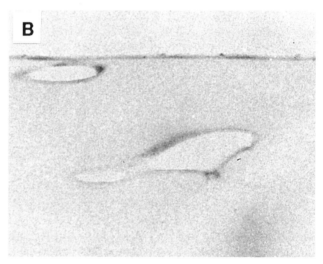

Figure 12.3 Human microvascular endothelial cells can be induced to form capillary tubes when they are grown on a fibrin matrix. In the presence of bFGF, TNF-α and VEGF formation of capillary tubes in the fibrin matrix by the microvascular endothelial cells is observed after 7 to 10 days by phase contrast microscopy (Panel A) and in cross-sections (Panel B).

1989). However, in transgenic mice lacking u-PA; PAI-1; or both u-PA and t-PA cell migration and development of the vascular system proceed normally (Carmeliet *et al.*, 1993, 1994a, 1994b, 1995). Therefore, alternative routes appear to exist which enable angiogenesis during embryo-development, or the association of u-PA and PAI-1 expression at areas of cell migration and angiogenesis does not reflect an involvement in these processes. Whether this also holds true for angiogenesis in adults is less clear. Angiogenesis in adults is observed during the formation of the corpus luteum, the formation of granulation tissue during wound healing and in many pathological conditions, such as tumor proliferation, rheumatoid arthritis, diabetic retinopathy (Folkman and Klagsbrun, 1987). Under these conditions fibrin is usually present and infiltration of mononuclear leucocytes occurs. Angiogenesis into a fibrin matrix or a mixed matrix of interstitial collagen fibers and fibrin (which is often present under these conditions) may have other requirements than angiogenesis during embryonic development. The observation that after vascular injury in transgenic mice lacking PAI-1 intima proliferation is accompanied by the formation of new intimal blood vessels supports this suggestion. However, the latter experiments do not yet allow conclusions as to whether the observed angiogenic response is a direct or an indirect reflection of the PAI-1 deficiency.

ROLE OF t-PA, u-PA AND u-PAR IN SMOOTH MUSCLE CELL MIGRATION

Vascular smooth muscle cells play an important role in the formation of atherosclerotic lesions and intimal hyperplasia causing restenosis (Ross, 1993). Migration of smooth muscle cells from the media into the intima followed by proliferation of these cells in the intima can contribute largely to cell accumulation and vessel wall thickening (Casscells *et al.*, 1993; O'Brien and Schwartz, 1994). In normal human arteries the majority of smooth muscle cells reside in the media, although a limited number of smooth muscle cells are present in the intima of arteries susceptible to atherosclerosis (Reidy *et al.*, 19931; Pauly *et al.*, 1994). The medial smooth muscle cells can become activated and start to migrate into the intima after mechanical injury of the vessel wall, or infiltration and accumulation of monocytes and T-lymphocytes (Ross, 1993). Both proliferation and migration of smooth muscle cells are processes tightly regulated by various growth factors and cytokines (Ferns *et al.*, 1991; Lindner and Reidy, 1991; Jawien *et al.*, 1992; Nabel *et al.*, 1993; Reidy, 1993; Ross, 1993). Recent data suggest that smooth muscle cell migration rather than proliferation is the major contributor to smooth muscle cell accumulation in the intima of atherosclerotic arteries (Katsuda *et al.*, 1993; O'Brien *et al.*, 1993).

Remodeling of the extracellular matrix is an essential step in migration of smooth muscle cells. During migration from the media to the intima smooth muscle cells have to cross various extracellular matrices (Burke and Ross, 1979; Moczar and Lafuma, 1986; Wight *et al.*, 1990). Cells have to pass their own surrounding matrix, mainly consisting of laminin, heparan sulphate proteoglycans and type IV collagen, and subsequently migrate through an interstitial matrix, composed of many fibrillar proteins including collagens I and III, fibronectin and proteoglycans, in the tunica media. The lamina elastica interna, which separates media and intima, is thought to be a significant barrier for invasion of smooth muscle cells into the intima, but it has fenestrations via which cells can migrate (Groves *et al.*, 1992). After passing the lamina elastica interna, the smooth muscle cells enter the interstitial matrix of the intima.

Migration of smooth muscle cells requires the continuous formation and degradation of cell-matrix contacts by which the cells can pull themselves through the fibrillar network. The interest in the mechanisms involved in smooth muscle cell migration is growing in particular regarding the role of proteases such as plasminogen activators and matrix-degrading metalloproteinases. Several lines of evidence support a role played by plasminogen activators in smooth muscle cell migration and accumulation. Most studies concern the involvement of plasminogen activators in smooth muscle cell migration. Recently Herbert *et al.*, (1994) suggested that t-PA may have a role in the regulation of smooth muscle cell proliferation *in vitro*.

An involvement of plasmin activity in smooth muscle cell migration was suggested by the *in vitro* observations of Schleef and Birdwell (1982) who found that smooth muscle cell migration was strongly reduced when the cells were deprived of plasminogen or when the plasmin activity was inhibited. Further evidence for an involvement of the plasmin/plasminogen activator system in smooth muscle cell migration comes from experiments with 'wounded' smooth muscle cell cultures, in which a strip of cells was removed. After removal of a strip of arterial smooth muscle cells, migration of cells into the denuded area can be partially inhibited by Trasylol, which inhibits plasmin. Migration was also inhibited by addition of anti-u-PA antibodies (Figure 12.4), which block the enzymatic activity of u-PA, or by addition of a soluble form of the u-PAR, which competes for the binding of u-PA to its cell surface receptor (Quax *et al.*, 1994). Cells at the migrating edge of the wound showed a marked increase in u-PA activity. Although these cultured cells produced large amounts of PAI-1, cell surface bound u-PA was active. Possibly rapid LRP-facilitated internalization of receptor-bound u-PA:PAI-1 complexes, and recycling of unoccupied u-PAR to the cell surface provides sufficient receptor molecules for continous binding and activation of single chain u-PA.

In animal models the putative role of plasminogen activation in smooth muscle cell migration is demonstrated in restenosis lesions induced by vascular injury. It has been demonstrated by Clowes *et al.*, (1990) that after removal of the endothelium by balloon injury in the rat carotid artery the expression of both u-PA and t-PA is induced. Determination of u-PA in extracts of these carotid arteries demonstrated that u-PA rapidly increases, its activity reaches a maximum between 16 and 24 hours after injury. t-PA activity appears after 3 days and is maximal at 7 days after injury, the time at which

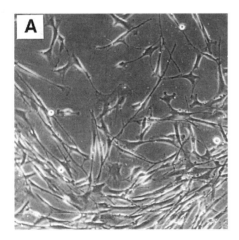 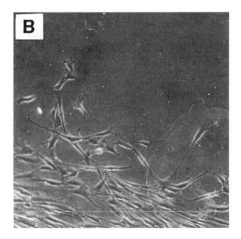

Figure 12.4   Migration of bovine smooth muscle cells in wounded cultures is inhibited in the presence of antibodies against u-PA. Migration 24 hours after wounding is shown in the absence (A) or presence (B) of anti-u-PA.

smooth muscle cell migration occurs. Heparin inhibited smooth muscle cell migration and intimal thickening, and, simultaneously, decreased t-PA activity in this system (Clowes *et al.*, 1992). Plasmin generation was necessary for migration of smooth muscle cells, since addition of tranexamic acid, an inhibitor of plasminogen activation, resulted in reduction of smooth muscle cell migration (Jackson *et al.*, 1993).

The best evidence for the role of the plasminogen activation system, in particular u-PA and PAI-1, in intimal thickening and smooth muscle cell migration is provided by the experiments with 'knock-out' mice deficient for u-PA, t-PA or PAI-1 (Carmeliet *et al.*, 1993, 1994a, 1994b, 1995). Preliminary analysis of neointima formation after vascular trauma in mice with a deficiency in PAI-1 shows a significant increase in the rate of neointima formation and neointimal cell accumulations (Carmeliet and Collen, 1994b, 1995). Mice deficient in u-PA show a significant decrease in neointima formation, whereas deficiency in t-PA had no effect on the neointima formation. These data suggest that u-PA rather than t-PA mediated plasmin generation is an absolute requirement for vascular wound healing and development of restenosis. The *in vitro* data mentioned above closely agree with the observations in deficient animals. The observation that in injured rat carotid artery smooth muscle cell migration is predominantly related to t-PA rather than to u-PA may reflect a species difference between rat and mouse, and needs further elucidation.

As discussed above for endothelial cells, other proteases, such as the matrix-degrading metalloproteinases, are also thought to contribute to the degradation of complex matrices by migrating smooth muscle cells. A role for matrix metalloproteinases in smooth muscle cell migration and the development of intimal hyperplasia is becoming more and more accepted. Evidence comes from experiments using specific inhibitors for matrix metallo-proteinases in balloon injured experimental animals *in vivo* (Bendeck *et al.*, 1994) and the presence of various MMPs in migrating smooth muscle cells in migration assays *in vitro* (Southgate *et al.*, 1992; Newby *et al.*, 1994; Pauly *et al.*, 1994) and *in vivo* (Zempo *et al.*, 1994).

COMPONENTS OF THE PLASMINOGEN ACTIVATION SYSTEM IN THE VESSEL WALL

In the Normal Vessel Wall

Although t-PA can be detected in many tissues including the ovary (Ny *et al.*, 1993; Peng *et al.*, 1993) and the central nervous system (Sappino *et al.*, 1992; Seeds *et al.*, 1992; Friedman and Seeds, 1994), it is more abundant in strongly vascularized tissues like the lung, liver and heart (Rickles and Strickland, 1988; Quax *et al.*, 1990) and in the vessel wall (Smokovitis *et al.*, 1989; Quax *et al.*, 1990; Levin and Delzoppo, 1993; Padro *et al.*, 1994; Emeis *et al.*, 1995). In the rat aorta vessel wall t-PA is produced by endothelial cells as well as by the smooth muscle cells in the media (Padro *et al.*, 1994). Levin and Delzoppo (1993) demonstrated by immunohistochemistry and in situ hybridization that t-PA was mainly present in the endothelium of smaller vessels like pre-capillary arterioles and post-capillary venules. Under normal conditions u-PA is not found in the walls of large vessels, such as the aorta (Padro *et al.*, 1994) although it has been reported that low levels of u-PA can be found in the vessel wall of the rat carotid artery (Clowes *et al.*,

1990). However, as will be discussed later, vascular cells can be induced by various stimuli to produce u-PA (Clowes *et al.*, 1990; Pepper *et al.*, 1990, 1991). The normal tissue distribution of PAI-1 protein and mRNA has been examined in humans as well as in rodent model systems by several groups (Lucore *et al.*, 1988; Quax *et al.*, 1990; Sawdey and Loskutoff, 1991; Simpson *et al.*, 1991; Fujii *et al.*, 1992) and is described in detail by Fearns *et al.*, (1995) in this book. In the human system the liver is a major source of PAI-1 (Simpson *et al.*, 1991; Chomiki *et al.*, 1994) although this is usually not found in animal models (Quax *et al.*, 1990; Sawdey and Loskutoff, 1991; Fearns *et al.*, 1995). The production of PAI-1 by the vessel wall, however, is found in all model systems studied (Quax *et al.*, 1990; Sawdey and Loskutoff, 1991; Simpson *et al.*, 1991; Fuji *et al.*, 1992; Schneiderman *et al.*, 1992; Lupu *et al.*, 1993; Chomiki *et al.*, 1994; Padro *et al.*, 1994). In the vessel wall both the endothelial cells and the smooth muscle cells are found to produce PAI-1, although not in all vessels the smooth muscle cells were found to produce PAI-1 (Clowes *et al.*, 1990; Chomiki *et al.*, 1994). No u-PAR was detectable in normal arterial tissues (Noda-Heiny *et al.*, 1995). The LRP is present on many tissues (Moestrup *et al.*, 1992; Lorent *et al.*, 1994). The presence of the LRP on the smooth muscle cells is clear (Moestrup *et al.*, 1992; Grobmeyer *et al.*, 1993). However, the presence of LRP on endothelial cells is uncertain.

Effect of Inflammatory Mediators on the Plasminogen Activation *in vivo*

Several mediators of inflammatory reactions have been shown to induce the production of plasminogen activators and their inhibitors in vascular cells not only *in vitro* but also *in vivo*. *In vitro*, the production of PAI-1 is stimulated by several factors involved in inflammatory and vascular diseases, such as the cytokines tumor necrosis factor-α (TNF-α) and interleukin-1 (IL-1), endotoxin (LPS), transforming growth factor-β (TGF-β), and also by oxidized lipoproteins and thrombin. *In vivo* the production of PAs and PAIs, and probably also u-PAR and LRP, is increased during inflammation, eg. at the inflammatory site in the vessel wall where infiltration of monocytes occurs. Administration of LPS to animals resulted in an increase of PAI-1 mRNA in vascularized tissues (Quax *et al.*, 1990). In such situations PAI-1 mRNA was not only elevated in the endothelium of various organs (Keeton *et al.*, 1993) but also in the smooth muscle cell containing medial layer of the aorta vessel wall (Padro *et al.*, 1994). An increase in t-PA mRNA has also been observed in several tissues.

In Atherosclerotic Lesions of the Vessel Wall.

The inflammatory factors TNF-α, IL-1 and TGF-β have been demonstrated in atherosclerotic lesions of the vessel wall (Nikol *et al.*, 1992; Tipping *et al.*, 1993). They are probably released from activated platelets and macrophages. These factors have been shown to influence the presence of PAI-1 and u-PAR on vascular cells. Analysis of the production of PAI-1 in atherosclerotic lesions in human aorta by Schneidermann *et al.*, (1992) revealed that PAI-1 gene expression is increased in atherosclerotic versus normal-appearing arterial tissues. In most studies the level of PAI-1 mRNA was found to correlate with the degree of atherosclerosis. Expression of PAI-1 in the atherosclerotic tissues was mainly localized in the neointimal region. Yorimitsu *et al.*, (1993) have demonstrated the presence of PAI-1 in endothelial cells, smooth muscle cells and on collagen fibers in coronary arterial stenotic lesions involved in an acute myocardial infarction. Lupu *et al.*, (1993) reported that in early atherosclerotic lesions PAI-1 was detected in association with vitronectin in the intimal smooth muscle cells and in extracellular areas. In advanced atheromatous plaques, PAI-1 mRNA expression in the smooth muscle cells within the fibrous cap was increased compared with smooth muscle cells located in the adjacent media. PAI-1 mRNA was also detected in macrophages located at the periphery of the necrotic core. In a recent study of Chomiki *et al.*, (1994) the presence of PAI-1 mRNA in the neointima in atherosclerotic lesions was found not only in some intimal cells and smooth muscle cells but also in neovessels scattering the lesions. It was suggested that the local increase in PAI-1 mRNA correlated with the abundant neovascularization present in the lesion.

The presence of the u-PAR in vascular smooth muscle cells and macrophages in neointima of atherosclerotic lesions in human tissue *in vivo* has been demonstrated recently (Noda-Heiny *et al.*, 1995). Also the LRP was detected in specimens of human atherosclerotic tissue (Luoma *et al.*, 1994; Lupu *et al.*, 1994).

In addition the matrix metalloproteinases stromelysin (MMP-3) (Henney *et al.*, 1991) as well as collagenase (MMP-1) and the gelatinases A and B (MMP-2 and MMP-9) (Galis *et al.*, 1994) have been demonstrated in the atherosclerotic lesions. Because of their expression in the macrophages in the shoulder of the plaque and in the core of the plaque the matrix metalloproteinases may contribute to destabilisation of the extracellular matrix, which may cause eventual plaque rupture. The expression of these matrix metalloproteinases in the smooth muscle cells, suggests an additional involvement of these enzymes in cell migration (Henney *et al.*, 1991; Galis *et al.*, 1994).

Summary

Plasminogen activators play a role in fibrinolysis, to dissolve thrombi, and in pericellular proteolysis. With respect to the vascular system, the latter occurs during matrix remodeling and cell migration in angiogenesis and neointima formation. The experiments suggesting a role of plasminogen activators in migration of endothelial cells and angiogenesis as well as the mechanism by which the various components of the plasminogen activator system interact in these processes are summarized in this chapter. A survey is given of the current evidence for a role of plasminogen activators, their receptors and inhibitors in smooth muscle cell migration in neointima formation. This evidence is coming from various experiments using *in vitro* migration assays and animal models in which neointima formation is induced by injury of the vessel wall. The expression of PAI-1 and u-PAR in atherosclerotic lesions of the vessel wall suggests a role for the plasminogen activation system in atherosclerosis. It should be realized, however, that also other proteolytic enzymes such as the matrix-degrading metalloproteinases are involved in these tightly regulated proteolytic processes in matrix remodeling.

The involvement of the plasminogen activator system in these processes and the various regulatory pathways involved in the complex modulation of the local plasminogen activator activity might provide powerful tools to interfere in uncontrolled matrix remodeling and cell migration processes in the vessel wall in order to reduce vascular complications.

Acknowledgement

We would like to acknowledge the financial support of the Netherlands Heart Foundation (grant MC93.001). We would like to thank W. de Vree and M. Wijnberg for their technical assistance with the experiments presented.

References

Bacharach, E., Itin, A. and Keshet, E. (1992). *In vivo* patterns of expression of urokinase and its inhibitor PAI-1 suggest a concerted role in regulating physiological angiogenesis. *Proc. Natl. Acad. Sci. USA*, **89**:10686–10690.

Bell, L., Luthringer, D.J., Madri, J.A. and Warren, S.L. (1992). Autocrine angiotensin system regulation of bovine aortic endothelial cell migration and plasminogen activator involves modulation of proto-oncogene pp60c-src expression. *J. Clin. Invest.*, **89**:315–320.

Bendeck, M., Zempo, N., Clowes, M.M., Galardy, R. and Reidy, M.A. (1994). Smooth muscle cell migration and matrix metalloproteinase expression after arterial injury in the rat. *Circ. Res.*, **75**:539–545.

Blasi, F. (1993). Urokinase and urokinase receptor — a paracrine/autocrine system regulating cell migration and invasiveness. *BioEssays*, **15**:105–111.

Blasi, F., Conese, M., Moller, L.B., Pedersen, N., Cavallaro, U., Cubellis, M.V., Fazioli, F., Hernandezmarrero, L., Limongi, P., Munozcanoves, P., Resnati, M., Riittinen, L., Sidenius, N., Soravia, E., Soria, M.R., Stoppelli, M.P., Talarico, D., Teesalu, T. and Valcamonica, S. (1994). The urokinase receptor: Structure, regulation and inhibitor-mediated internalization. *Fibrinolysis*, **8**:182–188.

Bosma, P.J., Rijken, D.C. and Nieuwenhuizen, W. (1988). Binding of tissue-type plasminogen activator to fibrinogen fragments. *Eur. J. Biochem.*, **172**:399–404.

Burke, J.M. and Ross, R. (1979). Synthesis of connective tissue macromolecules by smooth muscle. *Int. Rev. Connect. Tissue Res.*, **8**:119–157.

Busso, N., Masur, S.K., Lazega, D., Waxman, S. and Ossowski, L. (1994). Induction of cell migration by pro-urokinase binding to its receptor: Possible mechanism for signal transduction in human epithelial cells. *J. Cell Biol.*, **126**:259–270.

Carmeliet, P., Stassen, J.M., Schoonjans, L., Ream, B., Vandenoord, J.J., Demol, M., Mulligan, R.C. and Collen, D. (1993). Plasminogen activator inhibitor-1 gene deficient mice 2 effects on hemostasis, thrombosis, and thrombolysis. *J. Clin. Invest.*, **92**:2756–2760.

Carmeliet, P., Schoonjans, L., Kieckens, L., Ream, B., Degen, J., Bronson, R., Devos, R., Vandenoord, J.J., Collen, D. and Mulligan, R.C. (1994a). Physiological consequences of loss of plasminogen activator gene function in mice. *Nature*, **368**:419–424.

Carmeliet, P. and Collen, D. (1994b). Evaluation of the plasminogen/plasmin system in transgenic mice. *Fibrinolysis*, **8**:269–276.

Carmeliet, P. and Collen, D. (1995). Evaluation of the role of the fibrinolytic system in transgenic animals. in: *Vascular Control of Haemostasis*. edited by V.W.M. van Hinsbergh, pp 247–256, Camberwell, Australia, Gordon and Breach Science Publishers.

Casscells, W., Lappi, D.A. and Baird, A. (1993). Molecular Atherectomy for Restenosis. *Trends Cardiovasc. Med.*, **3**:235–243.

Castellino, F.J. (1988). Structure/function relationships of human plasminogen and plasmin. In: *Tissue-type plasminogen activator (t-PA): Physiological and clinical aspects*. Edited by C. Kluft, pp. 145–169, Boca Raton, Florida, USA, CRC Press.

Cesarman, G.M., Guevara, C.A. and Hajjar, K.A. (1994). An endothelial cell receptor for plasminogen/tissue plasminogen activator (t-PA) 2 Annexin II-mediated enhancement of t-PA-dependent plasminogen activation. *J. Biol. Chem.*, **269**:21198–21203.

Chomiki, N., Henry, M., Alessi, M.C., Anfosso, F. and Juhan-Vague, I. (1994). Plasminogen activator inhibitor-1 expression in human liver and healthy or atherosclerotic vessel walls. *Thromb. Haemost.*, **72**:44–53.

Clowes, A.W., Clowes, M.M., Au, Y.P.T., Reidy, M.A. and Belin, D. (1990). Smooth muscle cells express urokinase during mitogenesis and tissue-type plasminogen activator during migration in injured rat carotid artery. *Circ. Res.*, **67**:61–67.

Clowes, A.W., Clowes, M.M., Kirkman, T.R., Jackson, C.L., Au, Y.P.T. and Kenagy, R. (1992). Heparin inhibits the expression of tissue-type plasminogen activator by smooth muscle cells in injured rat carotid artery. *Circ. Res.*, **70**:1128–1136.

Conforti, G., Dominguez-Jimenez, C., Ronne, E., Hoyer-Hansen, G. and Dejana, E. (1994). Cell-surface plasminogen activation causes a retraction of *in vitro* cultured human umbilical vein endothelial cell monolayer. *Blood*, **83**:994–1005.

Cubellis, M.V., Wun, T.C. and Blasi, F. (1990). Receptor-mediated internalization and degradation of urokinase is caused by its specific inhibitor PAI-1. *Embo J.*, **9**:1079–1085.

Danø, K., Andreasen, P.A., Grøndahl-Hansen, J., Kristensen, P., Nielsen, L.S. and Skriver, L. (1985). Plasminogen activators tissue degradation and cancer. *Adv. Cancer Res.*, **44**:139–264.

Danø, K., Behrendt, N., Brunner, N., Ellis, V., Ploug, M. and Pyke, C. (1994). The urokinase receptor — Protein structure and role in plasminogen activation and cancer invasion. *Fibrinolysis*, **8**:189–203.

Dumler, I., Petri, T. and Schleuning, W.D. (1994). Induction of c-fos gene expression by urokinase-type plasminogen activator in human ovarian cancer cells. *FEBS Letters*, **343**:103–106.

Ellis, V., Behrendt, N. and Danø, K. (1991). Plasminogen activation by receptor-bound urokinase. A kinetic study with both cell-associated and isolated receptor. *J. Biol. Chem.*, **266**:12752–12758.

Emeis, J.J., van den Einden-Schrauwen, Y. and Kooistra, T. (1995). Tissue-type plasminogen activator and the vessel wall: Synthesis, storage and secretion. 2 in: *Vascular Control of Haemostasis*. edited by V.W.M. van Hinsbergh, pp 187–206, Camberwell, Australia, Gordon and Breach Science Publishers.

Estreicher, A., Muhlhauser, J., Carpentier, J.L., Orci, L. and Vassalli, J.D. (1990). The receptor for urokinase type plasminogen activator polarizes expression of the protease to the leading edge of migrating monocytes and promotes degradation of enzyme inhibitor complexes. *J. Cell Biol.*, **111**:783–792.

Fearns, C., Samad, F. and Loskutoff, D.J. (1995). Synthesis and localization of PAI-1 in the vessel wall. in: *Vascular Control of Haemostasis*. edited by V.W.M. van Hinsbergh, pp 207–226, Camberwell, Australia, Gordon and Breach Science Publishers.

Ferns, G.A.A., Raines, E.W., Sprugel, K.H., Motani, A.S., Reidy, M.A. and Ross, R. (1991). Inhibition of neointimal smooth muscle accumulation after angioplasty by an antibody to PDGF. *Science*, **253**:1129–1132.

Flaumenhaft, R., Abe, M., Mignatti, P. and Rifkin, D.B. (1992a). Basic fibroblast growth factor-induced activation of latent transforming growth factor-beta in endothelial cells — regulation of plasminogen activator activity. *J. Cell Biol.*, **118**:901–909.

Flaumenhaft, R. and Rifkin, D.B. (1992b). The extracellular regulation of growth factor action. *Molecular Biology of the Cell*, **3**:1057–1065.

Folkman, J. and Klagsbrun, M. (1987). Angiogenic factors. *Science*, **235**:442–447.

Friedman, G.C. and Seeds, N.W. (1994). Tissue plasminogen activator expression in the embryonic nervous system. *Develop. Brain Res.*, **81**:41–49.

Fujii, S., Sawa, H., Saffitz, J.E., Lucore, C.L. and Sobel, B.E. (1992). Induction of endothelial cell expression of the plasminogen activator inhibitor type-1 gene by thrombosis *in vivo*. *Circulation*, **86**:2000–2010.

Galis, Z.S., Sukhova, G.K., Lark, M.W. and Libby, P. (1994). Increased expression of matrix metalloproteinases and matrix degradation activity in vulnerable regions of human atherosclerotic plaques. *J. Clin. Invest.*, **94**:2493–2503:

Grobmyer, S.R., Kuo, A., Orishimo, M., Okada, S.S., Cines, D.B. and Barnathan, E.S. (1993). Determinants of binding and internalization of tissue-type plasminogen activator by human vascular smooth muscle and endothelial cells. *J. Biol. Chem.*, **268**:13291–13300.

Groves, P.H., Lewis, M.J., Newby, A.C., Cheadle, H.A. and Penny, W.J. (1992). Progressive intimal thickening after balloon angioplasty is associated with rupture of the internal elastic lamina. *Brit. H. Journal*, **68**:86.

Hajjar, K.A. (1991). The endothelial cell tissue plasminogen activator receptor — specific interaction with plasminogen. *J. Biol. Chem.*, **266**:21962–21970.

Hajjar, K.A., Jacovina, A.T. and Chacko, J. (1994). An endothelial cell receptor for plasminogen tissue plasminogen activator 1. Identity with annexin II. *J. Biol. Chem.*, **269**:21191–21197.

He, C., Wilhelm, S.M., Pentland, A.P., Marmer, B.L., Grant, G.A., Eisen, A.Z. and Goldberg, G.I. (1989). Tissue cooperation in a proteolytic cascade activating human interstitial collagenase. *Proc. Natl. Acad. Sci. USA*, **86**:2632–2636.

Hébert, C. and Baker, J.B. (1988). Linkage of extracellular plasminogen activator to the fibroblast cystoskeleton colocalization of cell surface urokinase with vinculin. *J. Cell Biol.*, **106**:1241–1247.

Henney, A.M., Wakeley, P.R., Davies, M.J., Foster, K., Hembry, R., Murphy, G. and Humphries, S. (1991). Localization of stromelysin gene expression in atherosclerotic plaques by in situ hybridization. *Proc. Natl. Acad. Sci. USA*, **88**:8154–8158.

Herbert, J.M., Lamarche, I., Prabonnaud, V., Dol, F. and Gauthier, T. (1994). Tissue-type plasminogen activator is a potent mitogen for human aortic smooth muscle cells. *J. Biol. Chem.*, **269**:3076–3080.

Herz, J., Hamann, U., Rogne, S., Myklebost, O., Gausepohl, H. and Stanley, K.K. (1988). Surface location and high affinity for calcium of a 500-kd liver membrane protein closely related to the LDL-receptor suggest a physiological role as lipoprotein receptor. *Embo J.*, **7**:4119–4127.

Holmes, W., Nelles, L., Lijnen, H.R. and Collen, D. (1987). Primary structure of human α2-antiplasmin a serine protease inhibitor serpin. *J. Biol. Chem.*, **262**:1659–1664.

Hoylaerts, M., Rijken, D.C., Lijnen, H.R. and Collen, D. (1982). Kinetics of the activation of plasminogen by tumor tissue plasminogen activator — Role of fibrin. *J. Biol. Chem.*, **257**:2912–2919.

Jackson, C.L., Raines, E.W., Ross, R. and Reidy, M.A. (1993). Role of endogenous Platelet-Derived Growth Factor in arterial smooth muscle cell migration after balloon catheter injury. *Arterioscl. Thromb.*, **13**: 1218–1226.

Jawien, A., Bowen-Pope, D.F., Lindner, V., Schwartz, Z. and Clowes, A.W. (1992). Platelet-derived Growth Factor promotes smooth muscle migration and intimal thickening in a rat model of balloon angioplasty. *J. Clin. Invest.*, **89**:507–511.

Katsuda, S., Coltrera, M.D., Ross, R. and Gown, A.M. (1993). Human Atherosclerosis — IV Immunocytochenical analysis of cell activation and proliferation in lesions of young adults. *Am. J. Pathol.*, **142**:1787–1793.

Keeton, M., Eguchi, Y., Sawdey, M., Ahn, C. and Loskutoff, D.J. (1993). Cellular localization of type-1 plasminogen activator inhibitor messenger RNA and protein in murine renal tissue. *Am. J. Pathol.*, **142**:59–70.

Koolwijk, P., de Vree, W., Hanemaaijer, R., van Erck, M., Vermeer, M., Zurcher, C., Weich, H. and van Hinsbergh, V. (1994). Cooperative effect of VEGF, bFGF, TNFα on pericellular u-PA expression and on the formation of capillary-like tubular structures by human microvascular endothelial cells *in vitro*. *Fibrinolysis*, 8 suppl 1, 145.

Kounnas, M.Z., Henkin, J., Argraves, W.S. and Strickland, D.K. (1993). Low Density Lipoprotein receptor-related protein/alpha(2)-macroglobulin receptor mediates cellular uptake of pro-urokinase. *J. Biol. Chem.*, **268**:21862–21867.

Kruithof, E.K.O. (1988). Plasminogen activator inhibitors — a review. *Enzyme*, **40**:113–121.

Levin, E.G. and Delzoppo, G.J. (1994). Localization of tissue plasminogen activator in the endothelium of a limited number of vessels. *Am. J. Pathol.*, **144**:855–861.

Lindner, V. and Reidy, M.A. (1991). Proliferation of smooth muscle cells after vascular injury is inhibited by an antibody against basic fibroblast growth factor. *Proc. Natl. Acad. Sci. USA*, **88**:3739–3743.

Liotta, L.A., Steeg, P.S. and Stetler-Stevenson, W.G. (1991). Cancer metastasis and angiogenesis: an imbalance of positive and negative regulation. *Cell*, **64**:327–336.

Lorent, K., Overbergh, L., Delabie, J., Vanleuven, F. and Vandenberghe, H. (1994). Distribution of mRNA coding for alpha-2-macroglobulin, the murinoglobulins, the alpha-2-macroglobulin receptor and the alpha-2-macroglobulin receptor associated protein during mouse embryogenesis and in adult tissues. *Differentiation*, **55**:213–223.

Lucore, C.L., Fujii, S., Wun, T.C., Sobel, B.E. and Billadello, J.J. (1988). Regulation of the expression of type 1 plasminogen activator inhibitor in Hep G2 cells by epidermal growth factor. *J. Biol. Chem.*, **263**:15845–15848.

Luoma, J., Hiltunen, T., Sarkioja, T., Moestrup, S.K., Gliemann, J., Kodama, T., Nikkari, T. and Yla-Herttuala, S. (1994). Expression of alpha(2)-macroglobulin receptor/low density lipoprotein receptor-related protein and scavenger receptor in human atherosclerotic lesions. *J. Clin. Invest.*, **93**:2014–2021.

Lupu, F., Bergonzelli, G.E., Heim, D.A., Cousin, E., Genton, C.Y., Bachmann, F. and Kruithof, E.K.O. (1993). Localization and production of plasminogen activator inhibitor-1 in human healthy and atherosclerotic arteries. *Arterioscl. Thromb.*, **13**:1090–1100.

Lupu, F., Heim, D., Bachmann, F. and Kruithof, E.K.O. (1994). Expression of LDL Receptor-related protein alpha2-macroglobulin receptor in human normal and atherosclerotic arteries. *Arterioscl. Thromb.*, **14**:1438–1444.

Mignatti, P., Morimoto, T. and Rifkin, D.B. (1991). Basic fibroblast growth factor released by single, isolated cells stimulates their migration in an autocrine manner. *Proc. Natl. Acad. Sci. USA*, **88**:11007–11011.

Miles, L.A., Dahlberg, C.M. and Plow, E.F. (1988). The cell-binding domains of plasminogen and their function in plasma. *J. Biol. Chem.*, **263**:11928–11934.

Miles, L.A., Dahlberg, C.M., Plescia, J., Felez, J., Kato, K. and Plow, E.F. (1991). Role of cell-surface lysines in plasminogen binding to cells: Identification of alpha-enolase as a candidate plasminogen receptor. *Biochemistry*, **30**:1682–1691.

Moczar, M. and Lafuma, C. (1986). Structural glycoproteins from aorta and lung. *Frontiers Matrix Biol.*, **11**:42–57.

Moestrup, S.K., Gliemann, J. and Pallesen, G. (1992). Distribution of the α2-macroglobulin receptor/low density lipoprotein receptro-related protein in human tissues. *Cell. Tissue Res.*, **269**:375–382.

Moestrup, S.K. (1994). The alpha(2)-macroglobulin receptor and epithelial glycoprotein-330: Two giant receptors mediating endocytosis of multiple ligands. *Biochim. Biophys. Acta*, **1197**: 197–213.

Montesano, R., Vasalli, J.D., Baird, A., Guillemin, R. and Orci, L. (1986). Basic fibroblast growth factor induces angiogenesis *in vitro*. *Proc. Natl. Acad. Sci. USA*, **83**:7297–7301.

Montesano, R. (1992). Regulation of angiogenesis *in vitro*. *Eur. J. Clin. Invest.*, **22**:504–515.

Møller, L.B., Ploug, M. and Blasi, F. (1992). Structural requirements for glycosyl phosphatidylinositol anchor attachment in the cellular receptor for urokinase plasminogen activator. *Eur. J. Biochem.*, **208**:493–500.

Moscatelli, D., Presta, M. and Rifkin, D.B. (1986). Purification of a factor from human placenta that stimulates capillary endothelial cell protease production, DNA synthesis and migration. *Proc. Natl. Acad. Sci. USA*, **83**:2091–2095.

Murphy, G., Atkinson, S., Ward, R., Gavrilovic, J. and Reynolds, J.J. (1992). The role of plasminogen activators in the regulation of connective tissue metalloproteinases. *Ann. N.Y. Acad. Sci.*, **667**:1–12.

Nabel, E.G., Shum, L., Pompili, V.J., Yang, Z.Y., San, H., Shu, H.B., Liptay, S., Gold, L., Gordon, D., Derynck, R. and Nabel, G.J. (1993). Direct transfer of transforming growth factor Beta1 gene into arteries stimulates fibrocellular hyperplasia. *Proc. Natl. Acad. Sci. USA*, **90**:10759–10763.

Newby, A.C., Southgate, K.M. and Davies, M. (1994). Extracellular matrix degrading metalloproteinases in the pathogenesis of arteriosclerosis. *Basic Res. Cardiol.*, **89**:59–70.

Niedbala, M.J. and Picarella, M.S. (1992). Tumor necrosis factor induction of endothelial cell urokinase-type plasminogen activator mediated proteolysis of extracellular matrix and its antagonism by gamma-Interferon. *Blood*, **79**:678–687.

Nieuwenhuizen, W., Voskuilen, M., Vermond, A., Hoegee N. and Traas, D.W. (1988). The influence of fibrin(ogen) fragments on the kinetic parameters of the tissue-type plasminogen-activator-mediated activation of different forms of plasminogen. *Eur. J. Biochem.*, **174**:163–169.

Nikol, S., Isner, J.M., Pickering, J.G., Kearney, M., Leclerc, G. and Weir, L. (1992). Expression of transforming growth factor beta-1 is increased in human vascular restenosis lesions. *J. Clin. Invest.*, **90**:1582–1592.

Noda-Heiny, H., Daugherty, A. and Sobel, B.E. (1995). Augmented urokinase receptor expression in atheroma. *Arterioscl. Thromb. Vasc. Biol.*, **15**:37–43.

Ny, T., Peng, X.R. and Ohlsson, M. (1993). Hormonal regulation of the fibrinolytic components in the ovary. *Thromb. Res.*, **71**:1–45.

Nykjaer, A., Petersen, C.M., Moller, B., Jensen, P.H., Moestrup, S.K., Holtet, T.L., Etzerodt, M., Thogersen, H.C., Munch, M., Andreasen, P.A. and Gliemann, J. (1992). Purified alpha2-Macroglobulin Receptor/LDL Receptor-Related protein binds urokinase activator inhibitor type-1 complex — evidence that the alpha2-Macroglobulin receptor mediates cellular degradation of urokinase receptor-bound complexes. J. Biol. Chem., **267**:14543–14546.

O'Brien, E.R., Alpers, C.E., Stewart, D.K., Ferguson, M., Tran, N., Gordon, D., Bensitt, E.P., Hinohara, T., Simpson, J.B. and Schwartz, S.M. (1993). Proliferation in primary and restenotic coronary atherectomy tissue. Implications for antiproliferative therapy. *Circ. Res.*, **73**:223–231.

O'Brien, E.R. and Schwartz, S.M. (1994). Update on the biology and clinical study of restenosis. *Trends Cardiovasc. Med.*, **4**:169–178.

Odekon, L.E., Sato, Y. and Rifkin, D.B. (1992). Urokinase-type plasminogen activator mediates basic fibroblast growth factor-induced bovine endothelial cell migration independent of its proteolytic activity. *J. Cell. Physiol.*, **150**:258–263.

Orth, K., Madison, E.L., Gething, M.J., Sambrook, J.F. and Herz, J. (1992). Complexes of tissue-type plasminogen activator and its serpin inhibitor plasminogen-activator inhibitor type-1 are internalized by means of the Low Density Lipoprotein Receptor-Related Protein/ alpha2-Macroglobulin Receptor. *Proc. Natl. Acad. Sci. USA*, **89**:7422–7426.

Orth, K., Willnow, T., Herz, J., Gething, M.J. and Sambrook, J. (1994). Low density lipoprotein receptor-related protein is necessary for the internalization of both tissue-type plasminogen activator-inhibitor complexes and free tissue-type plasminogen activator. *J. Biol. Chem.*, **269**:21117–21122.

Padro, T., Quax, P.H.A., van den Hoogen, C.M., Roholl, P., Verheijen. J.H. and Emeis, J.J. (1994). Tissue-type plasminogen activator and its inhibitor in rat aorta — Effect of endotoxin. *Arterioscl. Thromb.*, **14**:1459–1465.

Pauly, R.R., Passaniti, A., Bilato, C., Monticone, R., Cheng, L., Papadopoulos, N., Gluzband, Y.A., Smith, L., Weinstein, C., Lakatta, E.G. and Crow, M.T. (1994). Migration of cultured vascular smooth muscle cells through a basement membrane barrier requires type IV collagenase activity and is inhibited by cellular differentiation. *Circ. Res.*, **75**:41–54.

Peng, X.R., Hsueh, A.J.W. and Ny, T. (1993). Transient and cell-specific expression of tissue-type plasminogen activator and plasminogen-activator-inhibitor type-1 results in controlled and directed proteolysis during gonadotropin-induced ovulation. *Eur. J. Biochem.*, **214**:147–156.

Pepper, M.S., Vassalli, J.D., Montesano, R. and Ocri, L. (1987). Urokinase-type plasminogen activator is induced in migrating capillary endothelial cells. *J. Cell Biol.*, **105**:2535–2541.

Pepper, M.S., Belin, D., Montesano, R., Orci, L. and Vassalli, J.D. (1990). Transforming growth factor-beta-1 modulates basic fibroblast growth factor induced proteolytic and angiogenic properties of endothelial cells *in vitro*. *J. Cell Biol.*, **111**:743–755.

Pepper, M.S., Ferrara, N., Orci, L. and Montesano, R. (1991). Vascular endothelial growth factor (VEGF) induces plasminogen activators and plasminogen activator inhibitor-1 in microvascular endothelial cells. *Biochem. Biophys. Res. Comm.*, **181**:902–906.

Pepper, M.S., Sappino, A.P., Stocklin, R., Montesano, R., Orci, L. and Vassalli, J.D. (1993). Upregulation of urokinase receptor expression on migrating endothelial cells. *J. Cell Biol.*, **122**:673–684.

Ploug, M., Rønne, E., Behrendt, N., Jensen, A.L., Blasi, F. and Danø, K. (1991). Cellular receptor for urokinase plasminogen activator — carboxyl-terminal processing and membrane anchoring by glycosyl-phosphatidylinositol. *J. Biol. Chem.*, **266**:1926–1933.

Pöllänen, J., Saksela, O., Salonen, E.M., Andreasen, P.A., Nielsen, L., Danø, K. and Vaheri, A. (1987). Distinct localizations of urokinase type plasminogen activator and its 1 inhibitor under cultured human fibroblast and sarcoma cells. *J. Cell Biol.*, **104**:1085–1096.

Pöllänen, J., Hedman, K., Nielsen, L.S., Danø, K. and Vaheri, A. (1988). Ultrastructural localization of plasma membrane associated urokinase type plasminogen activator at focal contacts. *J. Cell Biol.*, **106**:87–95.

Quax, P.H.A., van den Hoogen, C.M., Verheijen, J.H., Padro, T., Zeheb, R., Gelehrter, T.D., van Berkel, T.J.C., Kuiper, J. and Emeis, J.J. (1990). Endotoxin induction of plasminogen activator and plasminogen activator inhibitor type 1 mRNA in rat tissues *in vivo*. *J. Biol. Chem.*, **265**:15560–15563.

Quax, P.H.A., Pedersen, N., Masucci, M.T., Weening-Verhoeff, E.J.D., Danø, K., Verheijen, J.H. and Blasi, F. (1991). Complementation between urokinase-producing and receptor producing cells in extracellular matrix degradation. *Cell Regul.*, **2**:793–803.

Quax, P.H.A., Khouw, I.M.S.L., Bakker, T.R., van Leeuwen R.T.J. and Verheijen, J.H. (1994). Urokinase-type plasminogen activator is involved in smooth muscle cell migration in wounded cultures. *Fibrinolysis* **8** suppl 1, 148.

Reidy, M.A. (1993). Neointimal Proliferation — The Role of Basic FGF on Vascular Smooth Muscle Cell Proliferation. *Thromb. Haemost.*, **70**:172–176.

Rickles, R.J. and Strickland, S. (1988). Tissue plasminogen activator mRNA in murine tissues. *FEBS Letters*, **229**:100–106.

Robbins, K.C., Summaria, L., Hsieh, B. and Shah, R.J. (1967). The peptide chains of human plasmin. Mechanism of activation of human plasminogen to plasmin. *J. Biol. Chem.*, **242**:2333–2342.

Ross, R. (1993). The pathogenesis of atherosclerosis: a perspective for the 1990s. *Nature*, **362**:801–809.

Saksela, O., Moscatelli, D. and Rifkin, D.B. (1987). The opposing effects of basic fibroblast growth factor and transforming growth factor beta on the regulation of plasminogen activator activity in capillary endothelial cells. *J. Cell Biol.*, **105**:957–963.

Sappino, A.P., Huarte, J., Belin, D. and Vassalli, J.D. (1989). Plasminogen activators in tissue remodeling and invasion — messenger RNA localization in mouse ovaries and implanting embryos. *J. Cell Biol.*, **109**:2471–2479.

Sappino, A.P., Madani, R., Huarte, J., Belin, D., Kiss, J.Z., Wohlwend, A. and Vassalli, J.D. (1993). Extracellular proteolysis in the adult murine brain. *J. Clin. Invest.*, **92**:679–685.

Sato, Y. and Rifkin, D.B. (1989). Inhibition of endothelial cell movement by pericytes and smooth muscle cells : activation of a latent transforming growth factor-beta1-like molecule by plasmin during co-culture. *J. Cell Biol.*, **109**:309–315.

Sawdey, M. and Loskutoff, D.J. (1991). Regulation of murine type 1 plasminogen activator inhibitor gene expression *in vivo*. Tissue specificity and induction by lipopolysaccharide, tumor necrosis factor-α and transforming growth factor-β. *J. Clin. Invest.*, **88**:1346–1353.

Schleef, R.R. and Birdwell, C.R. (1982). The effects of proteases on endothelial cell migration *in vitro*. *Exp. Cell Res.*, **141**: 503–508.

Schneiderman, J., Sawdey, M.S., Keeton, M.R., Bordin, G.M., Bernstein, E.F., Dilley, R.B. and Loskutoff, D.J. (1992). Increased type-1 plasminogen activator inhibitor gene expression in atherosclerotic human arteries. *Proc. Natl. Acad. Sci. USA*, **89**:6998–7002.

Seeds, N.W., Verrall, S., Friedman, G., Hayden, S., Gadotti, D., Haffke, S., Christensen, K., Gardner, B., Mcguire, P. and Krystosek, A. (1992). Plasminogen activators and plasminogen activator inhibitors in neural development. *Ann. N.Y. Acad. Sci.*, **667**:32–40.

Simpson, A.J., Booth, N.A., Moore, N.R. and Bennett, B. (1991). Distribution of Plasminogen Activator Inhibitor (PAI-1) in Tissues. *J. Clin. Pathol.*, **44**:139–143.

Smokovitis, A.A., Kokolis, N.A., Alexaki, E. and Binder, B.R. (1989). Demonstration of plasminogen activator activity in the intima and media of the normal human aorta and other large arteries: immunological identification of the plasminogen activator(s). *Thromb. Res.*, **55**:259–265.

Sprengers, E.D. and Kluft, C. (1987). Plasminogen activator inhibitors. *Blood*, **69**:381–387.

Southgate, K.M., Davies, M., Booth, R.F.G. and Newby, A.C. (1992). Involvement of extracellular-matrix-degrading metalloproteinases in rabbit aortic smooth-muscle cell proliferation. *Biochem. J.*, **288**:93–99.

Stephens, R.W., Pöllänen, J., Tapiovaara, H., Leung, K.C., Sim, P.S., Salonen, E.M., Rønne, E., Behrendt, N., Danø, K. and Vaheri, A. (1989). Activation of pro-urokinase and plasminogen on human sarcoma cells — a proteolytic system with surface-bound reactants. *J. Cell Biol.*, **108**:1987–1995.

Stoppelli, M.P., Corti, A., Soffientini, A., Cassani, G., Blasi, F. and Associan, R.K. (1985). Differentiation enhanced binding of the amino terminal fragment of human urokinase-type plasminogen activator to a specific receptor on U937 monocytes. *Proc. Natl. Acad. Sci. USA*, **82**:4939–4943.

Strickland, D.K., Kounnas, M.Z., Williams, S.E. and Argraves, W.S. (1994). LDL receptor-related protein (LRP): A multiligand receptor. *Fibrinolysis*, **8** suppl. 1:204–215.

Tipping, P.G., Davenport, P., Gallicchio, M., Filonzi, E.L., Apostolopoulos, J. and Wojta, J. (1993). Atheromatous plaque macrophages produce plasminogen activator inhibitor type-1 and stimulate its production by endothelial cells and vascular smooth muscle cells. *Am. J. Pathol.*, **143**:875–885.

Tsuboi, R., Sato, Y. and Rifkin, D.B. (1990). Correlation of cell migration, cell invasion, receptor number, proteinase production, and basic fibroblast growth factor levels in endothelial cells. *J. Cell Biol.*, **110**:511–517.

van Hinsbergh, V.W.M., van den Berg, E.A., Fiers, W. and Dooijewaard, G. (1990). Tumor necrosis factor induces the production of urokinase-type plasminogen activator by human endothelial cells. *Blood*, **75**:1991–1998.

van Hinsbergh, V.W.M., Vermeer, M., Koolwijk, P., Grimbergen, J. and Kooistra, T. (1994). Genistein reduces tumor necrosis factor alpha-induced plasminogen activator inhibitor-1 transcription but not urokinase expression in human endothelial cells. *Blood*, **84**:2984–2991.

Vassalli, J.D., Baccino, D. and Belin, D. (1985). A cellular binding site for the Mr 55, 000 form of the human plasminogen activator, urokinase. *J. Cell Biol.*, **100**:86–92.

Verheijen, J.H., Nieuwenhuizen, W. and Wijngaards, G. (1982). Activation of plasminogen by tissue activator is increased specifically in the presence of certain soluble fibrin(ogen) fragments. *Thromb. Res.*, **27**:377–385.

Waltz, D.A. and Chapman, H.A. (1994). Reversible cellular adhesion to vitronectin linked to urokinase receptor occupancy. *J. Biol. Chem.*, **269**:14746–14750.

Wight, T.N. (1990). The cell biology of arterial proteoglycans. *Arteriosclerosis*, **9**:1–20.

Yorimitsu, K., Saito, T., Toyozaki, T., Isshide, T., Ohnuma, N. and Inagaki, Y. (1993). Immunohistochemical localization of plasminogen activator inhibitor-1 in human coronary atherosclerotic lesions involved in acute myocardial infarction. *Heart Vessels*, **8**:160–162.

Zempo, N., Kenagy, R.D., Au, Y.P.T., Bendeck, M., Clowes, M.M., Reidy, M.A. and Clowes, A.W. (1994). Matrix metalloproteinases of vascular wall cells are increased in balloon-injured rat carotid artery. *J. Vasc. Surgery*, **20**:209–217.

13 Evaluation of the Role of the Fibrinolytic System in Transgenic Animals

Peter Carmeliet and Désiré Collen

The Center for Pagene Therapy Transgene Technology, University of Leuven, Leuven, B-3000, Belgium

Indirect evidence suggests a crucial role for the fibrinolytic system, and its physiological triggers tissue-type plasminogen activator and urokinase-type plasminogen activator in many proteolytic processes, including blood clot dissolution (thrombolysis), thrombosis, hemostasis, atherosclerosis, restenosis, reproduction, embryo implantation, embryogenesis, wound healing, malignancy and brain function. The implied role of the fibrinolytic system in vivo is, however, deduced from correlations between fibrinolytic activity and (patho) physiological phenomena, which does not allow to definitively establish a causal role of this system in these processes. Recently, several transgenic mice, over- or under-expressing fibrinolytic system components, have been generated. This article reviews briefly the physiological consequences of gain or loss of function of these fibrinolytic system components on thrombosis, hemostasis, neointima formation, brain function and the associated effects on reproduction, development, health and survival.

KEYWORDS: transgenic mice, homologous recombination, embryonic stem cells, tissue-type plasminogen activator, urokinase-type plasminogen activator and plasminogen activator inhibitor

THE PLASMINOGEN/PLASMIN SYSTEM

The fibrinolytic or plasminogen/plasmin system comprises an inactive proenzyme, plasminogen, that is activated to the proteolytic enzyme plasmin by two physiological plasminogen activators, tissue-type plasminogen activator (t-PA) and urokinase-type plasminogen activator (u-PA) (Collen and Lijnen 1991). Inhibition of the fibrinolytic system may occur at the level of plasmin, mainly by α_2-antiplasmin or at the level of the plasminogen activators by specific plasminogen activator inhibitors (PAIs) of which PAI-1 appears to be the principal inhibitor (Schneiderman and Loskutoff 1991). t-PA is believed to be primarily responsible for removal of fibrin from the vascular tree through its specific affinity for fibrin (Collen and Lijnen 1991). u-PA binds to a cellular receptor (u-PAR) and might participate in pericellular proteolysis via degradation of matrix components or via activation of latent proteinases or growth factors (Blasi *et al.*, 1987, Vassali 1994). Cell specific clearance of plasminogen activators (PA) by LDL Receptor-related Protein (LRP) or gp330 might constitute a mechanism to modulate pericellular plasmin proteolysis (Andreasen *et al.*, 1994).

247

DEVELOPMENT AND REPRODUCTION

Much circumstantial evidence based on expression of fibrinolytic system components, implicates the plasminogen/plasmin system in ovulation, sperm migration, fertilization, embryo implantation and embryogenesis, and the associated tissue remodeling of the ovary, prostate and mammary gland (Vassalli *et al.*, 1991). In addition, serine-proteinase inhibitors and/or plasminogen activator-specific antisera suppress ovulation and embryo implantation in rodents, supporting the implication of the fibrinolytic system in this phenomenon. Since no genetic deficiencies involving t-PA or u-PA have been described in man, inactivation of these genes in mice might have been anticipated to result in a lethal phenotype. We have generated mice with inactivation of the genes encoding tissue-type plasminogen activator (t-PA), urokinase-type plasminogen activator (u-PA) and plasminogen activator inhibitor-1 (PAI-1) (Carmeliet *et al.*, 1993a, 1993b and 1994a). Surprisingly, single- and double-deficient mice appeared normal at birth suggesting that neither t-PA nor u-PA, individually or in combination, are required for normal embryonic development (Carmeliet *et al.*, 1994a; 1994b). Furthermore, the observations that PAI-1 deficient mice produced normal offspring also suggest a non-essential role of PAI-1 in development.

Mice with single deficiency of t-PA, u-PA or PAI-1 were fertile (Carmeliet *et al.*, 1993a, 1994a). Normal fertility was also observed in a t-PA antisense transgenic mouse strain, expressing less then 50% of wild-type t-PA activity in oocytes (Richards *et al.*, 1993). Combined t-PA:u-PA deficient mice were able to reproduce but were significantly less fertile than wild-type mice or mice with a single deficiency of t-PA or u-PA. Although poor general health conditions (low body weight, dyspnea, anemia, rectal prolapse and cachexia) and the presence of large fibrin deposits in gonads (Carmeliet *et al.*, 1994a) might explain their reduced fertility, some apparently normal and healthy combined t-PA:u-PA deficient mice did not produce any litter at all, possibly suggesting a primary defect of reproduction. Inactivation of the LRP gene, which encodes a functional receptor involved in clearance of amongst others plasminogen activators, resulted in embryonic lethality at mid-gestation secondary to intra-abdominal bleeding (Herz *et al.*, 1992). Although LRP is involved in clearance of several molecules (Andreasen *et al.*, 1994), one possible explanation, which remains to be further examined, is that deficient clearance of plasminogen activators might result in local overexpression uncontrolled proteolysis. Collectively, these observations suggest that proteinases and proteinase inhibitors other than t-PA, u-PA or PAI-1 may be more essential in reproduction and embryonic development than previously suspected.

HEALTH AND SURVIVAL

Although certain species, including chicken, only possess u-PA and no t-PA, genetic deficiencies of t-PA or u-PA in man or mice have not been reported. Consequently, the role of the fibrinolytic system in general health and survival remained to be determined. No effects on health and survival were observed in t-PA deficient and PAI-1 deficient mice. A small percentage of u-PA deficient mice developed chronic (non-healing) ulcerations and rectal prolapse but without effect on survival. Although combined t-PA:u-PA deficient mice also developed such chronic ulcerations and rectal prolapse, these mice suffered significant growth retardation, developed a wasting-syndrome with anemia, dyspnea, lethargia and cachexia and had a significantly shorter life span (Carmeliet *et al.*, 1994a). Generalized thrombosis in the gastro-intestinal tract (with chronic ulcerations and rarely ischemic necrosis, possibly causing hypoalimentation), in the lungs (with lung atelectasis contributing to dyspnea) and in other organs (including gonads, liver and kidney) might contribute to the increased morbidity and mortality of combined plasminogen activator deficient mice.

THROMBOSIS/THROMBOLYSIS

Deficient fibrinolytic activity, e.g. resulting from increased plasma PAI-1 levels or reduced plasma t-PA or plasminogen levels, might participate in the development of thrombotic events (Schneiderman and Loskutoff 1991). Elevated plasma PAI-1 levels have indeed been correlated with a higher risk of deep venous thrombosis and of thrombosis during hemolytic uremic syndrome, disseminated intravascular coagulation, sepsis, surgery and trauma. PAI-1 plasma levels were also elevated in patients with ischemic heart disease, angina pectoris and recurrent myocardial infarction. However, the acute phase reactant behaviour of PAI-1 does not allow to deduce whether increased PAI-1 levels are cause or consequence of thrombosis.

Microscopical analysis of tissues from u-PA deficient mice revealed occasional minor fibrin deposits in liver and intestines but excessive fibrin deposits in chronic non healing skin ulcerations. No spontaneous fibrin deposits were observed in t-PA deficient mice. Mice with a combined deficiency of t-PA and u-PA revealed, however, extensive fibrin deposits in several normal and inflamed organs with ischemic necrosis, possibly resulting from thrombotic occlusions. Cellular, fibrin and platelet-rich venous occlusions in tail and hindlegs were also observed in transgenic mice, overexpressing human PAI-1 (Erickson *et al.*, 1990). Although mice with a single deficiency of t-PA or u-PA only had a minor spontaneous thrombotic phenotype, they were significantly more susceptible to development of venous thrombosis following local injection of proinflammatory endotoxin in the footpad (Carmeliet *et al.*, 1994a) or electrical injury of peripheral arteries (unpublished data). The increased susceptibility of t-PA deficient mice to endotoxin and the severe spontaneous thrombotic phenotype of combined t-PA:u-PA deficient mice could be explained by their significantly reduced rate of spontaneous lysis of ^{125}I-fibrin labelled plasma clots, injected via the jugular vein and embolized into the pulmonary arteries. On the contrary, PAI-1 deficient mice were virtually protected against development of venous thrombosis following injection of endotoxin (Carmeliet *et al.*, 1993b) or electrical injury (unpublished observations), consistent with their ability to lyse ^{125}I-fibrin labelled plasma clots at a significantly higher rate than wild-type mice. The increased susceptibility of u-PA deficient mice to endotoxin might be due to their impaired macrophage function. Indeed, thioglycollate-stimulated macrophages (which express increased cell-associated u-PA) from u-PA deficient mice, but not from t-PA deficient or PAI-1 deficient mice, lacked plasminogen-dependent breakdown of ^{125}I-labelled fibrin (fibrinolysis) or ^{3}H-labelled subendothelial matrix (mostly collagenolysis) (Carmeliet *et al.*, 1994a).

Collectively, these targeting studies confirm the importance of the plasminogen/ plasmin system in maintaining vascular patency and indicate that both plasminogen activators significantly cooperate in this process. Interestingly, u-PA appears to play a significant role in prevention of fibrin deposits during conditions of inflammation or injury, most likely through cell-associated plasmin proteolysis. Analysis of recently generated mice with deficiency of the urokinase-type plasminogen activator receptor (u-PAR) (Dewerchin *et al.*, 1994) might aid in resolving this issue. Somewhat surprisingly, the lack of a more severe phenotype in mice with single or combined deficiencies suggests that yet other plasminogen-dependent or -independent mechanisms might be involved in normal fibrin clot surveillance.

HEMOSTASIS

Hemostasis involves platelet deposition and coagulation factor-mediated fibrin deposition to stabilize the clot. Failure to stabilize the clot, e.g. as a result of hyperfibrinolytic activity might result in delayed rebleeding. A hemorrhagic tendency has indeed been observed in patients with absent or reduced plasma PAI-1 or α_2-antiplasmin activity levels and increased plasma t-PA levels (Aoki 1989, Schneiderman and Loskutoff 1991, Fay *et al.*, 1992). Delayed rebleeding might explain the hemorrhagic tendency in transgenic mice, expressing high levels of plasma u-PA (Heckel *et al.*, 1990) and in transgenic mice, overexpressing GM-CSF, with increased production of u-PA by peritoneal macrophages (Elliott *et al.*, 1992). LRP deficiency resulted in embryonic death with associated gastrointestinal bleeding, possibly due to increased proteolytic activity (Herz *et al.*, 1992). Contrary to patients with low or absent plasma PAI-1 levels, PAI-1 deficient mice did not reveal spontaneous or delayed rebleeding, even after trauma (Carmeliet *et al.*, 1993b). Lower plasma PAI-1 levels and the occurrence of alternative PAIs in murine plasma (unpublished data) might explain this species-specific difference in proteinase inhibitor control of plasmin proteolysis.

RESTENOSIS

Vascular reconstructions including coronary angioplasty, endarterectomy, bypass surgery, vascular stents and heart transplantation have become widely used treatments for patients with atherothrombotic disease. However, chronic restenosis in 30 to 50% of patients, necessitating costly and complicated reinterventions, remains a major limitation of these procedures. Elastic recoil, adventitial remodeling and thrombosis have been implicated in this process. Restenosis might, however, also result from excessive accumulation of smooth muscle cells (SMC) and deposition of matrix in the intimal layer as part of an hyperactive wound healing process in response to vascular trauma. Recently, evidence has been provided for a significant role of the plasminogen/plasmin system in vascular remodeling. In an uninjured vessel, expression of t-PA by endothelial cells (EC) and, to a variable extent, of PAI-1 by medial smooth muscle cells suggests a role in maintaining vascular patency and hemostasis, respectively (Simpson *et al.*, 1991, Lupu *et al.*, 1993, Chomiki *et al.*, 1994). Expression of u-PA and its cellular receptor appears to be undetectable whereas low levels of the PA-clearance receptor LRP are detected on SMC. Vascular trauma results, however, in activation of the plasminogen/plasmin system and net plasmin proteolysis. Following transient reduction of t-PA in the vessel wall as a result of EC damage, u-PA and t-PA activity in the vessel wall are significantly increased, coincident with the time of SMC proliferation and migration, respectively (Clowes *et al.*, 1990, Jackson and Reidy 1992, Jackson *et al.*, 1993, Reilly *et al.*, 1994). Whereas t-PA immunoreactivity is confined to SMC in the media adjacent to and migrating through the internal elastic membrane and to SMC in the neointima, u-PA might be produced by infiltrating macrophages, SMC or EC. *In vitro*, treatment of cultured EC, SMC and macrophages with basic Fibroblast Growth Factor (bFGF), Platelet Derived Growth Factor (PDGF), Tumor Necrosis Factor (TNFα), angiotensin II and thrombin, factors that are released after injury, induce expression of u-PA, its cellular receptor and occasionally of t-PA (Reuning and Bang 1992, van Leeuwen *et al.*, 1994 and reviewed in Vassali 1994) (Table 13.1). Induction of u-PA:u-PAR expression has also been observed after wounding

Table 13.1   Expression of the plasminogen/plasmin system in restenosis and atherosclerosis.

	Factors inducing	
Effector cell	*Profibrinolytic Activity*	*Antifibrinolytic Activity*
Smooth Muscle Cell	angiotensin II[1] PDGF[1,2] thrombin[2]	angiotensin II[3] PDGF[3] thrombin[3] TGFβ[3] TNFα[3] Heparin[1]
Endothelial cell	thrombin[1] bFGF[2] IL-1[2] TNFα[2] TGFβ[1,2] VEGF[1,2]	thrombin[3] bFGF[3] IL-1[1,3,4] TNFα[1,3,4] TGFβ[3] INFγ[2] VEGF[3] Lp(a)[1,3] LDL[1,3] ox LDL[1,3] VLDL, HDL[1,3]
Monocytes/Macrohages	thrombin[2] IL-1[2] TNFα[2] GM-CSF[2] INFγ[2] TGFβ[2] Heparin[2] acetylated-LDL[2]	thrombin[4] IL-1[4] TNFα[4] GM-CSF[4] TGFβ[3]

Legend: *In vitro* and *in vivo* studies have indicated that a variety of factors, produced or released in the vessel wall during restenosis or atherosclerosis, is able to induce pro- or anti-fibrinolytic activity by affecting expression of t-PA ([1]), u-PA or u-PAR ([2]), PAI-1 ([3]) or PAI-2 ([4]) by the indicated effector cells. Pro-fibrinolytic activity results from increased expression of t-PA, u-PA or u-PAR whereas anti-fibrinolytic activity results from increased expression of PAI-1, PAI-2 or reduced expression of t-PA.

PDGF: platelet derived growth factor; bFGF: basic fibroblast growth factor; IL-1: interleukin-1; TNFα: tumor necrosis factor alpha; TGFβ: transforming growth factor β; INFγ: interferon gamma; GM-CSF: granuloctye monocyte-colony stimulating factor; Lp(a): lipoprotein (a); ox-LDL: oxidized LDL; VEGF: vascular endothelial growth factor.

of EC and SMC *in vitro*. A variety of studies has implicated u-PA, and, to a lesser extent, t-PA in proteolytic degradation of and invasion through anatomical barriers by migrating EC and macrophages (Blasi *et al.*, 1987, Vassali 1994). t-PA might, however, also act as an autocrine mitogen for SMC (Herbert *et al.*, 1994). Control of excessive plasmin proteolysis may result from inhibition by PAI-1, released by platelets or adjacent endothelium following thrombosis (Sawa *et al.*, 1992) or by SMC following injury (Clowes *et al.*, 1990, Sawa *et al.*, 1992). *In vitro*, PAI-1 expression is induced in EC, SMC and macrophages in response to similar molecules that promote plasmin production (PDGF, thrombin, angiotensin II, TNFα and IL-1β), suggesting tight control of this proteolytic system (Reilly and McFall 1991, Noda-Heiny *et al.*, 1993) (Table 13.1). In addition, plasmin-mediated activation of latent TGFβ, which induces expression of PAI-1 may constitute another paracrine proteinase inhibitor control mechanism (Flaumenhaft *et al.*, 1992). Interestingly, balloon injury-induced production of PAI-1, is significantly higher in hypercholesterolemic than in normocholesterolemic rabbits (Sawa *et al.*, 1993) and has been reported to increase plasma PAI-1 levels to a variable extent (Shi *et al.*, 1992, Sawa *et al.*, 1993).

Local increases of plasmin proteolysis in the injured vessel may participate in clot lysis (a possible mediator of restenosis), passivation of the injured vessel lumen, matrix remodeling or in migration/proliferation of SMC, EC or macrophages. In fact, t-PA has been proposed to mediate the migratory response of SMC to PDGF (Jackson *et al.*, 1993) and treatment of rats with the anti-fibrinolytic drug tranexamic acid reduced migration of smooth muscle cells *in vivo* (Jackson and Reidy 1992). An inhibitory effect on t-PA production has also been proposed as a possible mechanism for the reduction of neointima formation by heparin in injured rat carotid artery (Clowes *et al.*, 1992).

In a recent analysis of neointima formation following vascular trauma in mice with deficiencies of t-PA, u-PA or PAI-1, we have observed that deficiency of t-PA does not affect the degree or rate of neointima formation nor neointimal cell accumulation, whereas deficiency of u-PA delayed and deficiency of PAI-1 accelerated neointima formation and neointimal cell accumulations (Carmeliet *et al.*, 1994b). Our data also suggest that u-PA- rather than t-PA-mediated plasmin proteolysis contributes to vascular wound healing and restenosis in mice. Further study is required to elucidate whether loss of plasminogen activator gene function affects cellular migration or proliferation. Another unresolved question is whether deposition or composition of the matrix are affected by these genetic manipulations, as suggested by our previous observations of impaired degradation of ^{3}H-proline labeled subendothelial matrix by u-PA deficient but not by t-PA deficient macrophages (Carmeliet *et al.*, 1994a).

ATHEROSCLEROSIS

The plasminogen/plasmin system may also be involved in the development and/or progression of atherosclerosis. Current evidence suggests that impaired fibrinolysis is correlated with coronary heart disease. Epidemiological studies indeed revealed a positive association of plasma PAI-1 activity not only with reinfarction but also with the degree of coronary artery disease (Hamsten and Eriksson 1994). Furthermore, known risk factors for atherosclerosis including obesity, noninsulin-dependent diabetes, hyperinsulinemia, hypertriglyceridemia and hypertension, all possibly related to an insulin resistance syndrome, have been correlated with increased plasma PAI-1 levels. In situ analysis of the atherosclerotic plaque also revealed increased expression of PAI-1 in intimal SMC and macrophages (Schneiderman *et al.*, 1992, Lupu *et al.*, 1993, Yorimitsu *et al.*, 1993, Chomiki *et al.*, 1994), coincident with expression of tissue factor, thrombin, fibrin and to a certain extent of vitronectin. A variety of growth factors, cytokines and lipids, that are present in plaques, might also contribute to impaired plasmin proteolysis by induction of PAI-1, suppression of t-PA expression or inhibition of plasminogen activation (Nachman 1992, Hamsten and Eriksson 1994, Liu and Lawn 1994) (Table 13.1). Genetic analysis of postinfarction patients has recently revealed a polymorphism in the PAI-1 promoter that might confer responsiveness to VLDL and render these individuals more prone to thrombotic complications (Hamsten and Eriksson 1994). In aggregate, impaired fibrinolysis, resulting from increased plasma or plaque PAI-1 levels, might contribute to the development or progression of atherosclerosis, by promoting thrombosis or matrix deposition.

It should be noticed however that, hitherto, most of the attention has been focused on PAI-1 and that information on expression levels of t-PA, u-PA, u-PAR or LRP in plaques is only fragmentary. Increased plaque levels of t-PA and u-PA mRNA and activity have indeed been observed (Smokovitis *et al.*, 1988, Underwood and de Bono. 1993). As shown in Table 13.1, several factors that induce anti-fibrinolytic activity, are also able to induce pro-fibrinolytic activity. Increased plasmin proteolysis, via its effects on cell migration/proliferation or on matrix degradation, might stimulate neovascularization of plaque lesions, destabilize the plaque and induce plaque rupture or facilitate formation of aneurysms (Reilly *et al.,* 1994). In aggregate, reduced or increased plasmin proteolysis might affect different aspects of atherosclerosis but, to date, a causal involvement of the plasminogen/plasmin system in any of these processes has not been conclusively established.

In a preliminary analysis of cholesterol feeding-induced atherosclerosis (unpublished data), we have observed that t-PA deficient mice develop fatty streak lesions to the same extent as their wild type littermates. However, whether, to what extent and at what stage the fibrinolytic system might affect atherosclerotic lesions remains to be further analyzed. This could be achieved by cross breeding t-PA, u-PA and PAI-1 deficient mice with other atherosclerosis-prone transgenic mice such as the apolipoprotein E deficient mice, the LDL Receptor deficient mice or the Lipoprotein(a) (Lp(a)) overexpressing mice.

An interesting but unresolved issue is whether the atherothrombotic activity of the plasminogen homologue Lp(a) might, at least in part, be attributed to an inhibitory role on plasmin formation (Nachman 1992, Liu and Lawn 1994). A significant correlation between high levels of apo(a), reduced in situ plasmin activity and active TGFβ levels was observed in atherosclerotic vessels of transgenic mice, overexpressing apo(a) (Grainger *et al.*, 1994). t-PA-, u-PA- and PAI-1-deficient mice and recently obtained u-PA receptor deficient (Dewerchin *et al.*, 1994) will serve as useful models to further elucidate whether reduced TGFβ activation (resulting from reduced plasmin activity) might constitute a growth stimulus for vascular smooth muscle cells.

BRAIN FUNCTION

Evidence has been provided that the plasminogen/plasmin system might also be involved in brain function based on expression of fibrinolytic system components in specialized areas of the brain during development or following different forms of brain activity (Qian *et al.*, 1993, Sappino *et al.*, 1993). In addition, *in vitro* studies with cultured neurons revealed that neurons are able to produce and respond to plasminogen activators (Krystosek and Seeds 1981). Restricted and temporal specific expression of t-PA in the nervous system during development has been also observed in transgenic mice, expressing the LacZ marker gene driven by various t-PA promotor constructs. Ectopic expression of murine u-PA in the brain (e.g. in the hippocampus and limbic system) was associated with impaired learning of tasks in transgenic mice (Meiri *et al.*, 1994). The ectopic u-PA expression experiments suggest that abnormal proteolysis in the brain may cause behavioral abnormalities, possibly due to an effect on tissue remodeling. Imbalanced plasmin proteolysis, such as in t-PA deficient mice, also resulted in abnormal brain function. Preliminary results indeed suggested that long term potentiation was specifically impaired in t-PA deficient but not in u-PA deficient mice (unpublished data). Further studies are being performed to examine possible learning deficits in t-PA deficient mice. No neuroanatomical abnormalities were, however, observed in t-PA deficient mice (unpublished data). Thus, although evidence for a physiological role of plasmin-mediated proteolysis in the brain is accumulating, the exact mechanisms underlying possible alterations in long term potentiation or learning need to be further defined.

Conclusions and Perspectives

Studies with transgenic mice over- or under-expressing components of the fibrinolytic system, have revealed a significant role of this system in fibrin clot surveillance, reproduction, (vascular) wound healing, brain function, health and survival. The distinct phenotypes associated with single loss and the more severe phenotype associated with combined loss of plasminogen activator gene function suggest that through evolution, both plasminogen activators have evolved with specific but overlapping biological properties. Interestingly, the role of the fibrinolytic system in thrombosis and vascular wound healing became more apparent after challenging mice with single deficiencies of plasminogen activators with an inflammatory or traumatic challenge, respectively. It therefore seems warranted to examine possible consequences of loss of plasminogen activator gene function in other processes including atherosclerosis, neoangiogenesis, inflammatory lung and kidney disease and malignancy.

The plasminogen activator knock-out mice with their thrombotic phenotypes are also valuable models to evaluate whether adenoviral mediated gene-transfer of wild-type or mutant plasminogen activator genes is able to restore normal thrombolytic function and to prevent thrombosis. Preliminary evidence suggests indeed that impaired thrombolysis of t-PA deficient mice can be completely restored using adenoviral mediated gene transfer of rt-PA (Carmeliet *et al.*, 1994c). In addition, analysis of neointima formation in plasminogen activator deficient mice suggests that controlled reduction of fibrinolytic activity in the vessel wall might be beneficial for the prevention or reduction of restenosis. Whether this can be achieved with gene transfer methodologies remains to be defined.

References

Andreasen, P.A. and Sottrup-Jensen, L.I. *et al.* (1994). Receptor-mediated endocytosis of plasminogen activators and activator/inhibitor complexes. *FEBS Letters*, **338**:239–245.

Aoki, N. (1989). Hemostasis associated with abnormalities of fibrinolysis. *Blood Rev.*, **3**: 11–17.

Blasi, F., Vassalli, J.D. and Dano, K. (1987). Urokinase-type plasminogen activator: proenzyme, receptor and inhibitors. *J. Cell Biol.*, **104**:801–804.

Carmeliet, P., Kieckens, L., Schoonjans, L. *et al.* (1993a). Plasminogen activator inhibitor-1 gene-deficient mice. I. Generation by homologous recombination and characterization. *J. Clin. Invest.*, **92**:2746–2755.

Carmeliet, P., Stassen, J.M., Schoonjans, L. *et al.* (1993b). Plasminogen activator inhibitor-1 gene-deficient mice. II. Effects on hemostasis, thrombosis and thrombolysis. *J. Clin. Invest.*, **92**:2756–2760.

Carmeliet, P., Schoonjans, L., Kieckens, L. *et al.* (1994a). Physiological consequences of loss of plasminogen activator gene function in mice. *Nature*, **368**:419–424.

Carmeliet, P., Stassen, J.M., De. Mol., M. *et al.* (1994b). Arterial neointima formation after trauma in mice with inactivation of the t-PA, u-PA or PAI-1 genes. *Fibrinolysis* **8**: Suppl 1: A280.

Carmeliet, P., Stassen, J.M., Collen, D. *et al.* (1994c). Adenovirus-mediated gene transfer of rt-PA restores thrombolysis in t-PA deficient mice. *Fibrinolysis* **8**, Suppl 1: A282

Chomiki, N., Henry, M., Alessi, M.C., Anfosso, F. and Juhan-Vague, I. (1994). Plasminogen activator inhibitor-1 expression in human liver and healthy or atherosclerotic vessel walls. *Thromb. Haemostas.*, **72**:44–53.

Clowes, A.W., Clowes, M.M., An, Y.P.T., Reidy, M.A. and Belin, D. (1990). Smooth muscle cells express urokinase during mitogenesis and tissue-type plasminogen activator during migration in injured rat carotid artery. *Circ. Res.*, **67**:61–67.

Clowes, A.W., Clowes, M.M., Kirkman, T.R., Jackson, C.L., Au., Y.P.T. and Kenagy, R. (1992). Heparin inhibits the expression of tissue-type plasminogen activator by smooth muscle cells in injured rat carotid artery. *Circ. Res.* **70**:1128–1136.

Collen, D. and Lijnen, H.R. (1991). Basic and clinical aspects of fibrinolysis and thrombolysis. *Blood*, **78**:3114–3124.

De Bono, D. (1994). Significance of raised plasma concentrations of tissue-type plasminogen activator and plasminogen activator inhibitor in patients at risk from ischaemic heart disease. *Br. Heart. J.*, **71**:504–507.

Dewerchin, M., Carmeliet, P., Van Nuffelen, A., Collen, D. and Mulligan, R.C.M. (1994). Inactivation of the mouse urokinase receptor gene. *Fibrinolysis* **8**, Suppl 1: A142

Elliott, M.J., Faulkner-Jones, B.E., Stanton, H., Hamilton, J.A. and Metcalf, D. (1992). Plasminogen activator in granulocyte-macrophage-CSF transgenic mice. *J. Immunol.*, **49**:3678–3681.

Erickson, L.A., Fici, G.J., Lund, J.E., Boyle, T.P., Polites, H.G. and Marotti, K.R. (1990). Development of venous occlusions in mice transgenic for the plasminogen activator inhibitor-1 gene. *Nature*, **346**:74–76.

Fay, W.P., Shapiro, A.D., Shih, J.L., Schleef, R.R. and Ginsburg, D. (1992). Complete deficiency of plasminogen activator inhibitor type 1 due to frameshift mutation. *N. Engl. J. Med.*, **327**:1729–1733.

Flaumenhaft, R., Abe, M., Mignatti, P. and Rifkin, D.B. (1992). Basic fibroblast growth factor-induced activation of latent transforming growth factor β in endothelial cells: regulation of plasminogen activator activity. *J. Cell Biol.*, **4**:901–909.

Grainger, D.J., Kemp, P.R., Liu, A.C., Lawn, R.M. and Metcalfe, J.M. (1994). Activation of transforming growth factor-β is inhibited in transgenic apolipoprotein (a) mice. *Nature*, **370**:460–462.

Hamsten, A. and Eriksson, P. (1994). Fibrinolysis and Atherosclerosis: and update. *Fibrinolysis* **8**, Suppl 1: 253–262

Heckel, J.L., Sandgren, E.P., Degen, J.L., Palmiter, R.D. and Brinster, R.L. (1990). Neonatal bleeding in transgenic mice expressing urokinase-type plasminogen activator. *Cell*, **62**:447–456.

Herbert, J.M., Lamarche, I., Prabonnaud, V., Dol, F. and Gauthier, (1994). T. Tissue-type plasminogen activator is a potent mitogen for human aortic smooth muscle cells. *J. Biol. Chem.*, **269**:3076–3080.

Herz, J., Clouthier, D.E. and Hammer, R.E. (1992). LDL receptor-related protein internalizes and degrades uPA-PAI-1 complexes and is essential for embryo implantation. *Cell*, **71**:411–421.

Jackson, C.L., Raines, E.W., Ross, R. and Reidy, M.A. (1993). Role of endogenous platelet-derived growth factor in arterial smooth muscle cell migration after balloon catheter injury. *Arterioscl. Thromb.*, **13**:1218–1226.

Jackson, C.L. and Reidy, M.A. (1992). The role of plasminogen activation in smooth muscle cell migration after arterial injury. *Ann. NY. Acad. Sci.*, **667**:141–150.

Krystosek, A. and Seeds (1981). NW Plasminogen activator release at the neuronal growth cone. *Science* **213**: 1532–1534.

Liu, A.C. and Lawn, R.M. (1994). Lipoprotein(a) and atherogenesis. *Trends Cardiovasc Medicine*, **4**:40–44.

Lupu, F., Bergonzelli, G.E., Heim, D.A., Cousin, E., Genton, C.Y., Bachmann, F. and Kruithof E.K.O. (1993). Localization and production of plasminogen activator inhibitor-1 in human healthy and atherosclerotic arteris. *Arterioscl Thromb.*, **13**:1090–1100.

Meiri, N., Masos, T., Rosenblum, K., Miskin, R. and Dudai, Y. (1994). Overexpression of urokinase-type plasminogen activator in transgenic mice is correlated with impaired learning. *Proc. Natl. Acad. Sci. USA,* **91**:3196–3200.

Nachman, R.L. (1992). Thrombosis and Atherogenesis: Molecular connections. *Blood,* **79**:1897–1906.

Noda-Heiny, H., Fujii, S. and Sobel, B.E. (1993). Induction of vascular smooth muscle cell expression of plasminogen activator inhibitor-1 by thrombin. *Circ. Res.,* **72**:36–43.

Qian, Z., Gilbert, M.E., Colicos, M.A., Kandel, E.R. and Kuhl, D. (1993). Tissue-type plasminogen activator is induced as an immediate-early gene during seizure, kindling and long-term potentiation. *Nature,* **361**:453–457.

Reilly, C.F. and McFall, R.C. (1991). Platelet-derived growth factor and transforming growth factor-β regulate plasminogen activator inhibitor-1 synthesis in vascular smooth muscle cells. *J. Biol. Chem.,* **266**:9419–9427.

Reilly, J.M., Sicard, G.A. and Lucore, C.L. (1994). Abnormal expression of plasminogen activators in aortic aneurysmal and occlusive disease. *J. Vasc. Surg.,* **19**:865–872.

Richards, W.G., Carroll, P.M., Kinloch, R.A., Wassarman, P.M. and Strickland, S. (1993). Creating maternal effect mutations in transgenic mice: antisense inhibition of an oocyte gene product. *Develop. Biol.,* **160**:543–553.

Sappino, A.P., Madani, R., Huarte, J., Belin, D., Kiss, J.Z., Wohlwend, A. and Vassalli, J.D. (1993). Extracellular proteolysis in the adult murine brain. *J. Clin. Invest.,* **92**:679–685.

Sawa, H., Fujii, S. and Sobel, B.E. (1992). Augmented arterial wall expression of type-1 plasminogen activator inhibitor induced by thrombosis. *Arterioscler. Thromb.,* **12**:1507–1515.

Sawa, H., Sobel, B.E. and Fujii, S. (1993). Potentiation by hypercholesterolemia of the induction of aortic intramural synthesis of plasminogen activator inhibitor type 1 by endothelial injury. *Circ. Res.,* **73**:671–680.

Schneiderman, J. and Loskutoff, D.J. (1991). Plasminogen activator inhibitors. *Trends Cardiovasc. Med.,* **1**:99–102.

Schneiderman, J., Sawdey, M.S., Keeton, M.R., Bordin, G.M., Bernstein, E.F., Dilley, R.B. and Loskutoff, D.J. (1992). Increased type 1 plasminogen activator inhibitor gene expression in atherosclerotic human arteries. *Proc. Natl. Acad. Sci. USA,* **89**:6998–7002.

Shi, Y., Nardone, D., Hernandez-Martinez, A., Walinsky, P., Bjornsson, T.D. and Zalewski, A. (1992). Fibrinolytic activity after vessel wall injury. *J. Am. Col. Cardiol.,* **19**:441–443.

Simpson, A.J., Booth, N.A., Moore, N.R., Bennett, B. (1991). Distribution of plasminogen activator inhibitor (PAI-1) in tissues. *J. Clin. Pathol.,* **44**:139–143.

Smokovitis, A., Kokolis, N. and Alexaki-Tzivanidou, E. (1988). Fatty streaks and fibrous plaques in human aorta show increased plasminogen activator activity. *Haemostasis,* **18**:146–153.

Underwood, M.J. and De Bono, D.P. (1993). Increased fibrinolytic activity in the intima of atheromatous coronary arteries: protection at a price. *Cardiovasc. Res.,* **27**:882–885.

van Leeuwen, R.T.J. Kol, A., Andreotti, F., Kluft, C., Maseri, A. and Sperti, G. (1994). Angiotensin II increases plasminogen activator inhibitor type 1 and tissue-type plasminogen activator messenger RNA in cultured rat aortic smooth muscle cells. *Circulation,* **90**:362–368.

Vassalli, J.D., Sappino, J.D. and Belin, D. (1991). The plasminogen activator/plasmin system. *J. Clin. Invest.,* **88**:1067–1072.

Vassalli, J.D. (1994). The Urokinase Receptor. *Fibrinolysis,* **8**: Suppl 1:172–181.

Yorimitsu, K., Saito, T., Toyozaki, T., Ishide, T., Ohnuma, N., Inagaki, Y. (1993). Immunohistochemical localization of plasminogen activator inhibitor-1 in human coronary atherosclerotic lesions involved in acute myocardial infarction. *Heart Vessels,* **8**:160–162.

14 Environmental Perturbation of Endothelium: Modulation of Vascular Properties by Hypoxia, Hyperglycemia and Tumor-Derived Cytokines

Ann Marie Schmidt, MD, David Pinsky, MD, Janet Kao, MD, Shi Du Yan, MD, Satoshi Ogawa, MD, Jean-Luc Wautier*, MD, and David Stern, MD

Department of Physiology and Cellular Biophysics, Columbia University, College of Physicians and Surgeons, 630 West 168th Street, New York, NY 10032

KEYWORDS: ischemia/transplantation/diabetes/vascular/complication/cytokine/thrombohemorrhage

INTRODUCTION

Endothelium is rapidly and directly reactive to changes in the vascular microenvironment, providing a critical link between the host response and perturbations in the intravascular milieu. The effects of inflammatory cytokines on the endothelium serve as a prototype of the impact of mediators on vessel wall functions (Old, 1986; Pober and Cotran 1990a; Simionescu and Simionescu, 1991; Dinarello and Wolff, 1993). Tumor necrosis factor, for example, has been shown to modulate critical properties of the vessel wall in part through its effects on endothelial cells (ECs[1]) (Old, 1986; Pober and Cotran, 1990b). Principally produced by mononuclear phagocytes following exposure to stimuli such as lipopolysaccharide (Beutler and Cerami, 1986), tumor necrosis factor-alpha (TNF) binds to specific EC receptors, resulting in changes in barrier function (permeability), vasomotor tone (nitric oxide production), expression of leukocyte adherence molecules, and changes in procoagulant and anticoagulant vessel wall properties (Simionescu and Simionescu, 1991). Each of these vascular functions (permeability, coagulant properties, regulation of vasomotor tone) is central to vascular homeostasis, as their perturbation results in a leaky vascular wall which contains adherent fibrin and

---

* Laboratoire de Recherche en Biologie Vasculaire et Cellulaire, Unite d'Immunohematologie, Hopital Lariboisiere, Universie Paris 7, Faculte de Medecine, Paris.
[1] Abbreviations: ECs, endothelial cells; TNF, tumor necrosis factor-alpha; Interleukin, IL; a/bFGF, acidic/basic fibroblast growth factor; PDGF, platelet-derived growth factor; MP, mononuclear phagocyte; PMN, polymorphonuclear leukocyte; ICAM, Intercellular Adhesion Molecule; AGE, advanced glycation endproduct; RAGE, receptor for AGE; ROI, reactive oxygen intermediate; TBARS, thiobarbituric acid-reactive substances; EMAP, endothelial-monocyte activating polypeptide; VEGF/VPF, vascular endothelial growth factor/vascular permeability factor; meth A, methylcholanthrene A-induced fibrosarcoma.

leukocytes and, is contracted. Delineation of the myriad effects of TNF, as well as similar studies with Interleukin (IL)-1 (Pober and Cotran, 1990a; Pober and Cotran, 1990b; Dinarello and Wolff, 1993), has provided a model for dissection of the EC response to diverse stimuli.

After strong stimulation, locally acting inflammatory cytokines (e.g., TNF, IL-1) can sometimes, after strong stimulation, spill over into the bloodstream sufficient to result in measurable plasma levels. Such inflammatory cytokines can then act on endothelium systemically throughout the vasculature whereas perturbations which are often systemic, such as hypoxia and hyperglycemia, can also act locally and may produce their most critical disturbances in particular vascular beds. In this chapter, we describe how three different, pathogenetically important disturbances in the endothelial environment affect the functions and properties of the vasculature.

PERTURBATION OF ENDOTHELIAL PROPERTIES

Hypoxia-Induced Modulation of Endothelial Cell Function. Hypoxia/hypoxemia is a common denominator of ischemia, and is thus a pathophysiologically important perturbation to which the endothelium must adapt. In contrast to neurons or cardiac myocytes, which undergo changes leading to cell death following oxygen deprivation, ECs maintain basic cellular metabolism (Loike *et al.*, 1992). After 48–72 hrs of severe oxygen deprivation ($pO_2 \approx 12$–14 torr), cultured bovine aortic ECs maintained protein synthesis at 70–80% the rate observed in normoxic controls, continued to produce ATP (levels were $\approx 75\%$ compared with normoxia), excluded trypan blue, retained cytosolic contents (e.g., lack of lactate dehydrogenase release), and adhered firmly to the growth substrate. A possible mechanism underlying this apparently facile endothelial adaptation to hypoxia is induction of the noninsulin-dependent glucose transporter, GLUT1, in ECs exposed to hypoxia. ECs maintained for 96 hrs under normoxic conditions consumed <0.6 μmoles glucose from the medium and produced about 1 μmole lactic acid (Figure 14.1). In contrast, exposure to hypoxia for 24 hrs resulted in 5 μmol glucose consumed and 8.4 μmol

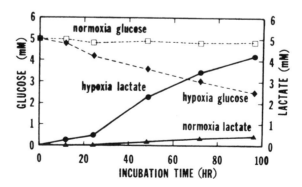

Figure 14.1 Glicose consumption and lactic acid production by cultured endothelial cells incubated for in the indicated time in hypoxia (diamonds and circles) or normoxia (squares and triangles). Glucose (dotted line) and lactic acid (solid line) determinations of the medium are shown.

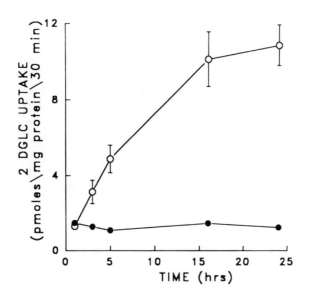

Figure 14.2 Time course of upregulation of glucose transport activity in hypoxic (open circles) and hormoxic ECs (closed circles). At the indicated times after exposure to hypoxia/normoxia, 2-deoxy-[³H]glucose uptake was measured for 30 min.

lactate produced, consistent with increased dependence on glycolysis. There are several means through which ECs could enhance their glycolytic capacity, including increasing their import of extracellular glucose. Uptake of 2-deoxyglucose by hypoxic ECs increased in a time dependent manner (Figure 14.2) compared with a relatively constant low level in normoxic cultures. Northern and Western analysis for mRNA and antigen, respectively, showed prominent up-regulation of GLUT1. Although the mechanism underlying increased GLUT1 expression is at present unclear, enhanced anaerobic glycolysis is an important factor in EC maintenance of energy charge during exposure to hypoxia.

Although central cellular metabolic processes continued during oxygen deprivation, the EC and its regulation of homeostasis were markedly perturbed. The effect of hypoxia on regeneration of endothelium and angiogenesis is illustrated in the sequence of events following injury of an EC monolayer (Figure 14.3; Shreeniwas *et al.*, 1991). When a wound was made in a confluent EC monolayer, the normoxic cells rapidly started to fill the gap by 24 hrs through induction of cell motility and proliferation (Figure 14.3A). In contrast, cultures grown to confluence in normoxia, wounded and placed in hypoxia failed to show significant repair over the same time interval (Figure 14.3B). Consistent with these data, rapidly growing EC cultures exposed to hypoxia slowed their growth and showed a reversible decreased entry of cells into S phase by flow cytometry. To search for a mechanism underlying these observations, the effect of hypoxia on EC expression of basic fibroblast growth factor (bFGF), a chemotactic and mitogenic agent for endothelium, was examined. Expression of bFGF mRNA (Figure 14.4- Northern) and immunoreactive polypeptide (Figure 14.4- Immunoblotting) was severely depressed in hypoxia, compared with normoxic controls. This suggested that diminished production of bFGF might be responsible for suppression of EC growth/motility in an hypoxic environment. The

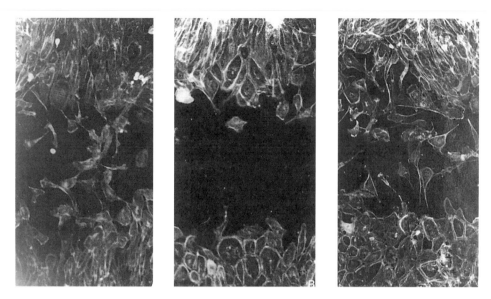

Figure 14.3 Confluent endothelial monolayers were wounded using a cell scraper and incubated for 24 hr in either normoxia (A), hypoxia (B), or hypoxia in the presence of added bFGF (5 ng/ml; C), and visualized using rhodamine phalloidin.

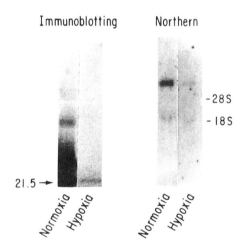

Figure 14.4 Expression of bFGF antigen (Immunoblotting) and mRNA (Northern) in lysates of ECs exposed to normoxia or hypoxia. The designation 21.5 on the far left demonstrates migration of a 21.5 kDa molecular weight marker run simultaneously on SDS-PAGE. The migration of 18S and 28S RNA is depicted on the far right. Equal total protein (immunoblotting) or equal total RNA (Northern) was loaded for normoxic and hypoxic samples.

response of hypoxic ECs to exogenous bFGF was also tested. First, radioligand binding studies with radioiodinated bFGF and hypoxic ECs showed high affinity binding sites whose number appeared to increase by ≈2–3-fold compared with their counterparts in normoxia (Shreeniwas, 1991). Addition of bFGF to hypoxic cultures stimulated endothelial

[3]H-thymidine incorporation and increased cell number, indicating a mitogenic response. The apparent functional integrity of bFGF receptors on hypoxic ECs was further confirmed by the enhanced response of wounded EC monolayers in hypoxia to which exogenous bFGF was added (Figure 14.3C).

These data posed an apparent paradox, as ECs must be able to proliferate and migrate in an hypoxic environment, the latter being the microenvironment in which angiogenesis occurs (Folkman and Klagsbrun, 1987; Risau, 1990). In view of the intact EC response to bFGF, we hypothesized that hypoxic ECs would respond to other cells capable of producing angiogenic factors under hypoxic conditions, i.e., via a paracrine mechanism. This led to an exploration of mitogenic activities released by hypoxic cells (Kuwabara *et al.*, 1994). As expected, since hypoxic ECs failed to proliferate, their conditioned media did not induce proliferation of other hypoxic EC cultures (Figure 14.5). Similar results were observed with supernatants from hypoxic vascular smooth muscle cells and fibroblasts (Figure 14.5). In contrast, media conditioned by hypoxic monocyte-derived macrophages (mononuclear phagocytes, MPs) released mitogenic activity for ECs, especially capillary ECs (Figure 14.5). MP release of mitogenic activity for hypoxic ECs occurred in a time-dependent manner, increasing up to 24 hr, and depended on the oxygen tension, requiring severe oxygen deprivation ($pO_2 < 20$ torr). Metabolic labelling studies of hypoxic MPs demonstrated enhanced synthesis and release of platelet-derived growth factor (Figure 14.6, PDGF), acidic fibroblast growth factor (Figure 14.6, aFGF), and basic FGF (Figure 14.6, bFGF). In each case, immunoprecipitation of the relevant band from supernatants of hypoxic MPs was prevented by addition of excess unlabelled growth factor or by cycloheximide (Figure 14.6, lanes designated + CX). In contrast, normoxic MPs did not produce in significant quantity any of the three polypeptide mitogens under these conditions. These data support the notion of a paracrine mechanism whereby macrophages or other

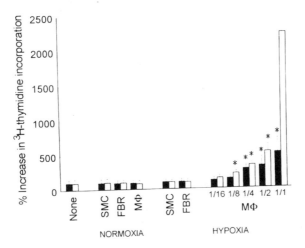

Figure 14.5 Effect of conditioned medium from hypoxic fibroblasts (FBR), smooth muscle cells (SMC), and macrophages (Mφ) on the growth of hypoxic aortic (specked bars) and capillary (open bars) ECs. Aliquots of serum-free conditioned medium from each of the above cells (following exposure to hypoxia for 24 hrs) were incubated with hypoxic ECs, and a proliferation assay was performed by assessing ^{3}H-thymidine incorporation (the fractions above the values for 3H-thymidine incorporation by ECs with Mφ-conditioned medium refer to the dilution of medium used. SMC and FBR conditioned media were utilized only at 1:1).

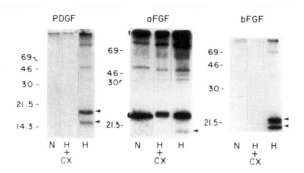

Figure 14.6 Immunoprecipitation of culture supernatants from hypoxic (H), or normoxic (N) macrophages to assess synthesis/release of PDGF, and acidic/basic (a/b) FGF. Macrophages were exposed to hypoxia for 24 hr, metabolically labelled, and cultured supernatants were immunoprecipitated with antibody to PDGF, aFGF or bFGF, followed by reduced SDS-PAGE and autoradiography. Where indicated, cycloheximide (+CX) was added. The migration of hypoxia-induced bands representing PDGF, aFGF and bFGF are indicated by the arrows. The migration of simultaneously electrophoresed standard proteins is shown on the far left in kDa.

non-endothelial cells produce growth factors which direct ingrowth of ECs, the latter being primed to respond, at least in the case of FGF, where the number of high affinity receptors is increased in the hypoxic environment. In wounds, macrophages may be the cell most efficiently producing growth factor, whereas in tumors or ischemic/hypoxic lesions, increased levels of mRNA for vascular permeability factor and/or bFGF have been observed in a range of cells (Chiba *et al.*, 1991; Jakeman *et al.*, 1992; Shweiki *et al.*, 1992).

Hypoxemic vasculature is known for increased permeability, thrombogenicity, and a propensity to attract leukocytes (Sevitt, 1967; Hultgren, 1978; Hamer *et al.*, 1981; Lockhart and Saiag, 1981; Mullane *et al.*, 1984; Kinasewitz *et al.*, 1986; Olesen, 1986; Crawford *et al.*, 1988; Stelzner *et al.*, 1988; Ma *et al.*, 1991). These seemingly diverse mechanisms are tied together by the evidence that hypoxia suppressed the cAMP second messenger signal transduction pathway. cAMP maintains barrier function in epithelium and can enhance barrier function of EC monolayers *in vitro* (Stelzner *et al.*, 1989; Ogawa *et al.*, 1992). Furthermore, agents which elevate cAMP, such as isoproterenol, attenuated thrombin-mediated pulmonary edema in animals (Minnear *et al.*, 1986, 1989). With respect to cellular coagulant properties, elevating intracellular cAMP enhances EC expression of the anticoagulant cofactor thrombomodulin and diminishes leukocyte EC interactions (Siflinger-Birnboim *et al.*, 1993). Exposure of ECs to hypoxia led to a time- and dose-dependent decrease in barrier function of the cultured monolayers in parallel with a fall in intracellular cAMP (Figure 14.7A-B) (Ogawa *et al.*, 1992). This was not due to extrusion of cyclic nucleotide into the medium or enhancement of phosphodiesterase activity. Rather, adenylate cyclase activity, basal as well as forskolin- and isoproterenol-stimulated activity, was diminished in hypoxia. The likelihood that decreased cAMP had an important role in hypoxia-induced increased EC monolayer permeability was supported by three lines of evidence: addition of dibutyryl-cAMP enhanced barrier function of hypoxic EC monolayers (Figure 14.8); pre-treatment of cultures with pertussis toxin prevented the increase in permeability and the fall in EC cAMP; and several different cyclic AMP analogs had enhanced barrier function as long as they retained activity as cAMP-dependent protein kinase stimulators (Ogawa *et al.*, 1992).

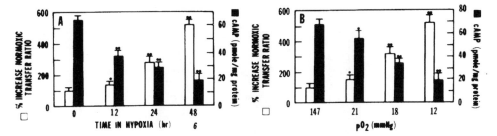

Figure 14.7 Effect of hypoxia on barrier function and intracellular cAMP levels of aortic ECs exposed to hypoxia ($pO_2 \approx 14$ torr) for the indicated times, or the indicated oxygen tension for 48 hr. Barrier function was determined by the diffusional transit of ^{3}H-inulin across the monolayer (open bars) and cAMP content (closed bars) of ECs was assessed. •, P < 0.05 and ••P < 0.01 from normoxia.

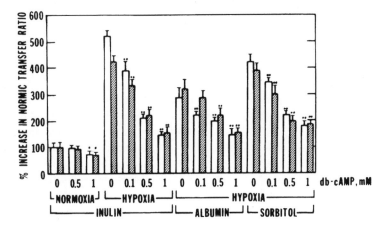

Figure 14.8 Addition of dibutyryl-cAMP (db-cAMP) to hypoxic/normoxic ECs modulates barrier function of aortic (open bars) and pulmonary (hatched bars) ECs. Endothelium was placed in normoxia of hypoxia for 48 hrs alone or in the presence of the indicated concentration of db-cAMP. A permeability study measuring diffusional transit of ^{3}H-inulin, ^{125}I-albumin or ^{3}H-sorbitol was performed four hours before the end of the experiment. •P < 0.05 and ••P < 0.01.

One situation in which the vasculature is subject to severe and prolonged hypoxemia is during the preservation period of an organ prior to transplantation (Pinsky *et al.*, 1993; Pinsky *et al.*, 1994). The vulnerability of the endothelium to preservation is well-known, especially in heart and lung transplantation, where vascular dysfunction is the principal limitation on the time for ischemic storage. The requirement for <6 hrs preservation time imposes severe limitations on the logistics of cardiac preservation, narrowing the radius of available donors, preventing adequate time for tissue typing, and making the procedure one that must be performed under emergency conditions thereby stressing physician and patient. Based on our studies with hypoxic ECs in culture, we hypothesized that cAMP levels in preserved hearts or lungs would fall during preservation resulting in vascular dysfunction during the reperfusion period. This could potentially explain leukostasis, edema, and thrombosis characteristic of transplants subjected to prolonged ischemia. If this concept was true, we reasoned that addition of cAMP to organ preservation solutions

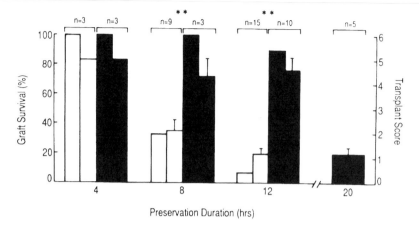

Figure 14.9 Rat hearts were explanted, flushed with cold lactated Ringer's (LR) alone (open bars) or LR + dibutyryl (db)-cAMP (4 mM; closed bars), and then stored in the same solution at 4°C for the indicated times. Data are shown as percent graft survival (left bar) or transplant score (right bar; the latter assessesgraft color, turgor and contractility) both determined 10 min after release of the aortic cross-clamp.

could maintain vascular function and prolong the preservation period. Using an hetero-topic rat heart transplant model (Ono and Lindsey, 1969), addition of dibutyryl-cAMP to lactated Ringer's solution greatly enhanced its efficacy as a preservation vehicle; the time for successful preservation was extended in a dose-dependent manner (Figure 14.9) (Pinsky *et al.*, 1993). Enhanced preservation in the presence of the cAMP analog was due to increasing levels of the adenine cyclic nucleotide and stimulation of cAMP-dependent protein kinase based on several lines of evidence: (1) although dibutyryl-cAMP was effective, sodium butyrate was not; (2) other cyclic nucleotide analogs, such as 8-bromo-cAMP, were effective whereas 8-bromoadenosine was not; (3) the stimulatory isomer of a sulfur-modified cAMP (Sp-cAMPS) was effective whereas the antagonist (Rp-cAMPS) blocked the beneficial effect of 8-bromo-cAMP; and (4) phosphodiesterase inhibitors, rolipram and indolidan, mimicked the effect of dibutyryl-cAMP. The beneficial properties of cAMP on cardiac preservation were also evident in University of Wisconsin solution, the current clinical standard for cardiac graft storage, extending preservation in a time- and dose-dependent manner (Pinsky *et al.*, 1993). Further experiments have demonstrated that the effect of cAMP on organ preservation is mediated, at least in part, through the vasculature; perfusion is enhanced and leukostasis in the transplant, a negative prognosti-cator of subsequent organ function, is diminished. These data support the concept that elevating levels of cAMP in cardiac grafts may promote restoration of vascular function following transplantation. Consistent with this, cyclic nucleotides have also been shown to enhance preservation in a baboon transplant model where considerations of cardiopul-monary bypass can be evaluated and an unprecedented storage time of 24 hrs was achieved (Oz *et al.*, 1993).

Although the most marked tissue injury during ischemia/reperfusion occurs during the reperfusion period, our studies in tissue culture and animal models suggest that mecha-nisms leading to vascular dysfunction are already set in motion during the period of hypoxia. One example of this is the production of IL-1alpha and IL-8 by hypoxic ECs

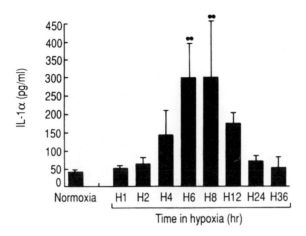

Figure 14.10 Mice were exposed to hypoxia ($pO_2 \approx 30\text{--}40$ torr) for the indicated times, and IL-1alpha in plasma was determined by radioimmunoassay. ••$P < 0.01$.

(Shreeniwas *et al.*, 1992; Karakurum *et al.*, 1994). Exposure of human ECs to hypoxia led to a time-dependent release of IL-1 activity which was neutralized by antibody to IL-1alpha. Generation of IL-1 was preceded by increased levels of IL-1 mRNA. EC production of IL-1 during hypoxia was followed by induction of E-selectin and enhanced expression of Intercellular Adhesion Molecule (ICAM)-1 (Pober and Cotran, 1990a) during subsequent reoxygenation, as the cellular response to IL-1 appeared to be blunted during hypoxia. Complementary results were obtained *in vivo*, as mice exposed to hypoxia showed a time-dependent increase in plasma IL-1alpha antigen (Figure 14.10), and polymerase chain reaction analysis of IL-1 transcripts in lung showed increased expression during hypoxia. A likely result of increased IL-1 in hypoxia was evidence of enhanced ICAM-1 expression in hypoxic lung. In addition to augmented IL-1 generation in hypoxia, ECs also produced IL-8 thereby providing an environment rich in a chemokine that promotes PMN activation, migration and adherence (Peveri *et al.*, 1988; Baggiolini *et al.*, 1989; Oppenheim *et al.*, 1991). IL-8 synthesis by hypoxic ECs was the result, at least in part, of increased transcription, as elevated levels of IL-8 mRNA were shown by nuclear run-on analysis to be associated with an increased rate of nascent transcripts (Karakurum *et al.*, 1994). The production of IL-8 by hypoxic mouse lung tissue probably underlies increased levels of the PMN marker enzyme myeloperoxidase in hypoxic lung tissue (Figure 14.11), consistent with leukostasis in response to oxygen deprivation. The impact of IL-8 in ischemia is further reinforced by the demonstration of further IL-8 production by reoxygenated monocytes (Metinko *et al.*, 1992). Taken together, these mechanisms of IL-8 involvement in ischemia are likely to underlie the protective effect of neutralizing anti-IL-8 IgG in a model of pulmonary ischemia (Sekido *et al.*, 1993).

These data indicate that hypoxic ECs potentially are subjected to autocrine (cytokine production) and paracrine (response to growth factors produced by other cells) stimulation which change their normally homeostatic role to one which facilitates adaptation to the ischemic milieu. Whereas the EC response to angiogenic stimuli produced by hypoxic

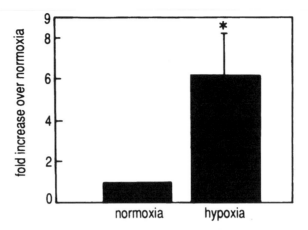

Figure 14.11 Mice were exposed to hypoxia (as in Figure 10 Above) or normoxia for 16 hours, and lung tissue was processed for myeloperoxidase activity. •P < 0.05 compared with normoxic control.

MPs may underlie wound repair, autocrine EC production of proinflammatory cytokines may set in motion elements of the host response which account for parallels between the pathologic picture in inflammation and ischemia. Gaining further insights into mechanisms underlying modulation of EC function in hypoxia, including means by which the cell senses oxygen deprivation resulting, for example, in diminished adenylate cyclase activity and increased transcription of IL-8, might serve as the basis for modifying these cellular properties.

Modulation of Endothelial Cell Properties by Hyperglycemia: Role of Advanced Glycation Endproducts

Proteins and lipids exposed to aldoses undergo nonenzymatic glycation and oxidation (Brownlee *et al.*, 1988; Sell and Monnier, 1989; Baynes, 1991; Ruderman *et al.*, 1992). Initially, early glycation products form: these constitute a group of reversibly modified proteins of which the best known is hemoglobin A_{1c}, which is used to monitor extended blood glucose levels in patients with diabetes (Klein *et al.*, 1989). Over longer exposure times of free amino groups to glucose (or other reducing sugars), further complex and incompletely understood irreversible molecular rearrangements occur and the advanced glycation endproducts (AGEs) are formed. These are heterogeneous, sharing in common a yellow-brown color, propensity to form cross-links, generation of reactive oxygen intermediates (ROIs), and interaction with specific cellular receptors (Ruderman *et al.*, 1992). Accumulation of AGEs in the vasculature and tissues has been linked to microvascular disease, accelerated atherosclerosis and other complications associated with diabetes suggesting a potentially etiologic role for AGEs (Brownlee *et al.*, 1988; Ruderman *et al.*, 1992). Formation of AGEs also occurs during the course of normal aging. Since AGE-modified proteins are present in the blood and accumulate in the basement membrane on long-lived extracellular matrix macromolecules (collagen, etc.), the EC is immersed in an AGE-rich environment.

Using AGE-modified albumin (AGE-albumin) as a prototypic ligand, we explored the interaction of AGEs with endothelium (Esposito *et al.*, 1989). Our first studies demonstrated that AGEs perturbed EC functions, including increased monolayer permeability and a shift in the balance of cell surface coagulant properties with decreased thrombomodulin and increased tissue factor expression. AGE-albumin bound to the EC surface in a saturable manner, and concentrations of ligand which occupied the cellular binding sites were comparable to those which altered EC properties. These data suggested that AGE-cellular interactions were mediated by specific cellular acceptor sites, and led us to isolate the putative receptor. By a series of chromatographic steps, a cell-associated polypeptide was isolated which bound AGEs in a manner comparable to ECs and MPs; the latter was termed Receptor for AGE or RAGE (Schmidt *et al.*, 1992; Schmidt *et al.*, 1994c). RAGE is a newly identified member of the immunoglobulin superfamily of cell surface molecules and is comprised of an extracellular domain, with one "V"type followed by two "C"-type immunoglobulin-like regions, a single putative transmembrane spanning domain, and a short, highly charged cytosolic tail having greatest homology to the B cell activation marker CD20 (Figure 14.12) (Neeper *et al.*, 1992; Schmidt *et al.*, 1994c). The receptor is expressed on endothelium and macrophages, as might be expected for a molecule mediating events in the vessel wall (Brett *et al.*, 1993). It was also found on smooth muscle cells, certain neurons, and mesangial cells, suggesting involvement in a range of cellular functions (Brett *et al.*, 1993). Expression of RAGE early in development, especially in brain, is consistent with the concept that there may be ligands for this receptor besides AGEs; it could then function in cell/cell or cell-matrix interactions, as a cytokine or a growth factor receptor (by analogy with other members of the immunoglobulin superfamily; Hunkapiller and Hood, 1989). Non-AGE ligands for RAGE have indeed been identified by our laboratory, suggesting that the receptor has functions in diverse situations. Other AGE binding proteins have been isolated from rat liver (Yang *et al.*, 1991).

RAGE has a central role in the interaction of AGEs with ECs and MPs (Schmidt *et al.*, 1992; Schmidt *et al.*, 1993). Binding of AGE albumin to cultured endothelium is blocked by antiRAGE IgG or by the extracellular domain of RAGE (the latter termed soluble [s]RAGE). Infusion of AGE albumin into mice demonstrates an initial rapid phase of

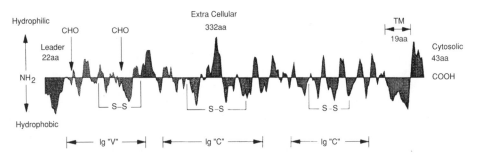

Figure 14.12 Hydrophilicity plot of bovine RAGE. The profile was generated from the Hopp and Woods program of intelligenetics. NH$_2$ amino terminus; COOH, carboxyl terminus; CHO, N-linked glycosylation sites; TM, transmembrane domain; S-S, disulfide-linked cysteine residues; IgV and IgC, immunoglobulin-like variable and constant domains, respectively.

clearance which is prevented by anti-RAGE IgG or sRAGE. Following infusion, EC-associated AGE albumin is found partly in multivesicular bodies and is also transported across the endothelium by receptor-mediated transcytosis (Schmidt *et al.*, 1994b), suggesting that RAGE is not a simple scavenger receptor; rather it can process the ligand with delivery to subendothelium where it interacts with smooth muscle cells. Further support for the potentially complex consequences of AGE-RAGE interaction derives from observations that ECs with cell-bound AGE albumin (via RAGE) undergo induction of oxidant stress (Schmidt *et al.*, 1994a; Yan *et al.*, 1994a). Exposure of cultured ECs to AGEs increases expression of thiobarbituric acid-reactive substances (TBARS), induces heme oxygenase type I mRNA, and activates the transcription factor NF-kB. Each of these events is blocked by anti-RAGE IgG, indicating a central role for RAGE, and by antioxidants (such as probucol or Nacetylcysteine), consistent with an underlying oxidant mechanism. The probable source of the ROIs is the AGE ligand itself (Mullarkey *et al.*, 1990; Sakurai and Tsuchiya, 1988; Hicks *et al.*, 1988; Hunt *et al.*, 1990): AGEs have been shown to generate ROIs, and, when tethered in close proximity to the cell surface by RAGE, AGEs can exert their effects on the cell membrane (Yan *et al.*, 1994a). The possibility that AGEs produce ROIs initially in the extracellular space is supported by the inhibitory effect of exogenous superoxide dismutase, catalase or glutathione peroxidase on subsequent induction of oxidant stress. *In vivo* experiments also indicate that AGEs in the intravascular space are associated with oxidant stress, as infusion of AGE albumin elevated TBARS, heme oxygenase mRNA, and activated NF-kB in a range of organs. In parallel with the results in tissue culture, AGE-mediated oxidant stress was blocked by anti-RAGE IgG and probucol (Yan *et al.*, 1994a).

The interaction of AGEs with RAGE on MPs further illustrates the range of consequences of AGE-mediated perturbation of cellular functions (Vlassara *et al.*, 1988; Kirstein *et al.*, 1990; Schmidt *et al.*, 1993). Both soluble AGEs prepared *in vitro* and AGEs isolated from patients with diabetes induce directional migration (i.e., chemotaxis) of MPs. The mechanism underlying cell movement involves AGE binding to RAGE with subsequent induction of cell motility, as antiRAGE IgG/F(ab')$_2$ or sRAGE are effective inhibitors of chemotaxis by AGEs (Schmidt *et al.*, 1993). However, if AGEs are immobilized on a surface, RAGE engagement of immobilized AGE ligands blocks MP migration in response to a different stimulus (such as the formylated peptide formyl-methionyl-leucinyl-phenylalanine). This is demonstrated in phagokinetic track assays (Albrecht-Buehler, 1977) with AGEs present in the underlying substrate (Figure 14.13). Note the long tracks made on the native matrix as MPs push gold particles out of their paths (Figure 14.13, left). In contrast, on the AGE-modified matrix, the tracks are much shorter suggesting inhibition of their movement (Figure 14.13, right). To model this situation *in vivo*, AGEs were adsorbed to polytetrafluorethylene mesh, the latter providing a slow release vehicle (Schmidt *et al.*, 1993). After subcutaneous implantation, the AGEs gradually diffused into the surrounding tissue, though much of the glycated protein remained on the graft. A striking mononuclear infiltrate was observed within several days, and the MPs trapped in the graft demonstrated features consistent with activation.

An example of the potential of RAGE on the EC surface to engage AGEs in the intravascular space to perturb vascular function is that of AGEs associated with diabetic red cells (Wautier *et al.*, 1981; Wautier *et al.*, 1994). In addition to the presence of glycated hemoglobin in diabetes, cell surface proteins on red cells also undergo AGE

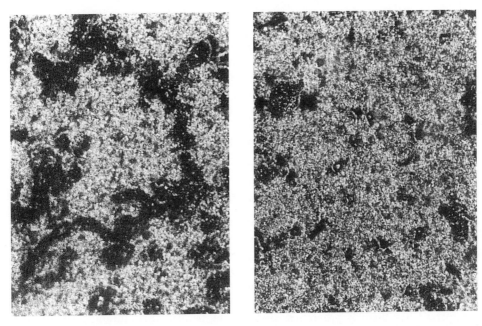

Figure 14.13 Phagokinetic track assay in which mononuclear phagocytes migrated for 6 hours on matrices of either native albumin (left) or AGE-albumin (right) which had been coated with colloidal gold particles. The dark tracks left by migrating mononuclear phagocytes are displayed by dark-field microscopy (magnification: × 125).

modification which results in their specific binding to endothelium via RAGE (the binding is prevented by anti-RAGE IgG/F[ab']$_2$ or sRAGE; Wautier *et al.*, 1994). Diabetic red cells infused into normal rats are cleared at an accelerated rate, which is blocked in large part by pretreatment of recipient animals with anti-RAGE IgG, indicative of diabetic red cell binding to RAGE *in vivo*. In view of the induction of cellular oxidant stress by AGE-modified proteinaceous ligands bound to RAGE (Yan *et al.*, 1994a), we considered it possible that AGE-modified diabetic red cells tethered to the endothelium via RAGE might also perturb these cellular properties. Consistent with this hypothesis, elevated levels of TBARS and activation of NF-kB, indicative of oxidant stress, were observed in the organs of rats treated with diabetic red cells, each of which was inhibited by anti-RAGE IgG. Pilot studies have suggested that these data can be extrapolated to include increased vascular permeability following infusion of diabetic red cells which is blocked by anti-RAGE IgG. Taken together, these data lead us to propose that the interaction of AGEs with RAGE could underlie the pathogenesis of certain diabetic complications, and design of agents which block this binding might provide a novel therapy.

Beyond the setting of diabetes, formation of AGEs is observed in other contexts in which proteins accumulate and display delayed turnover. An example of this is Alzheimer's disease in which there is increased expression of RAGE and deposition of AGEs. Glycation of amyloid βpeptide in the vasculature and in senile plaques (Yan *et al.*, 1993; Smith *et al.*, 1994; Vitek *et al.*, 1994) could promote their interaction with cellular elements via RAGE (certain neurons also express RAGE; Brett *et al.*, 1993). The micro-tubule-associated protein tau also accumulates in an altered form constituting the neu-rofibrillary tangles in Alzheimer's disease. Tau is an excellent substrate for nonenzymatic glycation as it is lysine-rich (about 10%; nonenzymatic glycation is initiated on free amino groups) and present in the cytosol where high concentrations of aldose phosphates cause rapid AGE formation (Giardino *et al.*, 1994). Paired helical filament tau (that present in neurofibrillary tangles) becomes AGE modified, and we have speculated that the AGEs generate oxygen free radicals thereby perturbing cellular functions (Yan *et al.*, 1994b). Thus, AGE formation may be relevant to a spectrum of disorders even beyond the context of diabetes.

Tumor-Derived Cytokines and Hemostatic Properties of Tumor Neovasculature

Systemic and developmental factors have an important impact on properties of the wide array of vascular beds present in specialized organs, but local mediators may also have a critical role. In tumor stroma the ingrowing neovasculature is completely immersed in a specialized microenvironment created by neoplastic cells of the tumor. The capacity of tumor cells to generate angiogenic factors and a stroma with characteristics which favors blood vessel growth has been extensively studied (Folkman, 1985; Dvorak, 1986). Tumor vasculature has distinct properties, in terms of permeability, thrombogenicity and response to certain agents (e.g., including cytokines, flavone acetic acid) (Senger *et al.*, 1983; Asher *et al.*, 1987; Nawroth *et al.*, 1988; Watanabe *et al.*, 1988; Bibby *et al.*, 1989; Constantinidis *et al.*, 1989; Karpati *et al.*, 1991), leading to the hypothesis that mediators made by the tumor could modulate not only the growth, but also the properties of the tumor vessels once formed. If one could understand the basis of differences between properties of tumor and normal vasculature and exploit these, tumor neovessels could provide a selective target for anti-tumor therapy.

A striking example of the distinctive properties of tumor vessels is indicated by the vascular response to infusion of tumor necrosis factor-alpha (TNF) (Old, 1986). Injection of a low concentration of TNF into the tail vein of mice bearing the transplantable methylcholanthrene A-induced (meth A) fibrosarcoma resulted in early fibrin deposition along the endothelial surface of tumor vasculature with progressive accumulation of thrombus and white cells over longer times (Old *et al.*, 1961; Old, 1986; Nawroth *et al.*, 1988). Although tumor vessels were undergoing thrombohemorrhage, the normal vascu-lature was unaffected and without evidence of intravascular thrombosis. This suggested the that tumor vasculature was demonstrating a heightened response to TNF because of the effects of adjacent neoplastic cells. In support of this concept, conditioned medium obtained from meth A cells applied to ECs in culture in the presence of TNF resulted in a synergistic enhancement of tissue factor induction (Figure 14.14A) (Nawroth *et al.*, 1988). That the tumor-derived mediator(s) which enhanced tissue factor was a polypep-tide was suggested by demonstrating that the activity was heat- and trypsin-sensitive, nondialyzable and could be separated from much of the protein in the conditioned medium by gel filtration (Figure 14.14B). Furthermore, neither antibody to TNF, IL-1 or other factors affected the activity of tumorconditioned medium suggesting that it was likely a novel polypeptide(s).

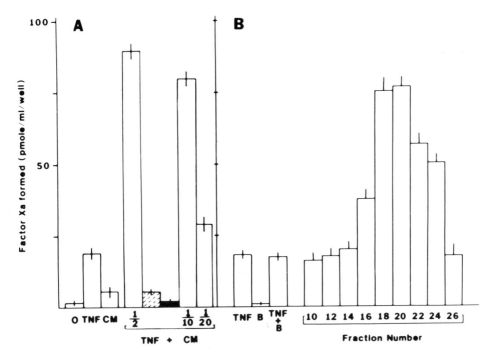

Figure 14.14 Induction of endothelial tissue factor by TNF and medium conditioned by meth A cells. A. ECs were incubated with either serum-free medium alone (0), conditioned medium from meth A cells at the indicated dilution (CM), TNF alone (0.1 nM) or TNF and conditioned medium (TNF + CM) for 7 hours at 37°C. Tissue factor activity was then determined with purified Factors VIIa and X. The cross-hatched bars shows a tissue factor assay performed in the presence of a blocking antibody to tissue factor, and the darkened bar shows a tissue factor assay from which Factor X was omitted. B. Tumor-conditioned medium was subjected to gel filtration chromatography (Sephadex G150), samples were then incubated with EC monolayers in the presence of TNF (0.1 nM), and the tissue factor assay was performed. TNF denotes cells incubated in TNF alone, and B denotes cells exposed to buffer alone.

After extensive study, we have resolved three different mediators in meth A cell supernatants which modulate properties of endothelium, and those of other cells involved in the inflammatory response to certain tumors, i.e., leukocytes and MPs. These are denominated Endothelial-Monocyte Activating Polypeptide (EMAP) I, vascular endothelial growth factor/vascular permeability factor (VEGF/VPF), and EMAP II (Clauss *et al.*, 1990a; Clauss *et al.*, 1990b; Kao *et al.*, 1992; Kao *et al.*, 1994a) .

EMAP I (Clauss *et al.*, 1990a) is a single-chain polypeptide Mr ≈40 kDa on nonreduced SDS-PAGE which potently modulates properties of endothelium; in the picomolar range, EMAP I induces EC expression of tissue factor and enhances the effects of TNF on EC accumulation of tissue factor mRNA and tissue factor procoagulant activity. EMAP I also increases permeability of EC monolayers, enhances adhesivity for leukocytes, and modulates properties of MPs as well.

VEGF/VPF. Further analysis of meth A-conditioned medium led to isolation of another polypeptide with Mr ≈40 kDa on nonreduced SDS-PAGE and which on reduction displayed a major band at ≈23 kDa (Clauss *et al.*, 1990b). The amino terminal sequence indicated that the latter was the murine homolog of VEGF/VPF, which was confirmed by studies with cross-reacting antibodies and experiments with purified VEGF/VPF. In each case, VEGF/VPF induced tissue factor activity in ECs, and also activated MPs with induction of cell migration and expression of tissue factor (Shen *et al.*, 1993). Thus, in addition to the well-known effects of VEGF/VPF to enhance vascular leakage and to induce angiogenesis (Senger *et al.*, 1983; Ferrara and Henzel, 1989; Keck *et al.*, 1989; Leung *et al.*, 1989), it also possesses properties of an inflammatory mediator. This is consistent with other studies which showed that VEGF/VPF can rapidly elevate cytosolic calcium (Brock *et al.*, 1991), thereby resulting in release of Weibel-Palade body contents and translocation of the adherence molecule P-selectin to the cell surface (Geng *et al.*, 1990; Birch *et al.*, 1992). These events render the vessel surface an attractive target for leukocytes, and could underlie tumor vascular thrombohemorrhage observed following administration of TNF to tumorbearing animals.

EMAP II (Kao *et al.*, 1992; Kao *et al.*, 1994a) was the third activity defined in supernatants of cultured meth A cells which could potently modulate properties of leukocytes, monocytes and ECs. Molecular cloning has shown EMAP II to be a novel mediator, not in any previously described cytokine or growth factor families. The proform of EMAP II is ≈34 kDa and possesses no signal peptide. The mature form, based on amino terminal sequence analysis of material in culture supernatants, has Mr 18–22 kDa, and is formed by proteolytic cleavage of the precursor. Based on the presence of an aspartic acid residue at the P1 site (in a region just prior to the start of mature EMAP II), it has been hypothesized that EMAP II may be a substrate for Interleukin-1β converting enzyme (Thornberry *et al.*, 1992; Cerretti *et al.*, 1992) or another similar enzyme. The only other limited region of sequence homology between EMAP II and previously described proteins is at the amino terminus of the mature form (Figure 14.15). The homology to IL-8 was particularly relevant in that it included the Glutamate-Leucine-Arginine region in IL-8 which is involved in recognition of cell surface receptors (Hebert *et al.*, 1991). This suggested that peptides derived from the amino terminal portion of mature EMAP II might bind to the cell surface and mediate some effects of the intact cytokine. Such peptides were prepared, and were indeed capable of mediating leukocyte activation as indicated by induction of chemotaxis, elevation of cytosolic calcium and release of myeloperoxidase (Kao *et al.*, 1994b). MPs were also affected by EMAP II derived peptides, which induced cell migration and cytosolic calcium flux. Furthermore, amino terminal peptides from EMAP II bound specifically to MPs (Figure 14.16) and cross-linked to an ≈73 kDa polypeptide. The latter cell surface polypeptide may be a novel receptor, as binding of [125]Ilabelled

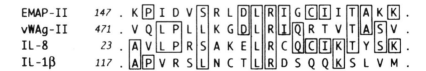

Figure 14.15 Comparison of EMAP II deduced amino acid sequence with the indicated residues from von Willebrand antigen II (vWAgII; Bonthron *et al.*, 1986; Fay *et al.*, 1986), IL-8 (Matsushima *et al.*, 1988; Lindley *et al.*, 1988) and IL-1β (March *et al.*, 1985). All sequences are human, and numbering is based on the precursor form of each. Identical residues in two or more sequences are boxed.

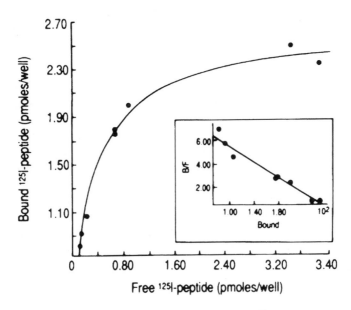

Figure 14.16 Binding of an amino terminal peptide from EMAP II (^{125}I-RIGRIVTAKY) to mononuclear phagocytes (Kao *et al.*, 1994). The experiment was performed at 4°C and specific binding is plotted versus the concentration of free peptide. Data were analyzed by nonlinear least squares analysis and the curve indicates the best-fit line. The Inset shows Scatchard analysis of the same data fit to a one-site model (B = bound; B/F = bound/free). Kd estimated from the Scatchard plot was ≈0.2 nM.

EMAP II peptide to MPs was not antagonized by IL-1, IL-8, TNF, formylated chemotactic peptide or other ligands.

Using recombinant EMAP II, experiments have been performed to determine if it can sensitize tumors to the effects of TNF. The murine mammary carcinoma is a tumor which is insensitive to TNF and does not express EMAP II. To test our hypothesis, mammary carcinomas were grown in mice, and EMAP II was injected locally at the site of the tumor (Kao *et al.*, 1994a). About 10–16 hrs later, a low concentration of TNF (one which in the absence of EMAP II would have no effect) was injected via tail vein and the response at the tumor site assessed. Thrombohemorrhage occurred after the regimen of EMAP II followed by TNF, and was followed by tumor regression. Clonogenic growth of cells isolated from tumors after EMAP II/TNF was dramatically reduced compared with controls. In order to achieve these effects, both active TNF and EMAP II were required, omission of either, or destruction of the cytokines by heat-treatment abrogated tumor regression. Systemic injection of TNF could be replaced by systemic injection of EMAP II with equivalent or even more striking results on tumor size. These data suggest an analogy to the Shwartzman reaction (Movat *et al.*, 1987) whereby locally produced cytokines, such as EMAP II, have a preparatory and localizing role, and the systemic cytokine infusion functions as a provocative stimulus. Recent studies have shown that a range of tumors, including human neoplasms grown in immunodeficient mice, initially insensitive to TNF can undergo TNF-induced tumor regression following local treatment with EMAP II. This suggests that EMAP II might potentially be exploited alone or along with TNF in regimens in the treatment of human tumors.

An important issue to consider in terms of the elaboration of proinflammatory cytokines by tumors is their possible role in tumor progression. The meth A tumor is well-known for its inflammatory features and inhomogeneity, with areas of focal necrosis. Studies are underway to determine if such pathologic features result from the expression of a mediator such as EMAP II. However, the teleologic question arises as to why any tumor produces EMAP II or other phlogogenic agents. On the one hand, EMAP II induces IL-8 production by MPs (Kao *et al.*, 1994b) which could promote tumor angiogenesis (Koch *et al.*, 1992; Strieter *et al.*, 1992) critical to the establishment of the neoplastic lesion. EMAP II-induced inflammation could also serve to isolate the tumor from host defense mechanisms through its induction of endothelial and monocyte tissue factor with activation of the procoagulant mechanism and resultant fibrin formation. The establishment of a protective fibrin "cocoon" as the result of local thrombus formation, could serve as an insulator for the tumor against incipient host defense mechanisms. We are studying these possibilities, as well as the conditions in which EMAP II may be produced by non-neoplastic cells as a part of the host response to other stimuli such as lipopolysaccharide.

EPILOGUE

Modulation of vascular function by local factors is critical for linking the vasculature to the host response to environmental perturbation. Hypoxia/hypoxemia and locally produced cytokines, as in the tumor bed, are likely candidates as important agents which can alter vascular properties both directly and by changing the response to other mediators. While hypoxia and local mediators can be produced rapidly, they are also removed/reversed over short time periods. In contrast, the accumulation of AGEs is irreversible and results in a vessel wall modified by the presence of structures which generate ROIs, attract monocytes, and modulate EC properties. The potential significance of AGE-induced priming of the vessel wall for subsequent interaction with other mediators is suggested by the synergistic enhancement of EC tissue factor expression on exposure to AGEs and TNF versus either agent alone (Esposito *et al.*, 1989). Thus, during normal aging or over shorter times in patients with diabetes the vasculature is already subject to a baseline change in critical properties, which may impact significantly on the ability to defend homeostasis against further challenges, such as hypoxemia. Although this is a complex situation, dissection of the key molecular interactions should provide future insights into the pathogenesis of vascular disorders.

Acknowledgements

This work was supported by grants from the PHS (HL42507, HL50629, HL21006, HL42833, AG00602), Juvenile Diabetes Foundation, Council for Tobacco Research, Alzheimer's Research Foundation, American Heart Association- New York affiliate (Grant-in-Aid; to AMS), American Heart Association (Grant-in-Aid; to DP). D. Pinsky completed this work during the tenure of a Clinician-Investigator Award from the American Heart Association. Dr. Gabriel Godman provided helpful suggestions during the course of our studies and invaluable suggestions for preparation of the manuscript.

References

Albrech-Buehler, G. (1977). The phagokinetic tracks of 3T3 cells. *Cell*, **11**:395–404.

Asher, A., Mule, J., Reichert, C., Shiloni, E. and Rosenberg, S. (1987). Studies on the antitumor efficacy of systemically administered recombinant tumor necrosis factor against several murine tumors *in vivo*. *Journal of Immunology*, **138**:963–974.

Baggiolini, M., Waltz, A. and Kunkel, S. (1989). Neutrophil-activating peptide-1/Interleukin-8, a novel cytokine that activates neutrophils. *Journal of Clinical Investigation*, **84**:1045–1049.

Baynes, J. (1991). Role of oxidative stress in development of complications in diabetes. *Diabetes*, **40**:405–412.

Beutler, B. and Cerami, A. (1986). Cachectin and tumor necrosis factor as two sides of the same biological coin. *Nature* (London), **32**:584–586.

Bibby, M., Double, J., Loadman, P. and Duke, C. (1989). Reduction of tumor blood flow by flavone acetic acid: a possible component of therapy. *Journal of the National Cancer Institute*, **81**:216–220.

Birch, K., Pober, J., Zavoico, G., Means, A. and Ewenstein, B. (1992). Calcium/calmodulin transduces thrombin-stimulated secretion: studies in intact and minimally permeabilized human umbilical vein endothelial cells. *Journal of Cell Biology*, **118**:1501–1510.

Bonthron, D., Handin, R., Kaufman, R., Wasley, L., Orr, E., Mitsock, L., Ewenstein, B., Loscalzo, J., Ginsburg, D. and Orkin, S. (1986). Structure of pre-pro- von Willebrand factor and its expression in heterologous cells. *Nature*, **324**:270–273.

Brett, J., Schmidt, A.M., Zou, Y.S., Yan, S.D., Weidman, E., Pinsky, D., Neeper, M., Przysiecki, M., Shaw,·A., Migheli, A. and Stern, D. (1993). Tissue distribution of the receptor for advanced glycation endproducts (RAGE): expression in smooth muscle, cardiac myocytes, and neural tissue in addition to the vasculature. *American Journal of Pathology*, **143**:1699–1712.

Brock, T., Dvorak, H. and Senger, D. (1991). Tumor secreted vascular permeability factor increases cytosolic calcium and von Willebrand factor release in human endothelial cells. *American Journal of Pathology*, **138**:213–221.

Brownlee, M., Cerami, A. and Vlassara, H. (1988). Advanced glycosylation endproducts in tissue and the biochemical basis of diabetic complications. *New England Journal of Medicine*, **318**:1315–1320.

Cerretti, D., Kozlisky, C., Mosley, B., Nelson, N., Van Ness, K., Greenstreet, T., March, C., Kronheim, S., Druck, T., Cannizzaro, L., Huebner, K. and Black, R., (1992). Molecular cloning of the Interleukin-1 B converting enzyme. *Science*, **256**:97–100.

Chiba, M., Sumida, E., Oka, N. and Nakata, M. (1991). The effect of hypoxia on bFGF synthesis of myocardial cells. *Circulation*, (Supplement) **84**:1573, 1991.

Clauss, C., Murray, C., Vianna, M., De Waal, R., Thurston, G., Nawroth, P., Gerlach, H., Gerlach, M., Bach, R., Familletti, P. and Stern, D. (1990a). A polypeptide factor produced by fibrosarcoma cells that induces endothelial tissue factor and enhances the procoagulant response to TNF. *Journal of Biological Chemistry*, **265** 7078–7083.

Clauss, M., Gerlach, M., Gerlach, H., Brett, J., Wang, F., Pan, Y-C., Familletti, P., Olander, J., Connolly, D. and Stern, D. (1990b). Vascular permeability factor: a tumor derived polypeptide which induces endothelial cell and monocyte procoagulant activity, and promotes monocyte migration. *Journal of Experimental Medicine*, **172**:1535–1545.

Connolly, D., Heivelman, D., Nelson, R., Olander, J., Eppley, B., Delfino, J., Siegel, N., Leimbruber, R. and Feder, J. (1989). Tumor vascular permeability factor stimulates endothelial cell growth and angiogenesis. *Journal of Clinical Investigation*, **84**:1470–1478.

Constantinidis, I., Braunscheweiger, J., Wehrele, J., Kumar, N., Johnson, C., Furmanski, P. and Glickson, J. (1989). *Cancer Research*, **49**:6379–6382.

Crawford, M., Grover, F., Kolb, W., McMahan, C., O'Rourke, R., McManus, L. and Pinckard, R. (1988). Complement and neutrophil activation in the pathogenesis of ischemic myocardial injury. *Circulation*, **78**:1449–1458.

Dinarello, C. and Wolff, S. (1993). The role of Interleukin 1 in disease. *New England Journal of Medicine*, **328**:106–113.

Dvorak, H. (1986). Tumors: wounds that do not heal. Similarities between tumor stroma generation and wound healing. *New England Journal of Medicine*, **315**:1650–1659.

Esposito, C., Gerlach, H., Brett, J., Stern, D. and Vlassara, H. (1989). Endothelial receptor mediated binding of glucose-modified albumin is associated with increased monolayer permeability and modulation of cell surface coagulant properties. *Journal of Experimental Medicine*, **170**:1387–1407.

Fay, P., Kawai, Y., Wagner, D., Ginsburg, D., Bonthron, D., Ohlsson-Wlhelm, B., Chavin, S., Abraham, G., Handin, R., Orkin, S., Montgomery, R. and Marder, V. (1986). Propolypeptide of von Willebrand Factor circulates in blood and is identical to von Willebrand antigen II. *Science*, **232**:995–998.

Ferrara, N. and Henzel, W. (1989). Pituitary follicular cells secrete a novel heparin-binding growth factor specific for vascular endothelial cells. *Biochemical Biophysical Research Communications*, **161**:851–858.

Folkman, J. and Klagsbrun, M. (1987). Angiogenic factors. *Science*, **235**:442–447.

Folkman, J. (1985). Tumor angiogenesis. *Advances in Cancer Research*, **43**:175–203.

Geng, J-G., Bevilacqua, M., Moore, K., McIntyre, T., Prescomtt, S., Kim, J., Bliss, G., Zimmerman, G., McEver, R. (1990). Rapid neutrophil adhesion to activated endothelium mediated by GMP-140. *Nature*, **343**:757–760.

Giardino, I., Edelstein, D. and Brownlee, M. (1994). Nonenzymatic glycosylation *in vitro* and in bovine endothelial cells alters basic fibroblast growth factor activity. *Journal of Clinical Investigation*, **94**:110–117.

Hamer, J., Malone, P. and Silver, I. (1981). The pO_2 in venous valve pockets: its possible bearing on thrombogenesis. *British Journal of Surgery*, **68**:166–170.

Hebert, C., Vitangcol, R. and Baker, J. (1991). Scanning mutagenesis of Interleukin-8 identifies a cluster of residues required for receptor binding. *Journal of Biological Chemistry*, **266**:18989–18994.

Hicks, M., Delbridge, L., Yue, D. and Reeve, R. (1988). Catalysis of lipid peroxidation by glucose and glycosylated proteins. *Biochemical Biophysical Research Communications*, **151**:649–655.

Hultgren, J. High altitude pulmonary edema. In *Lung Water and Solute Exchange*, N. Staub, (ed.), pp. 437–469. New York: Marcel Dekker, Inc. Marcel Dekker, Inc.

Hunkapiller, T. and Hood, L. (1989). Diversity of the immunoglobulin gene superfamily. *Advances in Immunology*, **44**:1–63.

Hunt, J., Smith, C. and Wolff, S. (1990). Autooxidative glycosylation and possible involvement of peroxides and free radicals in LDL modification by glucose. *Diabetes*, **30**:1420–1424.

Jakeman, L., Winer, J., Bennett, G., Altar, A. and Ferrara, N. (1992). Binding sites for vascular endothelial growth factor are localized on endothelial cells in adult rat tissues. *Journal of Clinical Investigation*, **89**: 244–253.

Kao, J., Ryan, J., Brett, J., Chen, J., Shen, H., Fan, Y-G., Godman, G., Familletti, P., Wang, F., Pan, Y-C., Stern, D. and Clauss, M. (1992). endothelial monocyte activating polypeptide (EMAP II): a novel tumor derived polypeptide which activates host-response mechanisms. *Journal of Biological Chemistry*, **267**:20239–20247.

Kao, J., Houck, K., Fan, Y., Haehnel, I., Libutti, S., Kayton, M., Grikscheit, T., Chabot, J., Nowygrod, R., Greenberg, S., Kuang, W-J., Leung, D., Hayward, J., Kisiel, W., Heath M., Brett, J. and Stern, D. 1994a). Characterization of a novel tumor-derived cytokine: endothelial monocyte activating polypeptide II (EMAP II), *Journal of Biological Chemistry*. **269**:25106–25119).

Kao, J., Fan, Y-G., Haehnel, I., Brett, J., Greenberg, S., Clauss, M., Kayton, M., Houck, K., Kisiel, W., Burnier, J. and Stern, D. (1994b). A peptide derived from the amino terminus of endothelial-monocyte activating polypeptide II (EMAP II) modulates mononuclear and polymorphonuclear leukocyte functions, defines an apparently novel cellular interaction site, and induces an acute inflammatory response. *Journal of Biological Chemistry*, **269**:9774–9782.

Karakurum, M., Shreeniwas, R., Chen, J., Sunouchi, J., Hamilton, T., Anderson, M., Kuwabara, K., Rot, A., Nowygrod, R. and Stern, D. (1994). Hypoxic induction of IL-8 gene expression in endothelial cells. *Journal of Clinical Investigation*, **93**:1564–1570, 1994.

Karpati, R., Banks, S., Malissen, B., Rosenberg, S., Sheard, M., Weber, J. and Hodes, R. (1991). Phenotypic characterization of murine tumor-infiltrating T lymphocytes. *Journal of Immunology*, **146**:2043–2051.

Keck, P., Hauser, S., Krivi, G., Sanzo, K., Warren, T., Feder, J. and Connolly, D. (1989). Vascular permeability factor, an endothelial cell mitogen related to PDGF. *Science*, **246**:1309–1312.

Kinasewitz, G., Groome, L., Marshall, R., Leslie,W. and Diana, H. (1986). Effect of hypoxia on permeability of pulmonary endothelium of canine visceral pleura. *Journal of Applied Physiology*, **61**:554–560.

Kirstein, M., Brett, J., Radoff, S., Ogawa, S., Stern, D. and Vlassara, H. (1990). Advanced glycosylation end-products induce selective monocyte migration across endothelium, and elaboration of growth factors. *PNAS(USA)*, **87**:9010–9014.

Klein, R., Kelin, B., Moss, S., Davis, M., DeMets, R. (1989). Glycosylated haemoglobin predicts the incidence and progression of diabetic retinopathy. *Journal of the American Medical Association*, **260**:2864–2868.

Koch, A., Polverini, P., Kunkel, S., Harlow, L., DiPietro, L., Elner, V., Elner, S. and Strieter, R. (1992). Interleukin-8 as a macrophage-derived mediator of angiogenesis. *Science*, **258**:1798–1801.

Kuwabara, K., Ogawa, S., Matsumoto, M., Koga, S., Clauss, M., Pinsky, D., Witte, L., Joseph-Silverstein, J., Furie, M., Torcia, G., Cozzolino, F., Kamada, T. and D. Stern. (1995) Hypoxia-mediated induction of acidic/basic fibroblast growth factor and platelet-derived growth factor in mononuclear phagocytes stimulates growth of hypoxic endothelial cells, *PNAS(USA)*. **92**:4606–4610.

Leung, D., Cachianes, G., Kuang, W-J., Goeddel, D. and Ferrara, N. (1989). Vascular endothelial growth factor is a secreted angiogenic mitogen. *Science*, **246**:1306–1309.

Lindley, I., Aschauer, H., Seifert, J-M., Lam, C., Brunowsky, W., Kownatzki, E., Thelen, M., Peveri, P., Dewald, B., von Tscharner, V., Walz, A. and Baggiolini, M. (1988). Synthesis and expression in escherichia coli of the gene encoding monocyte-derived neutrophil-activating factor: biological equivalence between natural and recombinant neutrophil-activating factor. *PNAS(USA)*, **85**:9199–9203.

Lockhart, A. and Saiag, B. Altitude and the human pulmonary circulation (1981). *Clinical Science (London)*, **60**:599–605.

Loike, J., Cao, L., Brett, J., Ogawa, S., Silverstein, S. and Stern, D. (1992). Induction of glucose transporters in hypoxic cultured endothelial cells. *American Journal of Physiology*, **263**:C326–C333.

Ma, X-L., Tsao, P. and Lefer, A. (1991). Antibody to CD-18 exerts endothelial and cardiac protective effects in myocardial ischemia and reperfusion. *Journal of Clinical Investigation*, **88**:1237–1243.

March, C., Mosley, B., Larsen, A., Cerretti, D., Braedt, G., Price, V, Gillis, S., Henney, C., Kronheim, S., Grabstein, K., Conlon, P., Hopp, T. and Cosman, D. (1985). Cloning, sequence and expression of two distinct human interleukin-1 complementary DNAs. *Nature*, **315**:641–647.

Matsushima, K., Morishita, K., Yoshimura, T., Lavu, S., Kobayashi, Y., Lew, W., Appella, E., Kung, H., Leonard, E. and Oppenheim, J. (1988). Molecular cloning of a human monocytederived neutrophil chemotactic factor (MDNCF) and the induction of MDNCF mRNA by interleukin 1 and tumor necrosis factor. *Journal of Experimental Medicine*, **167**:1883–1893.

Metinko, A., Kunkel, S., Sandiford, T. and Streiter, R. (1992). Anoxia-hyperoxia induces monocyte driven Interleukin 8. *Journal of Clinical Investigation*, **90**:791–798.

Minnear, F., Johnson, A. and Malik, A. (1986). Beta-adrenergic modulation of pulmonary transvascular fluid and protein exchange. *Journal of Applied Physiology*, **60**:266–274.

Minnear, F., DeMichele, M., Moon, D., Rieder, C. and Fenton, J. (1989). Isoproterenol reduces thrombin-induced pulmonary endothelial permeability *in vitro*. *American Journal of Physiology*, **257**:H1613–H1623.

Movat, H., Burrowes, C., Cybulsky, M. and Dinarello, C. (1987). Acute inflammation and a Shwartzman-like reaction induced by Interleukin-1 and tumor necrosis factor. *American Journal of Pathology*, **129**:463–476.

Mullane, K., Read, N., Salmon, J. and Moncada, S. (1984). Role of leukocytes in acute myocardial infarction in anesthetized dogs. *Journal of Pharmacology and Experimental Therapy*, **228**:510–522.

Mullarkey, C., Edelstein, D. and Brownlee, M. (1990). Free radical generation by early glycation products: a mechanism for accelerated atherogenesis in diabetes. *Biochemical and Biophysical Research Communications*, **173**:932–939.

Nawroth, P., Handley, D., Matsueda, G., De Waal, R., Gerlach, H., Blohm, D. and Stern, D. (1988). TNF-induced intravascular fibrin formation in meth A fibrosarcomas. *Journal of Experimental Medicine*, **168**:637–647.

Neeper, M., Schmidt, A.M., Brett, J., Yan, S.D., Wang, F., Pan, Y.C., Elliston, K., Stern, D. and Shaw, A. (1992). Cloning and expression of RAGE: a cell surface receptor for advanced glycation endproducts of proteins. *Journal of Biological Chemistry*, **267**:14998–15004.

Ogawa, S., Koga, S., Kuwabara, K., Brett, J., Morrow, B., Morris, S., Bilezikian, J., Silverstein, S. and Stern, D. (1992). Hypoxia-induced increased permeability of endothelial monolayers occurs through lowering of cellular cAMP levels. *American Journal of Physiology*, **262**:C546–C554.

Old, L., Benacerraf, B., Clarke, D., Carswell, D. and Stockert, E. (1961). The role of the reticuloendothelial system in the host reaction of neoplasia. *Cancer Research*, **21**:1281–1300.

Old, L. Tumor necrosis factor. (1986). *Science*, **230**:630–632.

Olesen, S-P. (1986). Rapid increase in blood-brain barrier permeability during severe hypoxia and metabolic inhibition. *Brain Research*, **368**:24–29.

Ono, K. and Lindsey, E. (1969). Improved technique of heart transplantation in rats. *Journal of Thoracic and Cardiovascular Surgery*, **57**:225–229.

Oppenheim, J., Zachariae, C., Mukaida, N. and Matsushima, K. (1991). Properties of the novel proinflammatory supergene "intercrine" cytokine family. *Annual Review of Immunology*, **9**:617–648.

Oz, M., Pinsky, D., Koga, S., Liao, H., Marboe, C., Han, D., Kline, R., Jeevanandam, V., Williams, M., Morales, A., Popilskis, S., Nowygrod, R., Stern, D., Rose, E. and Michler, R. (1993). Novel preservation solution permits 24 hr preservation in a rat and baboon cardiac transplant model. *Circulation*, **88** (part 2), 291–297.

Peveri, P., Walz, A., DeWald, B. and Baggiolini, M. (1988). A novel neutrophil-activating factor produced by human mononuclear phagocytes. *Journal of Experimental Medicine*, **167**:1547–1559.

Pinsky, D., Oz, M., Morris, S., Liao, H., Brett, J., Morales, A., Karakurum, M., Van Lookeren Camagne, M., Platt, J., Nowygrod, R., Koga, S. and Stern, D. (1993). Restoration of the cAMP second messenger pathway enhances cardiac preservation for transplantation in a heterotopic rat model. *Journal of Clinical Investigation*, **92**:2994–3002.

Pinsky, D., Oz, M., Koga, S., Taha, Z., Broekman, J., Marcus, A., Cannon, P., Nowygrod, R., Malinski, T. and Stern, D. (1994). Augmentation of the nitric oxide pathway enhances cardiac preservation for transplantation. *Journal of Clinical Investigation*, **93**:2291–2297.

Pober, J. and Cotran, R. (1990a). Cytokines and endothelial cell biology. *Physiological Reviews*, **70**:427–451.

Pober, J. and Cotran, R. (1990b). Overview: the role of endothelial cells in inflammation. *Transplant*, **50**:537–544.

Risau, W. (1990). Angiogenic Growth Factors. *Progress in Growth Factor Research,* **2**:71–79.

Ruderman, N., Williamson, J. and Brownlee, M. (1992). Glucose and diabetic vascular disease. *FASEB Journal,* **6**:2905–2914.

Sakurai, T. and Tsuchiya, S. (1988). Superoxide production from nonenzymatically glycated protein. *FEBS Letters,* **236**:406–410.

Schmidt, A-M., Vianna, M., Gerlach, M., Brett, J., Ryan, J., Kao, J., Esposito, C., Hegarty, H., Hurley, W., Clauss, M., Wang, F., Pan, Y.C., Tsang, T. and Stern, D. (1992). Isolation and characterization of binding proteins for advanced glycation endproducts from lung tissue which are present on the endothelial cell surface. *Journal of Biological Chemistry,* **267**:14987–14997.

Schmidt, A-M., Yan, S.D., Brett, J., Mora, R., Nowygrod, R. and Stern, D. (1993). Regulation of mononuclear phagocyte migration by cell surface binding proteins for advanced glycation endproducts. *Journal of Clinical Investigation,* **92**:2155–2168.

Schmidt, A-M., Mora, R., Cao, R., Yan, S.D., Brett, J., Ramakrishnan, R., Tsang, T.C., Simionescu, M. and Stern, D. (1994a). The endothelial cell binding site for advanced glycation endproducts consists of a complex: an integral membrane protein and a lactoferrin-like polypeptide. *Journal of Biological Chemistry,* **269**:9882–9888.

Schmidt, A-M., Hori, O., Brett, J., Yan, S.D., Wautier, J.L. and Stern, D. (1994c). Cellular receptors for advanced glycation endproducts: implications for induction of oxidant stress and cellular dysfunction in the pathogenesis of vascular lesion, *Arteriosclerosis and Thrombosis.* **14**:1521–1528.

Schmidt, A-M., Hasu, M., Popov, D., Zhang, J.H., Yan, S.D., J. Brett, J., Cao, R., Kuwabara, K., Costache, G., Simionescu, N., Simionescu, M. and Stern, D. (1994b). The receptor for advanced glycation endproducts (AGEs) has a central role in vessel wall interactions and gene activation in response to AGEs in the intravascular space, *PNAS (USA).* **91**:8807–8811.

Sekido, N., Mukaida, N., Harada, A., Nakanishi, I., Watanabe, Y. and Matsushima, K. (1993). Prevention of lung reperfusion injury in rabbits by a monoclonal antibody against Interleukin 8. *Nature,* **365**:654–657.

Sell, D. and Monnier, V. (1989). Structure elucidation of a senescence cross-link from human extracellular matrix: implication of pentoses in the aging process. *Journal of Biological Chemistry,* **264**:21597–21602.

Senger, D., Galli, S., Dvorak, A., Perruzii, C., Harvey, V. and Dvorak, H. (1983). Tumor cells secrete a vascular permeability factor that promotes accumulation of ascites fluid. *Science,* **219**:983–985.

Sevitt, S. (1967). The acutely swollen leg and deep vein thrombosis. *British Journal of Surgery,* **54**:886–890.

Shen, H., Clauss, M., Kao, J., Ryan, J., Schmidt, A-M., Tijburg, P., Borden, L. and Stern, D. (1993). Characterization of vascular permeability factor/vascular endothelial growth factor receptors on mononuclear phagocytes. *Blood,* **81**:2767–2773.

Shreeniwas, R., Ogawa, S., Cozzolino, F., Torcia, G., Braunstein, N., Butura, C., Brett, J., Lieberman, H., Furie, M. and Stern, D. (1991). Macrovascular and microvascular endothelium during long-term exposure to hypoxia: alterations in cell growth, monolayer permeability and cell surface coagulant properties. *Journal of Cellular Physiology,* **146**:8–17.

Shreeniwas, R., Koga, S., Pinsky, D., Kaiser, E., Brett, J., Wolitzky, B., Norton, C., Plocinski, J., Benjamin, W., Burns, D., Goldstein, A. and Stern, D. (1992). Hypoxiamediated induction of endothelial cell Interleukin 1 alpha: an autocrine mechanism promoting expression of leukocyte adhesion molecules on the vessel surface. *Journal of Clinical Investigation,* **90**:2333–2339.

Shweiki D., Itin, A., Soffer, D. and Keshet, E. (1992). Vascular endothelial growth factor induced by hypoxia may mediate hypoxia-initiated angiogenesis. *Nature,* **359**:843–845.

Siflinger-Birnboim, A., Bode, D. and Malik B. (1993). Adenosine 3',5'-cyclic monophosphate attenuates neutrophil-mediated increase in endothelial permeability. *American Journal of Physiology,* **264**:H370–H375.

Simionescu, N. and M. Simionescu. (1992). *Endothelial Cell Dysfunction.* New York: Plenum Corp.

Smith, M., Taneda, S., Richey, P., Miyata, S.,Yan, S.D., Stern, D., Monnier, V. and Perry, G. (1994). Advanced maillard reaction endproducts are associated with Alzheimer disease pathology. *Proceedings of the National Academy of Sciences (USA),* **91**:5710–5714.

Stelzner, T., O'Brien, R., Sato, K. and Weil, J. (1988). Hypoxia-induced increases in pulmonary transvascular protein escape in rats. *Journal of Clinical Investigation,* **82**:1840–1847.

Stelzner, T., Weil, J. and O'Brien, R. (1989). Role of cyclic adenosine monophosphate in the induction of endothelial barrier properties. *Journal of Cellular Physiology,* **139**:157–166.

Strieter, R., Kunkel, S., Elner, V., Martonyi, C., Koch, A., Polverini, P. and Elnser, S. (1992). A corneal factor that induces neovascularization. *American Journal of Pathology,* **141**:1279–1284.

Vitek, M., Bhattacharya, K., Glendening, J., Stopa, E., Vlassara, H., Bucala, R., Manogue, K. and Cerami, A. (1994). Advanced glycation endproducts contribute to amyloidosis in Alzheimer disease. *Proceedings of the National Academy of Sciences (USA),* **91**:4766–4770.

Vlassara, H., Brownlee, M., Manogue, K., Dinarello, C. and Pasagian, A. (1988). Cachectin/TNF and IL-1 induced by glucose-modified proteins: role in normal tissue remodeling. *Science,* **240**:1546–1548.

Watanabe, N., Niitsu, Y., Umeno, H., Kuriyama, H., Neda, H., Yamauchi, N., Maeda, M. and Urushizaki, I. (1988). Toxic effect of tumor necrosis factor on tumor vasculature in mice. *Cancer Research*, **48**:2179–2183.

Wautier, J-L., Paton, C., Wautier, M.P., Pintigny, D., Abadie, E., Passa, P. and Caen, J. (1981). Increased adhesion of erythrocytes to endothelial cells in diabetes mellitus and its relation to vascular complications. *New England Journal of Medicine*, **305**:237–242.

Wautier, J-L., Wautier, M.P., Schmidt, A.M., Anderson, G., Hori, O., Zoukourian, C., Capron, L., Chappey, O., Yan, S.D., Brett, J., Guillausseau, P.J. and Stern, D. (1994). Advanced glycation endproducts (AGEs) on the surface of diabetic red cells bind to the vessel wall via a specific receptor inducing oxidant stress in the vasculature: a link between surface-associated AGEs and diabetic complications. *Proceedings of the National Academy of Sciences (USA)*, **91**:7742–7746.

Yan, S-D., Schmidt, A.M., Chen, X., Zou, Y.S., Brett, J., Greene, L. and Stern, D. (1993). Increased levels of advanced glycation endproducts and their receptors in Alzheimer's brain tissue: a mechanism for induction of oxidative stress. *Clinical Research*, **41**:395A.

Yan, S-D., Schmidt, A.M., Anderson, G., Zhang, J., Brett, J., Zou, Y.S., Pinsky, D. and Stern, D. (1994a). Enhanced cellular oxidant stress by the interaction of advanced glycation endproducts with their receptors/binding proteins. *Journal of Biological Chemistry*, **269**:9889–9897.

Yan, S-D., Chen, X., Schmidt, A.M., Brett, J., Godman, G., Scott, C., Caputo, C., Frappier, T., Yen, S.H. and Stern, D. (1994b). The presence of glycated tau in Alzheimer's disease: a mechanism for induction of oxidant stress. *Proceedings of the National Academy of Sciences (USA)*, **91**:7787–7791.

Yang, Z., Makita, J., Horii, Y., Brunelle, S., Cerami, A., Sehajpal, P., Suthanthiran, M., Vlassara, H. (1991). Two novel rat liver membrane proteins that bind advanced glycosylation endproducts: relationship to macrophage receptor for glucose-modified proteins. *Journal of Experimental Medicine*, **174**:515–524.

15 Pathogenesis of the Altered Vascular Hemostasis Properties in Sepsis: *in vivo* Studies

Tom van der Poll, Hugo ten Cate, Sander J.H. van Deventer, Jan W. ten Cate

The Center of Hemostasis, Thrombosis, Atherosclerosis and Inflammation Research, Academic Medical Center, University of Amsterdam, Amsterdam, The Netherlands.

1 INTRODUCTION

Systemic infection is almost invariably associated with changes in the hemostatic mechanism, either at the clinical or subclinical level (Levi 1993). Patients with sepsis demonstrate evidence for activation of the common pathway of the coagulation system, as well as signs of stimulation of the intrinsic and the extrinsic pathway of the coagulation cascade, two separate routes that traditionally were considered to contribute to the development of disseminated intravascular coagulation (DIC)(Colman 1989, Levi *et al.,* 1993, Ten Cate *et al.,* 1993). Concurrently, in these patients the fibrinolytic system shows signs of early activation and subsequent inhibition. The net result of this disbalance in the hemostatic mechanism is widespread deposition of microthrombi in the vasculature of patients with generalized infection.

In recent years the insights into the mechanisms that underlie the hemostatic changes in sepsis have markedly increased. In this chapter we will review *in vivo* studies that investigated the endogenous factors and mediators involved in the development of the prethrombotic state that frequently accompanies critical infection.

2 REGULATION OF HEMOSTASIS *IN VIVO*

2.1 Present Concept of Coagulation

The end product of blood coagulation is a fibrin plug. The generation and degradation of fibrin is tightly regulated by a number of closely cooperating systems that include both cellular elements and plasma proteins. Historically, the coagulation system was divided into two separate pathways, the intrinsic and extrinsic routes, that merged into a common pathway at the level of clotting factor X (Colman *et al.,* 1987). In this traditional concept of coagulation the intrinsic route was initiated by autoactivation of factor XII (the Hageman factor), the first component of the contact system, when it adsorbed to negatively charged surfaces such as cell membranes, the extracellular matrix and heparin on endothelial cells. Factor XIIa can cleave factor XI to factor XIa, thereby initiating the classic intrinsic pathway of the coagulation system, and leading to the activation of factor X by the combined action of factor IXa and factor VIIIa in the tenase complex. Yet another substrate for factor XIIa is prekallikrein. Factor XIIa activates this zymogen to kallikrein, which in turn cleaves high molecular weight kininogen (HMWK) to liberate bradykinin. Bradykinin is a major end product of the contact system and one of the most potent vasoactive agents known. The extrinsic route of the coagulation system was considered to be initiated by tissue factor, the cofactor essential for rapid activation of factor X by factor VIIa. Factor Xa, once formed by either the intrinsic or extrinsic pathway, converts prothrombin to thrombin, the protease that activates fibrinogen to fibrin.

In the present concept of the coagulation system, however, the Hageman factor does not play a significant role. Instead, the coagulation cascade is viewed upon as one series of interrelated reactions that are driven by the generation of the factor VIIa-tissue factor complex (Ten Cate *et al.,* 1993). Indeed, this enzyme complex not only is able to activate factor X, but can also catalyze the conversion of factor IX to factor IXa, providing an additional route by which factor X activation can occur. In this concept the contact system does not contribute to the initiation of coagulation, but, as will be outlined below, is considered to be of importance in the pathogenesis of hypotension during sepsis.

Cell types that are important for plasmatic coagulative reactions include platelets, endothelial cells and monocytes. Platelets can provide a catalytic surface for clotting processes, markedly enhancing the activation rates of factors IX, X and prothrombin. The vascular endothelium plays a major role in the orchestration of local inflammatory reactions, including the regulation of the local hemostatic balance (Gerlach, Esposito and Stern 1990). Endothelial cells can express adhesion molecules that enable entrapping of leukocytes at sites of inflammation, and produce a number of factors that are actively involved in coagulant and anticoagulant mechanisms, including tissue-type plasminogen activator (tPA), urokinase type plasminogen activator (uPA), PAI-1, thrombomodulin, tissue factor and tissue factor pathway inhibitor (TFPI). Monocytes also express tissue factor at their surface upon stimulation with various stimuli. In addition, monocytes are a major source of cytokines such as tumor necrosis factor (TNF), interleukin 1 (IL-1) and IL-6.

2.2 Anticoagulant Mechanisms and Fibrinolysis

Several mechanisms exist to control and localize the formation of fibrin clots. Clotting factors can be bound and inhibited by plasma protease inhibitors. Antithrombin III (AT-III) is the major inhibitor of factors IXa, Xa and thrombin, and represents an important anticoagulant mechanism, as reflected by the fact that a decrease in AT-III levels to 40% predisposes to thrombotic disorders. The host has a another potent tool to inhibit coagulation factors Va and VIIIa: the protein C-protein S system (Figure 15.1) (Esmon 1987). Activation of the natural anticoagulant protein C is mediated by thrombin after its binding to endothelial cell thrombomodulin. Thrombomodulin serves as a receptor that binds thrombin, after which the latter loses its coagulative potential. The capacity of activated protein C to inhibit factors Va and VIIIa is markedly enhanced by its cofactor, protein S. Protein S circulates both in an active, free form (40%), and in an inactive form

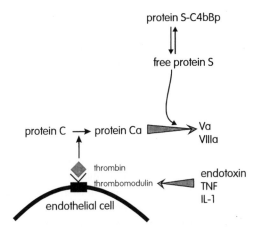

Figure 15.1 The Protein C-Protein S system and the effect of inflammatory mediators. Thrombin activates protein C after its binding to the endothelial cell receptor thrombomodulin. Endotoxin, TNF and IL-1 can impair protein C activation by downregulation of thrombomodulin (open arrow). Activated protein C (protein Ca) inactivates factors Va and VIIIa (open arrow), a process that is greatly enhanced by protein S. Protein S circulates in an active free form, and complexed with C4b binding protein (C4bBP).

(60%), complexed with complement factor 4b binding protein (C4bBP). The activity of the factor VIIa-tissue factor complex can be inhibited by TFPI, also called extrinsic pathway inhibitor or EPI, and lipoprotein-associated coagulation inhibitor or LACI. TFPI can bind factor Xa, and thereafter inhibit factor VIIa-tissue factor activity by forming a quaternary Xa-TFPI-VIIa complex, although recent investigations indicate that at high concentrations TFPI may also inhibit VIIa-tissue factor activity in the absence of factor Xa (Rappaport 1991).

Fibrinolysis regulates the degradation of fibrin. Plasmin is the key protease in this process, the generation and activity of which are tighly controlled by plasminogen activators, PAI-1 and α_2-antiplasmin.

2.3 Detection of Coagulation and Fibrinolysis *in Vivo*

Activation of coagulation and fibrinolysis *in vivo* can be monitored in several ways. The active proteases of both systems can not be detected in the circulation because of their extremely short half lifes. Zymogen proteins can be found in the circulation in high concentrations, and thus a decrease in zymogen levels is only expected to occur after massive conversion of zymogens to active proteases. Therefore, measurements of plasma zymogen concentrations is only useful in situations in which coagulation and fibrinolysis are strongly activated. More sensitive tools to detect coagulation and fibrinolytic activation include the measurement of protease-inhibitor complexes, and of so-called activation peptides of the coagulation system. Examples of the former are thrombin-AT-III (TAT) complexes and plasmin-α_2-antiplasmin (PAP) complexes, examples of the latter are factor IX peptide, factor X peptide, the prothrombin fragment F1+2 and fibrinopeptide A. Activation peptides are liberated from the inactive zymogen upon conversion to the active clotting factor, and therefore directly reflect activation of that particular zymogen. The development of immunoassays for these peptides has enabled the detection of coagulation activation *in vivo* at the picomolar level, and has greatly contributed to the current knowledge of physiological and pathophysiological regulation of the hemostatic mechanism.

3 CYTOKINES

3.1 General Properties

Cytokines are small proteins with molecular weights below 80 kDa that are produced and secreted by various cell types in response to various infectious and immunologic stimuli. Cytokines can exert a wide variety of biological effects at picomolar concentrations. Although frequently structurally unrelated, individual cytokines have multiple overlapping cell regulatory actions. They closely interact in a highly complex network, in which they influence each others production and action. Cytokines can induce other cytokines, can modulate the expression of specific cell surface receptors of other cytokines, and can synergistically, additively or antagonistically contribute to the actions of other cytokines. The complexicity of the cytokine network is further illustrated by the fact that the production of so-called proinflammatory cytokines, such as TNF and IL-1, is negatively controlled by so-called antiinflammatory cytokines, such as IL-4 and IL-10. Moreover, both types of cytokines can modulate the synthesis of naturally occurring inhibitors of proinflammatory cytokines, such as soluble TNF receptors and IL-1 receptor antagonist.

Cytokines are involved in immunity and inflammation, and are essential for the orchestration of the host response to local infection. During sepsis, however, the invasive generalized infection leads to excessive systemic production of cytokines, which results in tissue toxicity and injury. Indeed, ample evidence exists indicating that this "overproduction" of cytokines is the main event that initiates the sepsis cascade. Cytokines that have been implicated as possible mediators of the altered vascular hemostatic properties in infection and inflammation *in vivo* are TNF, IL-1, and IL-6.

We will first summarize studies that addressed the production of these cytokines in infection, and their putative roles in lethality associated with experimental infection.

3.2 Production of Cytokines in Infection

Both clinical and experimental studies have documented the enhanced production of TNF, IL-1, and IL-6 during systemic infection.

TNF was the first proinflammatory cytokine to be definitively detected in the circulation of patients with sepsis (Waage, Halstensen and Espevik 1987). In years thereafter, numerous studies confirmed the presence of TNF in patients with sepsis (Calandra *et al.*, 1990, Cannon *et al.*, 1990, Casey, Balk and Bone 1993, Girardin *et al.*, 1988, Munoz *et al.*, 1991, Wortel *et al.*, 1992). Notably, in most studies detection of TNF was largely confined to a subset of septic patients (16-100%) on admission to intensive care units. Several investigations comment upon a positive correlation between the serum concentration of TNF on admission and eventual mortality. Of the two forms of IL-1, IL-1α is rarely found in body fluids in soluble form. Indeed, investigators who have tried to measure IL-1α in patients with septic shock have been unsuccessful (Cannon *et al.*, 1990,

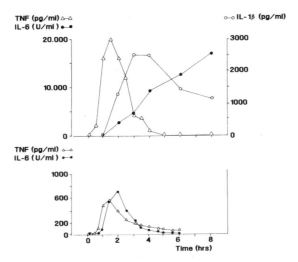

Figure 15.2 The appearance in the circulation of TNF, IL-6 and IL-1β after a lethal infusion of live *E. coli* in baboons (upper panel), and after an intravenous injection of a low dose of endotoxin into healthy humans (lower panel). In the latter experiment IL-1 can not be detected in serum.

Munoz *et al.,* 1991). IL-1β has been found more frequently in patients with sepsis, whereby the relationship of the detection of the cytokine with mortality was highly variable (Calandra *et al.,* 1990, Cannon *et al.,* 1990, Casey, Balk and Bone 1993, Girardin *et al.,* 1988, Munoz *et al.,* 1991). In comparison with other cytokines IL-6 has been detected most consistently in the circulation of septic patients (Calandra *et al.,* 1991, Casey, Balk and Bone 1993, Hack *et al.,* 1989, Waage *et al.,* 1989, Wortel *et al.,* 1992). In all studies published to date, the serum levels of IL-6 measured on admission showed a significant positive correlation with mortality.

Experimental investigations have provided insight into the kinetics of cytokine production during sepsis (Figure 15.2). In both lethal Escherichia coli sepsis in baboons, and after injection of a low dose of endotoxin (the toxic part of the outer membrane of gram-negative bacteria) into humans or chimpanzees, TNF is the first cytokine appearing in the circulation (Fong *et al.,* 1989, Hesse *et al.,* 1988, Levi *et al.,* 1994, Van der Poll *et al.,* 1994a, Van der Poll *et al.,* 1994b, Van Deventer *et al.,* 1990). In both sepsis models the release of TNF is transient, serum concentrations peaking after 90 minutes. The lethality of the baboon studies appears to be related to the magnitude of TNF secretion, which is much greater than in human and chimpanzee low grade endotoxemia. Shortly after the appearance of TNF, IL-6 can be detected in experimental sepsis and endotoxemia (Fong *et al.,* 1989, Levi *et al.,* 1994, Van der Poll *et al.,* 1994a, Van der Poll *et al.,* 1994b, Van Deventer *et al.,* 1990), while the detection of IL-1β, like IL-6 secreted shortly after TNF, is confined to lethal sepsis models (Fong *et al.,* 1989).

3.3 Role of Cytokines in Lethality of Sepsis

The mere detection of TNF, IL-1 and IL-6 in clinical and experimental sepsis does not prove their roles in the pathogenesis of the sepsis syndrome. This knowledge originates from investigations in septic animals treated with specific antibodies directed against TNF or IL-6, or with recombinant IL-1 receptor antagonist. A series of studies have shown that anti-TNF treatment, consisting either of purified antiserum or monoclonal antibodies, is highly protective against lethality when given before, simultaneously or very shortly (30 minutes) after intravenous infusion of a LD_{100} dose of endotoxin or live bacteria (Hinshaw *et al.*, 1990, Tracey *et al.*, 1987). Furthermore, passive immunization against TNF also strongly reduces the appearances of IL-1β and IL-6 in lethal bacteriaemia and sublethal endotoxemia in primates, indicating that TNF is an intermediate factor in the secretion of these other cytokines in sepsis (Fong *et al.*, 1989, Van der Poll *et al.*, 1994a).

The activity of IL-1 can be blocked by administration of the recombinant form of the naturally occurring inhibitor of IL-1, IL-1 receptor antagonist, which binds to both known IL-1 receptors without exerting any agonistic effect (Dinarello 1991). Recombinant IL-1 receptor antagonist strongly diminishes lethality in septic shock models in various species (Dinarello 1991, Fischer *et al.*, 1992, Ohlsson *et al.*, 1990). In baboons challenged with a lethal dose of live *E. coli* IL-1ra significantly attenuates hemodynamic collapse and improves survival (Fischer *et al.*, 1992). In addition, the IL-6 response is reduced by IL-1ra treatment, indicating that apart from TNF (see above), IL-1 also acts as an intermediate factor in the appearance of IL-6 in sepsis. IL-1ra does not affect TNF levels.

In contrast to the clear parts of TNF and IL-1 in the lethality of experimental sepsis, the role of IL-6 is less evident. One study has reported protection by an anti-IL-6 antibody against mortality after administration of a LD_{100} of endotoxin to mice; this protective effect disappeared after administration of endotoxin at doses slightly higher than the LD_{100} (Libert *et al.*, 1992). Other studies found no or only a marginal protection against endotoxin-induced death after passive immunization against IL-6 (Barton and Jackson 1993, Heremans *et al.*, 1992).

In accordance with the above cited studies in which neutralization of the activity of either TNF or IL-1 conferred significant protection in lethal sepsis, the administration of recombinant TNF or IL-1 induces a septic shock-like syndrome in animals (Okusawa *et al.*, 1988, Tracey *et al.*, 1986). Of interest, the simultaneous administration of TNF and IL-1 results in synergistic toxicity (Okusawa *et al.*, 1988). In contrast, infusion of high doses of IL-6 into animals is not associated with overt symptoms or hemodynamic changes (Preiser *et al.*, 1991).

4 ALTERED VASCULAR HEMOSTASIS PROPERTIES IN SYSTEMIC INFECTION

4.1 Hemostatic Changes in Clinical and Experimental Sepsis

Patients with septic shock almost always show evidence of activation of the coagulation system. Enhanced generation of thrombin is reflected by elevated plasma concentrations of F1+2 and TAT complexes, while in full-blown DIC the consumptive coagulopathy leads to decreased levels of clotting factors, AT-III and platelets. Concurrently, signs of activation of the contact system can be detected (i.e. low plasma levels of factor XII and prekallikrein)(Mason *et al.*, 1970, Nuijens *et al.*, 1988), as well as signs of activation of the extrinsic pathway (i.e. enhanced expression of tissue factor on circulating monocytes)(Osterud and Flaegstad 1983). The fibrinolytic system demonstrates evidence for

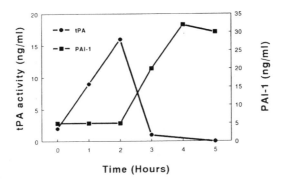

Figure 15.3 Activation (tissue type plasminogen activator activity) and subsequent inhibition (plasminogen activator inhibitor type 1) of fibrinolysis after a bolus intravenous injection of endotoxin into healthy humans. Adapted from Suffredini 1989 and Van Deventer 1990.

initial activation and subsequent inhibition, as reflected by elevated circulating antigenic levels of plasminogen activators, the absence of detectable systemic fibrinolytic activity, and increased plasma concentrations of PAI-1 (Brandtzaeg *et al.*, 1990, Voss *et al.*, 1990).

Investigations in healthy humans injected with a low dose of endotoxin have given insight into the kinetics by which activation of coagulation and fibrinolysis occur during a systemic inflammatory response (Suffredini, Harpel and Parillo 1989, Van Deventer *et al.*, 1990). Injection of endotoxin into humans results in a transient activation of the common pathway of the coagulation system, as reflected by rises in the plasma concentrations of the prothrombin fragment F1+2 and of TAT complexes, becoming evident from two hours postinjection (Van Deventer *et al.*, 1990). Interestingly, activation of coagulation is preceded by a rapid and transient activation of fibrinolysis. Endotoxin-induced fibrinolytic activation starts with the release of tPA into the circulation, which is followed in time by an abrupt rise in PAI-1 levels, indicating that the fibrinolytic response to endotoxin is highly regulated. The transient generation of active plasmin is confirmed by the detection of elevated plasma concentrations of PAP complexes (Suffredini, Harpel and Parillo 1989, Van Deventer *et al.*, 1990). Three hours after the administration of endotoxin fibrinolysis is completely offset, and coagulation activation is still proceeding (Figure 15.3). This hemostatic disbalance has also been observed in endotoxemic chimpanzees (Levi *et al.*, 1994, Van der Poll *et al.*, 1994a, Van der Poll *et al.*, 1994b). Thus, several hours after injection of endotoxin a net procoagulant state exists, a finding which may have relevance for the tendency towards microvascular thrombosis in sepsis. One study found no evidence of activation of the contact system after injection of endotoxin into humans at a dose of 2 ng/kg body weight, as indicated by unchanged levels of factor XIIa-C1-inhibitor and kallikrein-C1-inhibitor complexes (Van Deventer *et al.*, 1990). Another human study did find signs of contact system activation after administration of endotoxin at a dose 4 ng/kg body weight, demonstrating decreases in functional prekallikrein and factor XI, and an increase in kallikrein-α_2-macroglobulin complexes (DeLa Cadena *et al.*, 1993).

The kinetic pattern of early transient activation of fibrinolysis, and more sustained activation of coagulation also emerges from studies in baboons infused with a lethal dose of live *E. coli* (De Boer *et al.*, 1993a). In that model consumptive coagulopathy can be demonstrated by a profound decrease in plasma fibrinogen concentrations (Taylor 1994). In addition, in lethal *E. coli* sepsis in baboons both the extrinsic pathway of the coagulation system and the contact system become activated, as reflected by enhanced expression of tissue factor on circulating monocytes (Taylor 1994), and decreased HMWK levels and increased kallikrein-α_2-macroglobulin complexes (Pixley *et al.*, 1992, Pixley *et al.*, 1993) respectively.

4.2 Roles of the Extrinsic Pathway and the Contact System

There is now conclusive evidence that the activation of the coagulation system during sepsis is driven by the extrinsic tissue factor-mediated route. This evidence is derived from studies in primates in which antibodies directed against either tissue factor or factor VII/VIIa, or treatment with TFPI, prevent the activation of the common pathway of coagulation (Biemond *et al.*, 1995, Creasey *et al.*, 1993, Levi *et al.*, 1994, Taylor *et al.*, 1991b). Interestingly, blocking the tissue factor pathway in lethal *E. coli* sepsis in baboons not only prevents DIC, but also results in complete protection against lethality (Creasey *et al.*, 1993, Taylor *et al.*, 1991b). It is unlikely that anti-tissue factor or TFPI prevent death merely by an effect on the coagulation system, since more downstream intervention in the coagulation cascade, by administration of factor Xa blocked in its active center by Dansyl Glu Gly Arg chloromethyl ketone (DEGR-Xa), fails to block the lethal effects of *E. coli* in baboons, while completely inhibiting the development of DIC (Taylor *et al.*, 1991a). It is therefore likely that tissue factor and/or TFPI influence other inflammatory responses besides their effect on coagulation. In support of this hypothesis is the finding that treatment with TFPI reduces IL-6 levels in the circulation of septic baboons (Creasey *et al.*, 1993).

Activation of the contact system is now generally accepted not to contribute to the activation of the coagulation system during sepsis. Indeed, infusion of an antibody directed against factor XII does not prevent DIC in baboons with lethal *E. coli* sepsis, as manifested by unchanged decreases in the plasma concentrations of fibrinogen and factor V (Pixley *et al.*, 1993). Instead, anti-factor XII reversed the severe hypotension seen in untreated control animals, and extended survival time (Pixley *et al.*, 1993). This finding taken together with the positive correlation between contact system activation and hypotension in both clinical and experimental sepsis (Nuijens *et al.*, 1988, Pixley *et al.*, 1992), strongly argues for a role of contact system products (i.e. bradykinin) in the development of shock during generalized infection.

4.3 Role of the Protein C-Protein S System

Activation of protein C represents an important host defense mechanism against excessive fibrin formation. Infusion of activated protein C into septic baboons prevents hypercoagulability and death, while inhibition of activation of endogenous protein C by a monoclonal antibody exacerbates the response to a lethal *E. coli* infusion, and converts a sublethal model produced by a LD_{10} dose of *E. coli* into a severe shock response associated with DIC and death (Taylor *et al.*, 1987). Interference with the bioavailability of protein S, the cofactor for protein C, results in similar changes: administration of C4bBP, causing a decrease in free protein S levels, converts a non-lethal acute phase response to a sublethal dose of live *E. coli* into a lethal shock response with rapid consumption of fibrinogen, and systemic organ damage. Moreover, coinfusion of C4bBP results in detectable TNF in the circulation, not found in animals infused with a sublethal dose of *E. coli* only (Taylor *et al.,* 1991c). Hence, like the tissue factor mediated pathway, the protein C-protein S system may have other effects on host responses apart from its role in the coagulation system.

4.4 Activation of Fibrinolysis

As discussed above, in experimental endotoxemia in humans and chimpanzees activation of the fibrinolytic system preceeds that of the coagulation system (Levi *et al.,* 1993, Levi *et al.,* 1994, Van der Poll *et al.,* 1994a, Van der Poll *et al.,* 1994b, Van Deventer *et al.,* 1990). This led to the hypothesis that fibrinolytic activation is initiated independently from coagulation activation, and is not a mere reaction to the formation of fibrin. This hypothesis recently was confirmed in chimpanzees, in which blockade of coagulation activation by antibodies against either tissue factor or factor VII/VIIa did not influence the activation of the fibrinolytic system (Biemond *et al.,* 1995, Levi *et al.,* 1994). Present evidence indicates that TNF is an important mediator of the fibrinolytic response to infection (vide infra).

4.5 Role of Cytokines in Activation of Coagulation and Fibrinolysis

To date the involvement of TNF, IL-1 and IL-6 in the altered vascular hemostasis proper-ties in sepsis and endotoxemia has been investigated in *in vivo* studies. It should be noted, however, that it is highly likely that other members of the cytokine network also play a role in the activation of the hemostatic mechanism in systemic infection. Indeed, a number of cytokines have been demonstrated to affect tissue factor expression, as out-lined above considered to be a key event in the initiation of coagulation activation *in vivo*, on either endothelial cells or monocytes *in vitro* (table).

TNF is the cytokine most extensively investigated as a potential mediator of DIC. *In vitro* studies with cultured human umbilical vein endothelial cells have shown that TNF is able to directly influence coagulation and fibrinolysis. TNF stimulates the production and surface expression of tissue factor (Nawroth and Stern 1986, Scarpati and Sadler 1989, Van der Poll, Levi and Van Deventer 1991a). Apart from stimulating procoagulant properties of vascular endothelium, TNF inhibits its anticoagulant mechanisms, i.e. TNF directly reduces thrombomodulin activity on the surface of endothelial cells, primarily by decreasing thrombomodulin gene transcription (Lentz, Tsiang and Sadler 1991, Scarpati

Table 15.1 Cytokines influencing tissue factor expression *in vitro*

Cytokine	Endothelial cells	Monocytes
TNF	+	+
IL-1	+	+
IFN-γ	?	+
IL-4	–	–
IL-10	?	–
IL-13	–	–

+ = stimulation; – = inhibition of tissue factor expression induced by another stimulus (e.g. endotoxin)

and Sadler 1989), thereby impairing thrombin-mediated protein C activation (Figure 15.1). These procoagulant processes on endothelial cells may be potentiated by the effects of TNF on circulating monocytes, since this cytokine also stimulates mononuclear cell tissue factor activity (Conckling, Greenberg and Weinberg 1988). In addition, TNF affects the fibrinolytic properties of endothelial cells, the overall effect being an impairment of fibrinolysis, mainly by stimulation of the synthesis and release of PAI-1 (Scarpati and Sadler 1989, Van der Poll, Levi and Van Deventer 1991a).

Studies in human volunteers have confirmed that TNF potently influences coagulation and fibrinolysis. A single intravenous bolus injection of recombinant TNF induces an activation of the common pathway of the coagulation system (Van der Poll *et al.*, 1990). The formation of thrombin is sustained after TNF administration, as reflected by elevated plasma levels of the prothrombin fragment F1+2 for six to twelve hours after injection of TNF. The fibrinolytic response to intravenous TNF is characterized by a profound activation in the first hour postinjection, mediated by tPA, followed by a fast inhibition, mediated by PAI-1 (Van der Poll *et al.*, 1991b). Qualitatively similar hemostatic changes have been found in cancer patients infused with TNF for several to 24 hours (Bauer *et al.*, 1989, Logan *et al.*, 1992, Silverman *et al.*, 1990). A comparison of the kinetics of the procoagulant and fibrinolytic effects of endotoxin and TNF reveals the following important issues (Van der Poll *et al.*, 1991c) (Figure 15.4). First, TNF-induced changes in the coagulation

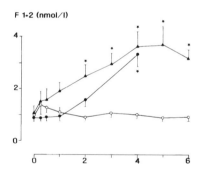

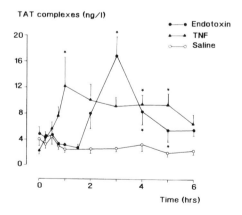

Figure 15.4 Comparison of the early kinetics of coagulation activation by intravenous administration of endotoxin or recombinant TNF in healthy humans. Adapted from Van der Poll 1990 and Van Deventer 1990.

and fibrinolytic systems completely resemble the changes provoked by endotoxin with the difference that the effects of TNF can be detected one to two hours earlier. Second, both endotoxin and TNF induce a net procoagulant state several hours after their administration, due to ongoing coagulation activation with concurrent inhibition of fibrinolysis.

Although these human data strongly suggest that TNF is crucial for activation of coagulation and fibrinolysis in endotoxemia, recent studies in chimpanzees have revealed that anti-TNF treatment does not affect endotoxin-induced coagulation activation, as reflected by unaltered rises in the plasma concentrations of both F1+2 and TAT complexes (Van der Poll *et al.*, 1994a) (Figure 15.5). Accordingly, in baboons infused with a lethal dose of *E. coli* treatment with an anti-TNF antibody has little or no effect on fibrinogen consumption, although it protects completely against lethality (Hinshaw *et al.*, 1990, Taylor 1994). Importantly, in the chimpanzee model of low grade endotoxemia anti-TNF does inhibit the activation of the fibrinolytic system, i.e. it virtually completely prevents the endotoxin-induced increase in PAP complexes (Van der Poll *et al.*, 1994a) (Figure 15.5). Thus, although TNF is capable of initiating a procoagulant response when administered to humans, endogenous TNF is not an essential factor in the activation of coagulation in sepsis and endotoxemia. Blockade of endogenous TNF in sepsis even may enhance the tendency to vascular thrombi depositions due to its specific inhibiting effect on fibrinolysis.

The role of IL-1 in the altered vascular hemostasis properties during sepsis is less clear. IL-1 affects vascular endothelium *in vitro* in a similar way as TNF (Van der Poll, Levi and Van Deventer 1991a). Preliminary results indicate that administration of recombinant IL-1 to cancer patients activates the common pathway of coagulation (C.E. Hack, personal communication), while treatment with IL-1ra transiently reduces coagulation activation in patients with sepsis (Boermeester *et al.*, 1995). Administration of IL-1α to

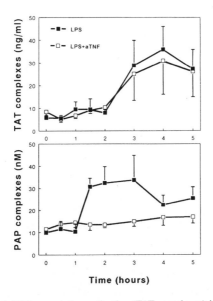

Figure 15.5 Anti-TNF fails to inhibit coagulation activation (TAT complexes) in low grade endotoxemia in chimpanzees, while it prevents endotoxin-induced fibrinolytic activation (PAP complexes). Adapted from Van der Poll 1994a.

baboons leads to activation of both the coagulation system and the fibrinolytic system (Jansen *et al.,* 1995).

Recent investigations point to a role for IL-6 in activation of the coagulation system *in vivo.* Infusion of recombinant IL-6 into patients with renal cell carcinoma is associated with rises in the plasma concentrations of F1+2 and TAT complexes, while fibrinolysis is not affected (Stouthard *et al.,* 1995). In accordance, treatment with an anti-IL-6 antibody prevents coagulation activation after administration of a low dose of endotoxin to chimpanzees, whereas it does not affect activation of the fibrinolytic system (Van der Poll *et al.,* 1994b). The potential role of IL-6 in coagulation activation is further supported by the finding that anti-IL-6 protects mice against the generalized Shwartzman reaction (Heremans *et al.,* 1992), a systemic inflammatory reaction characterized by thrombosis of renal glomeruli and other organs, and DIC (Edwards and Rickles 1992). IL-6 likely affects coagulation in an indirect way, since this cytokine has not been reported to influence the hemostatic properties of vascular endothelium or monocytes *in vitro.*

4.6 Other Possible Mediators of DIC

Several other mediators of inflammation can affect tissue factor expression *in vitro*; of these, complement products and C-reactive protein (CRP) may have relevance for induction of coagulation activation *in vivo.* Activation products of the complement system stimulate tissue factor expression by endothelial cells. It has been suggested that the initial activation of the coagulation system in septic baboons is at least in part mediated by induction of tissue factor by complement activation products, since both complement activation and coagulation activation can be detected before proinflammatory cytokines appear in the circulation in these animals, i.e. 30 minutes after starting the infusion of *E. coli* (De Boer *et al.,* 1993a, De Boer *et al.,* 1993b). Investigations examining the effect of specific inhibition of the complement system in sepsis are needed to confirm this hypothesis. Another factor that may contribute to ongoing coagulation activation during sepsis is the acute phase protein CRP. CRP is elevated in sepsis, and has been demonstrated to enhance tissue factor expression by monocytes (Cermak *et al.,* 1993). As IL-6 is the major cytokine regulating the classic acute phase protein response (Le and Vilcek 1989), it is conceivable that at least part of the effects of IL-6 on coagulation *in vivo* are mediated through CRP.

5 CONCLUSION

It is well established now that activation of coagulation in systemic infection proceeds through the extrinsic-tissue factor mediated pathway (Figure 15.6). This pathway is not only involved in coagulation activation, but likely has effects on other inflammatory systems yet to be defined. This hypothesis is based on the fact that inhibition of tissue factor function by either monoclonal antibodies or TFPI not only protects against DIC, but also against death in septic baboons, while the mere prevention of DIC by inhibition of factor Xa does not protect against lethality. Like the tissue factor pathway, the protein C-protein S system probably influences other inflammatory cascades besides its function as an important anticoagulant mechanism, since inhibition of normal protein C activation in sublethal sepsis with *E. coli* in baboons leads to fullblown DIC and death. In a recipro-

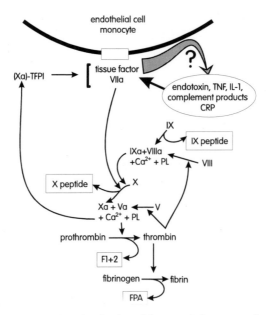

Figure 15.6 Diagrammatic presentation of activation of the coagulation system during sepsis. Enhanced expression of tissue factor at the surface of endothelial cells and monocytes plays a central role in coagulation activation during systemic infection. Tissue factor expression can be stimulated by mediators of other inflammatory systems (closed arrow), while the tissue factor-VIIa complex may exert a negative feedback effect on some of these (open arrow). The tissue factor-VIIa complex can be inhibited by tissue factor pathway inhibitor (TPHI) complexed with factor Xa. Tissue factor-VIIa can activate factor X directly, or indirectly via activation of factor IX. Both IXa and Xa act in catalytic complexes composed of calcium (Ca^{2+}) and phospholipids (PL), and either factor VIIIa (the IXa containing complex) or factor Va (the Xa containing complex). The classic common pathway starts with the conversion of X to Xa. The factor Xa-Va complex activates prothrombin to thrombin. Thrombin can activate fibrinogen, as well as factors V and VIII.

cal way, proinflammatory cytokines, complement factors and CRP may stimulate the activation of the tissue factor pathway, and TNF and IL-1 may inhibit activation of the protein C-protein S system by downregulation of thrombomodulin. Activation of the contact system does not contribute to DIC, but is involved in the development of hypotensive shock. Although TNF is a crucial factor in the lethality associated with infusion of live *E. coli* into baboons, it is not involved in DIC, neither does it mediate coagulation activation in low grade endotoxemia in chimpanzees. Thus, albeit TNF is able to initiate the coagulation cascade in humans, it is not a necessary component of coagulation activation or DIC in generalized infection. In contrast, neutralization of endogenous TNF in endotoxemia does completely prevent activation of the fibrinolytic system, indicating that coagulation and fibrinolysis are unlinked phenomena in endotoxemia, and that treatment with anti-TNF in sepsis may further shift the hemostatic balance towards a procoagulant state. IL-1 and IL-6 are possible cytokine mediators of initiation of coagulation activation *in vivo*, although their roles need to be explored further in models of DIC.

Current knowledge indicates that the coagulation cascade has close links with other mediator networks during an evolving systemic inflammatory response to a generalized infection. The coagulation system influences, as well as is influenced by, these other inflammatory mediator systems, such as the cytokine network and the complement system.

The unraveling of the interactions between coagulation and concurrently activated inflammatory systems in sepsis represents a major challenge for future investigations.

References

Barton, B.E. and Jackson, J.V. (1993). Protective role of interleukin 6 in the lipopolysaccharide-galactosamine septic shock model, *Infect. Immun.* **61**:1496–1499.

Bauer, K.A., Ten Cate, H., Barzegar, S., Spriggs, D.R., Sherman, M.L. and Rosenberg, R.D. (1989). Tumor necrosis factor infusions have a procoagulant effect on the hemostatic mechanism of humans, *Blood*, **74**:165–172.

Biemond, B., Ten Cate, H., Levi, M., Soule, H.R., Morris, L.D., Foster, D.L., Bogowitz, C.A., Van der Poll, T., Büller, H.R. and Ten Cate, J.W. (1995). Complete inhibition of endotoxin-induced coagulation activation in chimpanzees with a monoclonal Fab fragment against factor VII/VIIa. *Thromb. Haemostas.* **73**:223–230.

Boermeester, M.A., Van Leeuwen, P.A.M., Coyle, S.M., Houdijk, A.J.P., Eerenberg, A.M., Wolbink, G.J., Pribble, J.P., Stiles, D.M., Wesdorp, R.I.C., Hack, C.E., Lowry, S.F. (1995). Interleukin-1 receptor blockade in patients with sepsis syndrome: evidence that interleukin-1 contributes to the release of interleukin-6, elastase and phospholipase A_2 and to the activation of the complement, coagulation and fibrinolytic systems. *Arch. Surg.*, in press.

Brandtzaeg, P., Joo, G.B., Brusletto, B. and Kierulf, P. (1990). Plasminogen activator inhibitor 1 and 2 and α_2-antiplasmin and endotoxin levels in systemic meningococcal disease, *Thromb. Res.*, **57**:271–278.

Calandra, T., Baumgartner, J.D., Grau, G.E., Wu, M.M., Lambert, P.H., Schellekens, J., Verhoef, J., Glauser, M.P. and the Swiss-Dutch J5 Study Group (1990). Prognostic values of tumor necrosis factor/cachectin, interleukin-1, interferon-α and interferon-γ in the serum of patients with septic shock, *J. Infect. Dis.*, **161**:982–987.

Calandra, T., Gérain, J., Heumann, D., Baumgartner, J.D., Glauser, M.P. and the Swiss-Dutch J5 Immunoglobulin Study Group (1991). High circulating levels of interleukin-6 in patients with septic shock: evolution during sepsis, prognostic value and interplay with other cytokines, *Am. J. Med.*, **91**:23–29.

Cannon, J.G., Tompkins, R.G., Gelfand, J.A., Michie, H.R., tanford, G.G., Van der Meer, J.W.M., Endres, S., Lonnemann, G., Corsetti, J., Chernow, B., Wilmore, D.W., Wolff, S.M., Burke, J.F. and Dinarello, C.A. (1990). Circulating interleukin-1 and tumor necrosis factor in septic shock and experimental endotoxin fever, *J. Infect. Dis.*, **161**:79–84.

Casey, L.C., Balk, R.A. and Bone, R.C. (1993). Plasma cytokine and endotoxin levels correlate with survival in patients with the sepsis syndrome, *Ann. Intern. Med.*, **119**:771–778.

Cermak, J., Key, N.S., Bach, R.R., Balla, J., Jacob, H.S. and Vercelotti, G.M. (1993). C-reactive protein induces human peripheral blood monocytes to synthesize tissue factor, *Blood*, **82**:513–520.

Colman, R.W., Marder, V.J., Salzman, E.W. and Hirsh, J. (1987). Overview of hemostasis, In *Haemostasis and Thrombosis. Basic Principles and Clinical Practice*, 2nd edn, R.W. Colman, J. Hirsh, V.J. Marder, E.W. Salzman (ed.), pp. 3–17. Philadelphia: J.B. Lippincott.

Colman, R.W. (1989). The role of plasma proteases in septic shock, *N. Engl. J. Med.*, **320**:1207–1209.

Conckling, P.R., Greenberg, C.S. and Weinberg, J.B. (1988). Tumor necrosis factor induces tissue factor-like activity in human leukemia cell line U937 and peripheral blood monocytes, *Blood*, **72**:128–133.

Creasey, A.A., Chang, A.C.K., Feigen, L., Wün, T.C., Taylor Jr., F.B. and Hinshaw, L.B. (1993). Tissue factor pathway inhibitor reduces mortality from Escherichia coli septic shock, *J. Clin. Invest.*, **91**:2850–2860.

De Boer, J.P., Creasy, A.A., Chang, A., Roem, D., Brouwer, M.C., Eerenberg, A.J.M., Hack, C.E. and Taylor Jr., F.B. (1993a). Activation patterns of coagulation and fibrinolysis in baboons following infusion with lethal or sublethal dose of Escherichia coli, *Circ. Shock*, **39**:59–67.

De Boer, J.P., Creasey, .A., Chang, A., Roem, D., Eerenberg, A.J.M., Hack, C.E. and Taylor Jr., F.B. (1993b). Activation of the complement system in baboons challenged with live Escherichia coli: correlation with mortality and evidence for a biphasic pattern, Infect. *Immun.*, **61**:4293–4301.

DeLa Cadena, R.A., Suffredini, A.F., Page, J.D., Pixley, R.A., Kaufman, N., Parrillo, J.E. and Colman, R.W. (1993). Activation of the kallikrein-kinin system after endotoxin administration to normal human volunteers, *Blood*, **81**:3313–3317.

Dinarello, C.A. (1991). Interleukin-1 and interleukin-1 antagonism, *Blood*, **77**:1627–1652.

Edwards, R.L. and Rickles, F.R. (1992). The role of leukocytes in the activation of blood coagulation, Semin. *Haematol.*, **29**:202–212.

Esmon, C.T. (1987). The regulation of natural anticoagulant pathways, *Science*, **235**:1348–1352.

Fischer, E., Marano, M.A., Van Zee, K.J., Rock, C.S., Hawes, A.S., Thompson, W.A., DeForge, L., Kenney, J.S., Remick, D.G., Bloedow, D.C., Thompson, R.C., Lowry, S.F. and Moldawer, L.L. (1992). Interleukin-1 receptor blockade improves survival and hemodynamic performance in Escherichia coli septic shock, but fails to alter host responses to sublethal endotoxemia, *J. Clin. Invest.*, **89**:1551–1557.

Fong, Y., Tracey, K.J., Moldawer, L.L., Hesse, D.G., Manogue, K.R., Kenney, J.S., Lee, A.T., Kuo, G.C., Allison, A.C., Lowry, S.F. and Cerami, A. (1989). Antibodies to cachectin/tumor necrosis factor reduce interleukin 1β and interleukin 6 appearance during lethal bacteremia, *J. Exp. Med.*, **170**:1627–1633.

Gerlach, H., Esposito C. and Stern, D.M. (1990). Modulation of endothelial hemostatic properties: an active role in the host response, *Ann. Rev. Med.*, **41**:15–24.

Girardin, E., Grau, G.E., Dayer, J.M., Roux-Lombard, P., the J5 study group and Lambert, P.H. (1988). Tumor necrosis factor and interleukin 1 in the serum of children with severe infectious purpura, *N. Engl. J. Med.*, **319**:397–400.

Hack, C.E., De Groot, E.R., Felt-Bersma, R.J.F., Nuijens, J.H., Strack Van Schijndel, R.J.M., Eerenberg-Belmer, A.J.M., Thijs, L.G. and Aarden, L.A. (1989). Increased plasma levels of interleukin-6 in sepsis, *Blood*, **74**:1704–1710.

Heremans, H., Dillen, C., Put, W., Van Damme, J. and Billiau, A. (1992). Protective effect of anti-interleukin (IL)-6 antibody against endotoxin, associated with paradoxically increased IL-6 levels, *Eur. J. Immunol.*, **22**:2395–2401.

Hesse, D.G., Tracey, K.J., Fong, Y., Manogue, K.R., Palladino, M.A. Jr., Cerami, A., Shires, G.T. and Lowry, S.F. (1988). Cytokine appearance in human endotoxemia and primate bacteremia, *Surg. Gynecol. Obstet.*, **166**:147–153.

Hinshaw, L.B., Tekamp-Olson, P., Chang, A.C.K., Lee, P.A., Taylor, Jr. F.B., Murray, C.K., Peer, G.T., Emerson, Jr. T.E., Passey, B. and Kuo, G.C. (1990). Survival of primates in LD100 septic shock following therapy with antibody to tumor necrosis factor (TNF), *Circ. Shock*, **30**:279–292.

Jansen, P.M., Boermeester, M.A., Fischer, E., de Jong, I.W., Van der Poll, T., Moldawer, L.L., Hack, C.E., Lowry, S.F. (1995). Contribution of interleukin-1 to activation of coagulation and fibrinolysis, to neu-trophil degranulation and the release of sPLA₂ in sepsis. Studies in non-human primates following inter-leukin-1α administration and during lethal bacteremia. *Blood*, in press.

Le, J. and Vilcek, J. (1989). Interleukin 6: a multifunctional cytokine regulating immune reactions and the acute phase protein response, *Lab. Invest.*, **61**:588–602.

Lentz, S.R., Tsiang, M. and Sadler, J.E. (1991). Regulation of thrombomodulin by tumor necrosis factor-α: comparison of transcriptional and posttranscriptional mechanism. *Blood*, **77**:542–550.

Levi, M., Ten Cate, H., Van der Poll, T. and Van Deventer, S.J.H. (1993). Pathogenesis of disseminated intravas-cular coagulation in sepsis, *JAMA*, **270**:975–979.

Levi, M., Ten Cate, H., Bauer, K.A., Van der Poll, T., Edgington, T.S., Büller, H.R., Van Deventer, S.J.H., Hack, C.E., Ten Cate, J.W. and Rosenberg, R.D. (1994). Inhibition of endotoxin-induced activation of coagula-tion and fibrinolysis by pentoxifylline or by a monoclonal anti-tissue factor antibody in chimpanzees. *J. Clin. Invest.*, **93**:114–120.

Libert, C., Vink, A., Coulie, P., Brouckaert, P., Everaerdt, B., van Snick J. and Fiers, W. (1992). Limited involvement of interleukin-6 in the pathogenesis of lethal septic shock as revealed by the effect of mono-clonal antibodies against interleukin-6 or its receptor in various murine models, *Eur. J. Immunol.*, **22**:2625-2630.

Logan, T.F., Virji, M.A., Gooding, W.E., Bontempo, F.A., Ernstoff, M.S. and Kirkwood, J.M. (1992). Plasminogen activator and its inhibitor in cancer patients treated with tumor necrosis factor, *J. Natl. Cancer Instit.*, **84**:1802–1810.

Mason, J.W., Kleeberg, U., Dolan, P. and Colman, R.W. (1970). Plasma kallikrein and Hageman factor in gram-negative bacteremia, *Ann. Intern. Med.*, **73**:545–551.

Munoz, C., Misset, B., Fitting, C., Blériot, J.P., Carlet, J. and Cavaillon, J.M. (1991). Dissociation between plasma and monocyte-associated cytokines during sepsis. *Eur. J. Immunol.*, **21**:2177–2184.

Nawroth, P.P. and Stern, D.M. (1986). Modulation of endothelial cell hemostatic properties by tumor necrosis factor, *J. Exp. Med.*, **163**:740–745.

Nuijens, J.H., Huijbregts, C.C.M., Eerenberg-Belmer, A.J.M., Abbink, J.J., Strack Van Schijndel, R.J.M., Felt-Bersma, R.J.F., Thijs, L.G. and Hack, C.E. (1988). Quantification of plasma factor XIIa-C1-inhibitor complexes and kallikrein-C1-inhibitor complexes in sepsis, *Blood*, **72**:1841–1848.

Ohlsson, K., Björk, P., Bergenfeldt, M., Hageman, R. and Thompson, R.C. (1990). Interleukin 1 receptor antag-onist reduces mortality from endotoxin shock, *Nature*, **348**:550–552.

Okusawa, S., Gelfland, J.A., Ikejima, T., Connolly, R.J. and Dinarello, C.A. (1988). Interleukin 1 induces a shock-like state in rabbits. Synergism with tumor necrosis factor and the effect of cyclooxygenase inhibi-tion, *J. Clin. Invest.*, **81**:1162–1172.

Osterud, B. and Flaegstad, T. (1983). Increased tissue thromboplastin activity in monocytes of patients with meningococcal infections related to unfavourable prognosis, *Thromb. Haemostas.*, **49**:5–7.

Pixley, R.A., DeLa Cadena, R.A., Page, J.D., Kaufman, N., Wyshock, E.G., Colman, R.W., Chang, A. and Taylor Jr., F.B. (1992). Activation of the contact system in lethal hypotensive bacteremia in a baboon model, *Am. J. Pathol.*, **140**:897–906.

Pixley, R.A., De La Cadena, R., Page, J.D., Kaufman, N., Wyshock, E.G., Chang, A., Taylor Jr., F.B. and Colman, R.W. (1993). The contact system contributes to hypotension but not to disseminated intravascular coagulation in lethal bacteremia, *J. Clin. Invest.*, **91**:61–68.

Preiser, J.-C., Schmartz, D., Van der Linden, P., Content, J., Vanden Bussche, P., Buurman, W., Sebald, W., Dupont, E., Pinsky, M.R. and Vincent, J.L. (1991). Interleukin-6 administration has no acute hemodynamic or hematologic effect in the dog, *Cytokine*, **3**:1–6.

Rappaport, S.I. (1991). The extrinsic pathway inhibitor: a regulator of tissue factor-dependent blood coagulation, *Thromb. Haemostas.*, **66**:6–15.

Scarpati, E.M. and Sadler, J.E. (1989). Regulation of endothelial cell coagulant properties. Modulation of tissue factor, plasminogen activator inhibitors and thrombomodulin by phorbol 12-myristate 13-acetate and tumor necrosis factor. *J. Biol. Chem.*, **264**:20705–20713.

Silverman, P., Goldsmith, G.H., Spitzer, T.R. and Berger, N.A. (1990). Effect of tumor necrosis factor on the human fibrinolytic system, *J. Clin. Oncol.*, **8**:468–475.

Stouthard J.M.L., Levi M., Hack C.E., Veenhof C.H.N., Romijn J.A., Sauerwein H.P. and van der Poll T. (1995). Interleukin-6 stimulates coagulation, not fibrinolysis, in humans. In: J.M.L. *Stouthard, Biological and Clinical Effects of Interleukin-6*, Academic Thesis, University of Amsterdam, pp. 101–112.

Suffredini, A.F., Harpel, P.C. and Parrillo, J.E. (1989). Promotion and subsequent inhibition of plasminogen activation after administration of intravenous endotoxin to normal subjects, *N. Engl. J. Med.*, **320**: 1165–1172.

Taylor Jr., F.B., Chang, A., Esmon, T., D'Angelo, A., Vigano-D'Angelo, S. and Blick, K.E. (1987). Protein C prevents the coagulopathic and lethal effects of Escherichia coli infusion in the baboon, *J. Clin. Invest.*, **79**:918–925.

Taylor Jr., F.B., Chang A.C.K., Peer, G.T., Mather, T., Blick, K., Catlett, R., Lockhart, M.S. and Esmon, C.T. (1991a). DEGR-factor Xa blocks disseminated intravascular coagulation initiated by Escherichia coli without preventing shock or organ damage, *Blood*, **78**:364–368.

Taylor Jr., F.B., Chang, A., Ruf, W., Morrissey, J.H., Hinshaw, L., Catlett, R., Blick, K., Edgington, T.S. (1991b). Lethal E. coli septic shock is prevented by blocking tissue factor with monoclonal antibody, *Circ. Shock*, **33**:127–134.

Taylor Jr., F.B., Chang, A., Ferrell, G., Mather, T., Blick, K. and Esmon, C.T. (1991c). C4b-binding protein exacerbates the host response to Escherichia coli, *Blood*, **78**:357–363.

Taylor Jr., F.B. (1994). Studies on the inflammatory-coagulant axis in the baboon response to E. coli: regulatory roles of proteins C, S, C4bBP and of inhibitors of tissue factor, *Prog. Clin. Biol. Res.*, **388**:175–194.

Ten Cate, H., Brandjes, D.P.M., Wolters, H.J. and Van Deventer, S.J.H. (1993). Disseminated intravascular coagulation: pathophysiology, diagnosis and treatment, *New Horizons*, **1**:312–323.

Tracey, K.J., Beutler, B., Lowry, S.F., Merryweather, J., Wolpe, S., Milsark, I.W., Harir, R.J., Fahey III, T.J., Zentella, A., Albert, J.D., Shires, G.T. and Cerami, A. (1986). Shock and tissue injury induced by recombinant human cachectin, *Science*, **234**:470–474.

Tracey, K.J., Fong, Y., Hesse, D.G., Manogue, K.R., Lee, A.T., Kuo, G.C., Lowry, S.F. and Cerami, A. (1987). Anti-cachectin/TNF monoclonal antibodies prevent septic shock during lethal bacteraemia. *Nature*, **330**:662–664.

Van der Poll, T., Büller, H.R., Ten Cate, H., Wortel, C.H., Bauer, K.A., Van Deventer, S.J.H., Hack, C.E., Sauerwein, H.P., Rosenberg, R.D. and Ten Cate, J.W. (1990). Activation of coagulation after administration of tumor necrosis factor to normal subjects. *N. Engl. J. Med.*, **322**:1622–1627.

Van der Poll, T., Levi, M. and Van Deventer, S.J.H. (1991a). Tumor necrosis factor and the disbalance between coagulant and anticoagulant mechanisms in septicemia, In *Update in Intensive Care and Emergency Medicine*, Volume 14, J.L. Vincent (red), pp 269–273, Springer Verlag.

Van der Poll, T., Levi, M., Büller, H.R., Van Deventer, S.J.H., De Boer, J.P., Hack, C.E. and Ten Cate, J.W. (1991b). Fibrinolytic response to tumor necrosis factor in healthy subjects, *J. Exp. Med.*, **174**: 729–732.

Van der Poll, T., Van Deventer, S.J.H., Büller, H.R., Sturk, A. and Ten Cate, J.W. (1991c). Comparison of the early dynamics of coagulation activation after injection of endotoxin and tumor necrosis factor in healthy humans. *Prog. Clin. Biol. Res.*, **367**:55–60.

Van der Poll, T., Levi, M., Van Deventer, S.J.H., Ten Cate, H., Haagmans, B.L., Biemond, B.J., Büller, H.R., Hack, C.E. and Ten Cate, J.W. (1994a). Differential effects of anti-tumor necrosis factor monoclonal antibodies on systemic inflammatory responses in experimental endotoxemia in chimpanzees, *Blood*, **83**:446–451.

Van der Poll, T., Levi, M., Hack, C.E., Ten Cate, H., Van Deventer, S.J.H., Eerenberg, A.J.M., De Groot, E.R., Jansen, J., Gallati, H., Büller, H.R., Ten Cate, J.W. and Aarden, L.A. (1994b). Elimination of interleukin 6 attenuates coagulation activation in experimental endotoxemia in chimpanzees. *J. Exp. Med.*, **179**:1253–1259.

Van Deventer, S.J.H., Büller, H.R., Ten Cate, J.W., Aarden, L.A., Hack, C.E. and Sturk, A. (1990). Experimental endotoxemia in humans: analysis of cytokine release and coagulation, fibrinolytic and complement pathways. *Blood*, **76**:2520–2526.

Voss, R., Matthias, F.R., Borkowski, G. and Reitz, D. (1990). Activation and inhibition of fibrinolysis in septic patients in an internal intensive care unit, *B. J. Haematol.*, **75**:99–105.

Waage, A., Halstensen, A. and Espevik, T. (1987). Association between tumour necrosis factor in serum and fatal outcome in patients with meningococcal disease, *Lancet*, **I**:355–357.

Waage, A., Brandtzaeg, P., Halstensen, A., Kierulf, P. and Espevik, T. (1989). The complex pattern of cytokines in serum from patients with meningococcal septic shock, *J. Exp. Med.*, **169**:333–338.

Wakefield, T.W., Wrobleski, S.K., Sarpa, M.S., Taylor Jr., F.B., Esmon, C.T. and Greenfield, L.J., Deep venous thrombosis in the baboon generated through protein C inhibition, *J. Vasc. Surg.*, **14**:588–598.

Wortel, C.H., von der Möhlen M.A.M., Van Deventer, S.J.H., Sprung, C.L., Jastremski, M., Lubbers, M.J., Smith, C.R., Allen, I.E. and Ten Cate, J.W. (1992). Effectiveness of a human monoclonal anti-endotoxin antibody (HA-1A) in gram-negative sepsis: relation to endotoxin and cytokine levels. *J. Infect. Dis.*, **166**:1367–1374.

16 Viral Induction of Endothelial Cell Procoagulant Activity

Andrew C. Nicholson and David P. Hajjar

Departments of Pathology and Biochemistry, Cornell University Medical College,
1300 York Ave., New York, NY 10021. USA.

Hemostasis requires a balance between procoagulant activity, anticoagulant activity, fibrin assembly, and fibrinolysis. The vascular endothelium normally provides a thromboresistant surface. Perturbation of the endothelium by injury or activation in response to inflammatory mediators can shift this balance to one which promotes the assembly of the prothrombinase complex, thrombin generation and coagulation. *In vitro* experiments have shown that viral infection of vascular endothelial cells can inhibit anticoagulant function, induce the expression of receptors for coagulation proteins and thus, alter the balance of procoagulant and anticoagulant activity. In this review, we highlight data demonstrating that viral infection can directly (or indirectly via immune mechanisms) injure and activate the endothelium. In response, the endothelium can express receptors for coagulation proteins and inflammatory cells. We further speculate on how viral infection of the vascular endothelium and vessel wall may impact on the initiation and progression of atherosclerosis and summarize data implicating viral infection in this process.

KEYWORDS: atherosclerosis/coagulation/herpesviruses/adhesion receptors/platelet/thrombosis

INTRODUCTION

The normal vascular endothelium, by virtue of its location at the interface between the blood and vessel wall, plays a critical role in the regulation of coagulation and fibrinolysis. It forms a physical barrier between Factor VII in the plasma and tissue factor in the vessel. It separates platelets from underlying collagen preventing activation and aggregation. In addition to these passive functions, the endothelium actively inhibits clotting by producing prostacyclin (PGI2) (Pomerantz and Hajjar, 1992) and nitric oxide (NO) (Ignarro, 1989), potent inhibitors of platelet aggregation, cell-surface heparan sulfate proteoglycan which localizes and increases the activity of antithrombin III (ATIII), and thrombomodulin and protein S, important regulators of protein C, a protease that inactivates factors Va and VIIIa (Esmon, 1994). The endothelium also contributes to fibrinolysis by producing tissue plasminogen activator (tPA), urokinase plasminogen activator (uPA) and plasminogen activator inhibitor, regulators of plasminogen and subsequently the formation of plasmin (Tanaka and Sueishi, 1994).

When the vascular endothelium is injured or activated, it undergoes a phenotypic modulation resulting in the loss of anti-coagulant properties and the acquisition of procoagulant properties. Endothelial cell injury is a common feature of viral infection, and can alter hemostasis in two ways: directly, by altering endothelial cell function, and indirectly, via activation of immune and inflammatory pathways (Cosgriff, 1989). In this article, we review and interpret data which shows that herpesvirus infection can shift endothelial cell properties from an anti-thrombotic to a pro-thrombotic state. We highlight data from our laboratory and others demonstrating that herpesviral infection of endothelial cells *in vitro* can inhibit anti-coagulant functions and induce a pro-coagulant phenotype. The potential role of herpesviral infection as it relates to both thrombosis and atherosclerosis will be explored.

DO VIRUSES INFECT THE VASCULAR ENDOTHELIUM?

Viral infection can alter hemostatic balance resulting in either hemorrhage or coagulation. Thrombocytopenia is an occasional symptom of common viral infections, and is most likely immune mediated (Kelton and Neame, 1987). Severe hemorrhage is a hallmark of the hemorrhagic fever viruses. These viruses cause hemorrhage by multiple mechanisms including thrombocytopenia, platelet dysfunction, hepatic insult and reduction in the levels of coagulation factors, and direct and indirect endothelial cell damage (Cosgriff, 1989). Endothelial cell infection may represent a common pathway by which viruses alter hemostasis. Many human viruses have been shown to infect human endothelial cells *in vitro*. These include herpes simplex virus type 1 (HSV-1), adenovirus type 7, measles virus, parainfluenza type 3, mumps virus, poliovirus type 1, echovirus type 9, cytomegalovirus (CMV) Coxsackievirus B3, and Dengue and Junin viruses (Friedman *et al.*, 1981; Friedman *et al.*, 1986; Friedman, 1989). The *in vivo* consequences of endothelial cell infection by most of these viruses is undetermined. This review will document the *in vitro* and *in vivo* consequences of herpesvirus infection of vascular endothelium.

Three members of the herpesvirus family, herpes simplex virus type 1 (HSV-1), herpes simplex virus type 2 (HSV-2) and cytomegalovirus (CMV) have been shown to infect vascular endothelial cells. Herpesvirus infections are ubiquitous in the general population. By ten years of age, more than 50% of children demonstrate antibodies to herpes simplex virus type 1 (HSV-1) (Nachmias and Josey, 1978). The estimated incidence of HSV-2 in the United States is approximately 16% (Johnson *et al.*, 1986). CMV is an opportunistic pathogen causing disease in immunocompromised hosts. A majority of the population has been infected with CMV, but infection is usually asymtomatic in immunocompetent hosts. Herpesviral particles, viral inclusions or viral nucleic acids have been detected within endothelial cells or within vascular smooth muscle cells of the vascular wall. Herpesvirus nucleic acid sequences have been shown by *in situ* hybridization studies to be present in atherosclerotic plaques (Benditt *et al.*, 1983). Herpes simplex virus has been observed by electron microscopy in the aorta and coronary arteries of atherosclerotic patients (Gyorkey *et al.*, 1984; Yamashiroya *et al.*, 1988). CMV infection of endothelial cells was demonstrated by immunohistochemical methods in vessels of multiple tissues (Myerson *et al.*, 1984). CMV antigen (Melnick *et al.*, 1983) and CMV nucleic acid (Hendrix *et al.*, 1990; Hendrix *et al.*, 1989; Petrie *et al.*, 1987) have been detected in the carotid artery wall from humans undergoing bypass surgery in both atherosclerotic and non-atherosclerotic tissue.

VIRAL ACTIVATION OF THROMBOTIC PROCESSES

Herpesviral infection alters the normal thromboresistant surface formed by intact vascular endothelial cell surface by three mechanisms:

(1) inhibition of anti-coagulant/anti-thrombotic properties,
(2) induction of pro-coagulant/prothrombotic properties, and
(3) indirectly, by increasing binding sites for inflammatory cells which can further shift the endothelial surface from thromboresistance by secreting pro-thrombotic cytokines.

Although most experimental evidence demonstrating these effects are derived from *in vitro* studies using endothelial cells in monolayer culture, there is histologic evidence supportive of these phenomena *in vivo*. For example, HSV-1 can induce mucosal lesions which are often accompanied by a local vasculitis with fibrin deposition (McSorley *et al.*, 1974). Disseminated intravascular coagulation (DIC) is seen in fatal systemic neonatal HSV infections (Phinney *et al.*, 1982). DIC is thought to result, in part, from direct damage to the vessel wall, and exposure of sub-endothelial collagen (Phinney *et al.*, 1982).

One mechanism by which herpesvirus induce a prothrombotic endothelium is by inhibiting normal anti-coagulant and anti-thrombotic properties. Endothelial cells normally synthesize and express heparan sulfate proteoglycan (HSPG) on their surface. HSPG is a critical element for recruiting and binding antithrombin III, which is responsible for the inactivation of several coagulation proteases (thrombin and activated factors IX, X, XI, and XII). HSV infection of the endothelium markedly reduces HSPG synthesis and surface expression by endothelial cells (Kaner *et al.*, 1990). The expression of thrombomodulin on the endothelial surface is also reduced as a result of HSV-1 and HSV-2 infection (Key *et al.*, 1990). Loss of thrombomodulin is concomitant with a reduction in thrombin-dependent protein C activation. Inhibition of the protein C/protein S/thrombomodulin pathway is, therefore, another mechanism which could lead to thrombin generation by reducing the ability of protein C to inactivate factors Va and XIIIa.

In addition to inhibiting anti-coagulant mechanisms, herpesviruses can induce pro-coagulant/prothrombotic properties of the endothelium. Visser and his colleagues have demonstrated altered membrane topography on HSV-infected endothelial cells, i.e., is they have shown that the outer leaflet membrane conformation may be abnormal in HSV-infected endothelium (Visser *et al.*, 1988). They hypothesized that viral-induced changes in endothelial cell phospholipid may alter the efficiency of assembly of the prothrombinase complex. To test this hypothesis, they assessed the ability of HSV infected endothelium to support prothrombinase complex assembly using purified prothrombin and Factors Va and Xa and demonstrated enhanced (2–3 fold) thrombin generation. They further demonstrated enhanced thrombin-induced platelet accumulation on HSV infected endothelium. Thrombin-induced PGI_2 production by the infected endothelium was reduced by a factor of 20 (Visser *et al.*, 1988). Since thrombin-induced PGI$_2$ synthesis and release is thought to be a mechanism by which the endothelial cell may diminish thrombin-induced platelet adherence and aggregation, this may further compound platelet adhesion to the HSV-infected endothelium. HSV can also induce the transient expression of tissue factor on the endothelial cell surface. Tissue factor is not normally expressed by endothelial cells but can be induced by endotoxin or cytokines (Bevilacqua *et al.*, 1985; Adams *et al.*, 1993). Tissue factor expression in response to HSV was dependent on the magnitude of infection and increased linearly with increasing multiplicity of infection (MOI). Maximal expression (3–4 fold greater than mock-infected cells) was seen at 4 hr., but expression returned to baseline by 20 hr. (Key *et al.*, 1990). Tissue factor mRNA is also transiently induced (Key *et al.*, 1993). Tissue factor expression did not require replicative infection of HSV-1 since replication defective virus could also produce tissue factor procoagulant activity (Key *et al.*, 1993). In addition, CMV also has the capacity to induce procoagulant activity on human endothelial cells as measured by a reduction in clotting time (van Dam-Mieras *et al.*, 1992), suggesting a facilitated formation of the prothrombinase complex.

Our laboratory has extended these finding and has shown HSV infection of endothelial cells induces von Willebrand factor (vWF) secretion and that vWF mediates platelet adhesion to virally infected endothelial cells (Etingin *et al.*, 1993). Other types of endothelial cell injury, Rickettsial infection (Sporn *et al.*, 1991) and endotoxin (Schorer *et al.*, 1987) also cause vWF release. We hypothesize that thrombin is generated following assembly of the prothrombinase complex on the virally infected endothelium and subsequently mobilizes von Willebrand factor from the Weibel-Palade body to the endothelial cell surface where it acts as a platelet receptor. In contrast, CMV infection causes the disappearance of vWF from endothelial cells (Bruggeman *et al.*, 1988).

Our laboratory has demonstrated that specific virally encoded glycoproteins expressed on the surface of the HSV infected endothelium bind and promote activation of Factor X thereby contributing to thrombin generation (Etingin *et al.*, 1990). We found that HSV infection of endothelial cells promoted enhanced monocyte adhesion (Etingin *et al.*, 1990) and that this enhanced adhesion was dependent on EC surface expression of HSV glycoprotein C (gC) (Figure 16.1). Adhesion was blocked by monoclonal antibodies to gC but not by antibodies to glycoprotein D (gD) or glycoprotein E (gE) (Etingin *et al.*, 1990). Adhesion was dependent on local generation of thrombin and was blocked by treating endothelial cells with specific thrombin inhibitors or by growing cells in pro-thrombin-depleted serum. To support the hypothesis that gC was indeed involved in monocyte adhesion and could potentially be involved in thrombin activation, we used murine L cells which were stably transfected with the gene for herpesvirus gC (Etingin *et al.*, 1990). We found that Factor X bound to the transfected L cells but not to nontransfected cells (Etingin *et al.*, 1990). Furthermore, crosslinking and immunoprecipitation studies demonstrated that Factor X and gC formed a complex on the cell surface. In order to identify a site in Factor X which bound to gC we utilized a group of partially overlapping peptides representative of different regions of the Factor X molecule (Altieri *et al.*, 1991). Three synthetic Factor X peptides provided by Drs. Dario Altieri and Thomas Edgington of the Scripps Research Institute blocked Factor X mediated procoagulant activity and suppressed monocyte adhesion to HSV-infected endothelium. The three blocking peptides are in the catalytic domain of Factor X (Altieri *et al.*, 1991). In

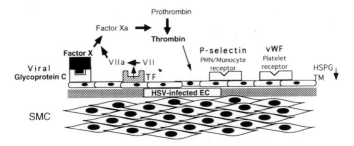

Figure 16.1 HSV induction of endothelial procoagulant activity. This model illustrates mechanisms by which herpes simplex virus (HSV) infection of the vascular endothelium can shift the hemostatic balance from an antithrombotic to a prothrombotic state. HSV infection induces the synthesis and expression of viral glycoprotein (C). This glycoprotein can serve as an Fc and C3b receptor and, in addition, a binding site for Factor X. Increased binding of Factor X and its subsequent conversion to the active form, Factor Xa, can lead to the conversion of prothrombin to thrombin. HSV can also increase surface expression of tissue factor and facilitate activation of the extrinsic pathway of the coagulation cascade. Thrombin can induce surface expression of P-selectin, a monocyte and neutrophil (PMN) receptor, and von Willebrand Factor (vWF), which acts as a platelet receptor. The binding of inflammatory cells and platelets and the release of cytokines and inflammatory mediators can further amplify this cascade. HSV can also reduce surface expression of heparan sulfate proteoglycan (HSPG) and thrombomodulin (TM) which, in turn, can lead to reduced antithrombin III (ATIII) binding and thrombin-dependent protein C activation, and inhibit normal anticoagulant surface properties.

summary, our data suggest that interaction of Factor X with gC on the surface of HSV infected cells leads to formation of Factor Xa, activation of thrombin, and enhanced binding of monocytes.

The third mechanism by which herpesvirus infection could contribute to a pro-thrombotic endothelium involves an increase in the number of binding sites for inflammatory cells. Adhesion of inflammatory cells (neutrophils and monocyte/macrophages) and the release of inflammatory cytokines could shift the endothelial surface balance further from thromboresistance to a more pro-thrombotic state. HSV infection of the endothelium induces the expression of two important neo-antigens on the endothelial surface, HSV gE and HSV gC. These virally encoded glycoproteins function as Fc and complement (C3b) receptors respectively (Cines *et al.*, 1982). The presence of these receptors suggested that the HSV-infected endothelium could bind Fc and C3b bearing granulocytes. In fact, granulocyte adherence was increased by about 2-fold to HSV infected endothelial cells (Macgregor *et al.*, 1980; Zajac *et al.*, 1988). This increased adherence did not require antibody or complement as increased adherence could be demonstrated when the granulocytes were suspended in serum-free media (Macgregor *et al.*, 1980). However, addition of IgG containing anti-HSV antibody further increased granulocyte adherence (Visser *et al.*, 1989). This data suggests that Fc or C3b receptors may act as granulocyte receptors on the HSV-infected endothelium but also suggest that receptors other than Fc or C3b (i.e. adhesion molecules) are acting as granulocyte receptors (Visser *et al.*, 1989).

Enhanced attachment of granulocytes to the virally-infected endothelium was associated with increased granulocyte-mediated lysis of HSV-infected endothelial cells (Visser *et al.*, 1989). CMV infection of endothelial cells also increases the adherence of granulocytes (Span *et al.*, 1989b). In fact, adherence was greater to the CMV infected endothelium (500% of control adherence) than had been reported for HSV infection (200% of control adherence). Tunicamycin, an agent that prevents glycosylation, abolished the effect of CMV infection on the increase of PMN adherence, suggesting that glycoproteins play a role in adhesion of granulocytes to the CMV-infected endothelium (Span *et al.*, 1989b). The increased binding of granulocytes could not be induced by supernatants from the CMV infected cells suggesting that adherence is a "cell-bound phenomena and is not induced by an adherence-stimulation factor"(Span *et al.*, 1989b). This is in contrast to the increased binding of monocytes to the HSV-1 infected endothelium which can be stimulated by a factor secreted into the medium (Span *et al.*, 1989a). This data is consistent with our model in which we propose that the enhanced generation and release of thrombin in response to HSV-1 infection of the endothelium subsequently results in expression of receptors for inflammatory cells (Figure 16.1).

Endothelial cells express several leukocyte receptors on their surface including E-selectin (ELAM-1) , ICAM-1, VCAM-1, and P-selectin (GMP140, PADGEM, CD62), in response to cytokines, phorbol ester or exposure to other agonists (McEver, 1991). E-selectin , ICAM-1, and VCAM-1 expression is induced in response to cytokines (TNF and IL-1) in a process requiring protein synthesis. P-selectin is a cytoplasmic protein found on the membrane of Weibel-Palade bodies of resting endothelial cells (Hattori *et al.*, 1989). After stimulation by thrombin, histamine or complement proteins, the Weibel-Palade body is rapidly translocated, and its membrane becomes incorporated into the plasma membrane of the cell resulting in surface expression (Hattori *et al.*, 1989). This translocation from a preformed intracellular compartment to the cell surface does not require *de novo* protein synthesis (Hattori *et al.*, 1989). Our recent data support the model that herpes infection induces endothelial cell surface expression of P-selectin and increased monocyte adhesion (Etingin *et al.*, 1990) (Figure 16.1). We propose the following mechanism. HSV gC acts as a binding site for Factor X. Concomitant generation of tissue factor converts bound Factor X to Factor Xa in an active prothrombinase complex leading to generation of thrombin. Thrombin then can act in an autocrine manner to induce expression of a leukocyte receptor, P-selectin (Etingin *et al.*, 1991). This concept is supported by data demonstrating that increased binding of monocytes to the HSV-1 infected endothelium can be stimulated by a factor secreted into the medium (Span *et al.*, 1989a). Our data indicate that monocyte adhesion induced by herpes infection is blocked by anti P-selectin but not by anti- ELAM or antibodies to other adhesive leukocyte integrins (LFA-1, MAC-1 and P150, 95) (Etingin *et al.*, 1991). This suggests that P-selectin is a major receptor for monocytes on the herpes infected endothelium (Etingin *et al.*, 1991). The adhesion of inflammatory cells to the HSV-infected endothelium can further amplify the prothrombotic phenotype of the endothelium. Release of cytokines such as IL-1 and TNF from adherent and activated inflammatory cells can induce tissue factor expression by endothelial cells (Schorer *et al.*, 1986; Bevilacqua *et al.*, 1985).

POTENTIAL LINKS BETWEEN HERPESVIRUSES, THROMBOSIS, AND ATHEROSCLEROSIS

We and others have suggested that viruses may have an etiologic role in the pathogenesis of atherosclerosis. As outlined above, herpesviral particles, viral inclusions, or viral nucleic acids have been detected within endothelial cells or within vascular smooth muscle cells of the vascular wall (Gyorkey *et al.*, 1984; Benditt *et al.*, 1983; Yamashiroya *et al.,* 1988; Myerson *et al.,* 1984; Hendrix *et al.,* 1990; Hendrix *et al.,* 1989; Petrie *et al.,* 1987). Chickens infected with Marek's disease herpesvirus develop accelerated atherosclerosis in the presence of a normo-cholesterolemic diet (Fabricant *et al.,* 1978; Minick *et al.,* 1978), and this atherosclerosis is associated with altered aortic cholesterol metabolism (Hajjar *et al.,* 1986; Hajjar *et al.,* 1985; Hajjar, 1986; Hajjar *et al.,* 1989) and decreased vascular cell prostacyclin production (Hajjar, 1986).

Several mechanisms are proposed by which herpesviruses could be involved in the initiation or progression of atherosclerosis (Hajjar, 1991; Benditt *et al.,* 1983). Primary viral infection or reactivation of latent infection could damage endothelial cells or induce expression of receptors for platelets, neutrophils or monocyte/macrophages as described above. This could lead to deposition of fibrin or release of growth factors or inflammatory cytokines from platelets, activated endothelial cells or inflammatory cells. Atherosclerosis has been compared to a chronic inflammatory process (Munro and Cotran, 1988). Inflammatory cytokines and growth factors are thought to participate in recruitment of macrophages, foam cell development, and smooth muscle cell proliferation, the hallmark lesions of atherosclerosis. The relationship between thrombosis and atherosclerosis is reviewed elsewhere (Loscalzo, 1992; Tanaka and Sueishi, 1994).

A potential link between CMV and p53 inactivation in coronary restenosis was recently proposed by Steven Epstein and colleagues at the NIH (Speir *et al.,* 1994) They demonstrated that IE84, a CMV protein, binds to and inhibits p53 function. Mutations in p53 which lead to loss of function are often accompanied by enhanced stability which allows the protein to be detectable by immunostaining. They demonstrated that there was a significant concordance between p53 immunoreactivity in human restenotic lesions and the presence CMV DNA; viral DNA was detected in 11 of 13 (85%) of the p53 immunopositive lesions but only 3 of 11 (27%) of the p53 immunonegative lesions. Conversely, almost 80 % of the CMV-positive lesions (11 of 14) were p53-immunopositive. They speculated that latent CMV could be reactivated following a procedure such as balloon angioplasty, IE84 could inhibit the function of p53, and the inhibition of p53 could contribute to smooth muscle cell proliferation seen in some post-angioplasty patients (Speir *et al.,* 1994). The potential relationship of CMV infection in the post-angioplasty setting and thrombosis has yet to be explored.

Epidemiological studies suggest a correlation between herpesvirus infection and atherosclerosis. Patients who underwent cardiovascular surgery were compared with a control group of subjects with similar cholesterol levels and epidemiological factors but who were not undergoing surgery (Adam *et al.,* 1987). In 160 pairs of patients, the prevalence of CMV antibodies was higher in the surgical group than the control group (Adam *et al.,* 1987). An association between asymptomatic carotid wall thickening consistent with early atherosclerosis and antibodies to CMV was reported (Sorlie *et al.,* 1994). Another study failed to demonstrate an overall association between having a history of fever blisters or cold sores and the incidence of coronary heart disease (Havlik *et al.,* 1989). However, a subgroup of women with recurrent cold sores had a 1.5-fold relative risk of developing coronary heart disease (Havlik *et al.,* 1989).

The strongest epidemiological link between infection with DNA viruses and atherosclerosis in humans is in the cardiac transplant population. Several recent studies have demonstrated a strong correlation between CMV infection and accelerated atherosclerosis (Gyorkey *et al.,* 1984; MacDonald *et al.,* 1989). Two hundred cardiac transplant patients who were treated with immunosuppressive agents were followed prospectively for seropositivity for CMV infection and the development of atherosclerosis. Of this group, 91 patients developed CMV infections as evidenced by one of three criteria:

(a) positive cultures for CMV,

(b) demonstration of characteristic CMV inclusions in tissue samples or

(c) four-fold rise in IgG CMV antibodies.

After a 5 year follow-up, the rate of graft loss due to accelerated atherosclerosis was 69% in CMV-infected patients compared to 37% in the non-CMV infected group (Gyorkey *et al.*, 1984). Similar results were reported from a smaller study at the University of Minnesota (MacDonald *et al.*, 1989). This study compared rates of CMV infection and atherosclerosis in 102 immunosuppressed patients who had received a cardiac transplant and survived for at least a year. Two years after transplant, 32% of the CMV positive patients had coronary artery disease as opposed to only 10% of the CMV negative patients (MacDonald *et al.*, 1989).

Summary

In summary, we have highlighted data from our laboratory, and others, demonstrating how viral infection of the vascular endothelium can alter the normal thromboresistant surface and alter hemostasis. Three major mechanisms were described:

(1) inhibition of anti-coagulant/anti-thrombotic properties,

(2) induction of pro-coagulant/prothrombotic properties, and

(3) induction of binding sites for inflammatory cells.

We believe that each of these mechanisms may either work alone or in concert to contribute to the pathophysiology of herpesvirus-induced thrombo-atherogenesis. The role of viral-induced changes in hemostasis is seen in several clinical settings, but the specific role of *in vitro* alterations of endothelial cell function and its relationship to *in vivo* thrombosis is still a matter of speculation. In addition, the etiologic role of viruses in the pathogenesis of atherosclerosis remains unclear. However, circumstantial evidence continues to accumulate suggesting a role for herpesvirus infections in the initiation and/or progression of this arteriopathy.

References

Adam, E., Melnick, J., Probesfield, J., Petrie, B., Burek, J., Bailey, K., McCollum, C. and DeBakey, M. (1987). High levels of cytomegalovirus antibody in patients requiring vascular surgery for atherosclerosis. *Lancet*, **2**:291.

Adams, D.H., Wyner, L.R. and Karnovsky, M.J. (1993). Experimental graft arteriosclerosis. 2. Immunocyto chemical analysis of lesion development. *Transplant.*, **56**:794–799.

Altieri, D., Etingin, O., Fair, D., Brunck, T., Geltosky, J., Hajjar, D. and Edgington, T. (1991). Structural homogolous ligand binding of integrin mac-1 and viral glycoprotein C receptors. *Science*, **254**:1200–1203.

Benditt, E., Barrett, T. and McDougall, J. (1983). Viruses in the etiology of atherosclerosis. *Proc. Natl. Acad. Sci. USA*, **80**:6386–6389.

Bevilacqua, M., Pober, J., Wheeler, M., Cotran, R. and Gimbrone, M. (1985). Interleukin-1 activation of vascular endothelium. Effects on procoagulant activity and leukocyte adhesion. *Amer. J. Pathol.*, **121**:393–403.

Bruggeman, C., Debie, W., Muller, A., Schutte, B. and van Dam-Mieras, M. (1988). Cytomegalovirus alters the von Willebrand factor content in human endothelial cells. *Thromb. Haemost.*, **59**:264–268.

Cines, D.B., Lyss, A.P., Bina, M., Corkey, R. and Kefalides, N.A. (1982). Fc and C3 receptors induced by Herpes simplex virus infection in cultured endothelial cells. *J. Clin. Invest.*, **69**:123.

Cosgriff, T. (1989). Viruses and hemostasis. *Reviews of Infectious Diseases*, **11**: 5672–5688.

Esmon, C. (1994). The regulation of natural anticoagulant pathways. *Science*, **235**:1348–1352.

Etingin, O., Silverstein, R., Friedman, H. and Hajjar, D. (1990). Viral activation of the coagulation cascade: molecular interactions at the surface of the infected endothelial cell. *Cell*, **61**:657–662.

Etingin, O., Silverstein, R. and Hajjar, D. (1991). Identification of a monocyte receptor on herpesvirus-infected endothelial cells. *Proc. Natl. Acad. Sci. USA*, **88**:7200–7203.

Etingin, O., Silverstein, R. and Hajjar, D. (1993). von Willeband factor mediates platelet adhesion to virally infected endothelial cells. *Proc. Natl. Acad. Sci. USA*, **90**:5153–5156.

Fabricant, C.G., Fabricant, J., Litrenta, M. and Minick, C. (1978). Virus induced atherosclerosis. *J. Exp. Med.*, **148**:335–340.

Friedman, H., Macarak, E., MacGregor, R., Wolfe, J. and Kefalides, N. (1981). Virus infection of endothelial cells. *J. Infect. Dis.*, **143**:266–273.

Friedman, H., Wolfe, J., Kefalides, N. and Macarak, E. (1986). Susceptibility of endothelial cells derived from different blood vessels to common viruses. *In Vitro Cell. Dev. Biol.*, **22**:397–401.

Friedman, H. (1989). Infection of endothelial cells by common human viruses. *Reviews of Infectious Diseases*, **11**:S700–S704.

Gyorkey, F., Melnick, J., Guinn, G., Gyorkey, P. and DeBakey, M. (1984). Herpes viridae in endothelial cells of the proximal aorta of atherosclerotic patients. *Expt. Mol. Pathol.*, **40**:328–339.

Hajjar, D., Falcone, D., Fabricant, C. and Fabricant, J. (1985). Altered cholesteryl ester cycle is associated with lipid accumulation in herpesvirus-infected arterial smooth muscle cells. *J. Biol. Chem.*, **260**:6124–6128.

Hajjar, D. (1986). Herpesvirus infection prevents activation of cytoplasmic cholesteryl esterase in arterial smooth muscle cells. *J. Biol. Chem.*, **261**:7611–7614.

Hajjar, D., Fabricant, C., Minick, C. and Fabricant, J. (1986). Virus-induced atherosclerosis. Herpesvirus infection alters arterial cholesterol metabolism and accumulation. *Am. J. Pathol.*, **122**:62–70.

Hajjar, D., Nicholson, A., Hajjar, K., Sando, G. and Summers, B. (1989). Decreased messenger RNA translation in herpesvirus-infected arterial cells: effects on cholesteryl ester hydrolase. *Proc. Natl. Acad. Sci. USA*, **86**:3366–3370.

Hajjar, D. (1991). Viral pathogenesis of atherosclerosis: impact of molecular mimicry and viral genes. *Am. J. Pathol.*, **139**:1195–1211.

Hattori, R., Hamilton, K., Fugate, R., McEver, R. and Sims, P. (1989). Stimulated secretion of endothelial cell von Willebrand factor is accompanied by rapid distribution of the intracellular granule membrane protein, GMP-140. *J. Cell. Biochem.*, **264**:7768–7771.

Havlik, R., Blackwelder, W., Kaslow, R. and Castelli, W. (1989). Unlikely association between clinically apparent herpesvirus infection and coronary incidence at older ages: The Framingham Heart Study. *Arteriosclerosis*, **9**:877–880.

Hendrix, M., Dormans, P., Kitslaar, P., Bosman, F. and Bruggeman, C. (1989). The presence of CMV nucleic acids in arterial walls of atherosclerotic and non-atherosclerotic patients. *Amer. J. Pathol.*, **134**:1151–1157.

Hendrix, M., Salimans, M., van Boven, C. and Bruggeman, C. (1990). High prevalence of latently present cytomegalovirus in artery walls of patients suffering grade III atherosclerosis. *Amer. J. Pathol.*, **136**:23–28.

Ignarro, L. (1989). Endothelium-derived nitric oxide: actions and properties. *FASEB J.*, **3**:31–36.

Johnson, R., Nahmias, A., Magder, L., Lee, F., Brooks, C. and Snowden, M. (1986). A seroepidemiologic survey of the prevalence of herpes simplex virus type 2 in the United States. *N. Engl. J. Med.*, **321**:7–12.

Kaner, R., Iozzo, R., Ziaie, Z. and Kefalides, N. (1990). Inhibition of proteoglycan synthesis in human endothelial cells after infection with herpes simplex virus type 1 in vitro. *Am. J. Respir. Cell Mol. Biol.*, **2**:423–431.

Kelton, J. and Neame, P. (1987). Hemorrhagic complications of infection in: Hemostasis and Thrombosis. J.B. Lippincott, Philadelphia, pp. 965–974.

Key, N., Vercellotti, G., Winkelmann, J., Moldow, C., Goodman, J., Esmon, N., Esmon, C. and Jacob, H. (1990). Infection of vascular endothelial cells with herpes simplex virus enhances tissue factor activity and reduces thrombomodulin expression. *Proc. Natl. Acad. Sci. USA*, **87**:7095–7097.

Key, N., Bach, R., Vercellotti, G. and Moldow, C. (1993). Herpes simplex virus type I does not require productive infection to induce tissue factor in human umbilical vein endothelial cells. *Lab. Invest.*, **68**:645–651.

Loscalzo, J. (1992). The relationship between atherosclerosis and thrombosis. *Circ.*, **86**[suppl III]:III 95-III 99.

MacDonald, K., Rector, T., Braunlan, E., Coubo, S. and Olivari, M. (1989). Association of coronary artery disease in cardiac transplant recipients with cytomegalovirus infection. *Amer. J. Pathol.*, **64**:359–362.

Macgregor, R.R., Friedman, H.M., Macarak, E.J. and Kefalides, N.A. (1980). Virus infection of endothelial cells increases granulocyte adherence. *J. Clin. Invest*, **65**:1469–1477.

McEver, R. (1991). GMP-140: A receptor for neutrophils and monocytes on activated platelets and endothelium. *J. Cell Biochem.*, **45**:156–161.

McSorley, J., Shapiro, L., Brownstein, M. and Hsu, K. (1974). Herpes simplex virus and varicella-zoster: comparative histology of 77 cases. *Intern. J. Dermatol.*, **13**:69–75.

Melnick, J., Dreesman, G., McCollum, C., Petrie, B., Burek, J. and DeBakey, M. (1983). Cytomegalovirus antigen within human arterial smooth muscle cells. *Lancet*, **2**:644–646.

Minick, C.R., Fabricant, C.G., Fabricant, J. and Litrenta, M.M. (1978). Atherosclerosis induced by infection by herpesvirus. *Amer. J. Pathol.*, **96**:673–706.

Munro, J. and Cotran, R. (1988). Biology of Disease: The pathogenesis of atherosclerosis: atherogenesis and inflammation. *Lab. Invest.*, **58**:249–261.

Myerson, D., Hackman, R., Nelson, J., Ward, D. and McDougall, J. (1984). Widespread occurance of histologically occult cytomegalovirus. *Hum. Pathol.*, **15**:430–439.

Nachmias, A. and Josey, K. (1978). Epidemiology of herpes simplex 1 and 2 in: *Viral infection of Humans-Epidemiology and Contol*. Plenum Medical Book Co., New York, pp. 253–271.

Petrie, B., Melnick, J., Adam, E., Burek, J., McCollum, C. and DeBakey, M. (1987). Nucleic acid sequence of cytomegalovirus in cells cultured from human arterial tissue. *J. Infect. Dis.*, **155**:158–159.

Phinney, P., Fligiel, S., Bryson, Y. and Porter, D. (1982). Necrotizing vasculitis in a case of disseminated neonatal herpes simplex infection. *Arch. Path. Lab. Med.*, **106**:64–67.

Pomerantz, K. and Hajjar, D. (1992). Signal transduction in atherosclerosis: integration of cytokines and the eicosanoid network. *FASEB J.*, **6**:2933–2941.

Schorer, A., Kaplan, M., Rao, G. and Moldow, C. (1986). Interleukin 1 stimulates endothelial cell tissue factor production and expression by a prostaglandin–independent mechanism. *Thromb. Haemo.*, **56**:256–259.

Schorer, A., Moldow, C. and Rick, M. (1987). Interleukin 1 or endotoxin increases the release of von Willebrand factro from human endothelial cells. *Br. J. Haematol.*, **67**:193–197.

Sorlie, P.D., Adam, E., Melnick, S.L., Folsom, A., Skelton, T., Chambless, L.E., Barnes, R. and Melnick, J.L. (1994). Cytomegalovirus herpesvirus and carotid atherosclerosis-the ARIC study. *J. Med. Virol.*, **42**:33–37.

Span, A., Endert, J., van Boven, C. and Bruggeman, C. (1989a). Virus induced adherence of monocytes to endothelial cells. FEMS *Microbiol. Immunol.*, **47**:237–244.

Span, A., van Boven, C. and Bruggeman, C. (1989b). The effect of cytomegalovirus infection on the adherence of polymorphonuclear leukocytes to endothelial cells. *Europ. J. Clin. Invest.*, **19**:542–548.

Speir, E., Modali, R., Huang, E., Leon, M., Shawl, F., Finkel, T. and Epstein, S. (1994). Potential role of human cytomegalovirus and p53 interaction in coronary atherosclerosis. *Science*, **265**:391–394.

Sporn, L., Shi, R., Silverman, D. and Marder, V. (1991). Rickettsia rickettsia infection of cultured endothelial cells induces release of large von Willebrand factor multimers from Weible-Palade bodies. *Blood*, **78**:2595–2602.

Tanaka, K. and Sueishi, K. (1994). The coagulation and fibrinolysis systems and atherosclerosis. *Lab. Invest.*, **69**:5–18.

van Dam-Mieras, M., Muller, A., van Hinsbergh, V., Mullers, W., Bomans, P. and Bruggeman, C. (1992). The procoagulant response of cytomegalovirus infected endothelial cells. *Thromb. Haemost.*, **68**:364–370.

Visser, M., Tracy, P., Vercellotti, G., Goodman, J., White, J. and Jacob, H. (1988). Enhanced thrombin generation and platelet binding on herpes simplex virus-infected endothelium. *Proc. Natl. Acad. Sci. USA*, **85**:8227–8230.

Visser, M., Jacob, H., Goodman, J., McCarthy, J., Furcht, L. and Vercellotti, G. (1989). Granulocyte-mediated injury to herpes simplex virus-infected human endothelium. . *Lab. Invest.*, **60**:296–304.

Yamashiroya, H., Ghosh, L., Yang, R. and Robertson, A. (1988). Herpesviridae in the coronary arteries and aorta of young trauma victims. *Amer. J. Pathol.*, **130**:71–79.

Zajac, B., O'Neill, K., Friedman, H. and MacGregor, R. (1988). Increased adherence of human granulocytes to herpes simplex type 1 infected endothelial cells. *In Vitro Cell. Dev. Biol.*, **24**:321–325.

INDEX

309